Age-Related Macular Degeneration

A Comprehensive Textbook

Age-Related Macular Degeneration
A Comprehensive Textbook

EDITORS

D. VIRGIL ALFARO, III, MD

Retina Consultants of Charleston
Chief of Retina Service
Trident Eye Surgery Center
Charleston, South Carolina

PETER E. LIGGETT, MD

New England Retina Associates
Clinical Professor
Cornell University Medical College
New York, New York

WILLIAM F. MIELER, MD

Professor and Chairman
Department of Ophthalmology
University of Chicago
Chicago, Illinois

HUGO QUIROZ-MERCADO, MD

Asociacion Para Evitar la Ceguera en Mexico
Hospital Dr. Luis Sanchez Bulnes
Mexico City, Mexico

RAMA D. JAGER, MD, MBA

University Retina and Macula Associates, P.C.
Oak Forest, Illinois
Clinical Assistant Professor
Department of Opthalmology and Visual Science
University of Chicago
Chicago, Illinois

YASUO TANO, MD

Professor and Chairman
Department of Opthalmology
Osaka University
Osaka, Japan

LIPPINCOTT WILLIAMS & WILKINS
A **Wolters Kluwer** Company
Philadelphia • Baltimore • New York • London
Buenos Aires • Hong Kong • Sydney • Tokyo

Acquisitions Editor: Jonathan Pine
Managing Editor: Joanne Bersin
Project Manager: Fran Gunning
Manufacturing Manager: Ben Rivera
Marketing Manager: Adam Glazer
Design Coordinator: Doug Smock
Production Services: TechBooks
Printer: Quebecor World Kingsport

© 2006 by LIPPINCOTT WILLIAMS & WILKINS
530 Walnut Street
Philadelphia, PA 19106 USA
LWW.com

Library of Congress Cataloging-in-Publication Data

Age-related macular degeneration : a comprehensive textbook / [edited by] D. Virgil Alfaro III . . . [et al.].
    p. ; cm.
  Includes bibliographical references and index.
  ISBN 0-7817-3899-7 (alk. paper)
 1. Retinal degeneration–Age factors. I. Alfaro, D. Virgil. II. Title.
  [DNLM: 1. Macular Degeneration–diagnosis. 2. Choroidal Neovascularization. 3. Macular Degeneration–complications. 4. Macular Degeneration–therapy. WW 270 A26493 2006] RE661.D3A32226 2006 618.97'7735–dc22

                                             2005020376

10 9 8 7 6 5 4 3 2

J. Donald Gass, MD
(1928–2005)

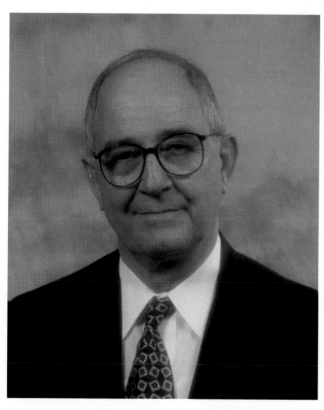

*J. Donald M. Gass, MD, outstanding
clinician, teacher, and colleague.*

It is fitting that this book on age-related macular degeneration (AMD) is dedicated to the memory of our friend and teacher, J. Donald M. Gass, MD, who passed away on February 26, 2005, at the age of 76, shortly after writing the foreword for this volume. No ophthalmologist has contributed more to our knowledge about and our understanding of this condition. From his early articles on the use of fluorescein angiography to characterize macular disease to his more recent manuscript classifying patterns of choroidal neovascularization, Dr. Gass's observations have been seminal, providing breakthrough insights into the pathogenesis of the disease and stimulating important advances in therapy.

J. Donald M. Gass was born in Charlottetown on Prince Edward Island, Canada, in 1928, and moved to Nashville,

Tennessee, as a child when his physician father became director of the Tennessee statewide tuberculosis program. He attended Vanderbilt University, graduating with a bachelor of arts degree in 1950. After serving in the United States Navy from 1950 to 1953, he entered the Vanderbilt School of Medicine, where he won the Founder's Medal as the top graduating student of the class of 1957.

At the urging of his mentors at Vanderbilt, Dr. Gass went to the University of Iowa for his internship and anticipated residency in ophthalmology. However, when a position opened at the Wilmer Eye Institute at Johns Hopkins, Don and his wife, Margy Ann, jumped at the opportunity to live and train closer to family. Dr. Gass's father-in-law, J. Carlton Loser, was a member of the US House of Representatives living in Washington, DC, at the time.

After his residency at Wilmer, Don spent a year at the Armed Forces Institute of Pathology under Dr. Lorenz Zimmerman and then returned to Hopkins as chief resident for the 1962–1963 academic year. Don's plans to return to Nashville were interrupted when Dr. Edward Norton recruited him to join the full-time faculty at the Bascom Palmer Eye Institute in Miami. For the next 30 years, Dr. Gass was one of the cornerstone physicians in the ascendancy of Bascom Palmer in becoming one of the premier eye centers in the world. There, he recognized the value of fluorescein angiography in describing lesions of the retina and specifically in AMD. He described the natural history of choroidal neovascularization and linked the relationship between drusen and what was then called "disciform macular detachment and degeneration." He made major contributions to our understanding of pigment epithelial detachments (PEDs), helping make the distinction between serous and hemorrhagic PEDs, as well as identifying the significance of a "notch" as a sign of occult choroidal neovascularization (CNV). Later, he evaluated the feasibility of submacular surgery for AMD, ultimately classifying CNV into type 1 and type 2, as designees of the location of the CNV relative to the neurosensory retina and the RPE. As well, this classification has served as probable indicators as to prognosis for a submacular surgical approach.

In 1995, Dr. Gass retired from Bascom Palmer and returned to Nashville. He joined the Vanderbilt faculty on a part-time basis, but remained the most sought-after consultant for challenging retinal cases. He continued to review fundus photographs and fluorescein angiograms sent in by physicians from all over the world. He continued to use his remarkable ability to recall similar cases, often leading to the description of a new syndrome.

Dr. Gass was an astounding teacher, be it one on one with a fellow, in a fluorescein conference with a group of residents, or at the podium of a large lecture hall. However, his greatest legacy, besides his family, will be his textbooks. His *Stereoscopic Atlas of Macular Disease* is the *sine qua non* of our field. The marvelous images and insights from this book, now in its fourth edition, have been shared with virtually every ophthalmologist in the world.

Thus, it is with great respect and deep humility that we dedicate this book on age-related macular degeneration to the memory of the man who has had the most profound influence on our field: our friend, our colleague, our teacher, J. Donald M. Gass, MD.

Paul Sternberg, Jr., MD
G. W. Hale Professor and Chair
Vanderbilt Eye Institute
Vanderbilt University Medical Center
Nashville, Tennessee

Contents

SECTION 6: FUTURE DIRECTIONS

Preface

The management of age-related macular degeneration remains a significant challenge for the retina specialist. While the Macular Photocoagulation Study provided useful data in the prevention of visual loss associated with certain choroidal neovascular membranes, its benefits do not apply to dry disease and many are reluctant to treat subfoveal lesions with argon laser photocoagulation.

The important contributions made in academia and by industry in the treatment of subfoveal choroidal neovascular membranes has breathed new hope into our beloved field. Clinical trials evaluating the use of photodynamic therapy with verteporfin have demonstrated that alternatives are possible in the management of subfoveal lesions—a scientific rationale that combines involution of a vascular complex with limited damage to the overlying photoreceptors.

The important contributions of Judah Folkman and Napoleane Ferrara have helped elucidate the importance of certain proteins integral to the formation of new blood vessels. This has resulted in novel and innovative approaches to treatment of subfoveal neovascular membranes through the use of intravitreally and intravenously injected medicines that have the capacity to neutralize various isoforms of vascular endothelial growth factor.

Our colleagues, Drs. David Guyer, Anthony Adamis, and Samir Patel, took lessons learned from the clinic and laboratories and applied them to industry, shouldering the burden of taking a novel compound, Macugen, from concept to approval by the U.S. Food and Drug Administration. Indeed, many patients today are benefiting from their hard work.

Repeated intravitreal therapy has become the norm, made so by the modern use of intravitreal triamcinolone for the treatment of a wide spectrum of diseases of the macula, including wet age-related macular degeneration. Most important is that the common intravitreal use of this steroid compound has cleared the way for other medicines (Macugen, Lucentis, and others to come) to be used intravitreally on a repeated basis.

Paralleling these developments has been the recent publication of the Submacular Surgery Trial, which showed little benefit from a pars plana approach to the treatment of submacular lesions associated with wet age-related macular degeneration. Gone, also, is the interest of most retinal specialists in the use of macular translocation as a means of treating this disease.

The editors of this textbook have chosen internationally acclaimed experts to provide a tome of information for the modern vitreoretinal specialist. *Age-Related Macular Degeneration: A Comprehensive Textbook* is the accumulation of collective efforts by those who have dedicated their professional lives to the diagnosis and treatment of patients suffering from this disease. The reader will find that each chapter can stand alone as a academic treatise dedicated to that topic. We imagine that the thirsty reader will open our textbook to a particular section and glean all the information available on that topic; each chapter is truly comprehensive.

The editors are very grateful to each co-author who took time away from family and patients and dedicated it to the difficult task of writing, an effort compensated only by the satisfaction of knowing that an outstanding work has been completed. Others have also been important in the process of bringing this book to fruition. I would like to thank Jonathan Pine, acquisitions editor at Lippincott Williams & Wilkins, who was personally involved in every step of the preparation of this textbook. Indeed, its very existence is a testament to his active involvement. Joanne Bersin, managing editor at Lippincott Williams & Wilkins, is deserving of great praise for her focus and dedication to this project and holding all of us to a high standard. Pamela Kilstein, our project manager at TechBooks, deserves warm and heartfelt thanks from all of us for her efforts in the very detailed process of production.

I also thank my international fellows who were at my side during the 4-year endeavor of completing this book: Simón Villalba, MD of Caracas; Mónica Rodríguez Fontal, MD, of Caracas; and Elizabeth Rodríguez Méndez, MD of Guadalajara.

D. Virgil Alfaro, III, MD
Charleston, South Carolina

Foreword

When Dr. Virgil Alfaro honored me with an opportunity to write the foreword for this textbook, I asked to review the table of contents and the list of contributors. I knew immediately that he and his team of co-editors had set their standard very high and planned to write, edit, and publish a truly outstanding textbook that would serve as an important reference for years to come.

The publication of *Age-Related Macular Degeneration: A Comprehensive Textbook* comes at an important time because improved diagnostic and treatment modalities appear to be part of the near future. I see three important entities providing pivotal and harmonious efforts in this regard: basic science research in academic centers, clinical trials performed by private practice and academic retina specialists, and the pharmaceutical industry.

Indeed it is interesting to note that the authors of this textbook represent the very best of what academic ophthalmology, private practice vitreoretinal specialists, and industry have to offer. Drs. Alfaro, Jager, Liggett, Mieler, and Tano deserve the collective applause from our field for publishing this important textbook.

J. Donald M. Gass, MD[†]
Professor of Ophthalmology
Vanderbilt University
School of Medicine

[†]Dr. Gass passed away on February 26, 2005. Please see the dedication page.

Contributors

Anthony P. Adamis, MD
Senior Vice President of Research and
   Development/Chief Scientific Officer
Eyetech Pharmaceuticals, Inc.
New York, New York

Ron Afshari Adelman, MD, MPH
Department of Ophthalmology
Yale University
New Haven, Connecticut

Everett Ai, MD
West Coast Retina Medical Group
San Francisco, California

D. Virgil Alfaro, III, MD
Retina Consultants of Charleston
Chief of Retina Service
Trident Eye Surgery Center
Charleston, South Carolina

J. Fernando Arévalo, MD
Clínica Oftalmológica Centro Caracas
Caracas, Venezuela

Richard M. Awdeh, MD
Yale University School of Medicine
New Haven, Connecticut

Colin J. Barnstable, PhD
Professor
Department of Ophthalmology and
   Visual Science
Yale University School of Medicine
New Haven, Connecticut

Lluis Arias Barquet, MD
Department of Ophthalmology
Hospital Universitari de Bellvitge
Barcelona, Spain

Dirk-Uwe Bartsch, PhD
Director of Retinal Imaging Laboratory
Jacobs Retina Center
Department of Ophthalmology
University of California San Diego
Shiley Eye Center
La Jolla, California

Suzanne Binder, MD
Professor and Chairman
Department of Ophthalmology
Krankenanstalt
Rudolfstiftung, Vienna

Alexander J. Brucker, MD
Professor of Ophthalmology
Penn Eye Care
Clinical Practices of the University
   of Pennsylvania
Philadelphia, Pennsylvania

Nauman Alam Chaudhry, MD
Clinical Assistant Professor of
   Ophthalmology
Department of Ophthalmology
Yale University School of Medicine
New England Retina Associates
New Haven, Connecticut

Antonio P. Ciardella, MD
Manhattan Eye, Ear and Throat
   Hospital
Department of Ophthalmology
New York, New York

Alfredo Domínguez Collazo, MD
Professor of Ophthalmology
Universidad Autónoma de Madrid
Madrid, Spain

Emmett Cunningham, MD, PhD
Vice President of Clinical and
   Research
Eyetech Pharmaceuticals, Inc
Department of Ophthalmology
New York University
New York, New York

Shane Dunne, MD
New York Eye and Ear Infirmary
New York, New York

Chiara M. Eandi, MD
Department of Ophthalmology
Universidad de Torino
Torino, Italy

Carlos F. Fernández, MD
Clínica Oftalmológica Centro Caracas
Caracas, Venezuela

Marta S. Figueroa, MD
Hospital Oftalmológico Internacional
   de Madrid
Madrid, Spain

Yale L. Fisher, MD
Vitreous-Retina-Macula Consultants of
   New York
Chief of Surgical Retina
Manhattan Eye and Ear Hospital
New York, New York

Mónica Rodríguez Fontal, MD
Retina Consultants of Charleston
Charleston, South Carolina

William R. Freeman, MD
Professor
University of California San Diego
Department of Ophthalmology
UCSD Shiley Eye Center
La Jolla, California

Thomas R. Friberg, MD
Director of Retina Service and Professor
   of Ophthalmology
University of Pittsburgh
Pittsburgh, Pennsylvania

Arthur D. Fu, MD
West Coast Retina Medical Group
San Francisco, California

Patricia M. C. Garcia, MD
New York Eye and Ear Infirmary
New York, New York

Bert Glaser, MD
The Bert M. Glaser National
   Retina Institute
Towson, Maryland

Francisco Gómez-Ulla, MD
Professor of Ophthalmology
Universidad de Santiago de Compostela
Santiago de Compostela, Spain

Evangelos S. Gragoudas, MD
Professor
Director of Retina Service
Massachusetts Eye and Ear Infirmary
Boston, Massachusetts

W. Richard Green, MD
Professor
Johns Hopkins Hospital
Wilmer Eye Institute
Baltimore, Maryland

David R. Guyer, MD
Chief Executive Officer and Founder
Eyetech Pharmaceuticals, Inc.
New York, New York

Nancy M. Holekamp, MD
Assistant Professor of Clinical
    Ophthalmology
Washington University School
    of Medicine
St. Louis, Missouri

Melanie Lynn Hom, MD
Department of Ophthalmology
California Pacific Medical Center
San Francisco, California

Mark S. Humayun, MD, PhD
Professor of Ophthalmology
Biomedical Engineering, Cell and
    Neurobiology
Doheny Retina Institute
Doheny Eye Institute
Keck School of Medicine
University of Southern California
Los Angeles, California

Mohan Iyer, MD
Baylor College of Medicine
Houston, Texas

Eric P. Jablon, MD
Retina Consultants of Charleston
Charleston, South Carolina

Rama D. Jager, MD, MBA
University Retina and Macula
    Associates, P. C.
Oak Forest, Illinois
Clinical Assistant Professor
Department of Opthalmology
    and Visual Science
University of Chicago
Chicago, Illinois

Robert N. Johnson, MD
Associate Clinical Professor
University of California-San Francisco
San Francisco, California

T. Mark Johnson, MD
Assistant Professor of Ophthalmology
George Washington University
Washington, D.C.

J. Michael Jumper, MD
West Coast Retina Medical Group
San Francisco, California

Motohiro Kamei, MD
Department of Ophthalmology
Osaka University Medical School
Osaka, Japan

Robert Kim, MD
Chief Clinical Scientist of
    Ophthalmic Medicine
Genentech, Inc.
South San Francisco, California

Christina M. Klais, MD
Department of Ophthalmology
Manhattan Eye, Ear and Throat
    Hospital
New York, New York

Frank H. J. Koch, MD
Department of Ophthalmology
University of Frankfurt
Frankfurt, Germany

Rohit R. Lakhanpal, MD
Fellow and Clinical Instructor
Doheny Retina Institute
Doheny Eye Institute
Keck School of Medicine
University of Southern California
Los Angeles, California

Alejandro J. Lavaque, MD
New England Retina and Education
    Foundation
Hamden, Connecticut

Peter E. Liggett, MD
New England Retina Associates
Clinical Professor
Cornell University Medical College
New York, New York

H. Richard McDonald, MD
Associate Clinical Professor
University of California-San Francisco
West Coast Medical Group
San Francisco, California

Elizabeth Rodríguez Méndez, MD
Retina Consultants of Charleston
Charleston, South Carolina

Arístides J. Mendoza, MD
Clínica Oftalmológica Centro Caracas
Caracas, Venezuela

William F. Mieler, MD
Professor and Chairman
Department of Ophthalmology
University of Chicago
Chicago, Illinois

Joan Miller, MD
Professor and Chairperson
Department of Ophthalmology
Massachusetts Eye and Ear Infirmary
Boston, Massachusetts

Jordi M. Monés, MD
Institut de Microcirugía Ocular
    de Barcelona
Barcelona, Spain

Siobhan E. Moriarty-Craige, MD
Nutrition and Health Sciences Program
Department of Medicine
Emory University
Atlanta, Georgia

Gene Ng, MD, MBA
Associate Director, Business Development
Eyetech Pharmaceuticals, Inc.
New York, New York

Michael D. Ober, MD
Department of Ophthalmology
Manhattan Eye, Ear and Throat Hospital
New York, New York

Stephen R. O'Connell, MD
Connecticut Retina Consultants
New Haven, Connecticut

Ana Pesce, MD
Department of Ophthalmology
The British Hospital
Montevideo, Uruguay

Adrian G. H. Podoleanu, MD
School of Physical Sciences
University of Kent
Canterbury, United Kingdom

Carmen Puliafito, MD, MBA
Bascom Palmer Eye Institute
Miami, Florida

Hugo Quiroz-Mercado, MD
Asociacion Para Evitar la Ceguera
    en Mexico
Hospital Dr. Luis Sanchez Bulnes
Mexico City, Mexico

Elias Reichel, MD
New England Eye Center
Boston, Massachusetts

Richard Rosen, MD
New York Eye and Ear Infirmary
New York, New York

Michelle Rothen, BS
Retina Consultants of Charleston
Charleston, South Carolina

Fernando de Santiago, MD
The British Hospital
Montevideo, Uruguay

Ursula Schmidt-Erfurth, MD
Department of Ophthalmology
University Eye Hospital Vienna
Vienna, Austria

Robin Singh, MBBS
University of Chicago
Chicago, Illinois

Jason S. Slakter, MD
Vitreous-Retina-Macula Consultants
   of New York
New York, New York

Lindsay M. Smithen, MD
Vitreous-Retina-Macula Consultants
   of New York
New York, New York

Richard Spaide, MD
Vitreous-Retina-Macula Consultants
   of New York
New York, New York

Paul Sternberg, Jr., MD
G. W. Hale Professor and Chair
Vanderbilt Eye Institute
Vanderbilt University Medical Center
Nashville, Tennessee

Yasuo Tano, MD
Professor and Chairman
Department of Ophthalmology
Osaka University
Osaka, Japan

Matthew A. Thomas, MD
Barnes Retina Institute
St. Louis, Missouri

Warren Thompson, MD
Vestavia Hills, Alabama

Joyce Tombran-Tink, PhD
Associate Professor
Department of Pharmaceutical
   Sciences
University of Missouri-Kansas City
Kansas City, Missouri

Simón J. Villalba, MD
Retina Consultants of Charleston
Charleston, South Carolina

James D. Weiland, PhD
Assistant Professor of Ophthalmology
   and Biomedical Engineering
Doheny Retina Institute
Doheny Eye Institute
Keck School of Medicine
University of Southern California
Los Angeles, California

James M. Weisz, MD
Connecticut Retina Consultants
New Haven, Connecticut

Daniel Will, MD
New York Eye and Ear Infirmary
New York, New York

Lawrence A. Yannuzzi, MD
Vitreous-Retina-Macula Consultants
   of New York
New York, New York

Akitoshi Yoshida, MD
New York Eye and Ear Infirmary
New York, New York

Normal Anatomy of the Macula

1

J. Fernando Arévalo   Carlos F. Fernández   Arístides J. Mendoza

INTRODUCTION

Francisco Buzzi in Milan, Italy, was the first to anatomically define the macula at the end of the 18th century (1782–1784). He described it as the yellow portion of the posterior retina, lateral to the optic nerve, with a depression in its center. Also in the 18th century (1797), Fragonard, a French ophthalmologist, made a very detailed description of the foveal zone, but he failed to mention the central foveola. In addition, Soemmering (1795–1798) described the macula lutea, however he thought that the foveola was a hole or foramen (foraminulum centrale retinae), and correlated it to the blind spot of the visual field. Finally, Michaelis in 1838 established the role of the macula, and it was confirmed by Müller in 1856. At the end of the 19th century, Tratuferi in Italy showed the first schematic drawings with the topographic localization of the retinal layers. The relationship between the retinal axonal layer, cones, and rods was established by Ramon y Cajal in 1894 (1).

The macula is recognized as the specialized region of the retina in charge of high-resolution visual acuity. Anatomically, it can be defined as the central part of the posterior retina that contains xanthophyll pigment and two or more layers of ganglion cells. In this chapter, we will focus primarily on the aspects of the normal anatomy of the macula as an introduction to the understanding and management of age-related macular degeneration.

EMBRYOLOGY

The neural components of the eye are an extension of the forebrain, and thus part of the central nervous system (Table 1.1).

The Neuroretina

The embryogenesis of the neuroretina occurs during the first month of life. The forebrain consists of a single layer of neuroectodermal cells. The optic vesicle extends laterally from the forebrain, and then invaginates to form the optic cup. There is a double layer of neuroectodermal cells in the optic cup; the apices are together and basal aspects apart. The macular area appears at the end of the fourth week.

The inner layer of neuroectoderm becomes the sensory retina posteriorly. Part of the inner limiting membrane is the basement membrane of the sensory retina, next to the vitreous. The foveal pit forms late in embryonic life, and morphologic maturity does not occur until the age when it is possible to obtain 20/20 visual acuity in small children (2). The induction of the foveal pit requires a normal pigment epithelium (3). The inner layer of neuroectoderm is divided into the inner neuroblastic layer (Müller, amacrine, and ganglion cells) and the outer neuroblastic layer (cones and rods, horizontal, and bipolar cells). Between the inner neuroblastic layer and the outer neuroblastic layer is the transient fiber layer of Chievitz, this layer will progressively disappear.

The central and peripheral retina start to differentiate between the first and third months. The ganglion cell layer becomes thicker, as so the inner plexiform layer and the amacrine cell layer. The cones appear at the fifth month. They are a protoplasmic extension of the outer neuroblastic layer (4,5,6). The rods appear in the sixth month (5). The macula becomes thinner at the seventh month because the cells of the different layers move laterally, and the foveal pit appears more evident (Fig. 1.1) (7,8).

The Retinal Pigmentary Epithelium

The outer layer of neuroectoderm (toward the sclera) becomes the retinal pigment epithelium (RPE), the

TABLE 1.1

DEVELOPMENT OF THE SENSORY RETINA[a]

4th–5th Week	6th Week–3rd Month	3rd–7th Month	Adult
Surface of marginal layer			Internal limiting membrane
	Superficial portion of marginal layer	Nerve fiber layer	Nerve fiber layer
		Ganglion cells	Ganglion cells
	Inner neuroblastic layer	Amacrine cells	
Primitive neuro-epithelium		Müllerian fiber nuclei	Inner nuclear layer
		Bipolar cells	
	Outer neuroblastic layer	Horizontal cells	
		Nuclei of rods and cones	Outer nuclear layer
Cilia		Primitive rods and cones	Rods and cones

[a] The marginal layer free from nuclei (not included) appears between the 4th–5th week, after which it disappears. In addition, the transient layer of Chievitz (not included) appears between the 6th week–3rd month and disappears after the 3rd month.

pigmented ciliary epithelium, and the iris dilator muscle. The basement membrane of the RPE forms the innermost part of Bruch's membrane (9).

Pigmentation of the neuroectodermal cells occurs early and is completed during embryonic life (10), whereas pigmentation of the uveal stroma, which is derived from the neural crest, starts much later and is not complete until several weeks after birth (9). The melanin granules of the neuroectoderm are larger and chemically different from those of the uveal stroma (11). Moreover, melanin content of the RPE is similar in all persons, regardless of race, in contrast to the amount of uveal stromal pigmentation, which corresponds to the racial pigmentation of the skin and hair (10).

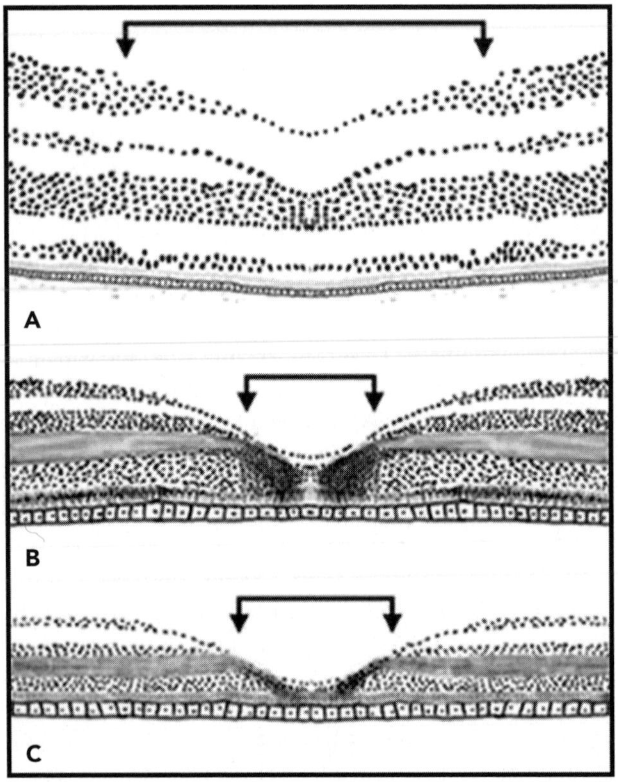

Vascularization

Vascularization of the retina begins during the 16th week of gestation at the optic nerve head (12), and normally reaches the ora serrata nasally by term. It is not quite complete temporally at term because the distance from the optic nerve head to the ora is greater.

There are differing theories as to how vascularization of the macula occurs. Some have proposed that the capillary-free zone (CFZ) develops by regression of previously formed capillaries, because the retina is thin enough in this area that sufficient oxygen can diffuse inward from the choroidal circulation (12). Others believe that the CFZ forms primarily, with the embryonic vessels gradually encircling the center of the fovea and with no evidence of regression (13).

The Choroid

In the first phase, at 4 weeks, the choroid begins to take form in the undifferentiated mesenchyma surrounding the optic cup. At 5 to 6 weeks, endothelial tubes near the pigment epithelium differentiate into capillaries. Simultaneously, Bruch's membrane and the vortex veins appear. With the appearance of the posterior ciliary arteries at 8 weeks, the choriocapillaris is fully established as a discrete layer.

During the growth phase in the third month, the anterior capillaries arrange themselves in a linear and radial

Figure 1.1   Diagram showing the development of the human fovea. **A.** Human fovea at birth. **B.** Human fovea at 45 months. **C.** Human fovea at 72 years of age. Black lines mark the width of the rod-free foveola; at birth the foveola is wider **(A)** than at 45 months **(B)**. Full foveal development is not complete until sometime between 15 and 45 months of age. G, ganglion cell layer; OS, outer segments of photoreceptors; P, photoreceptor nuclei.

pattern. The anterior supply of the choriocapillaris is complete by 3 months, even though the ciliary body and iris are not yet formed. The capillaries drain into the supra and infraorbital venous plexi.

The second phase of choroidal growth includes the formation of large vessels (Haller's layer) at 4 months. The third phase begins around the fifth month and is characterized by the formation of medium-sized vessels posterior to the equator. Anterior to the equator there are only two layers of vessels, the choriocapillaris and medium-sized vessels.

Pigmentation of the choroidal melanocytes commences in the fifth month and continues until after birth, beginning outward near the sclera and progressing inward towards Bruch's membrane. The peripapillary, intrascleral vascular circle of Haller and Zinn develops between 3 and 6 months. Between the sixth and tenth month the major arterial circle of the iris forms recurrent arterial branches that supply the anterior choroid during its rapid growth phase (14).

TOPOGRAPHIC ANATOMY

The terms *macula* and *fovea* are used in different ways by the anatomist and the clinician. Anatomically the macula (macula lutea or central retina) is defined as that portion of the posterior retina that contains xanthophyll and two or more layers of ganglion cells. This region is about 5.5 mm in diameter and is centered approximately 4 mm temporal and 0.8 mm inferior to the center of the optic disc (15). It corresponds clinically to the posterior pole, and is approximately bounded by the superior and inferior temporal vascular arcades. On the basis of microscopic anatomy, the macular area can be further subdivided into several zones (Fig. 1.2).

What is clinically referred as the macula corresponds to the anatomic fovea. The fovea (fovea centralis) is a depres-

sion in the inner retinal surface in the center of the macula. It measures approximately 1.5 mm, or one disc diameter in size, and it is more heavily pigmented than the surrounding retinal tissue. The central floor of the fovea is called the foveola. The anatomic foveola, often referred to clinically as the fovea, measures approximately 0.35 mm in diameter. It lies within the cfz, which measures approximately 0.5 mm in diameter in most patients. A small depression in the center of the foveola is called the umbo, where the retina is only 0.13 mm thick. A 0.5-mm-wide ring zone where the ganglion cell layer, inner nuclear layer, and outer plexiform layer of Henle are the thickest is called the parafoveal area. This zone is in turn surrounded by a 1.5-mm zone referred to as the perifoveal area (16).

CLINICAL APPEARANCE

The anatomic subdivisions of the macula are ill-defined ophthalmoscopically. The margins of either the 0.35-mm diameter foveola or the 1.5-mm diameter fovea are difficult to define. A poorly defined zone of greater pigmentation (one-fourth to one disc diameter in size) corresponds to the center of the macula, which is maximum in the foveolar area. The foveal reflex is present in most normal eyes and it lies just in front of the center of the foveola (Fig. 1.3). We can see the foveal depression with the narrow slit lamp beam.

The central retinal artery supplies the inner half of the retina. It usually divides into a superior and inferior trunk within the optic nerve head. These trunks divide into a nasal branch and a temporal branch. The corresponding retinal venous branches have much the same distribution as the arteries. They give off arteriolar and venular branches that posteriorly occur primarily at right angles to the parent vessel. They divide in a dichotomous way as they course peripherally. The right-angle branches are referred

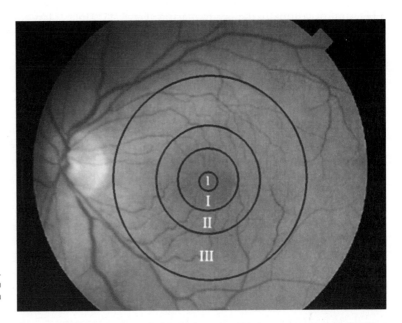

Figure 1.2 Topographic anatomy of normal macula. On the basis of microscopic anatomy, the macular area can be further subdivided into several zones. I. Fovea containing the foveola (1). II. Parafovea. III. Perifovea.

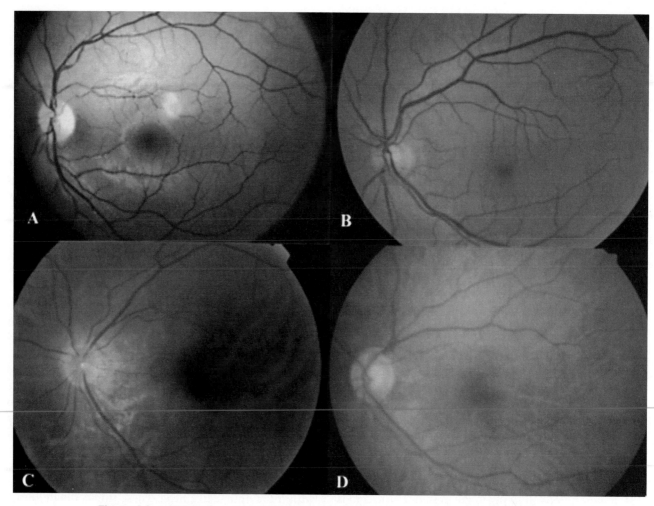

Figure 1.3   Clinical appearance of the normal macula. **A.** Fundus in a young patient. **B.** Fundus in an adult patient. **C.** Fundus in a moderately myopic patient. **D.** Tessellated fundus in older patient. Large choroidal vessels are visible in the macular area in **(D)** because of relative hypopigmentation of the retinal pigment epithelium. (Fig. 1.3-B and D courtesy of Dario Fuenmayor-Rivera and Enrique Murcia.)

to as first-order arterioles and venules. One or more cilioretinal arteries derived from the ciliary circulation supply the papillomacular area in approximately 20% of patients (17), and occasionally the entire macula (Fig. 1.4). The blood vessel walls are normally transparent (16,18).

GROSS ANATOMY

The retina loses its normal transparency within hours after death. Xanthophyll is a yellow pigment made up of two carotenoids (zeaxanthin and lutein) (22,23). It is apparent in the center of the macula and is highly concentrated in the foveolar area. The maximal concentration of xanthophyll pigment is in the outer nuclear and outer plexiform layers. However, we can find xanthophyll within the inner plexiform layer inside the foveal area (19,20,21,22). The greatest concentration of pigment is in the cones' central axons (21).

The entrance site for the short and long posterior ciliary arteries can be visualized after removal of the choroid.

There is no retinal circulation at the foveola. The short posterior ciliary arteries are concentrated in the macular area along the temporal margin of the fovea and the peripapillary area. The temporal long posterior ciliary artery and ciliary nerve enter about one and one-half disc diameters temporal to the center of the fovea (16).

HISTOLOGY

In the macula we find the thickest portion of the retina surrounding the thinnest portion, the foveolar area. At the umbo, the neural retina consists only of the inner limiting membrane, Henle's fiber layer, the outer nuclear layer, the external limiting membrane, and the photoreceptors outer and inner segments (Fig. 1.5). The typical neural-retinal histology is established out of the foveola (Fig. 1.6). The neural retina consists of the inner limiting membrane, the nerve fiber layer (NFL), the ganglion cell layer, the inner plexiform layer (synaptic processes between bipolar cells and ganglion cells), the inner nuclear layer (nuclei of bipolar,

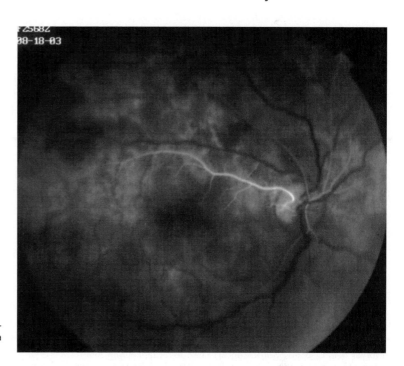

Figure 1.4 Fluorescein angiography shows a cilioretinal artery. (Courtesy of Dario Fuenmayor-Rivera and Enrique Murcia.)

horizontal, amacrine, and Müller cells), the outer plexiform layer (synaptic processes between bipolar cells and photoreceptors), the outer nuclear layer (nuclei of the rods and cones), the external limiting membrane (formed by cell junctions between photoreceptors and the terminal optical processes of Müller cells), and the photoreceptor layer (rod and cone cells). The bipolar cells, ganglion cells, fibers of the outer plexiform layer (Henle's fiber layer), and Müller cells are displaced circumferentially and show an oblique orientation in the macula that causes thickening of the marginal zone and a central thinning of the retina, forming the fovea.

Müller cells are modified glial cells. They span the region from the internal limiting membrane to the external limiting membrane and they give support to the neural elements of the retina. The internal limiting membrane consists of a basement membrane, which is a surface modification of the vitreous body, and the expanded vitreal

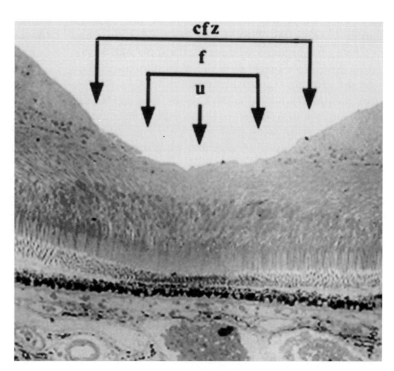

Figure 1.5 Histology of the normal macula. cfz, capillary-free zone; f, foveola; u, umbo. (Microphotograph courtesy of Dario Savino-Zari.)

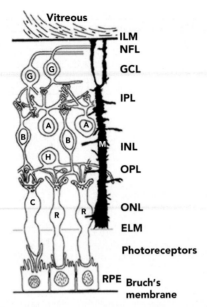

Figure 1.6 Schematic representation of the human retina illustrating its organization into discrete layers. A, amacrine cell; B, bipolar cell; C, cone photoreceptor; ELM, external limiting membrane; G, ganglion cell; GCL, ganglion cell layer; H, horizontal cell; ILM, internal limiting membrane; INL, inner nuclear layer; IPL, inner plexiform layer; M, Müller cell; NFL, nerve fiber layer; ONL, outer nuclear layer; OPL, outer plexiform layer of Henle; R, rod photoreceptor; RPE, retinal pigment epithelium.

processes of Müller cells. This membrane is relatively thick in the macular region except in the area of the foveola. The internal limiting membrane serves as an anchoring structure for the collagen framework of the vitreous. The outer limiting membrane is formed by junctional complexes between cell membranes of the Müller cells and inner segments of photoreceptors. Müller cells are connected to the visual cells by a system of terminal bars (24,25). These junctional complexes probably provide at least a partial barrier to the passage of large molecules in either direction.

The retinal blood vessels supply the inner half of the retina. The major branches of the retinal arterial system have the structure of small arteries, persisting even beyond the equator (15). Retinal arteries do not have an internal elastic lamina, however they have a well-developed muscularis (five to seven layers of smooth muscle cells posteriorly; one or two layers peripherally). Near the optic disc, the retinal veins have three to four layers of smooth muscle cells, and after a short distance the muscle cells are replaced by fibroblasts. There is controversy concerning the pattern of distribution of the capillary network in the retina (diffuse arrangement or a two- or three-tier arrangement) (15,26,27). The superficial network is predominantly postarteriolar and the deep network prevenular. There is a distinct radial peripapillary capillary network; this network richly interconnects with the inner retinal capillary layer (27). The large arterioles and venules of the retinal circulation travel in the NFL and ganglion cell layer. Close to the cfz (0.4 to 0.5 mm in diameter) the capillaries form a single layer, but elsewhere the capillaries are present

in two or more layers and extend into the inner nuclear layer. The cfz is normally vascularized during prenatal development of the retina. This vascularization undergoes spontaneous capillary obliteration just before or shortly after birth, forming the cfz (28).

The foveola is composed entirely of cones; the central 100 μm of the foveola contain only red and green cones (29). The peak foveal cone density averages nearly 200,000 per mm^2 and falls rapidly with increasing eccentricity, such that cone density decreases nearly tenfold within 1 mm of the umbo. Blue cone density is highest in a zone between 100 and 300 μm from the center of the fovea. The foveal cones take on a more rod-like shape; blue cones in the macula tend to have inner segments 10% taller, and more cylindrical shape than their red and green counterparts (29). Rod cells differ from cones, their outer segments consisting of stacks of flattened membrane discs that are separate from the plasma membrane.

The RPE is a monolayer of hexagonal cells densely adherent to one another by a system of tight cellular junctions or terminal bars that make up the blood–outer-retinal barrier, which maintains the subretinal space in a state of deturgescence. In the fovea there are 30 cones per RPE cell, while in the periphery there are 22 rods per RPE cell. Interdigitation of the RPE cells with the rod and cone outer segments provides only a tenuous adhesion of the RPE to the sensory retina. The RPE cells in the macular region are taller and contain increased amounts of melanin pigment than elsewhere (30,31). There is an inverse relationship between melanin and lipofuscin pigment concentration in the RPE. Lipofuscin concentration increases initially during the first two decades of life, and then again in the sixth decade. The concentration of lipofuscin in the RPE is significantly greater in light- than dark-skinned persons, whereas the concentration of melanin in the pigment epithelium is similar in light- and dark-skinned persons. The melanin content of the pigment epithelium and choroidal melanocytes decline with age (Fig. 1.3).

In young and middle-aged individuals the RPE is tightly adherent to the underlying Bruch's membrane by means of its own basement membrane. This adherence decreases with advancing age. Bruch's membrane consists of the basement membrane of the RPE, the inner collagenous layer, an elastic layer, an outer collagenous layer, and the basement membrane of the choriocapillaris. Because of its porous structure, it probably plays a minimal role in regulating movement of substances across it.

The choroid is the posterior aspect of the uveal tract, it is supplied by the short ciliary arteries, and they are concentrated in the macula and peripapillary region. These arteries form a rich anastomotic network that quickly empties large quantities of blood into the choriocapillaris (sinusoidal network). The choriocapillaris is fenestrated and arranged in a lobular pattern, with a feeding arteriole in the center of each lobule and several venules peripherally (Fig. 1.7) (32–40).

The prelaminar part of the optic nerve is supplied by the peripapillary branches of the short posterior ciliary

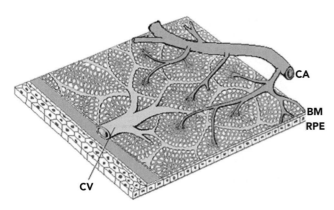

Figure 1.7 Schematic representation of the lobular pattern of the choriocapillaris. Each lobule is supplied by an arteriole. BM, Bruch's membrane; CA, choroidal artery; CV, choroidal vein; RPE, retinal pigment epithelium.

arteries. The choriocapillaris does not communicate directly with the optic disc capillaries. The prelaminar capillaries freely anastomose at the disc margin with those of the retina. Both capillary systems drain into the venules leading to the central retinal vein (33,40).

The RPE is an integral part of the visual cycle. It is an important component of photoreceptor renewal: new outer-segment discs are continually added proximal to the base and the oldest discs at the distal end of the outer segments are phagocytosed by the RPE cells. The RPE also transports metabolic wastes from the retina into the choriocapillaris. The melanin within the RPE cells absorbs light that has not been captured by the photoreceptors, thus preventing excessive light scattering within the eye. Melanin absorption may also confer protection from photo-oxidative stress (41). The RPE cells are also thought to secrete growth factors essential for proper differentiation of photoreceptors during development (42).

The macula has the highest rate of blood flow of any tissue in the body. It probably functions to stabilize the temperature environment of the retina (43) because blood flow is greatly in excess of that needed to meet the nutritional demands of the retina. The choriocapillaris supplies the RPE and outer retinal layers. The choriocapillaris has an endothelium with a pore size sufficient to allow some larger molecules, including proteins, to escape into the extravascular space. There are no lymphatic channels in the eye; the perivascular and perineural spaces in the sclera probably function as lymphatic channels. Thus the choriocapillaris endothelium controls the amount of extracellular fluid normally present in the choroid.

BLOOD-RETINAL BARRIERS

Retinal perfusion is accomplished by a non-overlapping, dual system of blood circulation. For each system there is a blood-retinal barrier analogous to the blood-brain barrier.

Both barriers confine even relatively small molecules, because of a non-leaky tight junction between cells (44).

The outer blood-retinal barrier is constituted by the RPE; it blocks the inward migration of small molecules from the choriocapillaris into the subretinal space. Anatomically, these junctions include a zonula adherens and adjacent zonula occludens of the RPE, both situated near the apex of the cell and encircling it (45). The inner blood-retinal barrier is the retinal vascular endothelium, including the capillary endothelium. The site of the barrier is the specialized tight junctions (zonulae occludentes) between individual endothelial cells (44,46).

NORMAL FLUORESCEIN ANGIOGRAPHIC FINDINGS

Fluorescein angiography (FA) was developed in the 1950s as a means of studying vascular flow. FA is still used for this purpose, but it provides much additional information. Sodium fluorescein is excited by a blue light (465–490 nm) and it emits a fluorescent yellow-green light (peak wave length of 520–530 nm). Because of its molecular weight (376 kd), it diffuses freely out of all the body capillaries except the retina. Approximately 80% of the dye is bound to plasma proteins (albumin), and it is the unbound fluorescein that is detected angiographically (16).

FA is performed using a fundus camera. Filters are used to produce the exciting wavelength. The FA is photographed digitally or with black and white film because of its superior resolution and speed. On the positive images, fluorescein appears white and nonfluorescent areas appear black (46). The normal FA shows the dual nature of the retinal circulation. The larger choroidal vessels fill first, with almost immediate filling of the choriocapillaris. Rapid perfusion of the choroid and leakage of the dye from the choriocapillaris give the fairly uniform background fluorescence.

The tight junctions of the retinal pigment epithelial cells (the outer blood-retinal barrier) block the fluorescein that leaks from the choriocapillaris and diffuses through Bruch's membrane. Normally the fluorescein does not gain access to the subsensory retinal space. The retinal vessels, including the capillaries (the inner blood-retinal barrier), normally do not leak fluorescein. Thus, the angiogram evaluates both of the blood-retinal barriers (44).

The normal macular region is hypofluorescent or has a barely visible fluorescence because of the greater density of the RPE in this area and the presence of xanthophyll in the outer retinal layers. In darkly pigmented individuals, the increased density of choroidal melanocytes in the macula helps obscure the background choroidal fluorescence. In addition, the capillaries appear particularly distinct, because there is only one capillary layer surrounding the foveal avascular zone (47). Only in the extramacular area, before the arteriovenous phase, can details of perfusion of the larger choroidal vessels be detected.

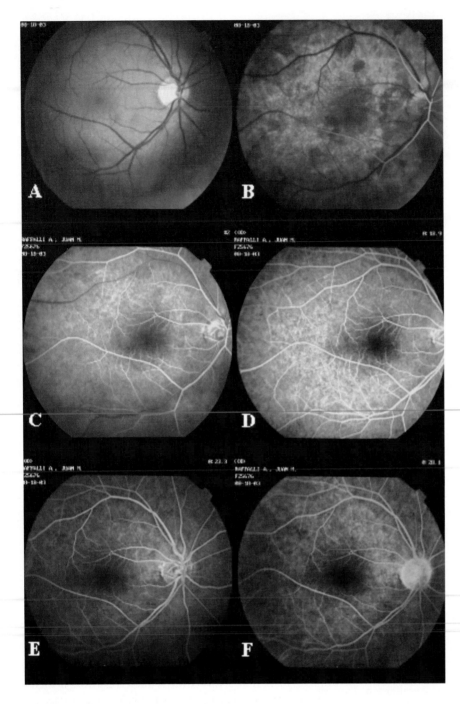

Figure 1.8 Fluorescein angiography of normal fundus. **A.** Red-free photograph. **B.** Arterial phase. **C.** Early arteriovenous phase. **D.** Intermediate arteriovenous phase. **E.** Venous phase. **F.** Recirculation phase. (Courtesy of Dario Fuenmayor-Rivera and Enrique Murcia.)

The FA consists of five phases (Fig. 1.8):

1. Prearterial phase: The choroid and choriocapillaris fill with dye. A cilioretinal vessel, if present, usually fills at the same time as the choroidal circulation, before fluorescein is detectable in the other retinal vessels, approximately 1 second before that of the proximal branches of the central retinal artery (Fig. 1.4).
2. Arterial phase: Lasts until the arteries are completely filled.
3. Arteriovenous phase: Characterized by complete filling of the arteries and capillaries and the first evidence of laminar flow in the veins.
4. Venous phase: Begins as the arteries are emptying and persists until the veins are filled with dye.
5. Recirculation phase: Follows the venous phase and represents the first return of blood to the eye after fluorescein has passed through the kidneys. During the recirculation phase the outer edges of the major retinal vessels appear relatively hyperfluorescent because of the greater amount of fluorescein in the tangential section of the plasma cuff near the edge of the blood vessels.

All abnormalities in the FA can be understood as the presence of either too much fluorescein (hyperfluorescence) or too little (hypofluorescence) in a specific location (48).

In evaluating diseases of the macula, FA can be of value in detecting alterations in blood flow, in permeability of the retinal blood vessels, in the retinal vascular pattern, in the density of the pigment epithelium, and other changes affecting the normal angiographic pattern in this area (16).

NORMAL INDOCYANINE GREEN ANGIOGRAPHY FINDINGS

Indocyanine green (ICG) is a dye that was originally used in the photographic industry. It was first used in ophthalmology by Flower and Hochheimer (49) in the early 1970s to image the choroidal circulation. Although both experimental and clinical investigations with ICG continued, it was not until the early 1990s that it became an established method of investigation. This was because of the increasing interest in the contribution of the choroid to retinal diseases and improvements in technology. ICG, a tricarbocyanine dye, is injected intravenously and is imaged as it passes through ocular vessels. An excitation filter with a peak at 805 nm and a barrier filter with a transmission peak of 835 nm, corresponding to the maximum fluorescence emitted by the dye in whole blood, are required. The standard technique is to inject 25 mg of ICG in 5 ml of water slowly and to begin photographs 7 to 10 minutes after injection with late photographs at 20 and 40 minutes. The circulating dye is rapidly excreted by the biliary system. A preinjection infrared fundus photograph showing pseudofluorescence or autofluorescence may help to avoid misinterpretation of the angiograms (50).

Adverse reactions to ICG are more rare than those with intravenous fluorescein. Mild reactions such as nausea, vomiting, sneezing, and transient itching occur in 0.15% of cases (51). More severe reactions such as urticaria, syncope, fainting, and pyrexia may also occur. Severe reactions such as hypotensive shock (52), anaphylactic shock (53), and death have been reported. Crossover allergy to iodine can occur in patients with seafood allergies, making iodine and seafood allergy a contraindication to ICG angiography. Because the liver primarily metabolizes ICG, it should be avoided in patients with hepatic disease. Those undergoing hemodialysis are also at increased risk of complications.

Photographic film with a conventional camera is not sensitive enough to acquire ICG images—more sensitive digital systems are required (54–57). Low-contrast individual images are digitally enhanced to allow better interpretation of choroidal structures (58,59). ICG and FA can each be performed and the images superimposed (60,61). New technologic developments now permit dynamic, simultaneous FA and ICG using the confocal scanning laser ophthalmoscope (62,63). The use of a wide-angle contact lens to visualize 160° of the fundus may help in the evaluation of flow characteristics and simultaneous assessment of the periphery and posterior pole (64).

Interpretation of ICG angiography is difficult because multiple vascular layers are displayed at one time. After choroidal arteries fill, the capillary phase is characterized by a rather diffuse hyperfluorescence resulting from the additive fluorescence effects of multiple crossing arterioles and venules. This fluorescence is brighter in the foveolar area. However, because xanthophyll does not efficiently absorb infrared light, the foveola cannot be located exactly during ICG angiography (Fig. 1.9). The choriocapillaris layer itself can only be sensed as a faint haze that becomes visible in the early venous phase. The images do not change significantly during the next several minutes. With reduction in dye fluorescence after about 5 minutes, discernibility of single choroidal vessels decreases and there is a fairly uniform background fluorescence on which larger retinal vessels are

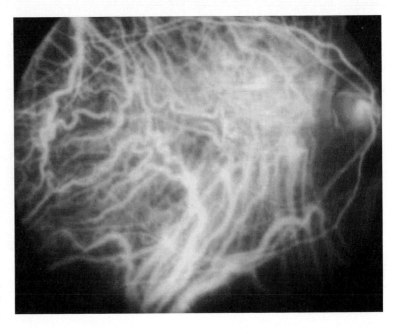

Figure 1.9 Indocyanine green video-angiography (ICG-V) of normal fundus. (Courtesy of Dario Fuenmayor-Rivera.)

visible as brighter structures; after 10 to 15 minutes, however, these vessels appear as darker structures. This rapid decrease in retinal vessel fluorescence reflects the fast hepatic extraction of the dye from the blood. In contrast, fluorescence in the choroid lasts much longer and could be interpreted as exudation of the dye. However, a comparative examination of ICG fluorescence demonstrates that plasma fluorescence of the dye is much brighter than that of whole blood and lasts much longer (65,66). In fact, it decreases at the same rate as background ICG fluorescence in the fundus. We therefore believe that plasma gaps in choroidal capillaries must be sufficiently large to become the main source of late choroidal fluorescence. As with fluorescein, ICG hyperfluorescence cannot always be attributed to extravasation of the dye. Focal, short-term hyperfluorescence is a common finding in the early venous phase and probably is caused by a plasma vortex in venous loops or additive fluorescence of crossing vessels. Though the pigment epithelium blocks only 10% of infrared light, that is still enough to create a window-like hyperfluorescence at the site of pigment epithelial atrophic defects (67).

NORMAL OPTICAL COHERENCE TOMOGRAPHY FINDINGS

Optical Coherence Tomography (OCT, Zeiss-Humphrey Instruments, Dublin, CA) uses a continuously emitting, optically coherent laser diode centered at 850 nm and focused at the retina. The superluminescence low-coherence

diode emits light with a 20 to 25 nm bandwidth. For thickness measurements, the time delay of reflected or backscattered light is determined using coherence interferometry. Reflectivity and distance information is contained in the interference signal between a probe beam, reflected from different structures within the investigated tissue, and light returning from a variable-reference optical delay path. The length of one scan is adjustable for 43 nm working distance up to 3 mm in air (in vivo approximately 6 mm), and one line can be measured within 1 second. The displayed image has a resolution of 500 × 500 pixels. The axial resolution of OCT is reported by the manufacturer to be 10 to 20 μm (68).

Wakitani et al. (69) reported a study of macular thickness measurements in 203 healthy subjects with different axial lengths using OCT. The thickness of three circular areas centered on the central fovea with diameters 350 μm, 1,850 μm, and 2,850 μm, were 167 ± 21 μm, 212 ± 17 μm, and 231 ± 15 μm, respectively. There was no significant difference in retinal thickness with age or with increasing axial length of the eye. However, the average thickness of the macula in females was significantly thinner than in males.

The contrast between different retinal layers is delineated by a narrow-field-of-view image of a normal fovea. The anterior and posterior margins of the retina are defined by highly reflective layers (the NFL and retinal pigmentary epithelium/choriocapillaris). In the area of the fovea, the retinal pigmentary epithelium/choriocapillaris appears distinct from the external segments of the photoreceptors. The stratified structure of the retina is composed of alternating layers of moderate and low reflectivity, and the

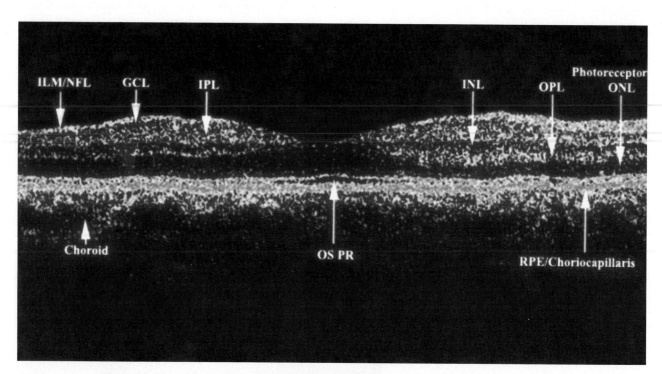

Figure 1.10 Optical coherence tomography (OCT) of normal macula. GCL, ganglion cell layer; ILM/NFL, internal limiting membrane/nerve fiber layer; INL, inner nuclear layer; IPL, inner plexiform layer; ONL, outer nuclear layer; OPL, outer plexiform layer of Henle; OS PR, photoreceptor's outer segments; RPE, retinal pigment epithelium.

photoreceptors appear minimally reflective. Moderate backscattering is observed from the inner and outer plexiform layers, which, like the NFL, consist of fibrous structures running perpendicular to the incident beam. In contrast, the nuclear layers show minimal backscattering because the cell bodies of the nuclear layers, like the photoreceptors, are oriented parallel to the incident light. The increased backscatter and the shadowing of the reflections from the RPE and choriocapillaris identify the retinal blood vessels. The larger choroidal vessels may also appear in the image and have minimally reflective dark lumens (70).

We can obtain information on three-dimensional structure thanks to the ability of OCT to acquire images of consecutive slices through the retina. Characteristic features of the retina appear consistently in the serial sections (Fig. 1.10). The anterior and posterior surfaces of the neural retina are defined by backscattering at the NFL and vitreoretinal interface, while the highly backscattering red layer represents the RPE and choriocapillaris. The development and resolution of the foveal depression, which reaches its maximum depth at the fovea centralis, are revealed by the sequence of tomograms. Retinal blood vessels derived from the superior and inferior branches of the central retinal artery are evident in the tomograms from the partial shadowing of the deep retinal structure beneath the vessels (70).

ACKNOWLEDGMENTS

Supported in part by the Fundacion Arevalo-Coutinho para la Investigacion en Oftalmologìa, Caracas, Venezuela.

REFERENCES

1. Amalric P. The macula: 50 years of study: from clinical aspects to genetics. *Points de Vue.* 1998;39:4–20.
2. Hendrickson AE, Yuodelis C. The morphological development of the human fovea. *Ophthalmology.* 1984;91:603–612.
3. Fulton AB, Albert DM, Craft JL. Human albinism. Light and electron microscopy study. *Arch Ophthalmol.* 1978;96:305–310.
4. Levenberger P. *Stèrèo-ultrastructure de la Retine: Ètude Comparative au Microscope Èlectronique ‡ TransmisiÙn et · Balayage.* Paris: Arch Ophthalmol; 1971.
5. Mann I. *Development of the Human Eye.* New York: Grune & Stratton; 1964.
6. Duke-Elder S, Cook C. Normal and abnormal development. In: *System of Ophthalmology,* vol 3, part 1. St. Louis: Mosby; 1963.
7. Streeten BW. Development of the human retinal pigment epithelium and the posterior segment. *Arch Ophthalmol.* 1969;81:383–394.
8. Provis JM, Van Driel D, Billson FA, et al. Development of the human retina: patterns of cell distribution and redistribution in the ganglion cell layer. *J Comp Neurol.* 1985;22:429–451.
9. Moore KL. *The Developing Human: Clinically Oriented Embryology.* 3rd. Ed. Philadelphia: WB Saunders; 1982:413–416.
10. Weiter JJ, Delori FC, Wing GL, et al. Retinal pigment epithelial lipofuscin and melanin and choroidal melanin in human eyes. *Invest Ophthalmol Vis Sci.* 1986;27:145–152.
11. Duvall J. Structure, function, and pathologic responses of pigment epithelium: a review. *Semin Ophthalmol.* 1987;2:130–140.
12. Garner A. Retinal angiogenesis: mechanism in health and disease. *Semin Ophthalmol.* 1987;2:71–80.
13. Engerman RL. Development of the macular circulation. *Invest Ophthalmol.* 1976;15:835–840.
14. Federman JL, Gouras P, Schubert H, et al. Retina and vitreous. In: Podos SM, Yanoff M, eds. *Textbook of Ophthalmology,* vol 9. London: Gower Medical; 1994.
15. Hogan MJ, Alvarado JA, Weddell JE. *Histology of the Human Eye: An Atlas and Textbook.* Philadelphia, WB Saunders; 1971:508–519.
16. Gass JD. *Stereoscopic Atlas of Macular Diseases: Diagnosis and Treatment.* 4th Ed, Vol 1. Mosby-Year Book Inc; 1997:1–17.
17. Justice J Jr, Lehmann RP. Cilioretinal arteries: a study based on review of stereo fundus photographs and fluorescein angiographic findings. *Arch Ophthalmol.* 1976;94:1,355–1,358.
18. Michaelson IC. *Retinal Circulation in Man and Animals.* Springfield: Charles C. Thomas; 1954.
19. Nussbaum JJ, Pruett RC, Delori FC. Historic perspectives: macular yellow pigment; the first 200 years. *Retina.* 1981;1:296–310.
20. Snodderly DM, Auran J, Delori FC. Localization of the macular pigment. *Invest Ophthalmol Vis Sci.* 1979;18:80.
21. Snodderly DM, Auran J, Delori FC. The macular pigment. II. Spatial distribution in primate retinas. *Invest Ophthalmol Vis Sci.* 1984;25:674–685.
22. Wald G. Human vision and the spectrum. *Science.* 1945;101:653–658.
23. Bone RA, Landrum JT, Hime GW, et al. Stereochemistry of the human macular carotenoids. *Invest Ophthalmol Vis Sci.* 1993;34:2033–2040.
24. Fine BS. Limiting membranes of the sensory retina and pigment epithelium: an electron microscopic study. *Arch Ophthalmol.* 1961;66:847–860.
25. Blanks JC. Morphology and topography of the retina. In: Ryan SJ. *Retina,* vol 1, 3rd Ed. St Louis: Mosby; 2001:32–53.
26. Marquardt R. Ein Beitrag zur Topographie and Anatomie der Netzhautgefasse des menschlichen Auges. *Klin Monatsbl Augenheilkd.* 1966;148:50–64.
27. Shimizu K, Ujiie K. *Structure of Ocular Vessels.* Tokyo: Igaku Shoin; 1978.
28. Henkind P, Bellhorn RW, Murphy ME, et al. Development of macular vessels in monkey and cat. *Br J Ophthalmol.* 1975;59:703–709.
29. Curcio CA, Allen KA, Sloan KR, et al. Distribution and morphology of human photoreceptors stained with anti-blue opsin. *J Comp Neurol.* 1991;312:610–624.
30. Tso MOM, Friedman E. The retinal pigment epithelium I. Comparative histology. *Arch Ophthalmol.* 1967;78:641–649.
31. Green WR. Retina. In: Spencer WH, *Ophthalmic Pathology: An Atlas and Textbook,* vol 2, 4th Ed. Philadelphia: W.B. Saunders Company; 1996:667–681.
32. Amalric PM. Choroidal vessel occlusive syndromes-clinical aspects. *Trans Am Acad Ophthalmol Otolaryngol.* 1973;77:OP291–OP299.
33. Hayreh SS. The choriocapillaris. *Albrecht von Graefes Arch Klin Exp Ophthalmol.* 1974;192:165–179.
34. Hayreh SS. Segmental nature of the choroidal vasculature. *Br J Ophthalmol.* 1975;59:631–648.
35. Hayreh SS. Submacular choroidal vasculature pattern: experimental fluorescein fundus angiographic studies. *Albrecht von Graefes Arch Klin Exp Ophthalmol.* 1974;192:181–196.
36. Krey HF. Segmental vascular patterns of the choriocapillaris. *Am J Ophthalmol.* 1975;80:198–206.
37. Dollery CT, Henkind P, Kohner EM, et al. Effect of raised intraocular pressure on the retinal and choroidal circulation. *Invest Ophthalmol.* 1968;7:191–198.
38. Hayreh SS. Recent advances in fluorescein fundus angiography. *Br J Ophthalmol.* 1974;58:391–412.
39. Perry HD, Hatfield RV, Tso MOM. Fluorescein pattern of the choriocapillaris in the neonatal rhesus monkey. *Am J Ophthalmol.* 1977;84:197–204.
40. Ernest JT, Stern WH, Archer DB. Submacular choroidal circulation. *Am J Ophthalmol.* 1976;81:574–582.
41. Sarna T. Properties and functions of the ocular melanin: a photobiophysical view. *J Photochem Photobiol B.* 1992;12:215–258.
42. Tombran-Tink J, Shivaram SM, Chader GJ, et al. Expresion, secretion, and age related down regulation of pigment epithelium-derived factor, a serpin with neurotrophic activity. *J Neurosci.* 1995;15:4,992–5,003.
43. Parver LM, Auker CR, Carpenter DO. The stabilizing effect of the choroidal circulation on the temperature environment of the macula. *Retina.* 1982;2:117–120.
44. Cunha-Vaz J. The blood-ocular barriers. *Surv Ophthalmol.* 1979;23:279–296.
45. Dubai J. Structure function, and pathologic responses of pigment epithelium: a review. *Semin Ophthalmol.* 1987;2:130–140.
46. Kincaid MC. Topographic anatomy, histology and fluorescein angiography. In: Grossniklaus HE, Kincaid, MC. *Ophthalmology Clinics of North America: Macular Diseases,* vol 6. WB Saunders Company; 1993:181–189.
47. Iwasaki M, Inomata H. Relation between superficial capillaries and foveal structures in the human retina. *Invest Ophthalmol Vis Sci.* 1986;27:1698–1705.
48. Rabb MF, Burton TC, Schatz H, et al. Fluorescein angiography of the fundus: a schematic approach to interpretation. *Surv Ophthalmol.* 1978;22:387–403.
49. Flower RW, Hochheimer BF. Clinical infrared absorption angiography of the choroid (letter). *Am J Ophthalmol.* 1972;73:458.
50. Piccolino FC, Borgia L, Zinicola E, et al. Pre-injection fluorescence in indocyanine green angiography. *Ophthalmology.* 1996;103:1837–1845.
51. Hope-Ross M, Yannuzzi LA, Gragoudas ED, et al. Adverse reactions due to indocyanine green. *Ophthalmology.* 1994;101:529–533.
52. Bonte CA, Ceuppens J, Leys AM. Hypotensive shock as a complication of indocyanine green injection. *Retina.* 1998;18:476–477.
53. Olsen TW, Lim JI, Capone A Jr, et al. Anaphylactic shock following indocyanine green angiography. *Arch Ophthalmol.* 1996;114:97.
54. Hyvärinen L, Flower RW. Indocyanine green fluorescence angiography. *Acta Ophthalmol (Copen)* 1980;58:528–538.
55. Bischoff PM, Flower RW. Ten years experience with choroidal angiography using indocyanine green dye: a new routine examination or an epilogue? *Doc Ophthalmol.* 1985;60:235–291.
56. Slakter JS, Yanuzzi LA, Guyer DR, et al. Indocyanine green angiography. *Curr Opin Ophthalmol.* 1995;6:25–32.
57. Bartsch DU, Weinreb RN, Zinser G, et al. Confocal scanning infrared laser ophthalmoscopy for indocyanine green angiography. *Am J Ophthalmol.* 1995;120:642–651.
58. Klein GJ, Baumgartner RH, Flower RW. An image processing approach to characterizing choroidal blood flow. *Invest Ophthalmol Vis Sci.* 1990;31: 629–637.

59. Maberly DAL, Cruess AF. Indocyanine green angiography: an evaluation of image enhancement for the identification of occult choroidal neovascular membranes. *Retina*. 1999;19:37–44.

60. Flower RW, Hochheimer BF. Indocyanine green dye fluorescence and infrared absorption choroidal angiography performed simultaneously with fluorescein angiography. *Johns Hopkins Med J*. 1976;138:33–42.

61. Bischoff PM, Niederberger HJ, Torok B, et al. Simultaneous indocyanine green and fluorescein angiography. *Retina*. 1995; 15:91–99.

62. Scheider A, Schroedel C. High resolution indocyanine green angiography with a scanning laser ophthalmoscope (letter). *Am J Ophthalmol*. 1989; 108:458–459.

63. Holz FG, Bellmann C, Rohrschneider K, et al. Simultaneous confocal scanning laser fluorescein and indocyanine green angiography. *Am J Ophthalmol*. 1998;125:227–236.

64. Spaide RF, Orlock DA, Herrmann-Delemazure B, et al. Wide angle indocyanine green angiography. *Retina*. 1998;18:44–49.

65. Scheider A, Voeth A, Kaboth A, et al. Fluorescence characteristics of indocyanine green in the normal choroid and in subretinal neovascular membranes. *Ger J Ophthalmol*. 1992;1:7–11.

66. Scheider A, Neuhauser L. Fluorescence characteristics of drusen during indocyanine green angiography and their possible correlation with choroidal perfusion. *Ger J Ophthalmol*. 1992;1:328–334.

67. Yannuzzi LA, Flower RW, Slakter JS, eds. *Indocyanine Green Angiography*. St. Louis: Mosby; 1997.

68. Neubauer AS, Priglinger S, Ullrich S, et al. Comparison of foveal thickness measured with the retinal thickness analyzer and optical coherence tomography. *Retina*. 2001;21:596–601.

69. Wakitani Y, Sasoh M, Sugimoto M, et al. Macular thickness measurements in healthy subjects with different axial lengths using optical coherence tomography. *Retina*. 2003;23:177–82.

70. Puliafito CA, Hee MR, Schuman JS, et al. *Optical Coherence Tomography of Ocular Diseases*. Thorofare, NJ: SLACK Inc; 1996.

Animal Disease Models

2

Melanie Lynn Hom   Ron Afshari Adelman

INTRODUCTION

Age-related macular degeneration (AMD) is diverse in its presentation. Pathological findings include deposition of abnormal material within Bruch's membrane, geographic atrophy, subretinal neovascularization, and detachment of the retinal pigment epithelium (RPE) (1). Studying AMD is complicated since the exact physiology remains unknown. To date, no animal model has been discovered that exactly replicates all of the features of clinical AMD. Despite this, animal disease models remain pivotal since they can closely mimic some aspects of the human disease. This enables the study of AMD pathology, cell biology, gene abnormalities, and gene products, all of which could lead to a better understanding of the disease or the development of a new treatment.

Initial studies to create an animal disease model used injections of enzymes such as collagenase and hyaluronidase delivered to the Bruch's membrane and the RPE (2). These models were occasionally successful at creating subretinal neovascularization, but failed to show reproducibility (3). Later, various animal models were created that reliably and consistently mimicked features of AMD, including subretinal neovascularization.

The majority of animal models to date have focused on exudative AMD and inducing choroidal and retinal neovascularization. The most extensively used models involve laser photocoagulation and transgenic animals. Since the presence of drusen and basal laminar deposits along the basement membrane of the RPE have been identified as important hallmarks of dry AMD, animal models have been developed to study the physiology and possible treatment of dry AMD. Specific animal models for dry AMD have been created using transgenic lines that have a predilection for drusen or basal laminar deposits.

In addition to the various techniques of creating an animal disease model, the species of animal studied have also greatly varied. Primates were the first subjects investigated and they remain the most extensively studied, since they most closely resemble the human eye in respect to size, anatomy, and physiology. Although the primate model is invaluable for the information that it is able to provide, it also has its disadvantages, given the animal's size, expense, and difficult care. Other models have been studied in animals that are smaller, have a shorter developmental cycle, more affordable, and can be studied in large numbers. Thus, the animal disease model has been extended from the primate to the rabbit, cat, pig, rat, mouse, chicken chorioallantoic membrane, and endothelial cells in tissue culture. Several of these animal models will be discussed for both exudative and dry AMD.

LASER PHOTOCOAGULATION MODEL

Laser photocoagulation successfully induces subretinal neovascularization (2,4–15). The basis of using laser photocoagulation to create an AMD animal model stems from the idea that laser photocoagulation induces microthrombi that result in neovascularization with endothelial cell proliferation (14–16). In addition, laser photocoagulation creates a breakdown in Bruch's membrane and an inflammatory response that may also play an important role in neovascularization (17,18).

Initial photocoagulation studies used a combination of retinal vein occlusion with argon laser photocoagulation (7,8), but it was found that the retinal branch vein occlusion was neither necessary nor reliable in creating subretinal neovascularization (4). The laser has been used to cause subretinal neovascularization in a reproducible manner in animal models (2,4,6–13,14–16,19–24). In the first studies using laser photocoagulation, the rhesus monkey (*Macaca mulatto*) was chosen because its macular anatomy and retinal and choroidal circulations are similar to those of humans. Also, the monkey has been extensively studied in vision research in the past and therefore its morphology is well known (25). This technique has been extended to establish subretinal neovascularization in rabbits (9,16,19), cats (14,15), rats (10,20–24), and mice (26,27).

The basis for using laser photocoagulation to create AMD in an animal model is based on work by Stephen Ryan (2,4,6). What follows is a description of his initial AMD animal model in the rhesus monkey using argon laser photocoagulation, but it is important to remember that a similar technique is now applied to other animals. The early study was done using 44 adult rhesus monkeys. For anesthesia during laser application, a combination of ketamine hydrochloride, phenothiazine, and atropine sulfate was administered intramuscularly followed by intravenous pentobarbital sodium. Topical 10% phenylephrine hydrochloride and 1% tropicamide were applied for pupillary dilation. A Coherent 900 argon laser was used through a slit lamp and a fundus contact lens to disrupt Bruch's membrane, which was evidenced by the appearance of a bubble during the procedure. The specific laser settings were a spot size of 100 μm, intensity of 600 to 900 mW (averaged approximately 700 mW), and duration of 0.1 seconds. These laser settings are higher than those for therapeutic laser photocoagulation, since the goal is to break the Bruch's membrane and produce neovascularization. The laser burns were applied as shown in Figure 2.1. In Ryan's

experiment, eight laser burns were applied in the macular region and at different distances from the center of the fovea, but both fovea were never treated in both eyes of the same animal. On the nasal side of the optic nerve head, the same grid pattern was applied in some animals, and the center of these eight points was approximately the same distance nasal to the optic nerve head as the fovea was temporal to the disc (Fig. 2.1). The periphery also had eight spots placed in a rectangular pattern. Some of the monkeys had treatment in all three areas, some in two areas, and others in only one the macula. The eyes were photographed and if an area had involuted or become quiescent, laser burns were subsequently placed in another location.

Overall a total of 779 laser burns were made in the 44 rhesus monkeys. This study found that 39% of the laser-induced lesions in the macular region showed subretinal neovascularization. Only 3% of the laser-induced lesions located nasal to the optic nerve head showed formation of subretinal neovascularization, and in the peripheral retina only 0.3% produced neovascularization. The average time for the development of neovascularization was 3 weeks and continued for approximately 13 weeks. The high incidence and predilection for subretinal neovascularization correlates with the findings of AMD.

This animal model provides a discrete and reproducible form of subretinal neovascularization in which basic pathogenic mechanisms can be studied and manipulated. Although this is an excellent animal model for subretinal neovascularization, there are limitations; spontaneous hemorrhages occurred in 28% of laser lesions and fluorescein leakage patterns varied (6). Despite its limitations, the

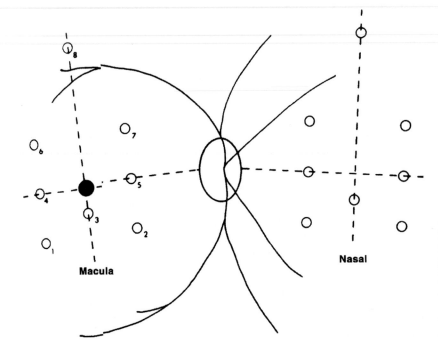

Macula

Nasal

Figure 2.1   Right eye. In macular pattern, horizontal dashed line bisects fovea (solid black circle) and optic disc. In nasal pattern, same grid is applied nasal to nerve head. Horizontal lines of both macular and nasal grids are slightly tilted to account for the inferior location of the fovea to the center of the disc. (Reprinted with permission from Ryan SJ. Subretinal neovascularization. Natural history of an experimental model. *Arch Ophthalmol.* 1982;100:1805.)

laser photocoagulation model has been extensively used in AMD studies.

Perry et al. have extended the technique to the domestic cat using argon laser retinal photocoagulation. The cats were anesthetized, pupils dilated, and argon laser spots were administered to the retina with 175 to 800 mW power, 0.2 second duration, and 500 μm spot size (14,15). Results obtained from vascular casts and scanning electron microscopy further support that argon laser photocoagulation induces microthrombi that result in subretinal neovascularization with proliferation of endothelial cells (14,15). Neodymium-YAG laser has been used in rabbits to produce choroidal and subretinal neovascularization (16,19). The laser setting was 35 to 150 mJ, 0.02 second duration, and 100 μm spot size (16,19). It should be noted that the neodymium-YAG laser light penetrates six-times deeper within the collagen tissue than argon laser light, but no significant differences were found in inducing neovascularization (16,19).

Laser-induced neovascularization in the rat model and the murine model have also been used. These models are similar to the primate model, though there are differences with respect to the laser parameters. For the rat, Pollack et al. used a krypton laser (630–647 nm) through a handheld cover slip serving as a contact lens (21–23). The laser parameters consisted of a power of 55 to 150 mW, an exposure duration of 0.05 second, and a spot size of 100 μm (10,20–23,28). Zacks et al. have used an argon dye pulsed laser with a power of 130 to 150 mW, applied for 0.1 second, and a spot size of 100 μm (29). Choroidal neovascularization was documented 3 weeks after laser induction with angiography (29). The rat model is affordable and reproducible.

Studies by Tobe et al. of the murine model have used krypton laser photocoagulation with a power of 350 to 400 mW, a duration of 0.05 seconds, and a spot size of 50 μm, delivered through a cover glass as a contact lens (26,30). Laser burns were in the 9, 12, and 3 o'clock positions (26,30). Murine models of neovascularization are efficient since neovascularization occurs rapidly (within 1 week), and highly reliable since neovascularization can be identified in over 80% of lesions. Additionally, the small size of mice allows for use of smaller amounts of drugs, which is an important consideration for testing new agents that may only be available in limited quantities.

Important treatments have recently been tested using the laser photocoagulation model, including photodynamic therapy (PDT) and rhuFab VEGF (discussed below). PDT is based on the use of photosensitizer drugs that are injected intravenously and activated by a non-thermal laser light to selectively occlude neovascular vessels. Early studies of PDT, were done in laser-induced neovascularization animal models with hematoporphyrin derivative (HPD) and rose bengal (31–34), but these have been limited by weak photosensitizing ability and prolonged cutaneous photosensitivity (35–37). The results obtained from verteporfin PDT in these animal models have been found to resemble the results in human studies.

Recently, Krzystolik et al. used laser-induce neovascularization to study the effects of an antigen binding fragment of a recombinant humanized monoclonal antibody directed toward vascular endothelial growth factor (VEGF) (31). This anti-VEGF antibody fragment, also known as rhuFab VEGF, was found to prevent formation of choroidal neovascularization as well as decrease leakage for already-present neovascularization (31).

TRANSGENIC MODEL

A number of growth factors and signaling molecules have been implicated in the regulation and development of retinal structure and function. Although the pathogenesis of AMD is not precisely known, studies of choroidal neovascular membranes from patients with AMD have demonstrated the presence of various growth factors, including fibroblast growth factor (FGF) (11,26–27,38–39), (VEGF) (27,31, 40–44), and transforming growth factor beta (TGF-beta) (45,46). Several methods have been studied to create transgenic models, including constructing a gene to overexpress the growth factor(s), blocking the growth factor(s) signal, and creating a dominant-negative receptor mutation (27,38,42–44,47). In addition to genetically altering the function or amount of growth factor available, other transgenic models have been created via alterations of other key genes or gene products that are thought to be involved in the disease process of AMD (11,41,48–51).

Vascular Endothelial Growth Factor (VEGF)

The hypoxia-regulated protein VEGF is one of the major stimulators of angiogenesis. It was first reported in 1983 in highly vascularized tumors (52). VEGF is a protein that is normally found in the RPE, ganglion cells, and the inner nuclear layer, and is thought to modulate retinal vascular permeability (53,54), vasculogenesis (55), and vascular proliferation (56). The protein is secreted as a polypeptide and has five isoforms that are formed by alternative mRNA splicing; two of these isoforms are commonly expressed in the ischemic retina (57–59). Studies have demonstrated high concentrations of VEGF and VEGF receptors in the subfoveal fibrovascular membranes, the surrounding tissues, and the RPE in patients with AMD (60,61). In addition, *in vitro* exposure to hypoxia and cytokines has been found to increase VEGF mRNA and VEGF protein concentration (62). Experiments have capitalized on these findings of VEGF to investigate its role in AMD by modulating VEGF expression.

Overexpression of VEGF in a transgenic murine model has been created to study its effects on neovascularization. VEGF overexpression has been induced by creating tissue-specific, gain-of-function transgenic mice in which a promoter is coupled to the gene for VEGF (27,42). Schwesinger et al. (27) used a murine RPE65 promoter to overexpress VEGF in the RPE, while Okamoto et al. (42) used a bovine rhodopsin promoter for overexpression of VEGF in the photoreceptors. These transgenic lines were studied with reverse transcription coupled to PCR and Southern blot analysis (27,42). Immunohistochemistry confirmed that the RPE and choroid both showed increased expression of VEGF protein (27,42). The findings from both studies confirm that the addition of a gain-of-function promoter to induce VEGF overexpression is useful in creation of an exudative AMD animal model. Figure 2.2 illustrates subretinal neovascularization that was present in the murine model with increased expression of VEGF.

Another technique to induce overexpression has been the introduction of a recombinant adenovirus vector expressing VEGF. Baffi et al. (43) and Spilsbury et al. (44) have constructed recombinant adenovirus-mediated delivery of VEGF to the subretinal space with resultant overexpression of VEGF in the RPE. Although transgene expression in the RPE from subretinally delivered adenovirus vectors in immunocompetent hosts is generally transient in nature (44,63–64), the short duration of VEGF expression from these studies have confirmed the development of choroidal neovascularization within 1 week. The transient expression of pathologic levels of VEGF is adequate to induce choroidal neovascularization but once the level decreases below a certain threshold, vascular growth also ceases and regression of growth is observed (56). Similar to the adenovirus vector model is the adeno-associated virus (AAV) vector encoding VEGF165, delivered to the subretinal space in the rat by Wang et al. (47). This method used an AAV vector with cloned human VEGF165 cDNA to induce overexpression of VEGF (47). This study established a rat model of neovascularization by AAV-induced VEGF overexpression in the RPE where vector dose could be titrated to control transgene expression and the development of choroidal neovascularization (47). Neovascularization was present at 5 weeks. Advantages of this method include a relatively long period of induced neovascularization (up to 20 months) and a very high induction rate (95%) (47).

Fibroblast Growth Factor (FGF)

The FGF family in both the retina and RPE consists of acidic FGF, basic FGF (bFGF), FGF2, and FGF5 (28,65–69). Some of these FGF factors have been found to promote the expression of differentiation markers in photoreceptors and RPE *in vitro* (28,70–71), and potentiate retinal progenitor cell fate differentiation (72). Despite many studies implicating their central role, one recent study has demonstrated that FGF2 expression is neither necessary nor sufficient for the development of retinal neovascularization (39).

Many diverse methods have been used to study FGF and its function. One approach is to alter the function of FGF receptors (FGFR). Neither gene knockouts nor disruption of the FGFR gene are viable methods for studying FGF function due to the induction of several developmental abnormalities and embryonic death (38). To avoid these problems, Campochiaro et al. (38) used dominant-negative receptor mutations that lack a functional ligand-induced tyrosine kinase domain for the FGFR. This is based on the idea that FGFRs are tyrosine kinase receptors that require dimerization for normal signaling, and that expression of a defective receptor can eliminate the ability of a cell to

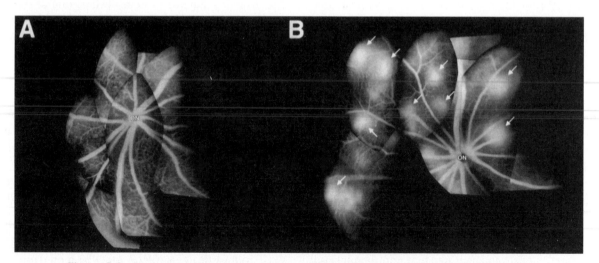

Figure 2.2 Fluorescein angiography in 3-month-old mice. **A.** This mouse had VEGF levels at baseline and has a normal appearing retinal vasculature. The central retinal artery enters at the optic nerve and divides into several branches that radiate out in all directions. Small discrete blood vessels are seen between the major vessels. Fluorescent dye is confined within blood vessels, because of tight junctions between normal retinal vacular endothelial cells. **B.** This mouse demonstrated sustained increased expression of VEGF in the retina and shows numerous hyperfluorescent spots with fuzzy borders throughtout the retina (arrows), indicating areas of fluorescein leakage. Histopathological evaluation of these areas demonstrates subretinal neovascularization. Hyperfluorescence occurs since experimental new vessels lack tight junctions between endothelial cells. ON, optic nerve. (Reprinted with permission from Ryan SJ. Subretinal neovascularization. Natural history of an experimental model. *Arch Ophthalmol.* 1982;100:1,805.)

respond to the ligand. By coupling a mutated FGFR gene to a tissue-specific promoter, the role of FGFs in a single cell type can be investigated while avoiding disruption of FGF signaling in other tissues. The bovine rhodopsin promoter was coupled to FGFR genes with deleted tyrosine kinase domains and generated transgenic mice that demonstrated photoreceptor-specific expression of the dominant-negative FGFR mutants. These FGFR mutants were found to have progressive photoreceptor degeneration, as occurs in AMD.

FGF modulation has also been achieved by implantation of bFGF-impregnated gelatin microspheres beneath the retina in rabbits to induce subretinal neovascularization (11). This study evolved from evidence that bFGF-impregnated gelatin hydrogels could induce neovascularization *in vivo* (73). This method provides an experimental disease model in the rabbit, where subretinal neovascularization with fluorescein leakage occurred in 83% of eyes that received the bFGF-impregnated gelatin microspheres (Fig. 2.3). Other studies using different modes of bFGF delivery have induce similar subretinal neovascularization in the minipig (48) and the rat (49).

Other Transgenic Models

Transgenic models are not only limited to exudative AMD, but have also been used for dry AMD models. Apolipoprotein-E (Apo-E) has been demonstrated to be present in drusen and basal laminar deposits (74). A decreased risk for AMD is seen in people carrying an Apo-E4 allele compared with those homozygous for Apo-E3 (74). An animal disease model was created with Apo-E3 Leiden transgenic mice (producing a dysfunctional form of human Apo-E3), using Apo-E knockout mice as controls (50,75–76). The mice were further divided into high-fat/cholesterol mouse chow versus standard mouse chow.

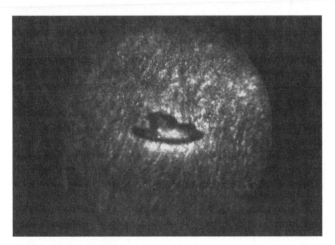

Figure 2.3 Fluorescein angiograms of the experimental eye with implanted bFGF-impregnated gelatin microspheres. Late-phase angiogram 3 weeks after implantation shows actively leaking fluorescein. (Reprinted with permission from Kimura H, Sakamoto T, Hinton DR, et al. A new model of subretinal neovascularization in the rabbit. *Invest Ophthalmol Vis Sci.* 1995;36:2,113.)

Basal laminar deposition was found in all eyes of the Apo-E3 Leiden transgenic mice on the high-fat/cholesterol diet and in 33% of those on the normal diet. The ultrastructural aspects of the mouse basal laminar deposits were found to be comparable with early basal laminar deposits in humans (50,77). These findings indicate that the Apo-E3 Leiden mice are a good animal disease model for basal laminar deposits and that a high-fat/cholesterol diet enhances the accumulation of these deposits.

Another transgenic model for dry AMD has been created by enzymatically inactivating cathepsin D (CatD), which is an aspartic protease (51). One theory for the etiology of dry AMD is the primary failure of the RPE cells due to abnormal build-up of photoreceptor outer segment (POS) breakdown products (50,77). To develop an animal model that might reproduce some features of AMD, the RPE cell lysosomal enzyme activity was modulated by producing a transgenic mouse line (mcd/mcd) expressing a mutated form of CatD that is enzymatically inactive, thus impairing processing of phagocytosed POS in the RPE cells (50,77). The model was found to have several AMD features, including RPE cell atrophy, RPE cell proliferation, photoreceptor degeneration, shortening of POS, and basal laminar and linear deposits (50,77). These findings occurred progressively with aging, as occurs with AMD.

Recently, a murine model deficient in either monocyte chemoattractant protein-1 (Ccl-2, also known as MCP-1) or its cognate C-C chemokine receptor-2 (Ccr-2) has been shown to develop features of both neovascular and dry AMD, including accumulation of lipofuscin and drusen, photoreceptor atrophy, and choroidal neovascularization (78). Ambati et al. used targeted gene disruption to create mice deficient in Ccl-2 and Ccr-2 (78). When these mice aged they were noted to have impairment in recruiting macrophages necessary for the clearance and degradation of drusen and other debris (78). C5a (the activated form of complement component C5) and IgG were allowed to accumulate without sufficient macrophage clearance. This is known to induce VEGF production by RPE, which, as noted previously, mediates the development of choroidal neovascularization (27,42-44,47,63–64,78). This animal model simulates features of both dry and neovascular AMD and further supports the role of inflammation and macrophage dysfunction in the pathogenesis of AMD. Although many investigations concerning the function and role of genes with regard to retinal abnormalities in AMD have shed some light on the complex pathogenesis and therapy, it is clear that more studies are needed.

OXYGEN-INDUCED MODEL

Varying oxygen exposure has been shown to cause retinal neovascularization. This is based on the idea that exposure to a hyperoxic environment and then return to room air probably causes relative ischemia in the non-perfused retina, which induces neovascularization. Most studies in this area have investigated retinopathy of prematurity and diabetic retinopathy. During the 1950s it was demonstrated that a high concentration of oxygen may lead to the production of a proliferative retinopathy (79). But until the last decade, the mouse model of oxygen-induced retinopathy remained inconsistent (80). Now with defined parameters for exposure to hyperoxia, a consistent, reproducible, and quantifiable neovascularization in the mouse retina can be obtained.

An oxygen-induced retinopathy model in the mouse has been described by Smith et al. (80). Neonatal mice at postnatal day 7 (P7) were chosen for the study after determining that this is the age where the balance between hyaloid regression and incomplete retinal vascularization is optimal. P7 mice were randomly assigned to hyperoxia (75% oxygen) or to room air. Seventy-five percent oxygen was found to be optimal from examining the effect of 50 to 95% oxygen on neovascularization. The oxygen-treated mice were housed in an incubator and the oxygen concentration was maintained at 75% ± 2%, using a flow rate of 1.5 L/min for 5 days. On P12 the hyperoxic-exposed animals were returned to room air. The greatest neovascular response occurred during P17 to P21 (Fig. 2.4). This was then followed by slow regression of the new vessels with reestablishment of a more normal, branching vascular pattern, which was observed in retinal flat mounts by P24. Quantification of the neovascular response was done by counting vascular nuclei in paraffin cross sections of retina. In addition, retinal flat mounts after fluorescein-dextran perfusion and glial fibrillary acidic protein (GFAP) immunohistochemistry were also used to quantify and confirm neovascularization (80).

In addition to the above study, multiple subtle variations to create retinopathy have been done by altering the amount and duration of oxygen exposure (81–83). A rat model for creating retinal neovascularization by varying oxygen exposure in a stepwise fashion has been studied by Penn et al. (82). Newborn rats were placed in an incubator and received oxygen exposure that was altered between 40% and 80% every 12 hours. Other groups were maintained for the same length of time, in either constant 80% oxygen or room air. Oxygen levels were maintained ±2%. Ink perfusion, ADPase staining, and light microscopy were used for evaluation. Rats maintained on a 40/80% oxygen cycle had more neovascularization, although rates maintained on 80% alone also had significant neovascularization (82).

With defined parameters for hyperoxic exposure, animal models of neovascularization are reliably created. This model has advantages since the creation of an ischemic event results in neovascularization without the dependence on technique of the investigator, as is necessary with laser photocoagulation.

DRY AMD MODELS

Several models have been created specifically for dry AMD. One of the early studies demonstrated drusen in aging rhe-

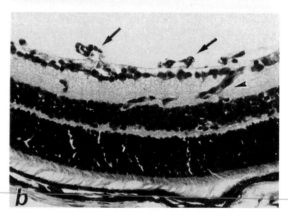

Figure 2.4   Comparison of room air and hyperoxia-exposed retinas in 6 μm cross section stained with PAS and hematoxylin. **A.** Postnatal day 21 (P21) retina exposed to room air. *Arrowhead* indicates normal intraretinal vessel. **B.** P21 retina exposed to hyperoxia from P7 to P12, before return to room air. *Arrows* indicate neovascular tufts extending into the vitreous. *Arrowheads* mark enlarged intraretinal vessel profiles. GCL, ganglion cell layer; ILM, internal limiting membrane; IPL, inner plexiform layer; V, vitreous (original magnification ×100). (Reprinted with permission from Smith LEH, Wesolowski E, McLellan A, et al. Oxygen-induced retinopathy in the mouse. *Invest Opthalmol Vis Sci.* 1994;35:106.)

sus monkeys after long-term administration of investigational oral contraceptive steroids (84). In the 1980s, a study by Tabatabay et al. (85) created an rabbit model for dry AMD using intravitreal injection of aminoglycoside antibiotics. This disease model is based on the idea that aminoglycosides have previously been used to induce experimental lipidosis of the RPE (86). One eye of each rabbit received an injection of an aminoglycoside (netilmicin 200, 400, or 800 μg; gentamicin 500 μg; or amikacin 2000 μg) while the contralateral eye received isotonic saline solution. The animals were examined with ophthalmoscopy and fluorescein angiography from 3 to 10 months. They were then sacrificed and the eyes were studied using light microscopy and transmission electron microscopy. The intravitreal injection of aminoglycoside induced focal RPE lesions 6 to 10 months after injection. Fluorescein angiography, histologic examination, and ultrastructural examination found the lesions to have characteristics of drusen.

Other models for dry AMD have been established by finding drusen via observation and examination of a

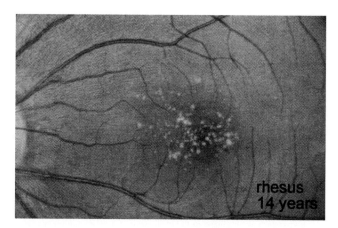

Figure 2.5 A primate model for age-related macular drusen. Fundus photograph of rhesus monkey retina with significant drusen spots. (Photo courtesy of Dr. GM Hope and Dr. WW Dawson.)

closed colony of semi-free-ranging rhesus monkeys that have been maintained in isolation since 1938 by the Caribbean Primate Research Center (CPRC) (87,88). The animals were examined by ophthalmoscopy, fundus photography, and fluorescein angiography. Of examined animals, 57.7% were found to have drusen (89), as seen in Figure 2.5. The prevalence and severity of drusen was found to be related to increasing age and was significantly higher in females and in specific maternal lineages. In fact, evidence indicates that the drusen in CPRC monkeys have the same histopathology as those seen in human AMD (89); however, the deposits differ from human drusen in both ultrastructural morphology and biochemical composition (88).

Most recently, transgenic models to study dry AMD have been created. The transgenic Apo-3 Leiden murine model (50), the transgenic CatD murine model (51), and the transgenic Ccl-2 and Ccr-2 murine model (78) previously discussed, all demonstrated basal laminar and linear deposits.

OTHER ANIMAL MODELS

Many animal models throughout the years have been created and studied as ideal or close-to-ideal models for investigation into the pathophysiology and therapy for AMD. While laser photocoagulation and transgenic animal models are the most extensively studied, many others have been used and will be discussed briefly.

Retinal vein occlusion in primates and pigs has been studied, but the incidence of retinal neovascularization has been low (90,91). Intravitreal injection of V-2 carcinoma cells in rabbits was found to cause retinal neovascularization, but the model has not been extensively used since the neovascularization can take 100 days to develop (92). Retinal detachment and intravitreal injection of fibroblasts in rabbits resulted in retinal neovascularization (93,94). Subretinal neovascularization has been induced in rabbits

by subretinal injection of autologous vitreous (95). Immunization in rats with synthetic interphotoreceptor retinoid-binding protein (IRBP) has also been shown to create subretinal neovascularization (96). Naphthalene applied directly onto the retina induced degeneration of the retina with subretinal neovascularization (97). An *ex ovo* chicken chorioallantoic membrane model has been used with laser ablation to induce leaky vessels representative of AMD (98). Although this model may be suboptimal, the chorioallantoic membrane has been used in several studies in investigating therapies for AMD (99–102) due to the similarity in size of the blood vessels compared to those of human eyes with AMD and the occurrence of rapid angiogenesis with leakage. A porcine model for the pathogenesis and treatment of AMD was created by using mitomycin C. This model demonstrated that loss of the RPE leads to secondary atrophy of the choriocapillaris; it is this concurrent atrophy of the RPE and choriocapillaris that leads to loss of the overlying outer retina and scotomas (4).

Spontaneous genetic models that mimic AMD have been identified. The spontaneous, autosomal semidominant mouse mutation, Belly spot and tail (Bst), has been suggested as an angiogenic model since subretinal neovascularization is found (103). The benefits of this model have been linked to its spontaneous occurrence. Additionally, angiogenesis was observed to occur with aging as it does in humans. Another genetically determined animal model is the senescence-accelerated mouse known as SAM P8, which exhibits some features of AMD, including lipoidal degeneration and atrophy of the RPE, abnormal deposits in the inner Bruch's membrane, thickened Bruch's membrane, and intra-Bruch's neovascularization (104). Both the Bst and SAM P8 mice are genetically determined, spontaneous aging models that may prove to be beneficial in future studies. Also, the Fas (CD95)-deficient (lpr) and FasL-defective (gld) mice have a significantly increased incidence of neovascularization compared with normal mice (105). FasL induces apoptosis in cells expressing the Fas receptor. Thus, FasL expressed on RPE cells may control the growth and development of new subretinal vessels, and warrants further investigation.

One of the newest models for AMD is an *in vitro* tissue-culture model. Renno et al. have demonstrated the use of cultured bovine retinal capillary endothelial and retinal pigment epithelial cells to study the effects of angiostatin and PDT (106). Bovine retinal capillary endothelial cells were used as a representative capillary endothelial line of the posterior segment. Tissue culture is thought to represent proliferating tissue/endothelium and may provide a useful disease model.

SUMMARY

Several animal models have been reviewed for both exudative and dry AMD. The majority of animal models for AMD have been focused on neovascular AMD. Although there are many animal models of neovascularization, the most extensively studied models involve laser photocoagulation and transgenic animals. These models have afforded reproducibility and continue to be the basis of many AMD studies today.

Also, dry AMD with its presence of drusen and basal laminar deposits along the basement membrane of the RPE have been replicated in animal models. Specifically, transgenic lines have been created that have a predilection for drusen or basal laminar deposit. Injection of aminoglycosides, use of oral steroids, and examination of an isolated primate colony for determination of spontaneous, age-related drusen are other models of dry AMD.

As varied as the techniques for animal disease models are, so are the subjects. Initially primates were the most extensively studied since their physiology and anatomy most closely resembles that of the human. Subsequently, investigators sought out other subjects that are smaller, easier to handle, and more affordable. Hence, the animal disease model has been extended from the primate to the rabbit, cat, pig, rat, mouse, chicken chorioallantoic membrane, and, most recently, endothelial cells in tissue culture.

An ideal or perfect animal model does not exist for AMD given its clinical complexity and lack of knowledge of its cause, genetic link, and pathomechanism. Each model has its flaws and no model has been found that mirrors AMD completely. It must be remembered that science and medicine are dynamic fields and new information is being gathered and discovered on a daily basis. The study of AMD is no different. Although many animal disease models have been created and improved upon, the ideal model has yet to be found and experiments will need to continue to be done to find this ideal model and to improve upon existing models. Regardless, the existing animal models for AMD have proven to be priceless for the information that they have provided.

REFERENCES

1. Hampton, GR, Nelson, PT. *Age-Related Macular Degeneration: Principles and Practice.* New York: Raven Press, Ltd.; 1992.
2. Ryan SJ. The development of an experimental model of subretinal neovascularization in disciform macular degeneration. *Trans Am Ophthalmol Soc.* 1979;77:707–745.
3. Ryan SJ, Mittl RN, Maumenee AE. Enzymatic and mechanically induced subretinal neovascularization. *Albrecht Von Graefes Arch Klin Exp Ophthalmol.* 1980;215:21–28.
4. Del Priore LV, Kaplan HJ, Hornbeck R, et al. Retinal pigment epithelial debridement as a model for the pathogenesis and treatment of macular degeneration. *Am J Ophthalmol.* 1996;122:629–643.
5. Ryan SJ. Subretinal neovascularization after argon laser photocoagulation. *Albrecht von Graefe's Arch Klin Exp Ophthalmol.* 1980;215:29–42.
6. Ryan SJ. Subretinal neovascularization: natural history of an experimental model. *Arch Ophthalmol.* 1982;100:1,804–1,809.
7. Archer DB, Gardiner TA. Morphologic fluorescein angiographic, and light microscopic features of experimental choroidal neovascularization. *Am J Ophthalmol.* 1981;91:297–311.
8. Archer DB, Gardiner TA. Electron microscopic features of experimental choroidal neovascularization. *Am J Ophthalmol.* 1981;91:433–457.
9. El Dirini AA, Ogden TE, Ryan SJ. Subretinal endophotocoagulation: a new model of subretinal neovascularization in the rabbit. *Retina.* 1991;11:244–249.
10. Dobi ET, Puliafito CA, Desto M. A new model of experimental choroidal neovascularization in the rat. *Arch Ophthalmol.* 1989;107:264–269.
11. Kimura H, Sakamoto T, Hinton DR, et al. A new model of subretinal neovascularization in the rabbit. *Invest Ophthalmol Vis Sci.* 1995;36:2,110–2,119.
12. Archer DB, Gardiner TA. Experimental subretinal neovascularization. *Tran Ophthalmol Soc UK.* 1980;100:363–368.
13. Brown GC, Green WR, Shah HG, et al. Effects of the Nd:YAG laser on the primate retina and choroids. *Ophthalmology.* 1984;91:1,397–1,405.
14. Perry DD, Risco JM. Choroidal microvascular repair after argon laser photocoagulation. *Am J Ophthalmol.* 1982;93:787–793.
15. Perry DD, Reddick RL, Risco JM. Choroidal microvascular repair after argon laser photocoagulation: ultrastructural observations. *Invest Ophthalmol Vis Sci.* 1984;25:1,019–1,026.
16. Van der Zypen E, Fankhauser F, Raess K. Choroidal reaction and vascular repair after chorioretinal photocoagulation with the free-running neodymium-YAG laser. *Arch Ophthalmol.* 1985;103:580–589.
17. Ishibashi T, Miki K, Sorgente N, et al. Effects of intravitreal administration of steroids on experimental subretinal neovascularization in the subhuman primate. *Arch Ophthalmol.* 1985;103:708–711.
18. Penforld P, Killingsworth M, Sarks S. An ultrastructural study of the role of leucocytes and fibroblasts in the breakdown of Bruch's membrane. *Aust J Ophthalmol.* 1984;12:23–31.
19. Van der Zypen E, Fankhauser F, Raess K, et al. Morphologic findings in the rabbit retina following irradiation with the free-running neodymium-YAG laser. *Arch Ophthalmol.* 1986;104:1,071–1,077.
20. Frank RN, Das A, Weber ML. A model of subretinal neovascularization in the pigmented rat. *Curr Eye Res.* 1989;8:239–47.
21. Pollack A, Heriot WJ, Henkind P. Cellular processes causing defects in Bruch's membrane following krypton laser coagulation. *Ophthalmology.* 1986;93:1,113–1,119.
22. Pollack A, Korte GE, Weitzner AL, et al. Ultrastructure of Bruch's membrane after krypton laser photocoagulation: I. Breakdown of Bruch's membrane. *Arch Ophthalmol.* 1986;104:1,372–1,376.
23. Pollack A, Korte GE, Weitzner AL, et al. Ultrastructure of Bruch's membrane after krypton laser photocoagulation: II. Repair of Bruch's membrane and the role of macrophages. *Arch Ophthalmol.* 1986;104:1,377–1,382.
24. Baurmann H, Sasaki K, Chioralia G. Investigation on laser coagulated rat eyes by fluorescence angiography and microscopy. *Graefes Arch Clin Exp Ophthalmol.* 1975;193:245–252.
25. Kluver H. *The Vertebrate Visual System.* Chicago: University of Chicago Press; 1957.
26. Tobe T, Ortega S, Luna LD, et al. Targeted disruption of the FGF2 gene does not prevent choroidal neovascularization in a murine model. *Am J Pathol.* 1998;153(5):1,641–1,646
27. Schwesinger C, Yee C, Rohan RM, et al. Intrachoroidal neovascularization in transgenic mice overexpressing vascular endothelial growth factor in the retinal pigment epithelium. *Am J Pathol.* 2001;158:1,161–1,172.
28. Zhang NL, Samadani EE, Frank RN. Mitogenesis and retinal pigment epithelial cell antigen expression in the rat after krypton laser photocoagulation. *Invest Ophthalmol Vis Sci.* 1993;34:2,412–2,424.
29. Zacks DN, Ezra E, Terada Y, et al. Verteporfin photodynamic therapy in the rat model of choroidal neovascularization. Angiographic and histologic characterization. *Invest Ophthalmol Vis Sci.* 2002;43:2,384–2,391.
30. Tobe T, Luna JD, Derevjanik NL, et al. Campochiaro PA. Experimental model of choroidal neovascularization in the mouse. *Invest Opthalmol Vis Sci.* 1996;37:S125.
31. Krzystolik MG, Afshari MA, Adamis AP, et al. Prevention of experimental choroidal neovascularization with intravitreal anti-vascular endothelial growth factor antibody fragment. *Arch Ophthalmol.* 2002;120:338–346.
32. Packer AJ, Tse DT, Gu X-Q, et al. Hematoporphyrin photoradiation therapy for iris neovascularization. *Arch Ophthalmol.* 1984;102:1,193–1,197.
33. Thomas EL, Langhofer M. Closure of experimental subretinal neovascular vessels with dihematoporphyrin ether augmented argon green laser photocoagulation. *Photochem Photobiol.* 1987;46:881–886.
34. Miller H, Miller B. Photodynamic therapy of subretinal neovascularization in the monkey eye. *Arch Ophthalmol.* 1993;111:5,855–5,860.
35. Moulton RS, Walsh AW, Miller JW, et al. Response of retinal and choroidal vessels to photodynamic therapy using benzoporphyrin derivative monoacid. *Invest Ophthalmol Vis Sci.* 1993;34:1,169. Abstract.
36. Miller JW, Walsh AW, Kramer M, et al. Photodynamic therapy of experimental choroidal neovascularization using lipoprotein-delivered benzoporphyrin. *Arch Ophthalmol.* 1995;113:810–818.
37. Kramer M, Miller JW, Michaud N, et al. Liposomal benzoporphyrin derivative verteporfin photodynamic therapy. Selective treatment of choroid neovascularization in monkeys. *Ophthalmol.* 1996;103:427–438.
38. Campochiaro PA, Chang M, Ohsato M, et al. Retinal degeneration in transgenic mice with photoreceptor-specific expression of a dominant-negative fibroblast growth factor receptor. *J Neurosci.* 1996;16:1,679–1,688.
39. Ozaki H, Okamoto N, Ortega S, et al. Basic fibroblast growth factor is neither necessary nor sufficient for the development of retinal neovascularization. *Am J Pathol.* 1998;153:757–765.
40. Robinson MR, Baffi J, Yuan P, et al. Safety and pharmacokinetics of intravitreal 2-Methoxyestradiol implants in normal rabbit and pharmacodynamics in a rat model of choroidal neovascularization. *Exp Eye Res.* 2002;74: 309–317.

41. Zhang D, Lai MC, Constable IJ, et al. A model for a blinding eye disease of the aged. *Biogerontology.* 2002;3:61–66.

42. Okamoto N, Tobe T, Hackett SF, et al. Transgenic mice with increased expression of vascular endothelial growth factor in the retina. *Am J Pathol.* 1997;151:281–291.

43. Baffi J, Byrnes G, Chan C, et al. Choroidal neovascularization in the rat induced by adenovirus mediated expression of vascular endothelial growth factor. *Invest Ophthalmol Vis Sci.* 2000;41:3,582–3,589.

44. Spilsbury K, Garrett KL, Shen W, et al. Overexpression of vascular endothelial growth factor (VEGF) in the retinal pigment epithelium leads to the development of choroidal neovascularization. *Am J Pathol.* 2000;157:135–144.

45. Amin R, Puklin JE, Frank RN. Growth factor localization in choroidal neovascular membranes of age-related macular degeneration. *Invest Ophthalmol Vis Sci.* 1994;35:3,178–3,188.

46. Reddy VM, Zamora RL, Kaplan HJ. Distribution of growth factors in subfoveal neovascular membranes in age-related macular degeneration and presumed ocular histoplasmosis syndrome. *Am J Ophthalmol.* 1995;129:291–301.

47. Wang F, Rendahl KG, Manning WC, et al. AAV-mediated expression of vascular endothelial growth factor induces choroidal neovascularization in rat. *Invest Ophthalmol Vis Sci.* 2003;44:781–790.

48. Soubrane G, Cohen SY, Delayre T, et al. Basic fibroblast growth factor experimentally induced choroidal angiogenesis in the minipig. *Curr Eye Res.* 1994;13:183–195.

49. Saito Y, Kitano S, Furukawa H, et al. Experimental subretinal neovascularization. ARVO abstracts. *Invest Ophthalmol Vis Sci.* 1993;34:1,168.

50. Kliffen M, Lutgens E, Daemen MJA, et al. The Apo*E3-Leiden mouse as an animal model for basal laminar deposit. *Br J Ophthalmol.* 2000;84:1,415–1,419.

51. Rakoczy PE, Zhang D, Robertson T, et al. Progressive age-related changes similar to age-related macular degeneration in a transgenic mouse model. *Am J Pathol.* 2002;161:1,515–1,524.

52. Senger DR, Galli SJ, Dvorak AM et al. Tumor cells secrete a vascular permeability factor that promotes accumulation of ascites fluid. *Science.* 1983;219:983–985.

53. Murata T, Nakagawa K, Khalil A, et al. The relation between expression of vascular endothelial growth factor and breakdown of the blood-retinal barrier in diabetic rat retinas. *Lab Invest.* 1996;74:819–825.

54. Aiello LP, Bursell SE, Clermont A, et al. Vascular endothelial growth factor-induced retinal permeability is mediated by protein kinase C in vivo and suppressed by an orally effective beta-isoform-selective inhibitor. *Diabetes.* 1997;46:1,473–1,480.

55. Murata T, Nakagawa K, Khalil A, et al. The temporal and spatial vascular endothelial growth factor expression in retinal vasculogenesis of rat neonates. *Lab Invest.* 1996;74:68–77.

56. Miller JW, Adamis AP, Shima DT, et al. Vascular endothelial growth factor/vascular permeability factor is temporally and spatially correlated with ocular angiogenesis in a primate model. *Am J Pathol.* 1994;145:574–584.

57. Ferrara N, Houck KA, Jakeman LB, et al. The vascular endothelial growth factor family of polypeptides. *J Cell Biochem.* 1991;47:211–218.

58. Veikkola T, Alitalo K. VEGFs, receptors and angiogenesis. *Semin Cancer Biol.* 1999;9:211–220.

59. Shima DT, Gougos A, Miller JW, et al. Cloning and mRNA expression of vascular endothelial growth factor in ischemic retinas of Macaca fascicularis. *Invest Ophthalmol Vis Sci.* 1998;39:180–188.

60. Kvanta A, Algvere PV, Berglin L, et al. Subfoveal fibrovascular membranes in age-related macular degeneration express vascular endothelial growth factor. *Invest Ophthalmol Vis Sci.* 1996;37:1,929–1,934.

61. Kliffen M, Sharma HS, Mooy CM, et al. Increased expression of angiogenic growth factors in age-related maculopathy. *Br J Ophthalmol.* 1997;81:154–162.

62. Kuroki M, Voest EE, Amano S, et al. Reactive oxygen intermediates increase vascular endothelial growth factor expression in vitro and in vivo. *J Clin Invest.* 1996;98:1,667–1,675.

63. Anglade E, Csaky KG. Recombinant adenovirus-mediated gene transfer into the adult rat retina. *Curr Eye Res.* 1998;17:316–321.

64. Rakoczy PE, Lai CM, Shen W, et al. Recombinant adenovirus-mediated gene delivery into the rat retinal pigment epithelium in vivo. *Aust N Z J Ophthalmol.* 1998;26:S56–S58.

65. Schweigerer L, Malerstein B, Neufeld G, et al. Basic fibroblast growth factor is synthesized in cultured retinal pigment epithelial cells. *Bichem Biophys Res Commun.* 1987;143:934–940.

66. Baudouin C, Fred-Reygrobellet D, Carvelle J-P, et al. Acidic fibroblast growth factor distribution in normal human eye and possible implications in ocular pathogenesis. *Ophthalmic Res.* 1990;22:73–81.

67. Connolly SE, Hjelmeland LM, LaVail MM. Immunohistochemical localization of basic fibroblast growth factor in mature and developing retinas of normal and RCS rats. *Curr Eye Res.* 1992;11:1,005–1,017.

68. Kitaoka T, Aotaki-Keen AE, Hjelmeland LM. Distribution of FGF-5 in the rhesus macaque retina. *Invest Ophthalmol Vis Sci.* 1994;35:3,189–3,198.

69. Gao H, Hollyfield JG. Basic fibroblast growth factor (bFGF) immunolocalization in the rodent outer retina demonstrated with an anti-rodent bFGF antibody. *Brain Res.* 1992;585:355–360.

70. Campochiaro PA, Hackett SF. Corneal endothelial cell matrix promotes expression of differentiated features of retinal pigmented epithelial cells:

71. implication of laminin and basic fibroblast growth factor as active components. *Exp Eye Res.* 1993;57:539–547.

71. Hicks D, Courtois Y. Fibroblast growth factor stimulates photoreceptor differentiation in vitro. *J Neurosci.* 1992;12:2,022–2,033.

72. Guillemot F, Cepko CL. Retinal fate and ganglion cell differentiation are potentiated by acidic FGF in an in vitro assay of early retinal development. *Development.* 1992;114:745–754.

73. Tabata Y, Hijikata S, Ikada Y. Enhanced vascularization and tissue granulation by basic fibroblast growth factor impregnated in gelatin hydrogels. *J Controlled Release.* 1994;31:189–199.

74. Klaver CC, Kliffen M, Van Duijn CM, et al. Genetic association of apolipoprotein E with age-related macular degeneration. *Am J Hum Genet.* 1998;63:200–206.

75. Van den Maagdenberg AM, Hofker MH, Krimpenfort PJ, et al. Transgenic mice carrying the apolipoprotein E3-Leiden gene exhibit hyperlipoproteinemia. *J Biol Chem.* 1993;268:10,540–10,545.

76. Van Ree JH, ven den Broek WJ, van der Zee A, et al. Inactivation of Apo-E and Apo-C1 by two consecutive rounds of gene targeting: effects on mRNA expression levels of gene cluster members. *Hum Mol Genet.* 1995;4:1,403–1,409.

77. Van der Schaft TL, de Bruijn WC, Mooy CM, et al. Basal laminar deposit in the aging peripheral human retina. *Graefes Arch Clin Exp Ophthalmol.* 1993;231:470–475.

78. Ambati J, Anand A, Fernandez S, et al. An animal model of age-related macular degeneration in senescent Ccl-1- or Ccr-2- deficient mice. *Nat Med.* 2003;9:1,390–1,397.

79. Gerschman R, Nadig PW, Snell AC, et al. Effect of high oxygen concentrations on eyes of newborn mice. *Am J Physiol.* 1954;179:115–118.

80. Smith LEH, Wesolowski, E, McLellan A, et al. Oxygen-induced retinopathy in the mouse. *Invest Ophthalmol Vis Sci.* 1994;35:101–111.

81. Gole GA, Browning J, Elts SM. The mouse model of oxygen-induced retinopathy: a suitable animal model for angiogenesis research. *Documenta Ophthalmologica.* 1990;74:143–149.

82. Penn JS, Tolman BL, Lower LA. Variable oxygen exposure causes preretinal neovascularization in the newborn rat. *Invest Ophthalmol Vis Sci.* 1993;34:576–585.

83. Berkowitz BA, Zhang W. Significant reduction of the panretinal oxygenation response after 38% supplemental oxygen recovery in experimental ROP. *Invest Ophthalmol Vis Sci.* 2000;41:1,925–1,931.

84. Fine BS, Kwapien RP. Pigment epithelial windows and drusen: an animal model. *Invest Ophthalmol Vis Sci.* 1978;17:1,059–1,068.

85. Tabatabay CA, D'Amico DJ, Hanninen LA, et al. Experimental drusen formation induced by intravitreal aminoglycoside injection. *Arch Ophthalmol.* 1987;105:826–830.

86. Lullmann-Rauch R. Experimentally induced lipidosis in cat retinal pigment epithelium. *Graefes Arch Clin Exp Ophthalmol.* 1981;215:297–303.

87. Ulshafer RJ, Engel HM, Dawson MM, et al. Macular degeneration in a community of rhesus monkeys. *Retina.* 1987;7:198–203.

88. Hirata A, Feeney-Burns L. Autoradiographic studies of aged primate macular-retinal pigment epithelium. *Invest Ophthalmol Vis Sci.* 1992;33:2,079–2,090.

89. Hope GM, Dawson WW, Engel HM, et al. A primate model for age related macular drusen. *Br J Ophthalmol.* 1992;76:11–16.

90. Miller JW, Stinson W, Folkman J. Regression of experimental iris neovascularization with systemic alpha-interferon. *Ophthalmology.* 1993;100:9–14.

91. Virdi P, Hayreh S. Ocular neovascularization with retinal vascular occlusion. I. Association with retinal vein vascular occlusion. *Arch Ophthalmol.* 1980;100:331–341.

92. Finkelstein D, Bren S, Patz A, et al. Experimental retinal neovascularization induced by intravitreal tumors. *Am J Ophthalmol.* 1977;83:660–664.

93. Tano T, Takeahashi K, Ohkuma H, et al. Experimental choroidal neovascularization after intravitreal fibroblast injection. *Am J Ophthalmol.* 1981;92:203–109.

94. Antoszyk A, Gottlieb J, Machemer R, et al. The effects of intravitreal triamcinolone acetonide on experimental pre-retinal neovascularization. *Graefe's Arch Clin Exp Ophthalmol.* 1993;231:34–40.

95. Zhu ZR, Goodnight R, Sorgente N, et al. Experimental subretinal neovascularization in the rabbit. *Graefe's Arch Clin Exp Ophthalmol.* 1989;227:257–262.

96. Sakamoto T, Sanui H, Ishibashi T, et al. Subretinal neovascularization in the rat induced by IRBP synthetic peptides. *Exp Eye Res.* 1994;58:155–160.

97. Orzalesi N, Migliavacca L, Miglior S. Subretinal neovascularization after naphthalene damage to the rabbit retina. *Invest Ophthalmol Vis Sci.* 1994;35:696–705.

98. Samkoe KS, Cramb DT. Application of an *ex ovo* chicken chorioallantoic membrane model for two-photon excitation photodynamic therapy of age-related macular degeneration. *J Biomed Optics.* 2003;8:410–417.

99. Gottfried V, Davidi R, Acerbuj C, et al. In vivo damage to chorioallantoic membrane blood vessels by porphycene-induced photodynamic therapy. *J Photochem Photobiol.* 1995;30:115–121.

100. Lange N, Ballini JP, Wagnieres G, et al. A new drug-screening procedure for photosensitizing agents used in photodynamic therapy for CNV. *Invest Ophthalmol Vis Sci.* 2001;42:38–46.

101. Hammer-Wilson MJ, Akian L, Espinoza J, et al. Photodynamic parameters in the chick chorioallantoic membrane (CAM) bioassay for topically applied photosensitizers. *J Photochem Photobiol.* 1999;53:44–52.

102. Hornung R, Hammer-Wilson MJ, Kimel S, et al. Systemic application of photosensitizers in the chick chorioallantoic membrane (CAM) model: photodynamic response of CAM vessels and 5-aminolevulinic acid uptake kinetics by transplantable tumors. *J Photochem Photobiol.* 1999;49:41–49.

103. Smith RS, John SWM, Zabeleta A. The Bst locus on mouse chromosome 16 is associated with age-related subretinal neovascularization. *Proc Natl Acad Sci USA.* 2000;97:2,191–2,195.

104. Majji AB, Hayashi A, Kim HC, et al. Age-related retinal pigment epithelium and Bruch's membrane degeneration in senescence-accelerated mouse. *Invest Ophthalmol Vis Sci.* 2000;41:3,936–3,942.

105. Kaplan HJ, Leibole MA, Tezel T, et al. Fas ligand (CD95 ligand) controls angiogenesis beneath the retina. *Nat Med* 1999;5:292–297.

106. Renno RZ, Delori FC, Holzer RA, et al. Photodynamic therapy using Lu-Tex induces apoptosis in vitro, and its effect is potentiated by angiostatin in retinal capillary endothelial cells. *Invest Ophthalmol Vis Sci.* 2000;41:3,963–3,971.

Etiology of Late-Age-Related Macular Disease

Richard Spaide

INTRODUCTION

Late-age-related macular degeneration (ARMD) is the largest cause of visual loss among older adults in industrialized countries. This disease entity is made up of two main components. Patients may develop choroidal neovascularization (CNV), which is marked by growth of vessels, proliferation of a number of cell types including those of the retinal pigment epithelium (RPE), and recruitment of inflammatory cells, such as neutrophils and macrophages. CNV by its very name highlights the vascular aspects of the process: the accompanying signs include leakage and bleeding, and the chief method of diagnosis is angiography. However, the temporal and spatial sequence of cytokine expression endothelial and inflammatory infiltration, endothelial cell proliferation, maturation, matrix remodeling, and apoptosis are quite similar to a wound healing response. The non-neovascular change that leads to significant loss of visual acuity is the development of geographic atrophy. Cell death in regions of the RPE occurs with atrophy of the overlying retina and underlying RPE. The shared epidemiological risk factors, common occurrence of one of these disorders in one eye with the other being present in the fellow eye, and the common occurrence of both forms of ARMD in one eye suggest they share some common etiobiologic phenomena. While control of some aspects of the neovascular forms of ARMD appears to be an attainable goal, the increasing prevalence and lack of any known treatment makes geographic atrophy an increasingly important public health problem.

EPIDEMIOLOGICAL FACTORS

The most significant risk factor for ARMD is age, but additional important risk factors have been identified. A positive family history (1–3), cigarette smoking (1,4,5), and hypertension (4,6,7) have been consistently found as risk factors for the development of exudative ARMD. Additional risk factors, found with varying degrees of consistency among studies (8) include increased C-reactive protein (9), increased white blood cell count (10), increased intake of vegetable fat, mono- and polyunsaturated fatty acids, linoleic acid (11,12), fat (13), and baked goods (13), female gender (5,14,15), hyperopia (16,17), and blue iris color (1,4). Black race (18,19), increased intake of docosohexanoic acid (11), which is curiously the most polyunsaturated fatty acid, higher intake of fish (12,13,20), nuts (13), and dark green leafy vegetables (21), and higher levels of serum carotenoids (4) have been associated with a lower risk. The Eye Disease Case-Control Study only had a handful of women using estrogen replacement, but these patients seemed to have a lower risk for neovascularization compared to women not using estrogen (4).

GENETIC FACTORS

There is a higher risk for the development of late-age-related maculopathy in people with a positive family history (1–3). This raises the possibility of finding a gene or genes that may be linked to macular degeneration. Genetic investigation into ARMD is hindered because the disease occurs in older individuals who are unlikely to have parents or grandparents alive for comparative testing. Mutation of the Stargardt disease gene (ABCR) was found by Allikmets et al. (22) to be associated with ARMD (in particular the non-neovascular subtype), but this same association was not found by others (23,24). The APOE-ε4 allele has been found to be associated with a decreased risk, and the ε2 allele was associated with a slight increase in risk for ARMD (25,26). This association was not found by others, however (27,28). Macular degeneration is a complex disease since there are a number of possible genetic, epigenetic, dietary, and environmental factors all interacting to confer a risk for the development of disease in any given individual. Because there are probably a large number of polymorphisms of many different genes that potentially could be related to the development of ARMD (in the context of various other genetic, epigenetic, and environmental factors), it is likely that there is no single gene defect responsible for more than a minority of cases of ARMD. It is also possible that with different genotypes there are different pathophysiologic mechanisms that produce a generic choroidal neovascular response.

STRUCTURALLY INDUCED CHANGES ASSOCIATED WITH AGING

Some cells in the body are capable of ongoing replication, while others, such as those of the RPE, have very limited ability to divide before reaching cellular senescence (29). Under most conditions, RPE cells persist for the life of the individual. Located between the choroid and the retina, the RPE acts in the absorption of light passing through the retina, regeneration of visual pigments, formation of the outer blood-ocular barrier, upkeep of the subretinal space including fluid and electrolyte balance, phagocytosis of spent outer segments discs (30), maintenance of the choriocapillaris, and formation of scar tissue. It is estimated that during a 70-year lifetime, each RPE cell will phagocytize three billion outer segment discs (31). Most of the discs appear to be degraded quickly in lysosomes of young healthy individuals. Over time, however, incompletely degraded membrane material builds up in the form of lipofuscin within secondary lysosomes or residual bodies (32,33). Lipofuscin is part of a diverse group of molecular species (34), yellow to brown in color and autofluorescent, that accumulate in all post-mitotic cells, especially in the RPE (Fig. 3.1) (35,36). The presence of lipofuscin may act as a cellular aging indicator (37–39), and its quantity in tissues may be estimated by the amounts of autofluorescence present (40,41). The topographical distribution of autofluorescence as an indicator of lipofuscin content shows that the macular region has much more lipofuscin than the periphery (42). Light irradiation of RPE cultures accelerates the formation of lipofuscin-like fluorophores, with a color and fluorescence similar to lipofuscin found in older cells. The formation of this pigment is nearly

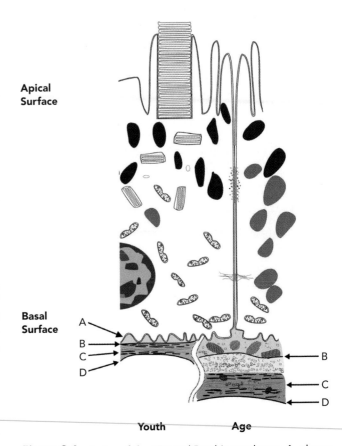

Figure 3.1 Aging of the RPE and Bruch's membrane. **A.** plasma membrane, **B.** basement membrane, **C.** trilaminar core of Bruch's membrane, **D.** basement membrane of choriocapillaris. Often times what is referred to as Bruch's membrane is a five layered structure comprised of B, C, and D. Bruch's membrane and associated structures undergo a number of changes with aging (right). In between the plasma membrane and the basement membrane an accumulation of material, including widespaced collagen occurs. This material is called basal laminar deposit. External to the basement membrane a material called basal linear deposit accumulates. This material has a high lipid content with membranous debris. Mounds of this material are visible as soft drusen. With age there is also an increased amount of lipofuscin in the RPE cell as well as thickening, calcification, and potential fracture (not shown) of Bruch's membrane.

eliminated in oxygen-free conditions (43). The formation of lipofuscin increases with vitamin E deficiency and reduces with vitamin A deficiency (44).

The structure of one component of lipofuscin, N-retinylidene-N-retinylethanolamine (A2E), has been characterized and appears to be formed from vitamin A and ethanolamine in a ratio of 2:1. Precursors to A2E are formed in the outer segments before phagocytosis (45,46). There appears to be numerous other components of lipofuscin, and many of these appear to be derived from free radical induced oxidation of macromolecules, particularly proteins and lipids, with subsequent molecular rearrangement and cross-linking to themselves or other macromolecules (47). The RPE is unusual in the amount of retinoids and polyunsaturated fatty acids that each of its cells must process through life. The indigestible portions of what is phagocytized daily contribute to the formation of lipofuscin. In older individuals, up to 25% of the volume of RPE cells may be occupied by lipofuscin. Room for normal cellular machinery is consequently limited. However, lipofuscin is not an inert filler material. Components of lipofuscin inhibit lysosomal protein degradation (48), are photoreactive (49,50), producing a variety of reactive oxygen species (ROS) and other radicals, have detergent properties, and lipofuscin may induce apoptosis of the RPE (51). Blue light damage to RPE cells is proportional to the amount of light given and the amount of lipofuscin within the RPE cells (52,53). There is an age-related loss in RPE cells, particularly in the fovea and mid-periphery (54). With time the RPE cells decline in function and number, forcing ever-hindered, lipofuscin-engorged cells to provide metabolic maintenance for the retina.

Deposition of material under the basal surface of the RPE contributes to Bruch's membrane thickening with age. Basal laminar deposit (BLD) accumulates between the RPE cell plasma membrane and its basement membrane (55–57). BLD is a complex composite that contains granular electron-dense material, coated membrane bodies, and wide- or long-spaced fibrous collagen (58–60). Although the characteristic material in BLD is collagen, transgenic mice with apo E3 formed BLD when fed a diet high in fat and cholesterol (61). Basal linear deposit, on the other hand, accumulates external to the basement membrane of the RPE and is comprised of vesicles and membranous debris. Accumulation of basal linear deposit is the most frequent histopathologic correlate of soft drusen (56,62). Contributing to the age-related thickening of Bruch's membrane is an increase in collagen, particularly in the outer collagenous layer (59,63). In a histologic study of 95 specimens of normal human maculae aged 6 to 100 years, Bruch's membrane thickness increased by 135%, from 2.0 to 4.7 μm over the 10 decades examined (64). In a study by Spraul et al., Bruch's membrane in eyes with exudative ARMD showed a greater degree of mineralization and fragmentation than did age-matched controls (65).

Analysis of Bruch's membrane specimens has shown an exponential increase in the amount of lipid present with age of the donor (Fig. 3.2) (66). There is also a decrease in the hydraulic conductivity (67,68) occurring somewhat earlier in age than the inflection point for the rise in extractable lipid from Bruch's membrane. Using eximer laser ablation, Starita et al. found the region accountable for the decreased hydraulic conductivity appeared to be located in the inner portion of Bruch's membrane, the same location of maximal lipid accumulation (69). The amounts of lipid, as well as the predominant decrease in hydraulic conductivity, occur more in Bruch's membrane specimens from the posterior pole than the periphery (66). Although Bruch's membrane has been found to contain neutral fats (70), the predominant class of lipids identified by one research group was phospholipids (66). Pauleikhoff et al. found that a high content of neutral fat was associated with a lack of fluorescein staining and fibronectin (71). In contrast, a high proportion of phospholipid was associated with strong fluorescein binding and the presence of fibronectin; the composition of the lipids found was consistent with a cellular rather than a blood origin (71). Pauleikhoff et al. (72) also found an age-related decrease in adhesion molecules, laminin and fibronectin that appeared to be inversely correlated with the lipid content of Bruch's membrane. The decrease in hydraulic conductivity may lead to the formation of serous RPE detachments, as the RPE cells pump fluid out toward the choroid, against a Bruch's membrane made more hydrophobic by the accumulation of lipid. Curcio et al. (71) found that the predominant lipid deposited in Bruch's membrane was esterified cholesterol, similar to deposition in other membranes throughout the body that occurs with age. They believed the high proportion of cholesterol esters indicated a blood rather than cellular origin for the lipid. Ultrastructural examination revealed the cholesterol accumulated in 80 nm particles densely packed within a thin layer external to the basement membrane of the RPE (74). The particle size appeared to be larger than the pore size of the basement membrane suggesting either that the particles probably did not pass as such from the RPE toward the choriocapillaris, or that they were inhibited from passing from the choriocapillaris to the RPE.

Histologic evaluation of choriocapillaris in aging eyes by Ramrattan et al. (64) has shown that there appeared to be an age-related decrease in the lumenal diameter and

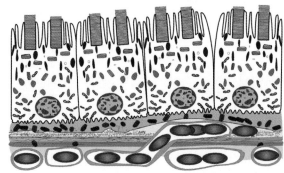

Increased Lipid in Bruch's

Possible VEGF/PEDF expression or diffusion abnormalities

Figure 3.2 Accumulation of lipids in Bruch's membrane as a potential cause of CNV in ARMD. Although the diffusion of growth factors secondary to lipid accumulation in Bruch's membrane has been proposed as a potential cause of CNV, the exact mechanism by which this is supposed to occur has not been defined.

vascular density. However, in a study by Spraul et al., eyes with ARMD showed fewer large choroidal vessels in the submacular choroid and a higher density of the submacular choriocapillaris than controls without ARMD (65). The RPE seems to play a role in maintaining the vitality of the choriocapillaris (75); perhaps with senescence of the RPE there is a corresponding degradation of the choriocapillaris.

PIGMENT EPITHELIUM-DERIVED FACTOR (PEDF)

The RPE constitutively expresses vascular endothelial growth factor (VEGF). It also produces another factor, PEDF (76) that has neutrophic, neuroprotective (77), and anti-angiogenic effects (78). Hypoxia is a well-known mechanism that results in increased VEGF expression. Retinal hypoxia can decrease the expression of PEDF by Muller cells (79). Intraocular injection of PEDF, directly or by a viral vector, thereby increasing local production of PEDF, results in inhibition of ocular neovascularization (80, 81). It has been proposed that the amounts or relative proportion of the expression of VEGF and PEDF may allow neovascularization to occur (82–85).

Experimental evidence to date does not support the contention that the ratio of PEDF to VEGF is the permissive event in the generation of ocular neovascularization. While some studies have shown decreased levels of PEDF in ocular tissues during various types of neovascularization (83,86), most studies have shown a simultaneous increase in VEGF and PEDF during active neovascularization (87–91). In addition, the concentration of PEDF measured in all studies appeared to be at least an order of magnitude higher than that required to inhibit neovascularization. There may be possible explanations for these observations. First, VEGF appears to upregulate secretion of PEDF in an autocrine manner (92). Many of the anti-angiogenic effects of PEDF were determined using fibroblast growth factor 2 (FGF2). In a study using VEGF, PEDF seemed to have a synergistic effect on endothelial proliferation (93). While VEGF is necessary and sufficient for angiogenesis, other factors, such as FGF2, are also commonly present. This suggests that if this effect is true, the control of angiogenesis is more complicated than the simple ratio of two different cytokines.

DOES THE SIMPLE ACCUMULATION OF LIPID EXPLAIN WHY CNV OCCURS?

A possible cause of CNV may be gleaned from the histopathologic observation of the deposition of basal laminar and basal linear deposit. The most common histopathologic correlate to soft drusen is the accumulation of membranous debris in basal linear deposit (56,57,63). Soft drusen are an ocular risk factor for the development of CNV in ARMD. There are several ways that

deposited material may play a role in the development of CNV. It is possible that the presence of deposits, particularly lipids, affects the ability of growth factors produced by the RPE to diffuse through Bruch's membrane. In particular, it is possible that the diffusion of factors could either selectively partition into the lipid layer or be blocked from passing through the lipid-rich area. The two possibly involved factors would be VEGF, which stimulates the growth of vessels, and PEDF, which inhibits neovascularization. Examination of the histopathology of CNV in ARMD and the topography of VEGF found in the eye would seem to argue against either of these two possibilities. CNV generally grows up to and into the inner portion of Bruch's membrane (94). If a mediator inhibiting neovascularization was selectively concentrated in this area, one would not expect the newly growing vessels to actively grow to, and then into the same layer. Histopathologic examination of CNV in ARMD shows that while the new vessels grow under the BLD, basal linear deposit is not commonly found in most specimens. This may imply that the basal linear deposit was never present; it was lost in processing; or that the CNV was growing into the layer previously occupied by the basal linear deposit, replacing or removing the deposit. Since the clinical correlate of mounds of basal linear deposit are soft drusen, and since soft drusen are known ocular risk factors for CNV, the latter interpretation seems more likely. Neovascularization may penetrate through the RPE or may start as vessels growing outward from the inner retina toward the subretinal space. In either of these two situations, the newly-growing vessels seem to proliferate in the outer retina as a separate plane, in contrast to the aforementioned vessels that grow in the region occupied by the basal linear deposit.

ISCHEMIA AND ANGIOGENESIS

Age-related decrease in delivery or diffusion of oxygen or metabolites to the macular region may occur, and has been theorized as the key event in the initiation of compensatory mechanisms that ultimately lead to the formation of new vessels in ARMD. Neovascularization is an important cause of blindness in a number of ocular diseases, such as diabetic retinopathy, neovascular glaucoma, and vein occlusions. In each case, neovascularization has been linked to ischemia. By logical extension, CNV has been theorized to be caused by ischemia.

Blood vessels grow in adult tissue by expansion of the vascular tree through angiogenesis, a process in which new vessels sprout from pre-existing vessels. The actual ischemic event is signaled by an increase in adenosine (95–97), which may bind to one of at least four receptors. This binding leads to increased VEGF in an action mediated by hypoxia-inducible factor-1 (HIF-1), a transcription factor that binds to one or more areas in the hypoxia response element (98–102). There are several hypoxia-inducible genes, including those for erythropoietin, VEGF, inducible nitric oxide synthase, glycolytic enzymes, and glucose transport proteins. The most important of these for vessel growth is VEGF (103–119). There are many different isoforms of VEGF caused by differential RNA splicing. Although VEGF is sufficient for new vessel growth, other growth factors are also commonly found in association (120).

At the initiation of angiogenesis, gaps begin to form between endothelial cells of the capillary wall, and the endothelial cells develop areas of fenestrations (103,104). These changes start within minutes after exposing vessels to VEGF. The capillary becomes more permeable allowing plasma proteins, particularly fibrinogen, to extravasate (121). Clotting of the fibrinogen leads to the creation of fibrin, which forms a provisional matrix to support the newly growing vessel. The endothelial cell forms a bud, with the advancing edge expressing integrins. With the aide of matrix metalloproteinases the endothelial cells degrade the extracellular matrix. The advancing cells move away from the pre-existing vessel toward the angiogenic stimulus. The endothelial cells in the vascular sprout proliferate, and a lumen forms. Anastomotic connections between neighboring sprouts form a capillary loop. At this stage, the cells form a thin-walled, pericyte-poor capillary that eventually starts to produce new basement membrane. Production of vessels starts with the secretion of VEGF, but a large number of different cytokines play a role in the development of a blood vessel. Withdrawal of VEGF, or blocking VEGF or the receptor, causes suppression of vascular growth and regression (122,123).

Hypoxia in retinal cell cultures induces VEGF (124). Animal models of neovascularization show increased VEGF levels from induced hypoxia, and these increased levels were spatially and quantitatively correlated with the resultant neovascularization (110,124,125). Inhibition of VEGF caused suppression of ocular neovascularization in an animal model (112). Many tested patients with ischemic retinal diseases leading to neovascularization had increased levels of VEGF in their vitreous, and these levels declined after successful laser photocoagulation (113). Autopsy specimens confirmed the presence of VEGF in diabetic eyes (114). Choroidal neovascular membranes that were surgically removed showed immunohistochemical evidence of VEGF (115). Experimental CNV induced by laser photocoagulation also shows VEGF expression (126). Injection of an adenoviral vector encoding VEGF into the subretinal space has caused experimental CNV in rats (127,128). One study showed that the indocyanine green angiographic grading of CNV activity was correlated with the amount of immunohistochemical staining for VEGF in excised specimens (117). Injection of an anti-VEGF aptamer and of an anti-VEGF antibody fragment caused angiographic regression of CNV (129,130). The mean visual acuity still declined in a randomized trial looking at the effects of the anti-VEGF aptamer, suggesting that anti-angiogenic treatment may not be a sufficient treatment for CNV.

ISCHEMIA AND CNV

Because of the weight of the basic and clinical science linking ischemia to VEGF production, and in turn, VEGF production to neovascularization, it may be very logical to presume the same factors may play a role in the development of CNV. Indeed, there are many clues suggesting decreased blood flow occurs in the aging choroid, especially in patients with ARMD (Fig. 3.3). Laser Doppler studies have shown that patients with ARMD, defined as having 10 or more large drusen, had decreased blood flow, but no change in velocity when compared with age-matched controls without 10 or more large drusen (131). In contradistinction, Mori et al., using a Langham Ocular Blood Flow (OBF) computerized tonometer, found no decrease in OBF in patients with non-exudative ARMD, but did find a statistically significant decrease in pulse amplitude and pulsatile

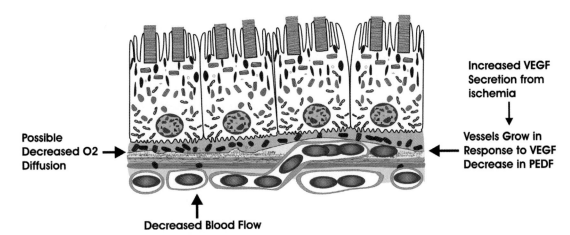

Figure 3.3 Ischemia as a potential cause of CNV in ARMD. Decreased diffusion of oxygen due to increased thickness and altered composition of Bruch's membrane has been proposed to lead to increased VEGF production. This would then lead to angiogenesis and neovascularization arising from the choriocapillaris.

OBF in patients with exudative ARMD as compared with age-matched controls (132). Tonographic methods of OBF measurement are based on assumptions about the relationship between intraocular volume and resultant intraocular pressure, from which OBF is estimated (133). Comparisons among individuals also assume that factors that may alter the pressure/volume relationship, such as scleral rigidity and axial length, do not vary. However, Yang et al. found the interindividual variation of peak OBF determined by the OBF tonography was so large that valid comparisons among individuals may not be possible (134).

Patients with ARMD are more likely to have choroidal watershed filling defects during fluorescein (135) and indocyanine green angiography (136,137) than controls, although the controls were not matched on important factors, such as hypertension (136). Besides the alterations in blood flow, it has been theorized that age-related changes in Bruch's membrane may also limit the diffusion of oxygen and therefore create an ischemic environment. The RPE cells lying on top of drusen were thought to be particularly ischemic (137); which would lead to VEGF secretion and formation of CNV (138).

There are some aspects of the physiology of the outer retina and RPE in which the histologic appearance and growth pattern of CNV do not appear to support the ischemic theory. In a prospective study of choroidal filling defects, patients were more likely to develop geographic atrophy, not CNV (139). A large histopathologic study found that the luminal cross-sectional area and choriocapillaris density is higher in ARMD patients than in non-ARMD controls (65). The blood flow through the choroid is the highest, and the oxygen extraction from hemoglobin is one of the lowest of any tissue in the body. In terms of volume, less than 1% of the oxygen in the blood is extracted from the choroidal blood flow. Consequently, the resultant $pO2$ at the choriocapillaris is maintained at a level higher than any other perfused tissue. The oxygen diffusion through the RPE and retina has been measured in several species (140–146), and follows a consistent pattern. The $pO2$ levels of the RPE are very high because of its close distance to the choriocapillaris. The $pO2$ decreases linearly with distance from the choriocapillaris to the inner portion of the photoreceptors. Under normal physiologic conditions, the $pO2$ at the inner portion of the photoreceptors approaches 0 mm Hg in the dark and somewhat higher in light. One possible reason for this design may be to lower the oxygen tension in the outer retina to decrease the amount of oxidative damage there, due to the inherently high susceptibility to oxidative damage conferred by the extraordinarily high proportions of both polyunsaturated fatty acids and retinoids in the outer segment membranes. In measurements of the constitutive secretion of VEGF in the eye, the RPE makes a prominent amount of VEGF (147). On the other hand, the photoreceptors make little VEGF. Under normal circumstances then, the RPE is exposed to an exceptionally high $pO2$, but secretes VEGF. The inner portions of the photoreceptors are exposed to a very low $pO2$, but do not produce much VEGF. This paradox cannot be explained by simple ischemia.

It is possible that lipid deposition in Bruch's membrane will limit the diffusion of oxygen. It has been theorized by some that this induces RPE ischemia with the subsequent production of VEGF. However, organisms are designed with the strategy, refined through evolution, of O2 diffusing through lipid membranes. Indeed, analysis has shown lipid membranes are not a rate-limiting step in oxygen diffusion (148–151), because the diffusion through lipid membranes approaches that of water (148). Although the lipids in Bruch's membrane are not necessarily in the form of lipid membranes, there is not much available evidence to support the assertion that the presence of lipids in Bruch's membrane leads to RPE ischemia. Thickening of Bruch's membrane may cause a decrease in the $pO2$ at the level of the RPE because of an increase in distance from the choriocapillaris to the RPE, but the RPE would still have a much higher $pO2$ than the photoreceptors. Even so, excessive VEGF production at the level of the photoreceptors as studied in transgenic mice showed that there was a growth of vessels extending from the middle retinal layers to the outer retina, but no development of CNV (152).

In one study, RPE cells exposed to 5% O_2 produced 1.3 times more VEGF than when exposed to normal atmospheric oxygen levels (116). In another study, human RPE cells exposed to 3% O_2 increased the secretion of VEGF approximately threefold as compared to atmospheric conditions, and the increase was statistically significant (124). (However, normal tissue levels of oxygen are far below that found in room air.) Bovine RPE cells cultured in the same conditions did not produce a statistically significant increase in VEGF (124). Studies examining O_2 delivery by the choroid have shown that as perfusion decreases, the oxygen extraction from the choriocapillaris increases (143). Under normal conditions, little of the O_2 in the choriocapillaris blood is extracted, so there is a significant reserve. Because of this process the change in oxygen flux at the level of the RPE shows much less change under conditions of decreased perfusion than what ordinarily is expected. Although experimental study has shown that RPE may increase VEGF production to a certain degree when exposed to levels of oxygen lower than room air, the O_2 levels used in experiments may not be physiologically relevant for understanding how CNV develops secondary to ARMD.

The growth patterns of CNV suggest there is more involved than just ischemia driven neovascularization. Excised choroidal neovascular "membranes" show significant participation by cells other than the vascular endothelium including a variety of inflammatory cells, such as lymphocytes, macrophages, and foreign body giant cells (153,154). The histopathologic picture of CNV in ARMD looks similar to granulation tissue or a wound-repair response (65). In one study, the amount of VEGF was found to be proportional to the number of macrophages in the specimen (155), a finding that is difficult to explain by any ischemia theory and suggests inflammation is important in CNV secondary to ARMD. In animal models of CNV, depletion of the monocyte cell lines inhibits experimental CNV (156–158). During the development of experimental CNV using a laser model, CD18 and ICAM-1 are expressed; targeted disruption of either of these inhibits the development of CNV (159). Animal models of CNV have been developed that mimic many aspects of CNV in ARMD. Mice expressing monocyte chemoattractant protein-1 (MCP-1) or its cognate, CC chemokine receptor-2, developed drusen, lipofuscin accumulation, geographic atrophy, and CNV (160). Depletion of neutrophils further inhibits the development of CNV (161). All of these factors strongly suggest integral involvement of inflammatory cells in the development of CNV. Finally, ischemia-based theories do not adequately explain the typical later stages of CNV in ARMD: the formation of scarring and regression of vessels. With time, the neovascularization appears to "burn out," leaving a cicatricial mass almost completely devoid of vessels. If ischemia is the only cause for the vessels to grow, then once the CNV does grow, the capillaries of the CNV recapitulate the anatomy of choriocapillaris and overlying neurosensory retina. One would not expect these vessels to make an abrupt regression, which would be expected to increase the amount of ischemia present. However, this growth pattern is analogous to a wound healing response (Fig. 3.4).

There is a strong link between ischemia and VEGF mediated angiogenesis. Patients with ARMD may have decreased blood flow as compared with those who do not have ARMD,

but the decrease in blood flow has yet to be firmly linked with a significant amount of ischemia. In addition, the growth patterns of CNV, the regression of active neovascularization later in the disease process, many of the histopathologic findings, and many findings in animal models are not explainable by ischemia. Readily identifiable ischemia, such as choroidal vascular occlusion seen in toxemia of pregnancy or malignant hypertension, is not associated with CNV. Ischemia of the retina is not associated with CNV either. The implication is that ischemia is not sufficient to explain CNV in ARMD, and there must be other factors involved.

OXIDATIVE STRESS

Although light-induced free radical oxidation in the photoreceptors has been known for almost 30 years, the full realization of the effects of oxidative damage is still being elucidated. There is tremendous interest in oxidative damage as an integral component in the etiology of several seemingly diverse diseases ranging from atherosclerosis to Alzheimer's disease to cancer. In the following section, successive steps in the progression of oxidation will be illustrated, along with responses from the cellular level to larger degrees of scale.

We are a carbon-based life form that burns carbon-based molecules to stay alive. In the process, free radicals are produced in a process designed to stay within mitochondria. For quantum mechanical reasons, atoms like to have paired electrons. A free radical is any atom or compound that has an unpaired electron; it is not necessarily an ion, which is an atom or compound with an excess positive or negative charge. Ordinarily, four electrons (and four associated protons) are required to reduce O_2 to form two molecules of water. In most interactions with organic molecules, oxygen preferentially accepts electrons one at a time. Each of these electron additions results in a potentially reactive molecule. The stepwise series of reductions produces metabolites of oxygen as electrons are donated to oxygen in the electron transport chain in the mitochondria.

Addition of one electron to oxygen results in the formation of the superoxide anion, represented as O_2^-. The walls of the mitochondria are curiously leaky to oxygen radicals produced during metabolism. Large amounts of superoxide leak from the walls of mitochondria, such that about 1% of oxygen used in respiration actually leaks from the mitochondria in the form of superoxide. In older subjects, the proportion is greater (162,163). This potentially exposes the cellular constituents to internally generated oxidative attack. Further reduction of the superoxide (with the addition of two hydrogen ions) produces hydrogen peroxide. Continued reduction leads to the formation of the hydroxyl radical, which is particularly reactive. The final reduction yields water.

When photosensitizers absorb light, they are elevated to a higher energy state called a triplet state. This excess

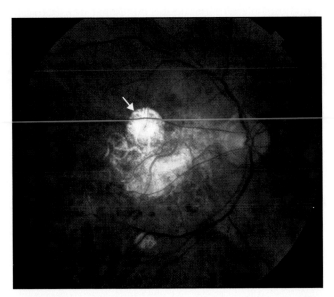

Figure 3.4 Endstage CNV. The recruitment of additional vessels as proposed by ischemia theories as the etiology of CNV in ARMD have a very difficult time explaining pictures such as these. **A.** There is a hyperplastic scar, but not much in the way of visible vessels. **B.** Spontaneous resolution of the CNV has lead to a complete absence of not only the CNV, but also the RPE. This process probably came about secondary to massive apoptosis. Although hyperplastic scarring, remodeling, and apoptosis are common events in a wound healing response, they are not expected as an angiogenic response to simple ischemia. This suggests that there are other factors in addition to, or other than, simple ischemia.

energy can be transferred to oxygen, creating singlet oxygen, which is another reactive species. Photosensitizers can be exogenous chemicals or endogenous compounds, such as porphyrin or lipofuscin. There are a number of protective enzymes that help to detoxify ROS. In addition to enzymes, various antioxidants may intercept ROS and chemically reduce them into less reactive molecules. The reason why the mitochondrial wall is leaky to ROS is not known, especially considering their toxic nature. The superoxide leaked may act as a chemical messenger. It is also possible that the ROS leak for some other purpose. It has been shown that there is an inverse correlation between the amount of superoxide leak and the expected life span of an organism across a large number of species. This has raised speculation that lifespan for a given species is intrinsically controlled, in part, by the amount of ROS leakage through mitochondria (164–166).

There are a number of sources of ROS in any organism besides the oxidative machinery in the mitochondria. The NADPH oxidase system, particularly the p47phox subunit, produces singlet oxygen and hydrogen peroxide as part of the respiratory burst in macrophages and neutrophils. A similar enzyme has been found in vascular endothelial cells. Superoxide can be produced by xanthene oxidase, nitric oxide synthase (167), as a byproduct in the production of prostaglandins, from exposure to light, ionizing radiation, pollution, cigarette smoke, and even ischemia (168). ROS are generated as a second messenger for some cytokines and hormones (169,170). ROS looks to find a source of electrons in cells in the form of nucleic acids, proteins, carbohydrates, and lipids; this reaction often leads to molecular damage.

ROS attack on proteins directly alters the chemical composition of the protein, may secondarily affect protein configuration, and can also lead to cross-link formation. Breakdown of these altered proteins is more difficult and can inhibit normal proteosome function. Inappropriate oxidation of lipids represents a special case for several reasons. The vulnerability of a fatty acid to oxidative damage is related to the number of double bonds that are present. One double bond increases the susceptibility by a factor of 100 (171). Each successive double bond increases the possibility in proportion to the total number of double bonds. The predominant polyunsaturated fatty acid (PUFA) found in the cell membrane of the photoreceptor outer segments, docosahexaneoic acid, is the most unsaturated fatty acid in the body with six double bonds. Peroxidized lipids can participate in reactions with other lipids to generate additional lipid peroxides in a process known as propagation reactions. Thus, one peroxidized lipid molecule may lead to a progeny of other peroxidized lipids. Each of these peroxidized PUFAs is reactive in their own right in a way analogous to ROS. Oxygen can attack any of the double bonds in a PUFA, and thereby create a reactive molecule capable of a large number of permutations of interactions and breakdown products. The result of lipid peroxidation is a diverse family of daughter molecules, many of which retain the ability to react with other molecules. In the process, though, they cross-link to the molecules they react with to produce abnormal conjugates.

These interactions may produce a number of untoward effects. For example, bonding to a protein may affect the functional ability of the protein if it binds to its active center, altering its tertiary or quaternary structure, or if it changes the hydrophobicity. The ability of a peroxidized lipid to attack a protein molecule is proportional to the number of double bonds in the fatty acid (172). Lipid peroxides lead to an increase in cell membrane rigidity, and contribute to aging of the membrane (173). Lipid peroxides may damage cellular organelles and membranes (173–175). Oxidatively damaged lipid may bind to more than one protein, creating large, interlinked molecules. Lipid derived molecules irreversibly altered by oxidative effects are known as advanced lipoxation end products or ALEs. Analogous end products derived from carbohydrates are known as advanced glycation end products or AGEs. Many AGEs may resemble and be quite similar to those formed from lipids, the ALEs (176–178). Because of the unusual structure caused by oxidative damage and cross-linking, and because these molecules have the potential to damage proteosomes, the cell may have a difficult time breaking these molecules down. The indigestible material, particularly lipid peroxides and their metabolites (179,180), are compartmentalized as lipofuscin granules (181–183), and the accumulation of lipofuscin is increased in proportion with greater RPE oxygen exposure (184). The production of lipofuscin in the RPE is compounded because of the high concentration of retinoids, molecules with double bonds that are used to capture energy from light, in the outer segments.

To help protect against inappropriate oxidation there are basically three levels of protection: molecular, cellular, and tissue. On the molecular level, the cell has antioxidant vitamins and enzymes. These include vitamins C and E, superoxide dismutase, catalase, glutathione transferase (185), glutathione reductase, and glutathione peroxidase. The antioxidants may limit inappropriate oxidation in the first place, or may terminate propagation reactions. Vitamin E, a lipophilic free-radical scavenger, may do both. In homogenous solutions, β-carotene is a potent free-radical scavenger, *in vitro*; the *in vivo* effects of β-carotene are less well defined.

On a cellular level, two main responses may occur. The cell may try to adapt to the oxidative stress by increased activation of such transcription factors as nuclear factor κB (NF-κB) (186) and Activator Protein 1, which help control gene expression of antioxidant enzymes. Oxidative stress itself alters the activity of matrix metalloproteinases and collagenases, possibly playing a role in tissue remodeling induced by oxidative stress (187). Exposure to ROS also may induce apoptosis, which can be blocked with antioxidants (188). Interestingly, the process of apoptosis is actually mediated by ROS; the mitochondria undergo a permeability transition and leak ROS into the cell, and the resultant oxidative damage causes cellular suicide (189).

Over larger levels of scale, increasingly sophisticated responses may occur. ROS and peroxidized lipids increase the production of VEGF (190,191), which is involved in supporting vascular endothelial cells as well as promoting the formation of new vessels. RPE cells show a dose related increase in VEGF mRNA levels when exposed to superoxide, and this response could be blocked with antioxidants (191). Exposure of cultured RPE cells to repeated doses of near ultraviolet light reduces RPE proliferation, similar to that seen in RPE senescence. These same cells showed increased lipofuscin content, an "age" pigment, and the cells also expressed less PEDF (43). The scavenger receptor system (192,193) is responsible for recognizing and binding to oxidatively damaged molecules, including AGEs and ALEs. It is involved in a diverse number of processes particularly in the recognition of old erythrocytes (194). When erythrocytes age, lipid peroxide products accumulate within the cell membrane, and because of the associated cross-linking, the cell membrane becomes more stiff. Scavenger receptors recognize these abnormalities and work to remove old erythrocytes from the circulation. A similar process to remove abnormally oxidized material may lead to atherosclerosis. Oxidation of LDL produces a variety of peroxidized molecules, which are recognized by the scavenger receptor system. Macrophages and smooth muscle cells bind oxidized LDL (oxLDL) as an initiating event in atheroma formation. Oxidatively damaged LDL may form under a number of different conditions, such as hypertension and exposure to cigarette smoke, transition metal ions, and pollutants; its oxidation may be inhibited by anti-oxidants (195). Under ordinary circumstances when a cell binds LDL through an LDL receptor, the receptor is down regulated through a negative feedback loop triggered by rising levels of intracellular cholesterol. When macrophages are exposed to oxLDL, they phagocytose the oxLDL through alternate receptors that are part of the scavenger receptor system, including CD36 (196–200).

Instead of down regulation of CD36, phagocytosis of oxLDL causes an increase of CD36 expression through a positive feedback loop (201). Important effects that occur on binding to CD36 are the secretion of VEGF, vascular cell adhesion molecule-1 (VCAM-1), and release of MCP-1 (202). Other receptors have been characterized, including a receptor for AGE, known as RAGE. Similar to CD36, RAGE binds its ligand, AGE, which causes an expression of more RAGE (203), the expression of a number of proinflammatory cytokines, evidence of increased oxidative stress, NF-κB activation (204), and expression of VEGF. These actions could be inhibited by administering a soluble receptor for RAGE or with antioxidants (205,206). This may have importance in ocular diseases (206–208). Excised CNV specimens have been found to not only express AGE, but also RAGE (209,210).

While it may seem counter-intuitive that ROS, lipid peroxides, and advanced end products can stimulate VEGF production, the response does seem to fit into a larger strategy in which the body takes aggressive steps to contain, neutralize, and rid itself of oxidatively damaged material. Not only do these molecules increase the secretion of VEGF, but also they can cause vascular endothelial cells to form capillary tubes much more efficiently, through a mechanism that apparently does not involve the upregulation or release of angiogenic growth factors (211).

OXIDATIVE DAMAGE AND CNV

Oxidized lipids are formed in the photoreceptor outer segments as a normal part of daily life. Scavenger receptors (212,213), in particular CD36, are present on the RPE cell and participate in phagocytosis of spent outer segments. It is possible that ordinary everyday exposure of the CD36 receptor to oxidized lipids in the photoreceptor outer segments help maintain the constitutive secretion of VEGF by RPE cells. Excessive secretion of VEGF by RPE cells, however, may be one factor responsible for the initiation of CNV. This raises the possibility that excessive exposure to oxidative damage may lead the RPE cells to secrete excessive VEGF. Animal models of increased excretion of VEGF by RPE cells can produce CNV (214,215).

Ueda et al. have previously shown that a 10 μg injection of linoleic hydroperoxide, a lipid peroxide derivative, into a corneal pocket leads to corneal neovascularization from the limbus (216). In addition, Armstrong et al. found injections of 50 to 600 μg of linoleic hydroperoxide into the vitreous cavity caused retinal neovascularization that persisted for four weeks (217). Following the injection of linoleic hydroperoxide, there was a cascade of cytokines secreted including VEGF. This brings us back to Bruch's membrane, which has an exponential increase in lipids with age. The lipid seems to preferentially accumulate in the same region where the neovascularization grows to; and Bruch's membrane has no known intrinsic mechanism offering protection against oxidative damage for the lipids accumulating there. Perhaps oxidative damage to lipids in Bruch's membrane is important in the etiology of CNV in ARMD.

The eye has a dioptric mechanism to focus light, which can stimulate photo-oxidative reactions, it has a high oxygen flux through Bruch's membrane, and there is a plethora of potentially susceptible lipids in the retina, and perhaps in Bruch's membrane, to enter into oxidative reactions. In Bruch's membrane, there is deposition of iron, which through redox cycling in the Fenton reaction can participate in oxidative injury to lipids, proteins, and other molecules (218). To evaluate this aspect, we looked at Bruch's membranes from autopsy eyes and measured the total amount of peroxidatively damaged molecules with the fluorometric thiobarbituric acid assay and characterized the lipids further with high pressure liquid chromatography (219). We found the total amount of peroxidized lipids increased exponentially in Bruch's membrane with age. We also found PUFAs occurred in Bruch's, and that peroxidation products of linoleic acid were the most common peroxidized PUFAs present, similar to those seen

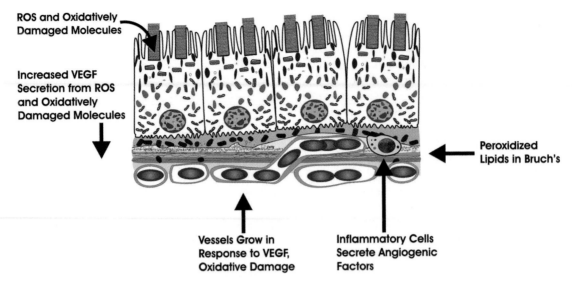

Figure 3.5 Oxidative damage as a potential cause of CNV. Exposure of RPE cells to ROS can lead to increased VEGF secretion. It is possible that CD36-mediated binding of outer segment discs does as well. Lipid peroxides, which can stimulate the formation of new vessels, increase in amount in Bruch's membrane with age.

in atherosclerotic lesions. Peroxidized docosahexaenoic acid was also found, indicating a cellular origin for at least some of the lipids present. In a study being prepared for publication, we found that although lipid peroxides are found in Bruch's membrane specimens from the macular region, those from the periphery of the same eyes contain very low levels. In a separate study, subretinal injection of linoleic hydroperoxide caused CNV in rabbits (Fig. 3.5) (220). Of interest is the finding that increased ingestion of zinc, a redox inactive metal, is associated with a decreased rate of progression to CNV in high-risk patients. There are several possibilities how increased levels of zinc may help prevent oxidative damage from iron, including displacement of iron by zinc (221–223), decreasing the number of redo-active sites available to participate in oxidative reactions in Bruch's membrane.

Lipid peroxides appear to increase with age in Bruch's membrane, but they do so in other tissues, principally in atherosclerotic lesions in arterial walls. Although by histopathology, cholesterol—both free and esterified—appears to be the predominant lipid present; the overwhelmingly large proportion of peroxidized lipid present is derived from PUFAs such as linoleic acid (224–225). In atherosclerotic vessels, the body mounts an aggressive cell-mediated approach to contain the oxidized material (226,227), principally using vascular endothelial cells and macrophages. The oxidized materials stimulate production of VEGF by these cells (228–231), in an effort that is thought to maintain the vitality of the vascular endothelial cells (232). VEGF may inhibit the apoptosis of a number of cell types (233). VEGF production leads to neovascularization of the plaque (198–230,234,235). It is thought the body's ability and tendency to aggressively remove oxidized lipids arises from an evolutionary derived process based on the strategy to remove old or oxidatively damaged cells,

using oxidatively damaged lipids in the plasma membrane as an identification system by the scavenger receptor system (227). Unfortunately an atherosclerotic plaque represents a mother lode of the same damaged lipids up to 30% of linoleic acid (the principle PUFA of cell membranes) contained in atherosclerotic plaques is in a peroxidized state (224). The presence of these lipids elicits a series of events, often self-reinforcing, in which the body tries to contain or remove the offending material. Perhaps some of the same sequence of events occurs in the eye as well. This is not to say that the stages leading to development of CNV in ARMD are identical to those seen in atherosclerosis. However, the body has a number of defined strategies and methods of dealing with degenerating cells and tissue, and many of the same strategies and methods that are used in atherosclerosis of vessel walls are also used in the eye. Perhaps these oxidatively damaged molecules help elicit the invasion of neovascularization in Bruch's membrane as they do in atherosclerotic lesions. Injection of these same lipids has lead to ocular neovascularization in the rabbit (216,217,220).

There are other oxidative mechanisms that may be operative at the level of the outer retina, RPE cell, or Bruch's membrane other than those involving inappropriate oxidation of lipids. However, if lifelong increase in oxidatively damaged molecules, particularly lipid peroxides, is a principle risk factor for the development of CNV, strategies to prevent CNV need to counter this build-up. One strategy may include a lifelong diet rich in carotenoids (4), which are selectively accumulated in the macula. These molecules function to absorb blue wavelengths and also as antioxidants. The Age-Related Eye Disease Study (236) found that supplementation with beta-carotene, vitamins C and E, copper, and zinc in patients at risk was associated with a reduction in neovascularization and visual acuity loss as compared with controls. Antioxidants may indeed scavenge free radicals and reduce inappropriately oxidized macro-molecules. They also function to alter gene expression (237–240), alter cell signaling proteins, such as protein kinase C (241), alter the valence of metal ions in the active center of enzymes (238), induce apoptosis in certain cell lines (242), cause maturation of other cell lines, reduce or induce expression of a variety of antioxidant enzymes (243), bind to structural proteins (244), and potentially displace pro-oxidant ions, such as iron in the case of zinc, so there may be other mechanisms to consider.

There are two established ocular findings that are risk factors for the development of CNV: focal hyperpigmentation and soft drusen. Recently a study of fundus autofluorescence, derived from lipofuscin has shown that fellow eyes of patients with CNV have higher mean levels of autofluorescence than do patients who do not have CNV (245). The focal areas of hyperpigmentation in these patients were found to have high levels of autofluorescence and had absorption characteristics suggesting the pigment seen was derived, at least in part, from lipofuscin. The histopathologic correlate to focal hyperpigmentation is detached pigment cells in the subretinal space. These areas of hyperpigmentation were autofluorescent suggesting lipofuscin accounted for at least some of the observed pigment. The finding of hyperautofluorescent, hyperpigmented spots in the fellow eye was particularly associated with retinal angiomatosis proliferation in the fellow eye. In a recent study imaging patients with retinal angiomatosis proliferation with optical coherence tomography and autofluorescence photography, the location of the angiomatosis proliferation was seen to be topographically associated with pigmented hyperautofluorescent structures in the outer nuclear layer (246). It was thought these structures were macrophages or detached RPE cells laden with lipofuscin. Since either of these cell-types can secrete VEGF when subjected to oxidative stress, it was theorized that these cells may be secreting VEGF in the outer retina. This would be expected to cause recruitment of the retinal vessels as they grow down the VEGF gradient, leading to formation of a RAP lesion. In rabbits, injection of lipid peroxide in the subretinal space caused migration of RPE cells into the subretinal space and outer retina and these RPE cells had phagocytized droplets of lipid peroxide (220). Optical coherence tomography suggests that either RPE cells detach or macrophages migrate into the subretinal space (Fig. 3.6).

The origin of drusen is a perplexing and contested issue. Analysis of the lipids in Bruch's membrane suggested to some that they were of cellular origin, while other investigators thought the lipids must have had a vascular origin. Through a very detailed analysis, Hageman et al. (247) determined that cellular remnants from degenerate RPE cells contribute to inflammatory stimulus, and these remnants may act as a nidus for drusen formation. In a proteomic analysis of drusen dissected from Bruch's membrane, oxidative protein modifications, including protein cross-links, were found. In particular, carboxyethyl

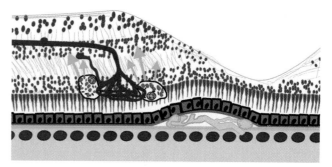

Figure 3.6 In patients with retinal vascular anastomosis to the neovascular process, which has a number of names including deep retinal vascular anomalous complexes (RVAC) and retinal angiomatous proliferation (RAP). These patients have focal hyperpigmentation that are hyperautofluorescent. Optical coherence tomography reveal particulate densities in the outer retina. It is proposed that these densities represent oxidatively stressed cells (icons in outer retina) containing lipofuscin that are producing VEGF (green arrows), something both oxidatively stressed macrophages or RPE cells do. The secretion of VEGF in the outer retina causes recruitment of new vessels from the retinal circulation. It has been proposed that these patients do not have concurrent occult CNV. However, careful inspection of late phase fluorescein and indocyanine green angiograms would suggest otherwise.

pyrrole adducts, which are formed from oxidation products of docosahexaenoic acid, were found more frequently in ARMD eyes than in age-matched controls (248). In addition, crystallins, which are nonsecreted heat shock proteins that are synthesized by the retina and RPE (248,249), were more likely to be found in drusen of eyes with ARMD. Many of the altered proteins could have been derived from either the blood or RPE cells. The accumulation of material in the first place may be related to altered Bruch's membrane physiology from accumulated cross-links with oxidatively damaged lipid and protein, and subsequent inflammatory sequela (247–249). One would expect that there is a bidirectional flux of lipid through Bruch's membrane over time and that there may be a selective partitioning of molecules within the altered Bruch's membrane, contributing to the formation of drusen, particularly those containing lipid, such as soft drusen. The principle material leading to the formation of soft drusen, basal linear deposit, represents a cache of lipids and other materials that could be the target of oxidative attack. There are no intrinsic cellular mechanisms to counter this attack. However, it is certainly possible that vitamins and antioxidants may offer some protection.

While there is compelling evidence, some of which is circumstantial, linking CNV in ARMD to oxidative stress and damage, other mechanisms are certainly operative. Once the invasion of tissue begins, especially if it reaches the subretinal space, will experience the physiologically normal, but low oxygen tension and may itself produce growth factors to perpetuate endothelial proliferation. In addition, hypoxia promotes migration and tube formation by the bone marrow derived endothelial progenitor cells (Fig. 3.7).

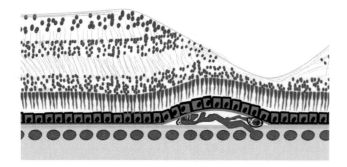

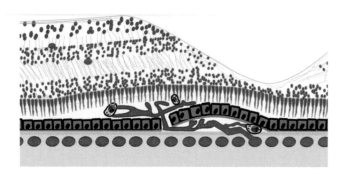

Figure 3.7 Invasion of CNV. Once the invading tissue reaches the inner portion of Bruch's membrane and potentially the outer retina space there may be some influence on VEGF production by the oxygen tension there.

OXIDATIVE DAMAGE AND GEOGRAPHIC ATROPHY

More than 100 different types of oxidative lesions to DNA have been described, including single and double-strand breaks and the development of a variety of cross-link lesions (250,251). The maintenance of genome integrity is extremely important in not only avoiding the production of mutations in progeny of the organism, but also in the potential progeny of the cell. Many types of DNA damage can be fixed through the coordinated action of a number of different proteins, but other types cannot be repaired with guaranteed fidelity. The cell responds to genomic damage through repair processes employing a large number of proteins. In addition, the cell may turn off growth and replication until the repair process is complete (252).

Some cells may be permanently induced into a senescent state or may die through apoptosis. Cellular senescence occurs in most cell lines as a consequence of increasingly limited proliferative potential and eventual growth arrest with shortening of the telomeres (252). Induced cellular senescence causes a premature decline in replicative potential from cell cycle arrest without death (253). Senescent cells are not responsive to growth factors and have altered gene expression, protein synthesis, and cellular morphologies as compared with non-senescent cells (253,254). Induction of senescence occurs with the production of

tumor suppressor proteins, in particular p53 and pRb (mutation of the Rb gene can lead to retinoblastoma), which among other things arrests the affected cells at check points in their cell cycle. Continued oxidative injury can cause senescent cells to undergo apoptosis, or cellular suicide. Induced cellular senescence and apoptosis are seen as adaptive responses to the onslaught of genomic damage, where the organism trades cell death to prevent the possibility of replication of mutated cells (cancer). This has been called the Samurai law of biology: It is better to be dead than wrong (255). Production or activation of p53 encourages senescence, while inactivation of p53 can lead to rescue from senescence, with an increase in the tendency for carcinogenesis (256). Oxidative stress increases the activation of p53 and pRb and also increases the rate of telomere shortening (257). Oxidative damage not only affects nuclear DNA, but also mitochondrial DNA, where mutation affects the efficiency of energy production and increases the propensity for additional ROS production (161,162,258).

Extension of these concepts to ARMD may explain a number of factors. The accumulation of oxidative damage has been suggested as a cause of CNV, but the same oxidative damage may induce senescence (259) and an aging phenotype, with possible apoptosis (260) in RPE cells as well. Oxidative damage can lead to an increased accumulation of lipofuscin within RPE cells, a finding linked with the development of geographic atrophy. This series of events may explain geographic atrophy, where there is a localized well demarcated area of "atrophy" of the retina and choriocapillaris sandwiching a region of absent RPE cells. This hypothesis may explain the seemingly illogical response, in which adjacent RPE cells do not replicate and fill in areas vacated by apparently dying fellow RPE cells. It is possible that in the area of atrophy, affected RPE cells have been lost through apoptosis and cannot be replaced by adjacent RPE cells because they themselves are in senescence. Of interest is that the autofluorescence of the RPE cells immediately adjacent to geographic atrophy are increased, indicating a larger lipofuscin load, and in follow-up, these areas of increased autofluorescence are more likely to undergo "atrophy" (261). Geographic atrophy is frequently seen in fellow eyes with CNV, also implying a common etiologic link.

CONCLUSIONS

This review critically examined a number of different theories in light of known physiologic concepts. No one specific theory by itself explains all aspects of the development of CNV in ARMD. Integration of a number of aspects from differing theories, particularly oxidative damage, as delineated, appears to explain many aspects, however. There are still a number of questions that face all of these diseases in terms of prevention and treatment.

Although aging, in part, may be the result of an accumulation of genetic defects that do not necessarily inhibit reproduction, there is increasing evidence that much of the aging phenotype is also the result of oxidative stress and the induced cellular adaptation responses. A principle risk factor for degenerative aspects of aging appears to be life itself. Aging is a problem that has challenged biologists and philosophers for centuries. Aging has deterministic and stochastic aspects, something the most ancient of philosophers knew. Clearly there are numerous factors involved and many of these are coded into our genetic structure. Certainly genes are powerful navigators of our fate, but the course can be modified by our interventions. ARMD affects the quality of life, particularly in aged people who may have other infirmities. With increasing life spans and increasing number of aged people, the incidence of macular degeneration is expected to rise. Development of a comprehensive hypothesis for the etiology of late ARMD is an iterative process over time, but is central to developing treatments for this debilitating disorder.

REFERENCES

1. Hyman LG, Lilienfeld AM, Ferris FL III, et al. Senile macular degeneration: a case-control study. *Am J Epidemiol.* 1983;118:213–227.
2. Klaver CC, Wolfs RC, Assink JJ, et al. Genetic risk of age-related maculopathy. Population-based familial aggregation study. *Arch Ophthalmol.* 1998;116:1,646–1,651.
3. Smith W, Mitchell P. Family history and age-related maculopathy: the Blue Mountains Eye Study. *Aust N Z J Ophthalmol.* 1998;26:203–206.
4. Risk factors for neovascular age-related macular degeneration. The Eye Disease Case–Control Study Group. *Arch Ophthalmol.* 1992;110:1,701–1,708.
5. Smith W, Assink J, Klein R, et al. Risk factors for age-related macular degeneration: Pooled findings from three continents. *Ophthalmology.* 2001;108:697–704.
6. Risk factors for choroidal neovascularization in the second eye of patients with juxtafoveal or subfoveal choroidal neovascularization secondary to age-related macular degeneration. Macular Photocoagulation Study Group. *Arch Ophthalmol.* 1997;115:741–747.
7. Risk factors associated with age-related macular degeneration. A case–control study in the age-related eye disease study: age-related eye disease study report number 3. Age-Related Eye Disease Study Research Group. *Ophthalmology.* 2000;107:2,224–2,232.
8. Klein R, Peto T, Bird A, et al. The epidemiology of age-related macular degeneration. *Am J Ophthalmol.* 2004;137:486–495.
9. Seddon JM, Gensler G, Milton RC, et al. Association between C-reactive protein and age-related macular degeneration. *JAMA.* 2004;11;291:704–710.
10. Klein R, Klein BE, Tomany SC, et al. Association of emphysema, gout, and inflammatory markers with long-term incidence of age-related maculopathy. *Arch Ophthalmol.* 2003;121:674–678.
11. Cho E, Hung S, Willett WC, et al. Prospective study of dietary fat and the risk of age-related macular degeneration. *Am J Clin Nutr.* 2001;73:209–218.
12. Seddon JM, Rosner B, Sperduto RD, et al. Dietary fat and risk for advanced age-related macular degeneration. *Arch Ophthalmol.* 2001;119:1,191–1,199.
13. Seddon JM, Cote J, Rosner B. Progression of age-related macular degeneration: association with dietary fat, transunsaturated fat, nuts, and fish intake. *Arch Ophthalmol.* 2003;121:1,728–1,737.
14. Klein R, Klein BE, Jensen SC, et al. The five-year incidence and progression of age-related maculopathy: the Beaver Dam Eye Study. *Ophthalmology.* 1997;104:7–21.
15. Smith W, Mitchell P, Wang JJ. Gender, estrogen, hormone replacement and age-related macular degeneration: results from the Blue Mountains Eye Study. *Aust N Z J Ophthalmol.* 1997;25(Suppl 1):S13–S15.
16. Wang JJ, Mitchell P, Smith W. Refractive error and age-related maculopathy: the Blue Mountains Eye Study. *Invest Ophthalmol Vis Sci.* 1998;39:2,167–2,171.
17. Risk factors associated with age-related macular degeneration. A casecontrol study in the age-related eye disease study: age-related eye disease study report number 3. Age-Related Eye Disease Study Research Group. *Ophthalmology.* 2000;107:2,224–2,232.
18. Chumbley LC. Impressions of eye diseases among Rhodesian Blacks in Mashonaland. *S Afr Med J.* 1977 Aug 13;52:316–318.
19. Gregor Z, Joffe L. Senile macular changes in the black African. *Br J Ophthalmol.* 1978;62:547–550.
20. Smith W, Mitchell P, Leeder SR. Dietary fat and fish intake and age-related maculopathy. *Arch Ophthalmol.* 2000;118:401–404.
21. Seddon JM, Ajani UA, Sperduto RD, et al. Dietary carotenoids, vitamins A, C, and E, and advanced age-related macular degeneration. Eye Disease CaseControl Study Group. *JAMA.* 1994 9;272:1,413–1,420.
22. Allikmets R, Shroyer NF, Singh N, et al. Mutation of the Stargardt disease gene (ABCR) in age-related macular degeneration. *Science.* 1997;19;277 (5333):1,805–1,807.
23. Webster AR, Heon E, Lotery AJ, et al. An analysis of allelic variation in the ABCA4 gene. *Invest Ophthalmol Vis Sci.* 2001;42:1,179–1,189.
24. De La Paz MA, Guy VK, AbouDonia S, et al. Analysis of the Stargardt disease gene (ABCR) in age-related macular degeneration. *Ophthalmology.* 1999;106:1,531–1,536.
25. Klaver CC, Kliffen M, van Duijn CM, et al. Genetic association of apolipoprotein E with age-related macular degeneration. *Am J Hum Genet.* 1998;63:200–206.
26. Souied EH, Benlian P, Amouyel P, et al. The epsilon4 allele of the apolipoprotein E gene as a potential protective factor for exudative age-related macular degeneration. *Am J Ophthalmol.* 1998;125:353–359.
27. Pang CP, Baum L, Chan WM, et al. The apolipoprotein E epsilon4 allele is unlikely to be a major risk factor of age-related macular degeneration in Chinese. *Ophthalmologica.* 2000;214:289–291.
28. Schmidt S, Saunders AM, De La Paz MA, et al. Association of the apolipoprotein E gene with age-related macular degeneration: possible effect modification by family history, age, and gender. *Mol Vis.* 2000 31;6:287–293.
29. Gao H, Hollyfield JG. Aging of the human retina. Differential loss of neurons and retinal pigment epithelial cells. *Invest Ophthalmol Vis Sci.* 1992;33:1–17.
30. Young RW, Bok D. Participation of the retinal pigment epithelium in the rod outer segment renewal process. *J Cell Biol.* 1969;42:392–403.
31. Marshall J. The ageing retina: physiology or pathology. *Eye.* 1987;1:282–295.
32. Boulton M, McKechnie NM, Breda J, et al. The formation of autofluorescent granules in cultured human RPE. *Invest Ophthalmol Vis Sci.* 1989;30:82–89.
33. Rakoczy PE, Baines M, Kennedy CJ, et al. Correlation between autofluorescent debris accumulation and the presence of partially processed forms of cathepsin D in cultured retinal pigment epithelial cells challenged with rod outer segments. *Exp Eye Res.* 1996;63:159–167.
34. Eldred GE, Katz ML. Fluorophores of the human retinal pigment epithelium: separation and spectral characterization. *Exp Eye Res.* 1988;47:71–86.
35. Wolf G. Lipofuscin, the age pigment. *Nutr Rev.* 1993;51:205–206.
36. Eldred GE, Lasky MR. Retinal age pigments generated by selfassembling lysosomotropic detergents. *Nature.* 1993;25;361:724–726.
37. Boulton M, Marshall J. Effects of increasing numbers of phagocytic inclusions on human retinal pigment epithelial cells in culture: a model for aging. *Br J Ophthalmol.* 1986;70:808–815.
38. FeeneyBurns L, Berman ER, Rothman H. Lipofuscin of human retinal pigment epithelium. *Am J Ophthalmol.* 1980;90:783–791.
39. Wing GL, Blanchard GC, Weiter JJ. The topography and age relationship of lipofuscin concentration in the retinal pigment epithelium. *Invest Ophthalmol Vis Sci.* 1978;17:601–607.
40. Delori FC, Dorey CK, Staurenghi G, et al. In vivo fluorescence of the ocular fundus exhibits retinal pigment epithelium lipofuscin characteristics. *Invest Ophthalmol Vis Sci.* 1995;36:718–729.
41. von Ruckmann A, Fitzke FW, Bird AC. Distribution of fundus autofluorescence with a scanning laser ophthalmoscope. *Br J Ophthalmol.* 1995;79:407–412.
42. Hayasaka S. Aging changes in lipofuscin, lysosomes and melanin in the macular area of human retina and choroid. *Jpn J Ophthalmol.* 1989;33:36–42.
43. Li W, Yanoff M, Li Y, et al. Artificial senescence of bovine retinal pigment epithelial cells induced by nearultraviolet in vitro. *Mech Ageing Dev.* 1999;22;110:137–55.
44. Yin D. Biochemical basis of lipofuscin, ceroid, and agepigmentlike fluorophores. *Free Radic Biol Med.* 1996;21:871–888.
45. Liu J, Itagaki Y, Ben-Shabat S, et al. The biosynthesis of A2E, a fluorophore of aging retina, involves the formation of the precursor, A2PE, in the photoreceptor outer segment membrane. *J Biol Chem.* 2000;275(38):29,354–29,360.
46. Fishkin N, Jang YP, Itagaki Y, et al. A2-rhodopsin: a new fluorophore isolated from photoreceptor outer segments. *Org Biomol Chem.* 2003;1:1,101–1,105.
47. Yin D. Biochemical basis of lipofuscin, ceroid, and agepigmentlike fluorophores. *Free Radic Biol Med.* 1996;21:871–888.
48. Eldred GE. Lipofuscin fluorophore inhibits lysosomal protein degradation and may cause early stages of macular degeneration. *Gerontology.* 1995;41 (Suppl 2):15–28.
49. Wihlmark U, Wrigstad A, Roberg K, et al. Lipofuscin accumulation in cultured retinal pigment epithelial cells causes enhanced sensitivity to blue light irradiation. *Free Radic Biol Med.* 1997;22:1,229–1,234.
50. Gaillard ER, Atherton SJ, Eldred G, et al. Photophysical studies on human retinal lipofuscin. *Photochem Photobiol.* 1995;61:448–453.
51. Suter M, Reme C, Grimm C, et al. Age-related macular degeneration. The lipofuscin component n-retinyl-n-retinylidene ethanolamine detaches proapoptotic proteins from mitochondria and induces apoptosis in mammalian retinal pigment epithelial cells. *J Biol Chem.* 2000 15;275:39,625–630.

52. Shaban H, Richter C. A2E and blue light in the retina: the paradigm of age-related macular degeneration. *Biol Chem.* 2002;383:537–545.
53. Sparrow JR, Zhou J, Cai B. DNA is a target of the photodynamic effects elicited in A2Eladen RPE by bluelight illumination. *Invest Ophthalmol Vis Sci.* 2003;44:2,245–2,251.
54. PandaJonas S, Jonas JB, Jakobczyk et al. Retinal pigment epithelial cell count, distribution, and correlations in normal human eyes. *Am J Ophthalmol.* 1996;121:181–189.
55. Green WR, Enger C. Age-related macular degeneration histopathologic studies. The 1992 Lorenz E. Zimmerman Lecture. *Ophthalmology* 1993;100:1,519–1,535.
56. Green WR. Histopathology of age-related macular degeneration. *Mol Vis.* 1999 3;5:27.
57. Grossniklaus HE, Green WR. Histopathologic and ultrastructural findings of surgically excised choroidal neovascularization. Submacular Surgery Trials Research Group. *Arch Ophthalmol.* 1998;116:745–749.
58. Ishibashi T, Sorgente N, Patterson R, et al. Aging changes in Bruch's membrane of monkeys: an electron microscopic study. *Ophthalmologica.* 1986;192:179–190.
59. van der Schaft TL, de Bruijn WC, Mooy CM, et al. Is basal laminar deposit unique for age-related macular degeneration? *Arch Ophthalmol.* 1991;109:420–425.
60. van der Schaft TL, Mooy CM, de Bruijn WC, et al. Immunohistochemical light and electron microscopy of basal laminar deposit. *Graefes Arch Clin Exp Ophthalmol.* 1994;232:40–46.
61. Karwatowski WS, Jeffries TE, Duance VC, et al. Preparation of Bruch's membrane and analysis of the age-related changes in the structural collagens. *Br J Ophthalmol.* 1995;79:944–952.
62. Sarks JP, Sarks SH, Killingsworth MC. Evolution of soft drusen in age-related macular degeneration. *Eye.* 1994;8(Pt 3):269–283.
63. Holz FG, Owens SL, Marks J, et al. Ultrastructural findings in autosomal dominant drusen. *Arch Ophthalmol.* 1997;115:788–792.
64. Ramrattan RS, van der Schaft TL, Mooy CM, et al. Morphometric analysis of Bruch's membrane, the choriocapillaris, and the choroid in aging. *Invest Ophthalmol Vis Sci.* 1994;35:2,857–2,864.
65. Spraul CW, Lang GE, Grossniklaus HE, et al. Histologic and morphometric analysis of the choroid, Bruch's membrane, and retinal pigment epithelium in postmortem eyes with age-related macular degeneration and histologic examination of surgically excised choroidal neovascular membranes. *Surv Ophthalmol.* 1999;44(Suppl):S10–S32.
66. Holz FG, Sheraidah G, Pauleikhoff D, et al. Analysis of lipid deposits extracted from human macular and peripheral Bruch's membrane. *Arch Ophthalmol.* 1994;112:402–406.
67. Morre DJ, Hussain AA, Marshall J. Age-related variation in the hydraulic conductivity of Bruch's membrane. *Invest Ophthalmol Vis Sci.* 1995;36:1,290–297.
68. Starita C, Hussain AA, Marshall J. Decreasing hydraulic conductivity of Bruch's membrane: Relevance to photoreceptor survival and lipofuscinoses. *American J Med Genetics.* 1995;57:235–237.
69. Starita C, Hussain AA, Patmore A, et al. Localization of the site of major resistance to fluid transport in Bruch's membrane. *Invest Ophthalmol Vis Sci.* 1997;38:762–767.
70. Sheraidah G, Steinmetz R, Maguire J, et al. Correlation between lipids extracted from Bruch's membrane and age. *Ophthalmology.* 1993;100:47–51.
71. Pauleikhoff D, Zuels S, Sheraidah GS, et al. Correlation between biochemical composition and fluorescein binding of deposits in Bruch's membrane. *Ophthalmology.* 1992;99:1,548–1,553.
72. Pauleikhoff D, Wojteki S, Muller D, et al. Adhesive properties of basal membranes of Bruch's membrane. Immunohistochemical studies of agedependent changes in adhesive molecules and lipid deposits. *Ophthalmologe.* 2000;97:243–250.
73. Curcio CA, Millican CL, Bailey T, et al. Accumulation of cholesterol with age in human Bruch's membrane. *Invest Ophthalmol Vis Sci.* 2001; 42:265–274.
74. Ruberti JW, Curcio CA, Millican CL, et al. Quickfreeze/deepetch visualization of age-related lipid accumulation in Bruch's membrane. *Invest Ophthalmol Vis Sci.* 2003;44:1,753–1,759.
75. Korte GE, Pua F. Choriocapillaris regeneration in the rabbit: a study with vascular casts. *Acta Anat (Basel).* 1988;133:224–228.
76. Dawson DW, Volpert OV, Gillis P, et al. Pigment epitheliumderived factor: a potent inhibitor of angiogenesis. *Science.* 1999;285:245–248.
77. Imai D, Yoneya S, Gehlbach PL, et al. Intraocular gene transfer of pigment epithelium-derived factor rescues photoreceptors from lightinduced cell death. *J Cell Physiol.* 2005;202(2):570–578.
78. Barnstable CJ, TombranTink J. Neuroprotective and antiangiogenic actions of PEDF in the eye: molecular targets and therapeutic potential. *Prog Retin Eye Res.* 2004;23:561–577.
79. Eichler W, Yafai Y, Keller T, et al. PEDF derived from glial Muller cells: a possible regulator of retinal angiogenesis. *Exp Cell Res.* 2004;10;299:68–78.
80. Mori K, Duh E, Gehlbach P, et al. Pigment epitheliumderived factor inhibits retinal and choroidal neovascularization. *J Cell Physiol.* 2001;188:253–263.
81. Gehlbach P, Demetriades AM, Yamamoto S, et al. Periocular injection of an adenoviral vector encoding pigment epitheliumderived factor inhibits choroidal neovascularization. *Gene Ther.* 2003;10:637–646.
82. OhnoMatsui K, Morita I, TombranTink J, et al. Novel mechanism for age-related macular degeneration: an equilibrium shift between the angiogenesis factors VEGF and PEDF. *J Cell Physiol.* 2001;189:323–333.
83. Holekamp NM, Bouck N, Volpert O. Pigment epitheliumderived factor is deficient in the vitreous of patients with choroidal neovascularization due to age-related macular degeneration. *Am J Ophthalmol.* 2002;134:220–227.
84. Spaide RF, Armstrong D, Browne R. Continuing medical education review: choroidal neovascularization in age-related macular degenerationwhat is the cause? *Retina.* 2003;23:595–614.
85. Holz FG, Pauleikhoff D, Klein R, et al. Pathogenesis of lesions in late age-related macular disease. *Am J Ophthalmol.* 2004;137:504–510.
86. Renno RZ, Youssri AI, Michaud N, et al. Expression of pigment epitheliumderived factor in experimental choroidal neovascularization. *Invest Ophthalmol Vis Sci.* 2002;43:1,574–1,580.
87. Duh EJ, Yang HS, Haller JA, et al. Vitreous levels of pigment epitheliumderived factor and vascular endothelial growth factor: implications for ocular angiogenesis. *Am J Ophthalmol.* 2004;137:668–674.
88. Martin G, Schlunck G, Hansen LL, et al. Differential expression of angioregulatory factors in normal and CNVderived human retinal pigment epithelium. *Graefes Arch Clin Exp Ophthalmol.* 2004;242:321–326.
89. Matsuoka M, Ogata N, Otsuji T, et al. Expression of pigment epithelium derived factor and vascular endothelial growth factor in choroidal neovascular membranes and polypoidal choroidal vasculopathy. *Br J Ophthalmol.* 2004;88:809–815.
90. McColm JR, Geisen P, Hartnett ME. VEGF isoforms and their expression after a single episode of hypoxia or repeated fluctuations between hyperoxia and hypoxia: relevance to clinical ROP. *Mol Vis.* 2004 21;10:512–520.
91. Ogata N, Wada M, Otsuji T, et al. Expression of pigment epitheliumderived factor in normal adult rat eye and experimental choroidal neovascularization. *Invest Ophthalmol Vis Sci.* 2002;43:1,168–1,175.
92. OhnoMatsui K, Yoshida T, Uetama T, et al. Vascular endothelial growth factor upregulates pigment epitheliumderived factor expression via VEGFR1 in human retinal pigment epithelial cells. *Biochem Biophys Res Commun.* 2003;303:962–967.
93. Hutchings H, Maitre-Boube M, TombranTink J, et al. Pigment epitheliumderived factor exerts opposite effects on endothelial cells of different phenotypes. *Biochem Biophys Res Commun.* 2002;294:764–769.
94. Killingsworth MC. Angiogenesis in early choroidal neovascularization secondary to age-related macular degeneration. *Graefes Arch Clin Exp Ophthalmol.* 1995;233:313–323.
95. Shryock JC, Belardinelli L. Adenosine and adenosine receptors in the cardiovascular system: biochemistry, physiology, and pharmacology. *Am J Cardiol.* 1997 19;79:2–10.
96. Hashimoto E, Kage K, Ogita T, et al. Adenosine as an endogenous mediator of hypoxia for induction of vascular endothelial growth factor mRNA in U937 cells. *Biochem Biophys Res Commun.* 1994 14;204:318–324.
97. Takagi H, King GL, Robinson GS, et al. Adenosine mediates hypoxic induction of vascular endothelial growth factor in retinal pericytes and endothelial cells. *Invest Ophthalmol Vis Sci.* 1996;37:2,165–2,176.
98. Minchenko A, Salceda S, Bauer T, et al. Hypoxia regulatory elements of the human vascular endothelial growth factor gene. *Cell Mol Biol Res.* 1994;40(1):35–39.
99. Wang GL, Semenza GL. Characterization of hypoxiainducible factor 1 and regulation of DNA binding activity by hypoxia. *J Biol Chem.* 1993 15;268:21,513–21,518.
100. Yin JH, Yang DI, Ku G, et al. iNOS expression inhibits hypoxiainducible factor1 activity. *Biochem Biophys Res Commun.* 2000 9;279:30–34.
101. Sandau KB, Faus HG, Brune B. Induction of hypoxiainduciblefactor 1 by nitric oxide is mediated via the PI 3K pathway. *Biochem Biophys Res Commun.* 2000 11;278:263–267.
102. Melillo G, Musso T, Sica A, et al. A hypoxiaresponsive element mediates a novel pathway of activation of the inducible nitric oxide synthase promoter. *J Exp Med.* 1995 1;182:1,683–1,693.
103. Dvorak HF, Brown LF, Detmar M, et al. Vascular permeability factor/vascular endothelial growth factor, microvascular hyperpermeability, and angiogenesis. *Am J Pathol.* 1995;146:1,029–1,039.
104. Roberts WG, Palade GE. Increased microvascular permeability and endothelial fenestration induced by vascular endothelial growth factor. *J Cell Sci.* 1995;108:2,369–2,379.
105. Berse B, Brown LF, Van de Water L, et al. Vascular permeability factor (vascular endothelial growth factor) gene is expressed differentially in normal tissues, macrophages, and tumors. *Mol Biol Cell.* 1992;3:211–220.
106. Zachary I, Mathur A, YlaHerttuala S, et al. Vascular protection: A novel nonangiogenic cardiovascular role for vascular endothelial growth factor. *Arterioscler Thromb Vasc Biol.* 2000;20:1,512–1,520.
107. Senger DR, Ledbetter SR, Claffey KP, et al. Stimulation of endothelial cell migration by vascular permeability factor/vascular endothelial growth factor through cooperative mechanisms involving the alphavbeta3 integrin, osteopontin, and thrombin. *Am J Pathol.* 1996;149:293–305.
108. Kubo H, Fujiwara T, Jussila L, et al. Involvement of vascular endothelial growth factor receptor3 in maintenance of integrity of endothelial cell lining during tumor angiogenesis. *Blood.* 2000 15;96:546–553.
109. Pierce EA, Avery RL, Foley ED, et al. Vascular endothelial growth factor/vascular permeability factor expression in a mouse model of retinal neovascularization. *Proc Natl Acad Sci USA.* 1995 31;92:905–909.

110. Dorey CK, Aouididi S, Reynaud X, et al. Correlation of vascular permeability factor/vascular endothelial growth factor with extraretinal neovascularization in the rat. *Arch Ophthalmol.* 1996;114:1,210–1,217.

111. Shima DT, Adamis AP, Ferrara N, et al. Hypoxic induction of endothelial cell growth factors in retinal cells: identification and characterization of vascular endothelial growth factor (VEGF) as the mitogen. *Mol Med.* 1995;1:182–193.

112. Aiello LP, Pierce EA, Foley ED, et al. Suppression of retinal neovascularization in vivo by inhibition of vascular endothelial growth factor (VEGF) using soluble VEGFreceptor chimeric proteins. *Proc Natl Acad Sci USA.* 1995 7;92:10,457–10,461.

113. Aiello LP, Avery RL, Arrigg PG, et al. Vascular endothelial growth factor in ocular fluid of patients with diabetic retinopathy and other retinal disorders. *N Engl J Med.* 1994 1;331:1,480–1,487.

114. Lutty GA, McLeod DS, Merges C, et al. Localization of vascular endothelial growth factor in human retina and choroid. *Arch Ophthalmol.* 1996;114: 971–977.

115. Lopez PF, Sippy BD, Lambert HM, et al. Transdifferentiated retinal pigment epithelial cells are immunoreactive for vascular endothelial growth factor in surgically excised age-related macular degenerationrelated choroidal neovascular membranes. *Invest Ophthalmol Vis Sci.* 1996;37:855–868.

116. Blaauwgeers HG, Holtkamp GM, Rutten H, et al. Polarized vascular endothelial growth factor secretion by human retinal pigment epithelium and localization of vascular endothelial growth factor receptors on the inner choriocapillaris. Evidence for a trophic paracrine relation. *Am J Pathol.* 1999;155:421–428.

117. Asayama N, Shimada H, Yuzawa M. [Correlation of indocyanine green angiography findings and expression of vascular endothelial growth factor in surgically excised age-related macular degenerationrelated choroidal neovascular membranes]. *Nippon Ganka Gakkai Zasshi.* 2000; 104:390–395.

118. Enholm B, Paavonen K, Ristimaki A, et al. Comparison of VEGF, VEGFB, VEGFC and Ang1 mRNA regulation by serum, growth factors, oncoproteins and hypoxia. *Oncogene.* 1997 22;14:2,475–2,483.

119. Schott RJ, Morrow LA. Growth factors and angiogenesis. *Cardiovasc Res.* 1993;27:1,155–1,161.

120. Folkman J. Angiogenesis and angiogenesis inhibition: an overview. *EXS.* 1997;79:1–8.

121. Connolly DT, Heuvelman DM, Nelson R, et al. Tumor vascular permeability factor stimulates endothelial cell growth and angiogenesis. *J Clin Invest.* 1989;84:1,470–1,478.

122. Kendall RL, Thomas KA. Inhibition of vascular endothelial cell growth factor activity by an endogenously encoded soluble receptor. *Proc Natl Acad Sci USA.* 1993;15;90:10,705–10,709.

123. Kondo S, Asano M, Suzuki H. Significance of vascular endothelial growth factor/vascular permeability factor for solid tumor growth, and its inhibitionby the antibody. *Biochem Biophys Res Commun.* 1993 16;194:1,234–1,241.

124. Aiello LP, Northrup JM, Keyt BA, et al. Hypoxic regulation of vascular endothelial growth factor in retinal cells. *Arch Ophthalmol.* 1995;113: 1,538–1,544.

125. Miller JW, Adamis AP, Shima DT, et al. Vascular endothelial growth factor/vascular permeability factor is temporally and spatially correlated with ocular angiogenesis in a primate model. *Am J Pathol.* 1994;145:574–584.

126. Kwak N, Okamoto N, Wood JM, et al. VEGF is major stimulator in model of choroidal neovascularization. *Invest Ophthalmol Vis Sci.* 2000;41: 3,158–3,164.

127. Baffi J, Byrnes G, Chan CC, Csaky KG. Choroidal neovascularization in the rat induced by adenovirus mediated expression of vascular endothelial growth factor. *Invest Ophthalmol Vis Sci.* 2000;41:3,582–3,589.

128. Spilsbury K, Garrett KL, Shen WY, et al. Overexpression of vascular endothelial growth factor (VEGF) in the retinal pigment epithelium leads to the development of choroidal neovascularization. *Am J Pathol.* 2000;157:135–144.

129. Eyetech Study Group. Antivascular endothelial growth factor therapy for subfoveal choroidal neovascularization secondary to age-related macular degeneration: phase II study results. *Ophthalmology.* 2003;110:979–986.

130. Barouch FC, Miller JW. Antivascular endothelial growth factor strategies for the treatment of choroidal neovascularization from age-related macular degeneration. *Int Ophthalmol Clin.* 2004;44:23–32.

131. Grunwald JE, Hariprasad SM, DuPont J, et al. Foveolar choroidal blood flow in age-related macular degeneration. *Invest Ophthalmol Vis Sci.* 1998; 39:385–390.

132. Mori F, Konno S, Hikichi T, et al. Pulsatile ocular blood flow study: decreases in exudative age related macular degeneration. *Br J Ophthalmol.* 2001;85:531–533.

133. Krakau CE. A model for pulsatile and steady ocular blood flow. *Graefes Arch Clin Exp Ophthalmol.* 1995;233:112–118.

134. Yang YC, Hulbert MF, Batterbury M, et al. Pulsatile ocular blood flow measurements in healthy eyes: reproducibility and reference values. *J Glaucoma.* 1997;6:175–179.

135. Chen JC, Fitzke FW, Pauleikhoff D, et al. Functional loss in age-related Bruch's membrane change with choroidal perfusion defect. *Invest Ophthalmol Vis Sci.* 1992;33:334–340.

136. Ross RD, Barofsky JM, Cohen G, et al. Presumed macular choroidal watershed vascular filling, choroidal neovascularization, and systemic vascular disease in patients with age-related macular degeneration. *Am J Ophthalmol.* 1998;125:71–80.

137. Pauleikhoff D, Spital G, Radermacher M, et al. A fluorescein and indocyanine green angiographic study of choriocapillaris in age-related macular disease. *Arch Ophthalmol.* 1999;117:1,353–1,358.

138. Ryan SJ, Hinton DR, Murata T. Choroidal Neovascularization. In: Ryan SJ, ed. *Retina.* 3rd Ed. St. Louis: Mosby; 2001: vol 3;1,005–1,006.

139. Piguet B, Palmvang IB, Chisholm IH, et al. Evolution of age-related macular degeneration with choroidal perfusion abnormality. *Am J Ophthalmol.* 1992;15;113:657–663.

140. Yancey CM, Linsenmeier RA. The electroretinogram and choroidal PO2 in the cat during elevated intraocular pressure. *Invest Ophthalmol Vis Sci.* 1988;29:700–707.

141. Yancey CM, Linsenmeier RA. Oxygen distribution and consumption in the cat retina at increased intraocular pressure. *Invest Ophthalmol Vis Sci.* 1989;30:600–611.

142. Haugh LM, Linsenmeier RA, Goldstick TK. Mathematical models of the spatial distribution of retinal oxygen tension and consumption, including changes upon illumination. *Ann Biomed Eng.* 1990;18(1):19–36.

143. Linsenmeier RA, Braun RD. Oxygen distribution and consumption in the cat retina during normoxia and hypoxemia. *J Gen Physiol.* 1992;99:177–197.

144. Ahmed J, Braun RD, Dunn R, et al. Oxygen distribution in the macaque retina. *Invest Ophthalmol Vis Sci.* 1993;34:516–521.

145. Braun RD, Linsenmeier RA, Goldstick TK. Oxygen consumption in the inner and outer retina of the cat. *Invest Ophthalmol Vis Sci.* 1995;36:542–554.

146. Linsenmeier RA, PadnickSilver L. Metabolic dependence of photoreceptors on the choroid in the normal and detached retina. *Invest Ophthalmol Vis Sci.* 2000;41:3,117–3,123.

147. Kim I, Ryan AM, Rohan R, et al. Constitutive expression of VEGF, VEGFR1, and VEGFR2 in normal eyes. *Invest Ophthalmol Vis Sci.* 1999;40:2,115–2,121.

148. Subczynski WK, Hopwood LE, Hyde JS. Is the mammalian cell plasma membrane a barrier to oxygen transport? *J Gen Physiol.* 1992;100:69–87.

149. Subczynski WK, Hyde JS, Kusumi A. Oxygen permeability of phosphatidylcholine–cholesterol membranes. *Proc Natl Acad Sci USA.* 1989;86:4,474–4,478.

150. Subczynski WK, Hyde JS, Kusumi A. Effect of alkyl chain unsaturation and cholesterol intercalation on oxygen transport in membranes: a pulse ESR spin labeling study. *Biochemistry.* 1991;30:8,578–8,590.

151. Subczynski WK, Renk GE, Crouch RK, et al. Oxygen diffusionconcentration product in rhodopsin as observed by a pulse ESR spin labeling method. *Biophys J.* 1992;63:573–577.

152. Vinores SA, Derevjanik NL, Vinores MA, et al. Sensitivity of different vascular beds in the eye to neovascularization and bloodretinal barrier breakdown in VEGF transgenic mice. *Adv Exp Med Biol.* 2000;476:129–138.

153. Penfold PL, Killingsworth MC, Sarks SH. Senile macular degeneration: the involvement of immunocompetent cells. *Graefes Arch Clin Exp Ophthalmol.* 1985;223:69–76.

154. Penfold PL, Killingsworth MC, Sarks SH. Senile macular degeneration. The involvement of giant cells in atrophy of the retinal pigment epithelium. *Invest Ophthalmol Vis Sci.* 1986;27:364–371.

155. Kvanta A, Algvere PV, Berglin L, Seregard S. Subfoveal fibrovascular membranes in age-related macular degeneration express vascular endothelial growth factor. *Invest Ophthalmol Vis Sci.* 1996;37:1,929–1,934.

156. Espinosa-Heidmann DG, Suner IJ, Hernandez EP, et al. Macrophage depletion diminishes lesion size and severity in experimental choroidal neovascularization. *Invest Ophthalmol Vis Sci.* 2003;44:3,586–3,592.

157. Sakurai E, Anand A, Ambati BK, et al. Macrophage depletion inhibits experimental choroidal neovascularization. *Invest Ophthalmol Vis Sci.* 2003;44:3,578–3,585.

158. Ishida S, Usui T, Yamashiro K, et al. VEGF164-mediated inflammation is required for pathological, but not physiological, ischemiainduced retinal neovascularization. *J Exp Med.* 2003;198:483–489.

159. Sakurai E, Taguchi H, Anand A, et al. Targeted disruption of the CD18 or ICAM1 gene inhibits choroidal neovascularization. *Invest Ophthalmol Vis Sci.* 2003;44:2,743–2,749.

160. Ambati J, Anand A, Fernandez S, et al. An animal model of age-related macular degeneration in senescent Ccl2- or Ccr2deficient mice. *Nat Med.* 2003;9:1,390–1,397.

161. TsutsumiMiyahara C, Sonoda KH, Egashira K, et al. The relative contributions of each subset of ocular infiltrated cells in experimental choroidal neovascularisation. *Br J Ophthalmol.* 2004;88:1,217–1,222.

162. Hagen TM, Yowe DL, Bartholomew JC, et al. Mitochondrial decay in hepatocytes from old rats: membrane potential declines, heterogeneity and oxidants increase. *Proc Natl Acad Sci USA.* 1997;94:3,064–3,069.

163. Brierley EJ, Johnson MA, Lightowlers RN, et al. Role of mitochondrial DNA mutations in human aging: implications for the central nervous system and muscle. *Ann Neurol.* 1998;43:217–223.

164. Ku HH, Brunk UT, Sohal RS. Relationship between mitochondrial superoxide and hydrogen peroxide production and longevity of mammalian species. *Free Radic Biol Med.* 1993;15:621–627.

165. Ku HH, Sohal RS. Comparison of mitochondrial prooxidant generation and antioxidant defenses between rat and pigeon: possible basis of variation in longevity and metabolic potential. *Mech Ageing Dev.* 1993;72:67–76.

166. Harman D. The biologic clock: the mitochondria? *J Am Geriatr Soc.* 1972;20:145–147.

167. Vasquez-Vivar J, Kalyanaraman B, Martasek P, et al. Superoxide generation by endothelial nitric oxide synthase: the influence of cofactors. *Proc Natl Acad Sci USA.* 1998;4;95:9,220–9,225.

168. Bonne C, Muller A, Villain M. Free radicals in retinal ischemia. *Gen Pharmacol.* 1998;30:275–280.

169. Thannickal VJ, Fanburg BL. Reactive oxygen species in cell signaling. *Am J Physiol Lung Cell Mol Physiol.* 2000;279(6):L1,005–L1,028.

170. Nose K. Role of reactive oxygen species in the regulation of physiological functions. *Biol Pharm Bull.* 2000;23:897–903.

171. Fukuzumi K. Relationship between lipoperoxides and diseases. *J Environ Pathol Toxicol Oncol.* 1986;6:25–56.

172. Refsgaard HH, Tsai L, Stadtman ER. Modifications of proteins by polyunsaturated fatty acid peroxidation products. *Proc Natl Acad Sci USA.* 2000;97:611–616.

173. Choe M, Jackson C, Yu BP. Lipid peroxidation contributes to age-related membrane rigidity. *Free Radic Biol Med.* 1995;18:977–984.

174. Hruszkewycz AM. Evidence for mitochondrial DNA damage by lipid peroxidation. *Biochem Biophys Res Commun.* 1988;153:191–197.

175. Ardelt BK, Borowitz JL, Maduh EU, et al. Cyanideinduced lipid peroxidation in different organs: subcellular distribution and hydroperoxide generation in neuronal cells. *Toxicology.* 1994;89:127–137.

176. Kislinger T, Fu C, Huber B, et al. N(epsilon)(carboxymethyl)lysine adducts of proteins are ligands for receptor for advanced glycation end products that activate cell signaling pathways and modulate gene expression. *Biol Chem.* 1999;29;274:31,740–749.

177. Fu MX, Requena JR, Jenkins AJ, et al. The advanced glycation end product, Nepsilon(carboxymethyl)lysine, is a product of both lipid peroxidation and glycoxidation reactions. *J Biol Chem.* 1996;26;271:9,982–9,986.

178. Reddy S, Bichler J, Wells-Knecht KJ,et.al. N epsilon(carboxymethyl)lysine is a dominant advanced glycation end product (AGE) antigen in tissue proteins. *Biochemistry.* 1995;29;34:10,872–10,878.

179. Kikugawa K, Beppu M. Involvement of lipid oxidation products in the formation of fluorescent and crosslinked proteins. *Chem Phys Lipids.* 1987; 44:277–296.

180. Kikugawa K, Kato T, Beppu M. Fluorescent and crosslinked proteins formed by free radical and aldehyde species generated during lipid oxidation. *Adv Exp Med Biol.* 1989;266:345–356.

181. Bazan HE, Bazan NG, FeeneyBurns L, et al. Lipids in human lipofuscinenriched fractions of two age populations. Comparison with rod outer segments and neural retina. *Invest Ophthalmol Vis Sci.* 1990; 31:1,433–1,443.

182. Wiegand RD, Giusto NM, Rapp LM, et al. Evidence for rod outer segment lipid peroxidation following constant illumination of the rat retina. *Invest Ophthalmol Vis Sci.* 1983;24:1,433–1,435.

183. Katz ML, Gao CL, Rice LM. Formation of lipofuschinlike fluorophores by reaction of retinal with photoreceptor outer segments and liposomes. *Mech Ageing Dev.* 1996;92:159–174.

184. Wihlmark U, Wrigstad A, Roberg K, et al. Lipofuscin formation in cultured retinal pigment epithelial cells exposed to photoreceptor outer segment material under different oxygen concentrations. *APMIS.* 1996;104: 265–271.

185. Singhal SS, Godley BF, Chandra A, et al. Induction of glutathione Stransferase hGST 5.8 is an early response to oxidative stress in RPE cells. *Invest Ophthalmol Vis Sci.* 1999;40:2,652–2,659.

186. Sasaki H, Ray PS, Zhu L, et al. Oxidative stress due to hypoxia/reoxygenation induces angiogenic factor VEGF in adult rat myocardium: possible role of NFkappaB. *Toxicology.* 2000;30;155:27–35.

187. Siwik DA, Pagano PJ, Colucci WS. Oxidative stress regulates collagen synthesis and matrix metalloproteinase activity in cardiac fibroblasts. *Am J Physiol Cell Physiol.* 2001;280:C53–C60.

188. Ishikawa Y, Kitamura M. Antiapoptotic effect of quercetin: intervention in the JNK and ERKmediated apoptotic pathways. *Kidney Int.* 2000;58: 1,078–1,087.

189. Jabs T. Reactive oxygen intermediates as mediators of programmed cell death in plants and animals. *Biochem Pharmacol.* 1999;57:231–245.

190. Monte M, Davel LE, Sacerdote de Lustig E. Hydrogen peroxide is involved in lymphocyte activation mechanisms to induce angiogenesis. *Eur J Cancer.* 1997;33:676–682.

191. Kuroki M, Voest EE, Amano S, et al. Reactive oxygen intermediates increase vascular endothelial growth factor expression in vitro and in vivo. *J Clin Invest.* 1996;98:1,667–1,675.

192. Horiuchi S, Higashi T, Ikeda K, et al. Advanced glycation end products and their recognition by macrophage and macrophagederived cells. *Diabetes.* 1996;Jul;45 Suppl 3:S73–S76.

193. Smedsrod B, Melkko J, Araki N, et al. Advanced glycation end products are eliminated by scavengerreceptormediated endocytosis in hepatic sinusoidal Kupffer and endothelial cells. *Biochem J.* 1997 1;322:567–573.

194. Sambrano GR, Parthasarathy S, Steinberg D. Recognition of oxidatively damaged erythrocytes by a macrophage receptor with specificity for oxidized low density lipoprotein. *Proc Natl Acad Sci USA.* 1994;91:265– 269.

195. YlaHerttuala S, Palinski W, Rosenfeld ME, et al. Low density lipoprotein undergoes oxidative modification in vivo. *Proc Natl Acad Sci USA.* 1989; 86:1,372–1,376.

196. Wintergerst ES, Jelk J, Rahner C, et al. Apoptosis induced by oxidized low density lipoprotein in human monocytederived macrophages involves CD36 and activation of caspase3. *Eur J Biochem.* 2000;267:6,050–6,059.

197. Janabi M, Yamashita S, Hirano K, et al. Oxidized LDLinduced NFkappa B activation and subsequent expression of proinflammatory genes are defective in monocytederived macrophages from CD36deficient patients. *Arterioscler Thromb Vasc Biol.* 2000;20:1,953–1,960.

198. Gillotte KL, Horkko S, Witztum JL, et al. Oxidized phospholipids, linked to apolipoprotein B of oxidized LDL, are ligands for macrophage scavenger receptors. *J Lipid Res.* 2000;41:824–833.

199. Chawla A, Barak Y, Nagy L, et al. PPAR–gamma dependent and independent effects on macrophagegene expression in lipid metabolism and inflammation. *Nat Med.* 2001;7(1):48–52.

200. Nicholson AC, Febbraio M, Han J, et al. CD36 in atherosclerosis. The role of a class B macrophage scavenger receptor. *Ann N Y Acad Sci.* 2000; 902:128–131.

201. Han J, Hajjar DP, Febbraio M, et al. Native and modified low density lipoproteins increase the functional expression of the macrophage class B scavenger receptor, CD36. *J Biol Chem.* 1997 22;272:21,654–21,659.

202. Shi W, Haberland ME, Jien ML, et al. Endothelial responses to oxidized lipoproteins determine genetic susceptibility to atherosclerosis in mice. *Circulation.* 2000;4;102:75–81.

203. Tanaka N, Yonekura H, Yamagishi S, et al. The receptor for advanced glycation end products is induced by the glycation products themselves and tumor necrosis factoralpha through nuclear factorkappa B, and by 17betaestradiol through Sp1 in human vascular endothelial cells. *J Biol Chem.* 2000;18;275:25,781–25,790.

204. Yan SD, Schmidt AM, Anderson GM, et al. Enhanced cellular oxidant stress by the interaction of advanced glycation end products with their receptors/binding proteins. *J Biol Chem.* 1994 1;269:9,889–897.

205. Bierhaus A, Chevion S, Chevion M, et al. Advanced glycation end productinduced activation of NF-kappaB is suppressed by alpha-lipoic acid in cultured endothelial cells. *Diabetes.* 1997;46:1,481–1,490.

206. Segawa Y, Shirao Y, Yamagishi S, et al. Upregulation of retinal vascular endothelial growth factor mRNAs in spontaneously diabetic rats without ophthalmoscopic retinopathy. A possible participation of advanced glycation end products in the development of the early phase of diabetic retinopathy. *Ophthalmic Res.* 1998;30:333–339.

207. Hirata C, Nakano K, Nakamura N, et al.Advanced glycation end products induce expression of vascular endothelial growth factor by retinal Muller cells. *Biochem Biophys Res Commun.* 1997;30;236:712–715.

208. Murata T, Nagai R, Ishibashi T, et al. The relationship between accumulation of advanced glycation end products and expression of vascular endothelial growth factor in human diabetic retinas. *Diabetologia.* 1997;40:764–769.

209. Ishibashi T, Murata T, Hangai M, et al. Advanced glycation end products in age-related macular degeneration. *Arch Ophthalmol.* 1998;116:1,629–1,632.

210. Hammes HP, Hoerauf H, Alt A, et al. N(epsilon)(carboxymethyl)lysin and the AGE receptor RAGE colocalize in age-related macular degeneration. *Invest Ophthalmol Vis Sci.* 1999;40:1,855–1,859.

211. Lelkes PI, Hahn KL, Sukovich DA, et al. On the possible role of reactive oxygen species in angiogenesis. *Adv Exp Med Biol.* 1998;454:295–310.

212. Duncan KG, Bailey KR, Kane JP, et al. Human retinal pigment epithelial cells express scavenger receptors BI and BII. *Biochem Biophys Res Commun.* 2002;292:1,017–1,022.

213. Ryeom SW, Sparrow JR, Silverstein RL. CD36 participates in the phagocytosis of rod outer segments by retinal pigment epithelium. *J Cell Sci.* 1996; 109:387–395.

214. Spilsbury K, Garrett KL, Shen WY, et al. Overexpression of vascular endothelial growth factor (VEGF) in the retinal pigment epithelium leads to the development of choroidal neovascularization. *Am J Pathol.* 2000; 157:135–144.

215. Baffi J, Byrnes G, Chan CC, et al. Choroidal neovascularization in the rat induced by adenovirus mediated expression of vascular endothelial growth factor. *Invest Ophthalmol Vis Sci.* 2000;41:3,582–3,589.

216. Ueda TO, Ueda TA, Fukuda S, et al. Lipid peroxide induced TNFa, VEGF, and neovascularization in the rabbit cornea, effect of TNF inhibition. *Angiogenesis.* 1998;2:174–184.

217. Armstrong D, Ueda TO, Ueda TA, et al. Lipid peroxide stimulates retinal neovascularization in rabbit retina through expression of TNFa, VEGF, and PDGF. *Angiogenesis.* 1998;2:93–104.

218. Hahn P, Milam AH, Dunaief JL. Maculas affected by age-related macular degeneration contain increased chelatable iron in the retinal pigment epithelium and Bruch's membrane. *Arch Ophthalmol.* 2003;121:1,099–1,105.

219. Spaide RF, Ho-Spaide WC, Browne R, et al. Characterization of lipid peroxides in Bruch's membrane. *Retina.* 1999;19:141–147.

220. Tamai K, Spaide RF, Ellis EA, et al. Lipid hydroperoxide stimulates subretinal choroidal neovascularization in the rabbit. *Exp Eye Res.* 2002;74: 301–308.

221. Shinar E, Rachmilewitz EA, Shifter A, et al. Oxidative damage to human red cells induced by copper and iron complexes in the presence of ascorbate. *Biochim Biophys Acta.* 1989;30;1014:66–72.

222. Chevion M. Protection against free radicalinduced and transition metalmediated damage: the use of "pull" and "push" mechanisms. *Free Radic Res Commun.* 1991;12–13 Pt 2:691–696.

223. Jin S, Kurtz DM Jr., Liu ZJ, et al. Displacement of iron by zinc at the diiron site of Desulfovibrio vulgaris rubrerythrin: Xray crystal structure and anomalous scattering analysis. *J Inorg Biochem.* 2004;98:786–796.

224. Suarna C, Dean RT, SouthwellKeeley PT, et al. Separation and characterization of cholesteryl oxo and hydroxy-linoleate isolated from human atherosclerotic plaque. *Free Radic Res.* 1997;27:397–408.

225. Piotrowski JJ, Shah S, Alexander JJ. Mature human atherosclerotic plaque contains peroxidized phosphatidylcholine as a major lipid peroxide. *Life Sci.* 1996;58:735–740.

226. Terpstra V, Bird DA, Steinberg D. Evidence that the lipid moiety of oxidized low density lipoprotein plays a role in its interaction with macrophage receptors. *Proc Natl Acad Sci USA.* 1998;17;95:1,806–1,811.

227. Boullier A, Bird DA, Chang MK, et al. Scavenger receptors, oxidized LDL, and atherosclerosis. *Ann N Y Acad Sci.* 2001;947:214–222.

228. Ramos MA, Kuzuya M, Esaki T, et al. Induction of macrophage VEGF in response to oxidized LDL and VEGF accumulation in human atherosclerotic lesions. *Arterioscler Thromb Vasc Biol.* 1998;18:1,188–1,196.

229. Inoue M, Itoh H, Tanaka T, et al. Oxidized LDL regulates vascular endothelial growth factor expression in human macrophages and endothelial cells through activation of peroxisome proliferatoractivated receptorgamma. *Arterioscler Thromb Vasc Biol.* 2001;21:560–566.

230. Inoue M, Itoh H, Ueda M, et al. Vascular endothelial growth factor (VEGF) expression in human coronary atherosclerotic lesions: possible pathophysiological significance of VEGF in progression of atherosclerosis. *Circulation.* 1998;17:2,108–2,116.

231. Khan BV, Parthasarathy SS, Alexander RW, et al. Modified low density lipoprotein and its constituents augment cytokineactivated vascular cell adhesion molecule1 gene expression in human vascular endothelial cells. *J Clin Invest.* 1995;95:1,262–1,270.

232. Kuzuya M, Ramos MA, Kanda S, et al. VEGF protects against oxidized LDL toxicity to endothelial cells by an intracellular glutathionedependent mechanism through the KDR receptor. *Arterioscler Thromb Vasc Biol.* 2001;21:765–770.

233. Katoh O, Tauchi H, Kawaishi K, Kimura A, Satow Y. Expression of the vascular endothelial growth factor (VEGF) receptor gene, KDR, in hematopoietic cells and inhibitory effect of VEGF on apoptotic cell death caused by ionizing radiation. *Cancer Res.* 1995;1;55:5,687–5,692.

234. Jeziorska M, Woolley DE. Neovascularization in early atherosclerotic lesions of human carotid arteries: its potential contribution to plaque development. *Hum Pathol.* 1999;30:919–925.

235. O'Brien ER, Garvin MR, Dev R, et al. Angiogenesis in human coronary atherosclerotic plaques. *Am J Pathol.* 1994;145:883–894.

236. A randomized, placebocontrolled, clinical trial of highdose supplementation with vitamins C and E, beta carotene, and zinc for age-related macular degeneration and vision loss: AREDS report no. 8. *Arch Ophthalmol.* 2001;119:1,417–1,436.

237. Linnane AW, Kopsidas G, Zhang C, et al. Cellular redox activity of coenzyme Q10: effect of CoQ10 supplementation on human skeletal muscle. *Free Radic Res.* 2002;36:445–453.

238. DemmigAdams B, Adams WW 3rd. Antioxidants in photosynthesis and human nutrition. *Science.* 2002;13;298:2,149–2,153.

239. Visala Rao D, Boyle GM, Parsons PG, et al. Influence of ageing, heat shock treatment and in vivo total antioxidant status on geneexpression profile and protein synthesis in human peripheral lymphocytes. *Mech Ageing Dev.* 2003;124:55–69.

240. Gohil K, Packer L. Bioflavonoidrich botanical extracts show antioxidant and gene regulatory activity. *Ann N Y Acad Sci.* 2002;957:70–77.

241. Gopalakrishna R, Jaken S. Protein kinase C signaling and oxidative stress. *Free Radic Biol Med.* 2000;28:1,349–1,361.

242. Muller K, Carpenter KL, Challis IR, et al. Carotenoids induce apoptosis in the Tlymphoblast cell line Jurkat E6.1. *Free Radic Res.* 2002;36:791–802.

243. Gohil K, Moy RK, Farzin S, et al. mRNA Expression profile of a human cancer cell line in response to ginkgo biloba extract: induction of antioxidant response and the golgi system. *Free Radic Res.* 2001;33:831–849.

244. Bernstein PS, Balashov NA, Tsong ED, et al. Retinal tubulin binds macular carotenoids. *Invest Ophthalmol Vis Sci.* 1997;38:167–175.

245. Spaide RF. Fundus autofluorescence and age-related macular degeneration. *Ophthalmology.* 2003;110:392–399.

246. Spaide RF. Focal hyperpigmented autofluorescent particles in the outer retina are associated with retinal angiomatous proliferation. In preparation.

247. Anderson DH, Mullins RF, Hageman GS, et al. A role for local inflammation in the formation of drusen in the aging eye. *Am J Ophthalmol.* 2002;134:411–431.

248. Crabb JW, Miyagi M, Gu X, et al. Drusen proteome analysis: an approach to the etiology of age-related macular degeneration. *Proc Natl Acad Sci USA.* 2002;99:14,682–14,687.

249. Bok D. New insights and new approaches toward the study of age-related macular degeneration. *Proc Natl Acad Sci USA.* 2002 99:14,619–14,621.

250. Nilsson I, Shibuya M, Wennstrom S. Differential activation of vascular genes by hypoxia in primary endothelial cells. *Exp Cell Res.* 2004;299:476–485.

251. Hasty P, Campisi J, Hoeijmakers J, et al. Aging and genome maintenance: lessons from the mouse? *Science.* 2003 28;299:1,355–1,359.

252. Soussi T. The p53 tumor suppressor gene: from molecular biology to clinical investigation. *Ann N Y Acad Sci.* 2000;910:121–137.

253. Chen QM. Replicative senescence and oxidantinduced premature senescence. Beyond the control of cell cycle checkpoints. *Ann N Y Acad Sci.* 2000; 908:111–125.

254. Chen Q, Fischer A, Reagan JD, et al. Oxidative DNA damage and senescence of human diploid fibroblast cells. *Proc Natl Acad Sci USA.* 1995;92:4,337–4,341.

255. Skulachev VP. Programmed death phenomena: from organelle to organism. *Ann N Y Acad Sci.* 2002;959:214–237.

256. Chin L, Artandi SE, Shen Q, et al. p53 deficiency rescues the adverse effects of telomere loss and cooperates with telomere dysfunction to accelerate carcinogenesis. *Cell.* 1999;97:527–538.

257. Saretzki G, Von Zglinicki T. Replicative aging, telomeres, and oxidative stress. *Ann N Y Acad Sci.* 2002;959:24–29.

258. Miquel J. An update on the oxygen stressmitochondrial mutation theory of aging: genetic and evolutionary implications. *Exp Gerontol.* 1998; 33:113–126.

259. Honda S, Hjelmeland LM, Handa JT. Senescence associated beta galactosidase activity in human retinal pigment epithelial cells exposed to mild hyperoxia in vitro. *Br J Ophthalmol.* 2002;86:159–162.

260. Zhang C, Baffi J, Cousins SW, et al. Oxidantinduced cell death in retinal pigment epithelium cells mediated through the release of apoptosisinducing factor. *J Cell Sci.* 2003;116:1,915–1,923.

261. Holz FG, Bellman C, Staudt S, et al. Fundus autofluorescence and development of geographic atrophy in age-related macular degeneration. *Invest Ophthalmol Vis Sci.* 2001;42:1,051–1,056.

Histopathology of Age-Related Macular Degeneration

4

Ana Pesce   *Fernando de Santiago*   *W. Richard Green*

Age-related macular degeneration (AMD) is a degenerative and progressive condition involving the retinal pigmentary epithelium (RPE), Bruch's membrane, and choriocapillaris. It is the leading cause of severe visual acuity loss in people over 65 years in the Western world. Changes in the RPE, Bruch's membrane, and choroid can be an expression of normal aging with minimal functional symptoms, but in AMD these structures may show several pathologic characteristics with clinical expression of central visual loss.

Most of the visual loss is due to choroidal neovascularization (CNV) in the exudative form of the disease. Many histopathologic studies identified the tissue changes associated with AMD, the effects of different treatments available for this condition, and the causes of the high incidence of treatment failure and recurrence of CNV.

NORMAL CHANGES OF THE AGING MACULA

Changes resulting from normal aging in the outer retina, RPE, Bruch's membrane, and choriocapillaris include a decrease in the number and density of photoreceptors (1), RPE hyperpigmentation (2), formation of lipofuscin granules, accumulation of residual bodies in RPE, basal laminar deposits (BLD) between plasma membrane and the basement membrane of RPE (1), and modifications of choroidal vessels that affect the retinal nutrition (3). These

abnormalities are not representative of AMD, and usually, they are not clinically detectable.

HISTOPATHOLOGY OF AMD

Tissue changes associated with AMD can be classified into non-neovascular and neovascular.

Non-Neovascular Changes

The earliest morphologic feature in AMD is the abnormal accumulation of extracellular material under the RPE. BLD are composed of granular material with wide-spaced collagen that are located between the plasma membrane and the basal lamina of the RPE. The basal linear deposits are composed of phospholipid vesicles and electron-dense granules. They are located in the inner collagenous zone of Bruch's membrane (4–7). These deposits are not ophthalmoscopically evident, but they can cause retinal dysfunction and angiographic changes in late phases. The localized accumulation of basal linear and basal laminar material leads to the development of soft drusen, the second feature of AMD (5,8), and the first manifestation of the disease that is ophthalmoscopically evident. This is seen clinically as pigmentary mottling (3).

Histologically, soft drusen corresponds to the abnormal thickening of the inner aspect of Bruch's membrane (7). Localized accumulation of basal linear material is emerging as the most frequent form of soft drusen (5,8). Different types of soft drusen described also include localized detachments of BLD with or without basal linear deposits (5).

Clinically, soft drusen are round yellow lesions larger than nodular drusen with poorly demarcated boundaries, located under the RPE. The thickened inner aspect of Bruch´s membrane and the RPE may separate from the rest of the Bruch´s membrane and represent a localized pigment epithelial detachment—seen as a large drusen when the detachment is small or as a RPE detachment when it involves a large area (7). This type of drusen may produce serous detachments of RPE and collaborate in the development of CNV (3,9,10).

Other types of drusen have been described and studied histopathologically. These include hard or nodular, calcified, and diffuse. Hard drusen appear to be a consequence of material extrusion from RPE cells, and are composed of hyalin material (1,9). Eyes with hard drusen are less likely to progress to atrophy or CNV in comparison to eyes containing soft, confluent drusen (7,9). Calcified drusen are sharply demarcated lesions usually associated with RPE atrophy (1).

Several changes of the RPE can be seen as another non-neovascular feature of AMD, and they include depigmentation, hypertrophy and cellular hyperplasia (2), attenuation, and severe atrophy of the RPE (4,5,11). When the atrophy covers a mottled area, it is called nongeographic atrophy; when it covers a contiguous area, it is known as geographic atrophy of the RPE, with frequent atrophy of the underlying choriocapillaris (3,7,12). In this area, a loss of about 90% of RPE cells and a decreased density of blood vessels have been demonstrated (11). Photoreceptors may be attenuated or absent in areas overlying atrophied RPE (1–3).

These changes are thought to be a response to decreased nutrients and increased metabolic abnormalities, namely accumulation of extracellular debris (3,6). In addition, a reticulated pattern of hyperpigmentation of RPE may be recognizable because of the pigmented cells (RPE cells and macrophages) (7,12) that are present—hemorrhages may also be present (3). These non-neovascular changes may be present in the dry or nonexudative form of AMD. The presence of non-neovascular changes associated with AMD increase the likelihood of CNV to develop, the third major feature of the disease.

Neovascular Changes

CNV in the macula is a major cause of severe central vision loss, especially when it is located subfoveally. Once the neovascularization involves the fovea, visual results are poor. Neovascular tissue and disciform scars are both features of the exudative or wet form of AMD. CNV growth is associated with an increased expression of angiogenic growth factors in the RPE and in the outer nuclear layer of the macula, independent of the etiologic cause (3,13,14). Although the precise pathogenesis of neovascular macular degeneration is still unknown, it is the objective of several studies (15).

Histopathologic studies have shown that areas of choroidal ischemia are seen often near CNV in AMD patients, and in response to this, surviving RPE cells may elaborate substances that lead to CNV growth (3,6). CNV originates from the choriocapillaris predominantly (3,5) and goes into the sub-RPE and subretinal spaces through cellular breakdown in the inner aspect of Bruch's membrane (1,2,4,5). The presence of diffuse and soft drusen and large serous detachments is associated with the development of CNV (9).

BLD were shown in excised CNV membranes (1). During early stages of AMD, these vessels are capillary-like, and with time evolve into arteries and veins (5). Vascular endothelium and RPE cells are constituents of CNV (10,11,16), and macrophages surrounding neovascularization areas have been shown in histopathologic studies (17,18). In surgically excised CNV membranes, nonuniform distribution of blood vessels, avascular areas at the margins of the membranes, photoreceptor outer segments, basal laminar and linear deposits, and hyperplastic RPE were found (1,7,19). CNV may leak fluid or bleed and lead to a serous or hemorrhagic RPE or retinal detachment (1,3,5). This is directly related to visual loss.

Choroidal neovascular membranes in AMD may be extrafoveal, juxtafoveal, or subfoveal. Each type is classified as classic or occult, following the guidelines of the Macular Photocoagulation Study Group. Membranes with both components, classic and occult, are considered mixed membranes (4,20). Occult membranes have a fibrovascular sub-RPE component, while classic CNV membranes have a major subretinal fibrovascular component. Mixed membranes contain fibrovascular tissue on both sides of the RPE. The inner surface of occult CNV is covered by fibrin and remains of outer segments that are located in the lateral edges of classic membranes (21). Excised CNV membranes associated with AMD were found to be larger than those associated with other etiologies (10). With the new vessels from the choroid, fibrous tissue may grow within Bruch's membrane, resulting in a fibrovascular complex that proliferates within the inner aspect of Bruch's membrane and may disrupt the normal architecture of the choriocapillaris, Bruch's membrane, and RPE (5) (Figs. 4.1 and 4.2).

Bleeding from neovascular tissue leads to a disciform scar (9), the fourth major feature of AMD and the last stage of the exudative form. If a disciform scar is present in one eye, the probability of an exudative lesion developing in the fellow eye is 12% to 34% (4). Vascularized scars with subretinal and sub-RPE components and BLD (4) were described in most cases, although non-vascularized scars with single subretinal or sub-RPE components may be present (5).

Areas of neovascular channels with surrounding macrophages (17), fibrocellular tissue, RPE atrophy, and photoreceptor loss and degeneration have been shown in disciform scars; and they are frequently associated to sub-RPE or subretinal serous or serosanguineous detachments and hemorrhages (3–5). Tears in RPE and defects in BLD

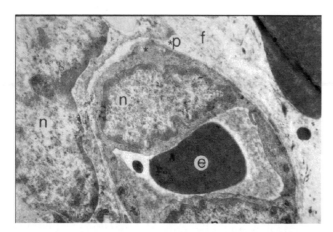

Figure 4.1 Electron microscopy of an excised neovascular membrane associated to AMD. E, erythrocyte; F, collagen fibers; N, nuclei; P, pericyte. (Courtesy of Professor Juan Verdaguer T., Juan I. Verdaguer D., and Luis Strozzi.)

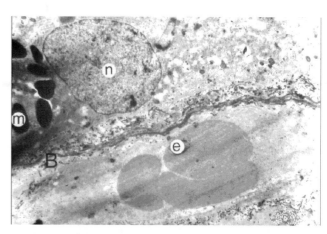

Figure 4.2 Electron microscopy of an excised neovascular membrane associated to AMD. B, Bruch's membrane; E, erythrocyte; M, melanin granules; N, nuclei. (Courtesy of Professor Juan Verdaguer T., Juan I. Verdaguer D., and Luis Strozzi.)

may be present in eyes with scars and blood vessels may extend through them (5). The relationship of disciform scars and defects of Bruch's membrane with CNV and photoreceptor cell degeneration extending beyond the area of BLD were shown in clinicopathologic studies (4).

HISTOPATHOLOGY OF TREATED CNV

Laser photocoagulation was the only proven treatment for selected cases of CNV for several years, until other treatments appeared. Available treatments for CNV secondary to AMD include conventional laser photocoagulation, photodynamic therapy, transpupillary thermotherapy, choroidal feeder vessel photocoagulation therapy, radiation therapy, pneumatic displacement of submacular hemorrhages, submacular surgery, macular translocation surgery, and pharmacologic therapies. The goal of AMD treatments today is to delay or reduce the risk of visual acuity loss, but there is still a high incidence of persistence and recurrence of CNV shown in histopathologic studies of excised, previously treated CNV membranes (7).

Histopathologic findings after laser photocoagulation, photodynamic therapy, and radiation therapy of exudative AMD, have been useful to improve the understanding of their mechanism of action and the reason why the high incidence of failure exists.

Histopathology of CNV after Conventional Laser Photocoagulation

The Macular Photocoagulation Study Group showed that although laser photocoagulation does nothing to alter the basic disease process, laser treatment of well-defined extrafoveal, subfoveal, and juxtafoveal CNV secondary to AMD could delay the visual acuity loss (4). Microscopic examinations of eyes with laser-treated CNV revealed loss

of RPE, photoreceptor cell layer, outer plexiform, and inner nuclear and inner plexiform layers, as well as the presence of basal laminar and linear deposits, fibrocellular tissue, and scarring of the choroid. Photoreceptor loss in the treated area was shown. No CNV in the Bruch's defects were shown in the treated area, but other areas of early CNV with new vessels in small defects of Bruch's membrane were described (4,22,23). In excised subfoveal, laser-treated, CNV membranes, large areas of avascular margin were shown, suggesting that angiograms underestimate the true size of subfoveal membranes and that the lesion may be incompletely treated, leading to a recurrence (19).

Histopathology of CNV After Photodynamic Therapy

Photodynamic therapy is a relatively new modality of treatment for subfoveal CNV secondary to AMD that may reduce the risk of moderate to severe visual loss. Benefits of this therapy are greater in patients presenting lesions up to four disk areas and low levels of visual acuity before treatment (20/50 or less) (24). The mechanism of action of this modality derives from activation of a photosensitizing drug administered systemically followed by diode laser irradiation to the affected tissue. This incites a photochemical reaction that in turn activates the clotting cascade, which leads to capillary endothelial cell and CNV occlusion (3,25).

Histopathologic findings in excised recurrent membranes of patients treated with photodynamic therapy that did not respond to it, were useful to understand the mechanism of action and the reason of CNV recurrences and progression after treatment (25–27). Metaplastic RPE cells with highly vacuolated cytoplasm, vascular damage evidenced by vacuolization, fragmentation and disintegration of endothelial cell layer, and extravasated erythrocytes and fibrocellular tissue were shown in excised treated membranes. Platelet aggregation and thrombus formation in CNV were described (27–29). Patent vessels within CNV complex, thought to occur due to recanalization, reperfusion, or regeneration of previously occluded or partially occluded vessels were noted. Macrophages may play a role in the resorption of occluded vessels. New vessel formation may lead to fluorescein leakage in patients after photodynamic therapy and these cases require retreatment (25,27,28).

Histopathology of CNV After Radiation Therapy

The role of radiation therapy in AMD is in question now that other options are available. The mechanism of ionizing radiation on CNV is still unknown, but a direct effect from toxicity to the endothelium leading to capillary closure, or an indirect effect from attenuation of the macrophage-mediated response have been proposed (3,30). The goal of this modality is to slow or delay the progress of the disease.

In low dose irradiated eyes, three years after radiation, histopathologic studies found little effect that included presence of fibrocellular and fibrovascular tissue, RPE and BLD, photoreceptor loss, or patent vessels in choriocapillaris and in CNV membrane with no wall thickness changes. Macrophages in CNV and underlying choroid were present (30). Ocular side effects of low dose radiation therapy include radiation-associated choroidal neovasculopathy, which leads to a poor visual prognosis (30).

ACKNOWLEDGMENTS

We specially thank Professor Juan Verdaguer Taradella and Dr. Juan Ignacio Verdaguer, from Fundación Oftalmológica Los Andes in Santiago, Chile, who excised the neovascular membrane shown on the photographs, and Dr. Luis Strozzi, from the Ocular Pathology Laboratory of José J. Aguirre Hospital in Santiago, Chile, who did the histopathologic study.

REFERENCES

1. The Foundation of the American Academy of Ophthalmology. *Basic and Clinical Science Course 4. Ophthalmic Pathology and Intraocular Tumors.* 2001–2002;141–144.
2. Quiroz-Mercado H. *Retina. Diagnóstico y Tratamiento.* McGraw-Hill Interamericana; 1996.
3. Alezzandrini A. *Enfermedad Macular Tratable. Etiopatogenia, Diagnóstico y Tratamiento.* Buenos Aires: Ediciones Científicas Argentinas; 2001.
4. Schneider S, Greven C, Green R. Photocoagulation of well-defined choroidal neovascularization in age-related macular degeneration. Clinicopathologic correlation. *Retina.* 1998;18:242–250.
5. Green R. Histopathology of age-related macular degeneration. *Molecular Vision.* 1999;5:27.
6. Zarbin MA. Age-related macular degeneration: review of pathogenesis. *Eur J Ophthalmol.* 1998;8(4):199–206.
7. The Foundation of the American Academy of Ophthalmology. *Basic and Clinical Science Course 12. Retina and Vitreous.* 2001–2002.
8. Curcio C, Leigh Millican C. Basal linear deposit and large drusen are specific for age-related maculopathy. *Arch Ophthalmol.* 1999;117:329–339.
9. Green WR, McDonnell PJ, Yeo JH. Pathologic features of senile macular degeneration. *Ophthalmology.* 1985;92:615–627.
10. Grossnikalus H, Green WR. For the Submacular Surgery Trials Research Group. Histopathologic and ultrastructural findings of surgically excised choroidal neovascularization. *Arch Ophthalmol.* 1998;116:745–749.
11. Mc Leod DS, Taomoto M, Otsuji T, et al. Quantifying changes in RPE and choroidal vasculature in eyes with age-related macular degeneration. *Invest Ophthalmol Vis Sci.* 2002;43:1,986–1,993.
12. Bressler SB, Bressler NM, Gragoudas ES. Age-related macular degeneration: drusen and geographic atrophy. In: Albert DM, Jakobiec FA, ed. *Principles and Practice in Ophthalmology.* 2nd Ed. Philadelphia: Saunders; 1999.
13. Tsutsumi C, Sonoda KH, Egashira K, et al. The critical role of ocular-infiltrating macrophages in the development of choroidal neovascularization. *J Lekoc Biol.* 2003;74:25–32.
14. Shikun H, Man Lin J, Worpel V, et al. A role of connective tissue growth factor in the pathogenesis of choroidal neovascularization. *Arch Ophthalmol.* 2003;121:1,283–1,288.
15. Kliffen M, Sharma H, Mooy C, et al. Increased expression of angiogenic growth factors in age-related maculopathy. *Br J Ophthalmol.* 1997;81:154–162.
16. Castellarin AA, Nasir MA, Sugino IK, et al. Clinicopathological correlation of primary and recurrent choroidal neovascularization following surgical excision in age-related macular degeneration. *Br J Ophthalmol.* 1998;82:480–487.
17. Grossniklaus H, Cingle K, Doo Yoon Y, et al. Correlation of histologic 2-dimensional reconstruction and confocal scanning laser microscopic imaging of choroidal neovascularization in eyes with age-related maculopathy. *Arc Ophthalmol.* 2000;118:625–629.
18. Hinton D, Shikun He, Lopez P. Apoptosis in surgically excised choroidal neovascular membranes in age-related macular degeneration. *Arch Ophthalmol.* 1998;116:203–209.
19. Bynoe L, Chang TS, Funatta M, et al. Histopathologic examination of vascular patterns in subfoveal neovascular membranes. *Ophthalmology.* 1994;101;(6):1,112–1,117.
20. Macular Photocoagulation Study Group. Five year-follow up of fellow eyes of patients with age-related macular degeneration and unilateral extrafoveal choroidal neovascularization. *Arch Ophthalmol.* 1993;111:1,189–1,199.
21. Lafaut BA, Bartz-Scmidt KU, Vanden Broecke C, et al. Clinicopathological correlation in exudative age-related macular degeneration: histological differentiation between classic and occult choroidal neovascularization. *Br J Ophthalmol.* 2000;84:239–243.
22. Lauer AK, Wilson DJ, Klein ML. Clinicopathologic correlation of fluorescein and indocyanine green angiography in exudative age-related macular degeneration. *Retina.* 2000;20(5):492–499.
23. Hsu JK, Thomas MA, Ibañez H, et al. Clinicopathologic studies of an eye after submacular membranectomy for choroidal neovascularization. *Retina.* 1995;15:43–52.
24. Verteporfin in Photodynamic Study Group. Verteporfin therapy of subfoveal choroidal neovascularization in age-related macular degeneration: two years results of a randomized clinical trial including lesions with occult with no classic choroidal neovascularization- Verteporfin in photodynamic therapy report 2. *Am J Ophthalmol.* 2001;131(5):541–560.
25. Moshfeghi D, Kaiser P, Grossniklaus H, et al. Clinicopathologic study after submacular removal of choroidal neovascular membranes treated with verteporfin ocular photodynamic therapy. *Am J Ophthalmol.* 2003;135(3):343–350.
26. Staurenghi G, Massacesi A, Musicco I, et al. Combining photodynamic therapy and feeder vessel photocoagulation: a pilot study. *Seminars in Ophthalmology.* 2001;16(4):233–236.
27. Schnurrbusch UE, Welt K, Horn LC, et al. Histological findings of surgically excised choroidal neovascular membranes after photodynamic therapy. *Br J Ophthalmol.* 2001;85(9):1,086–1,091.
28. Ghazi NG, Jabbour NM, De La Cruz ZC, et al. Clinicopathologic studies of age-related macular degeneration with classic subfoveal choroidal neovascularization treated with photodynamic therapy. *Retina.* 2001;21(5):478–486.
29. Michels S, Schmidt-Erfurth U. Sequence of early vascular events after photodynamic therapy. *Invest Ophthalmol Vis Sci.* 2003;44(5):2,147–2,154.
30. Lambooij A, Kuijpers R, Mooy C, et al. Radiotherapy of exudative age-related macular degeneration: a clinical and pathologic study. *Graefe's Arch Clin Exp Ophthalmol.* 2001;239:539–543.

Classification of Age-Related Macular Degeneration

Warren Thompson

Age-related macular degeneration (AMD) was originally described by Haab in 1885 (1). Numerous names and classification schemes have since been used to describe what is now considered by most to be the same degenerative process. Historically, the disciform lesions were attributed to disturbances of the inner retinal layers, outer retinal layers, retinal vasculature, Bruch's membrane, choriocapillaris, choroidal vasculature, and choroiditis (2).

The modern era of AMD began during the 1960s. Gass described in detail the clinical findings associated with AMD in a series published in the *American Journal of Ophthalmology* in 1967 (2). He coined the term senile macular choroidal degeneration because he believed that the source of pathology was at the level of the choroid.

Macular degeneration is conveniently divided into the non-exudative or dry type and the exudative or wet type. In addition to simplicity, the two types also offer a natural division in prognosis, as up to 88% of vision loss attributed to macular degeneration is found in the exudative form (3). Our discussion will begin with the non-exudative form, as it is the most prevalent.

NONEXUDATIVE AMD

AMD is characterized by the deposition of basal laminar deposits (BLD) of debris at the level of Bruch's membrane. The debris is thought to originate from incomplete metabolism of degenerating retinal pigment epithelium (RPE) cells. It is the degeneration of the RPE and the accumulation

of metabolic byproducts from RPE dysfunction that defines the clinical manifestations of AMD.

Sarks demonstrated that the histologic and clinical manifestations of the aging macula and AMD are a continuous spectrum (1). He followed a series of 216 patients/378 eyes for nine years in the Lidcombe Hospital. The patients ranged in age from 43 to 97 years old. Data collected included full ocular exams, fundus photography, and selected fluorescein angiography. At the time of death, the eyes were submitted for histologic examination by microscopy. The results were stratified by age, visual acuity, presence or absence of clinical AMD, and histology. The analysis demonstrated that the normal eye develops BLD throughout life and that only when the deposits become continuous do the clinical manifestations of AMD become apparent.

The earliest stage of dry AMD begins when the BLD have formed a thin continuous layer (4). The clinicopathologic correlate of this stage is loss of the macular reflex, pigment dispersion, and pigment clumping (5). The RPE layer continues to degenerate, and two other hallmark findings of AMD, drusen and retinal thinning, become manifest clinically (Fig. 5.1).

Drusen

Drusen have long been associated with AMD and its various clinical outcomes (6). Drusen are localized deposits of membranous debris that lie between the basement membrane of the RPE and the remainder of Bruch's membrane (6).

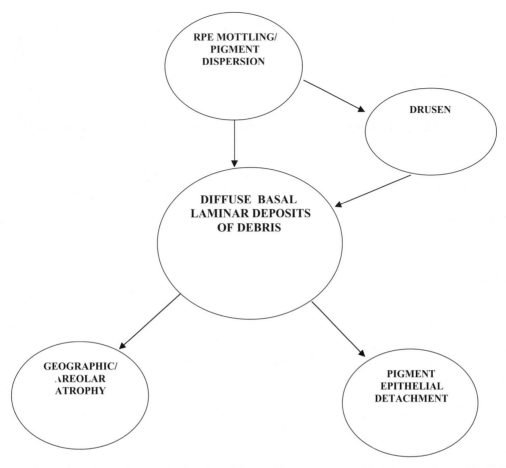

Figure 5.1 Nonexudative age-related macular degeneration. RPE, retinal pigment epithelium.

Drusen can be divided clinically into hard or cuticular drusen, soft or granular drusen, and diffuse or confluent drusen (6).

Hard drusen are thought to represent a localized area of RPE dysfunction. They are normally smaller than 50 μm and have been shown to be unrelated to increasing age (7). Further evidence suggests that the presence of small drusen does not increase the risk of progression to late maculopathy (7). In the Beaver Eye Dam Study 95.5% of subjects over age 43 had drusen present in their macula region (8).

Soft drusen display ill-defined borders and tend to be variable in size and shape (8). Typically, soft drusen are larger than 50 μm and increase with age. In the Beaver Eye Dam Study, 20% of the population had at least one soft drusen in their macula region (7). Soft drusen also tend to coalesce and become confluent drusen.

Drusen are classified as confluent if two or more soft drusen touch or merge into one another. This clinical finding is thought to represent a more diffuse pattern of RPE dysfunction (6). Green proposes that the coalescence of several soft drusen is all that is necessary for the apparent clinical progression from drusen to serous RPE detachment or exudative AMD (6). In fact, it is difficult to differentiate by fluorescein angiography a small pigment epithelial detachment from an area of soft confluent drusen.

Geographic Atrophy

Geographic atrophy of the RPE is the end-stage maculopathy in non-exudative AMD (9). Gass applied the term to one or more circumscribed areas of atrophy that slowly enlarge and coalesce such that the spreading lesion is often irregular (9,10) (Fig. 5.2). Fluorescein angiography demonstrates a transmission defect that appears in the early phase and does not alter in size or shape. Staining is present during the late phase from adjacent choroidal capillaries.

Retinal function in the area of geographic atrophy is severely compromised. The loss of visual acuity is variable because the area of fixation is sometimes spared, even when large areas of atrophy are present. Geographic atrophy accounts for 12% to 21% of legally blind eyes in AMD (11,12).

The Classification Systems

Our understanding of the prevalence, natural history, and risk factors for AMD has increased exponentially in the last three decades. The main reasons for this advancement are the large population-based studies. To allow multi-center participation there had to be a common system of terminology, grading, and classification in place. Several systems have been developed to facilitate these large studies. The

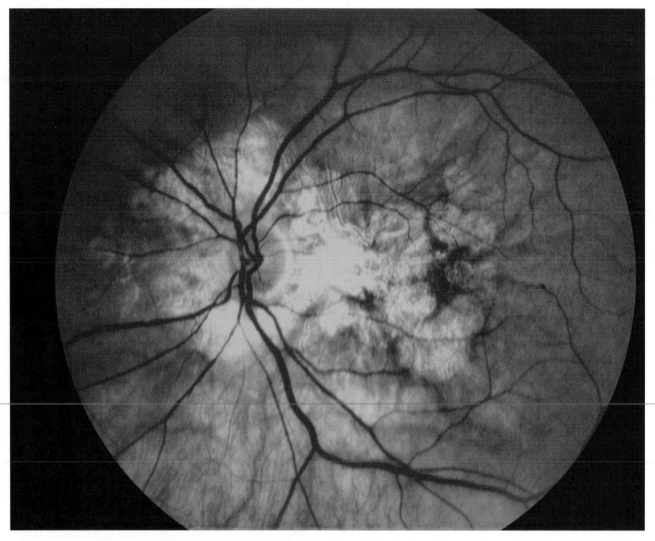

Figure 5.2 Red-free photograph of a macula with geographic atrophy.

following section outlines the basic principles of the systems used in the more prominent studies. It is not a substitute for the studies themselves but rather is a supplement to understand how the studies were designed.

The Wisconsin Age-Related Maculopathy Grading System

The Wisconsin Grading System was developed to reliably classify AMD in clinical studies and trials. The Framingham Eye Study and Beaver Dam Eye Study are two large population-based studies that have utilized the Wisconsin Grading System (7,11). The following is a brief synopsis of the Wisconsin Grading System.

Stereoscopic fundus photographs centered on the disc and macula are developed. The photographs are visualized on a light box with a Kelvin rating of 6,200. This light has a bluer hue than sunlight, which is thought to allow easier and more reliable observation of subtle drusen (13). The photographs are then graded using a standard magnification of ×15. A grid consisting of three concentric circles of 500, 1,500, and 3,000 μm with four radial lines that divide

it into nine separate fields is placed on one of the stereo photos during examination (Fig. 5.3).

The Grading System identifies three sections: drusen, other lesions typical of AMD, and other abnormalities. Drusen are further characterized by maximum size, predominant type, area, and degree of confluence. Lesions typical of AMD include increased pigmentation, presence and extent of RPE degeneration, pigment epithelial detachment, sensory retinal detachment, retinal hard exudates, subretinal and/or sub-RPE hemorrhage, subretinal/sub-RPE fibrous tissue, geographic atrophy, retinal edema, and retinal hemorrhages (13). Other abnormalities can include surface wrinkling retinopathy, branch and central retinal venous or arterial occlusions, chorioretinal scars or degenerations, and asteroid hyalosis.

The advantages of the Wisconsin Grading System over others are the ability to specify the presence or absence, as well as extent and location of the principal abnormalities of AMD (13). This allows for the objective quantification of the entire spectrum of AMD, from mild pigmentary disturbance to geographic atrophy and disciform scars. Large

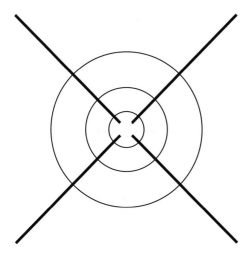

Figure 5.3 Wisconsin Grading System grid used to define subfields in macula. (Reprinted with permission from Klein R, Davis MD, Magli YL, et al. The Wisconsin age-related maculopathy grading system. *Ophthalmology*. 1991;98:1128–1134.)

multicenter trials are able to analyze patients in a reliable and reproducible format.

The disadvantage of the Wisconsin Grading System is that it is very complex. In a private practice setting, it is impractical to apply the system to a group of individual patients.

The Chesapeake Bay Watermen Grading System

The goal of the Chesapeake Bay Waterman Grading System is to include the earliest fundus changes associated with macular degeneration, as well as the drusen characteristics felt to be associated with an increased risk of developing exudative AMD.

Stereographic fundus photographs were also used, as was an overlying grid template with concentric circles of 1,500 and 3,000 μm centered on the fovea. A magnification of ×5 was used to examine the photographs.

The first criterion recorded is the presence of exudative disease. These are separated because the presence of exudative disease can alter or obscure the drusen characteristics (14). Drusen are then measured using the two concentric circles. Drusen are labeled as having high risk characteristics if they are larger than a 50-μm circle, confluence of drusen is greater than the standardized photograph, morphologic borders are ill defined, or focal hyperpigmentation associated with the drusen is greater than the standardized photograph (14). The final criteria recorded are the presence of geographic atrophy and whether the greatest diameter of the atrophy is more or less than 700 μm.

The data is then stratified into the following grades of macular degeneration: grade 4—presence of geographic atrophy or exudative AMD; grade 3—presence of large or confluent drusen, or eyes with focal hyperpigmentation; grade 2—presence of at least 20 small drusen within 1,500 μm of the foveal center; grade 1—presence of five small drusen within 1,500 μm of the foveal center or at least ten small drusen between 1,500 and 3,000 μm from the foveal center (14).

The advantage of the Chesapeake Bay Watermen Grading System is that it is easy to understand and apply in a clinical setting.

The Age-Related Eye Disease Study (AREDS) Grading System

AREDS is a large case-control study involving more than 4,500 patients at 11 different retina centers. The aim of the study is to investigate possible risk factors for AMD and to assess nutritional supplementation as a possible intervention. The grading system is adapted from the Wisconsin Grading System (15).

Subjects are divided into five groups, ranging from no discernible signs of AMD to neovascular AMD (Table 5.1).

The investigators have created a system that is very user friendly by limiting the number of groups and the criteria that are graded. In doing so, they claim to have combined the reliability of the original Wisconsin system with the simplicity of the Chesapeake Bay Waterman System.

The Health and Nutrition Examination Survey (HANES) Grading System

The HANES survey was conducted between 1971 and 1974 at 35 centers on subjects ranging from 1 to 74 years of age. The objective of the survey was to examine the prevalence of cataracts and macular degeneration in a noninstitutionalized U.S. population. The classification scheme used in the HANES survey to identify subjects with macular degeneration was unique. It allowed for the diagnosis of macular degeneration in the absence of drusen (5). It also required a loss of visual acuity of 20/25 or worse (5). The following is a brief synopsis of the three groups identified in HANES as having macular degeneration.

The first group, labeled "senile macular degeneration," is analogous to nonexudative AMD and is characterized by loss of macular reflex, pigment dispersion and clumping, and drusen associated with visual acuity of 20/25 or worse believed to be due to this disease (5).

The second group, "senile disciform macular degeneration," is analogous to exudative AMD and is characterized by choroidal hemorrhage and connective tissue proliferation between RPE and Bruch's membrane. It must be differentiated from other disease processes that result in disciform scars (5).

The third group, senile circinate macular degeneration, is analogous to the Coat's response that is sometimes seen with exudative AMD. It is characterized by perimacular accumulation of lipoid material within the retina (5).

EXUDATIVE AMD

Pigment Epithelial Detachment

Exudative AMD is distinguished from nonexudative AMD when the integrity of the Bruch's membrane/RPE complex

TABLE 5.1

DEFINITION OF AGE-RELATED MACULAR DEGENERATION CATEGORIES 1 THROUGH 4

Category 1:	No drusen or nonextensive small drusen only in both eyes
Category 2:	Extensive small drusen, nonextensive intermediate drusen, or pigment abnormalities in at least one eye
Category 3:	Large drusen, extensive intermediate drusen, or noncentral geographic atrophy in at least one eye
Category 4:	Advanced age-related macular degeneration, or visual acuity less than 20/32 attributable to lesions of nonadvanced age-related macular degeneration, such as large drusen in the fovea, in only one eye
Definitions	
Drusen size	Based on largest drusen diameter as follows (relative to the size of an average optic disc, considered by convention to be 1,500 μm): small drusen <63 μm (1/24 disc diameter, standard circle C-0), intermediate drusen ≥63 μm but <125 μm, and large drusen ≥125 μm (1/12 disc diameter, standard circle C-1).
Drusen extent	Variability in drusen size required so that total drusen area, rather than drusen number, be considered when defining extent of drusen. Small drusen were considered extensive when their cumulative area within two disc diameters of the center of the macula was at least that of the Age-Related Eye Disease Study (AREDS) standard circle C-1 (with diameter 1/12 that of the average disc). This corresponds to approximately 15 small drusen from stereo photographs and probably 5 to 10 small drusen by ophthalmoscopic examination. Intermediate drusen were considered extensive when soft indistinct drusen were present and the total area occupied by the drusen was equivalent to the area that would be occupied by 20 drusen, each having a diameter of 100 μm. If no soft indistinct drusen were present, intermediate drusen were considered extensive when they occupied an area equivalent to at least 1/5 disc area (approximately 65 100-μm-diameter drusen).
Advanced age-related macular degeneration	
	Defined by the presence of at least one of the following features: geographic atrophy, retinal pigment epithelial detachment in one eye (nondrusenoid retinal pigment epithelial detachment, serous sensory, or hemorrhagic retinal detachment), choroidal neovascularization (subretinal hemorrhage, subretinal pigment epithelial hemorrhage, subretinal fibrosis), or scars of confluent photocoagulation for neovascular age-related macular degeneration. Other features of age-related macular degeneration are specified in detail in the fundus photograph grading protocol (AREDS Manual of Operations, The EMMES Corporation, Potomac, MD).

(Reprinted with permission from Age-Related Eye Disease Study Research Group. Risk factors associated with age-related macular degeneration. *Ophthalmology.* 2000;107:2,224–2,232.)

separates and forms a pigment epithelial detachment. When this occurs, the sub-RPE and sub-retinal potential spaces are exposed to the rich vascular milieu of the choriocapillaris. The result is the formation of a pigment epithelial detachment (PED) and exudative AMD (Fig. 5.4). The exudative form of AMD is responsible for 88% of patients who are legally blind from the disease.

PEDs are classified by their clinical appearance and angiographic characteristics. Clinically there are confluent drusen, serous, hemorrhagic, and vascular pigment epithelial detachments associated with AMD (4). The visual prognosis is poor for all groups if the foveal region is involved (16).

Confluent drusen PEDs consist of multiple, large, and confluent exudative drusen. They are usually shallow and irregular in outline (16). Angiographically, they fluoresce faintly during the early phase and do not progress to the bright hyperfluorescence seen in the other groups (16). Drusen PEDs are also the least likely to progress to disciform scars (16).

Serous PEDs are sharply demarcated, dome-shaped elevations of the RPE (17). The fluid contained within the serous PED can be clear, turbid, or lipid laden. Angiographically, they fluoresce rapidly with a uniform border. In the late phase serous PED stain but do not leak (17). A variant of the serous PED found in AMD can be present in patients under age 55 that do not have signs of AMD. This is thought to be a variant of central serous choroidopathy, and therefore it has a much better prognosis (17,18).

Hemorrhagic and vascular PED are closely related since all hemorrhagic PEDs are assumed to have choroidal neovascularization (CNV), and all vascular PED have demonstrable CNV. However, the angiographic characteristics of hemorrhagic and vascular PED are vastly different. The hemorrhage in hemorrhagic PED prevents the identification of the CNV membrane. The CNV membrane is normally visible within a vascular PED.

Once a PED forms, there are four potential outcomes: persistent PED, spontaneous flattening of the PED, spontaneous RPE tear, or choroidal neovascularization (Fig. 5.2).

Persistent PED is categorized only because it frequently is present for several years and often can enlarge (16,18). Invariably, the PED will flatten spontaneously, develop a tear, or develop choroidal neovascularization.

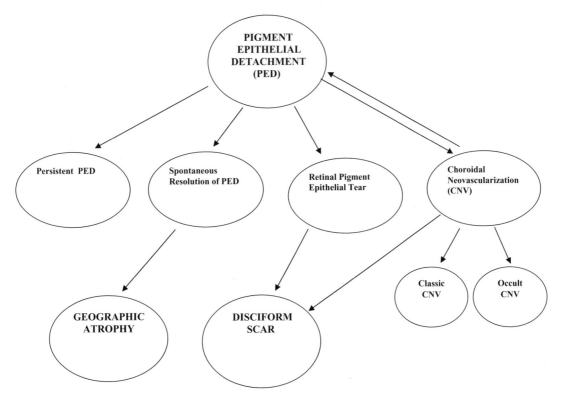

Figure 5.4 Exudative age-related macular degeneration.

Spontaneous flattening of PEDs has been reported to lead to geographic atrophy (19,20). Other investigators suggest that a more common outcome is incomplete loss of RPE pigmentation (18).

Tears of the RPE are a visually devastating complication of PEDs. The tears occur at the margin of the PED between attached and detached RPE (19,21). The edge of the tear retracts under the elevated RPE and forms a fold that is parallel to the tear (19) (Fig. 5.5). The exposed Bruch's membrane and choriocapillaris frequently hemorrhage into the subretinal space, although CNV is not a

common finding (19). The etiology of RPE tears is unknown; two existing hypothesis are weak atrophic margins of chronic PEDs and sub-RPE fibrovascular scar tissue contraction (4,19).

The most common complication of PED is the formation of CNV, which occurs frequently with all of the PED groups except confluent drusen (16). It is ubiquitous in the hemorrhagic and vascular groups (4). Meredith et al. found that patient age and PED size were predictive of conversion to CNV (18). In their study, no one under age 56 developed CNV, 29% of those between 56 and 75 developed CNV, and 62.5% over 75 developed CNV (18). In addition, CNV did not develop when the PED was smaller than one disc diameter. Other studies have demonstrated that older patients tend to have larger PEDs, with more turbid fluid, lipid, hemorrhage, and subretinal neovascularization, than younger patients (18,22).

CNV

CNV develops when a defect occurs in Bruch's membrane and new capillaries from the choriocapillaris grow through towards the pigment epithelium (23). When the neovascularization is confined to the sub-RPE space, it is known as type I (24). The new capillaries often hemorrhage or produce a serous exudate that clinically appears as a PED. The CNV will frequently penetrate the RPE to enter the subretinal space. When this occurs the CNV is known as type II (24). Cystoid macular edema can evolve as the pressure from the serous exudation enters the retinal tissue (23).

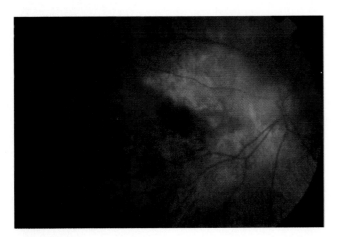

Figure 5.5 Color photograph of a retinal pigment epithelial detachment with linear tear.

The ingrowth of choroidal capillaries is eventually accompanied by fibrous scar tissue, which damages the overlying RPE (25). The result of the fibrovascular scar formation is the classic disciform scar.

Classification of CNV

In 1986, the Macular Photocoagulation Study Group (MPS) began randomizing patients into a clinical trial to test the effectiveness of laser ablation of subfoveal choroidal neovascularization from AMD (26). By the end of 1988, the investigators realized that the old methods of angiogram interpretation were inadequate. Beginning in 1989, a new method for interpretation was applied both for previous and current angiograms in the study. The classification scheme that evolved is still used today, with new studies involving CNV in AMD. The following section, derived from the MPS protocol, is an overview of the basic principles used in classifying CNV in AMD (26,27).

Classic CNV

Classic CNV is characterized by an area of choroidal hyperfluorescence with well-demarcated boundaries that can be discerned in the early phase of the angiogram. Rarely in AMD, the capillary network can be identified during the early phase of the angiogram. This is in sharp contrast to CNV associated with ocular histoplasmosis. During the late phases of the angiogram, progressive pooling of dye leakage occurs in the subretinal space and obscures the borders of the CNV complex (Fig. 5.6).

A slow-filling subset of classic CNV has been described, in which the boundaries of the CNV are not visualized until two minutes after dye injection. The late-phase leakage and pooling in this subset does correspond with the boundaries defined after two minutes.

Occult CNV

Occult CNV is divided into two categories. The first, fibrovascular PED, is not to be confused with the serous PED that was discussed previously. Fibrovascular PED is

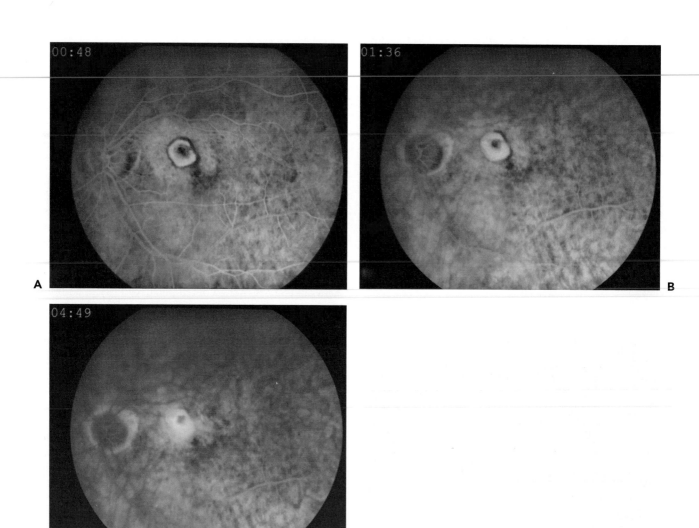

Figure 5.6 Red-free photograph and fluorescein angiogram of a patient with "classic" choroidal neovascularization. The photographs are taken at 48 seconds (**A**), 96 seconds (**B**), and five minutes (**C**).

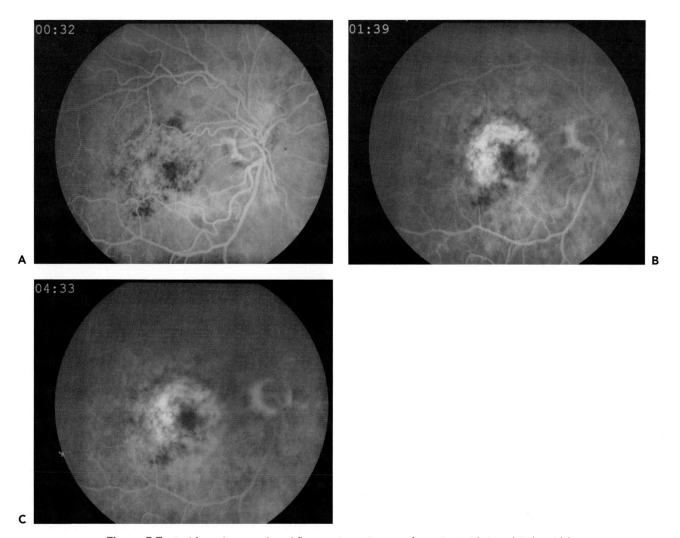

Figure 5.7 Red-free photograph and fluorescein angiogram of a patient with "occult" choroidal neovascularization. The photographs are taken at 32 seconds **(A)**, 99 seconds **(B)**, and four minutes **(C)**.

characterized by areas of irregular elevation of RPE detectable on stereoscopic frames of the angiogram. In stark contrast from classic CNV, the borders are neither as discrete nor as bright during the early phase of the angiogram. Stippled areas of hyperfluorescence manifest during the first one to two minutes of the angiogram. Persistent staining or leakage within a sensory retinal detachment follows during the late phase of the angiogram. The precise boundaries of the fibrovascular PED are rarely discernible. Frequently, the borders of the CNV are irregular with areas of hyperfluorescence mixed with areas that fade as the angiogram progresses. In addition, the borders will frequently slope from areas of elevation to flat RPE, further complicating the exact determination of the lesion boundary (Fig. 5.7).

The second category established within the occult CNV division is late-phase choroidal fluorescein leakage of undetermined source. It appears as a speckled hyperfluorescence with pooling of dye in the overlying subsensory retinal space. The precise source of the leakage cannot be determined during the early phase of the angiogram. The hyperfluorescence becomes manifest between two and

five minutes following injection. A discernible, discrete, well-demarcated area of hyperfluorescence that could be considered the source of the leakage is not identifiable. The borders of late-phase choroidal fluorescein leakage of undetermined source are never well demarcated.

Disciform Scar

The end-stage maculopathy in exudative AMD, especially the hemorrhagic form, is the formation of a disciform scar. Gass described the resolution of hemorrhage as a source of fibrous metaplasia and proliferation of the pigment epithelium (2). Hemosiderin has been detected in some of the scars, lending further evidence to the mechanism described by Gass (6).

The majority of scar-tissue formation occurs between the thickened inner layer of Bruch's membrane and the remainder of Bruch's membrane (6). A second layer of scar tissue can develop in the subretinal layer. In larger disciform lesions, a tear can develop in the RPE, and the two scar layers become contiguous (6).

Angiographically, the disciform scar stains in the early phase, with minimal leakage in the late phase.

The retinal function overlying a disciform scar is absent. This is a common and debilitating finding when exudative AMD has reached the end stage.

CONCLUSION

Our systems of classifying AMD are continuing to evolve as our understanding of this common yet devastating condition progresses. It is possible that in the future a single system will be adopted by the worldwide ophthalmologic community.

REFERENCES

1. Sarks SH. Ageing and degeneration in the macular region: a clinico-pathological study. *Br J Ophthalmia*. 1976;60:324–340.
2. Gass JDM. Pathogenesis of disciform detachment of the neuroepithelium. III. Senile disciform macular degeneration. *Am J Ophthalmol* 1967;63:617–644.
3. Berkow JW. Subretinal neovascularization in senile macular degeneration. *Amer J Ophthalmol*. 1984;97:143–147.
4. Gitter KA, Schatz H, Yannuzi LA, et al., eds. *Laser Photocoagulation of Retinal Disease. Classification of Retinal Pigment Epithelial Detachments in Age-Related Macular Degeneration.* San Francisco: Pacific Medical Press; 1988.
5. Klein BE, Klein R. Cataracts and macular degeneration in older Americans. *Arch Ophthalmol*. 1982;100:571–573
6. Green WR, McDonnell PJ, Yeo JH. Pathologic features of senile macular degeneration. *Ophthalmology*. 1985;92:615–627.
7. Klein R, Klein B, Linton K. Prevalence of age-related maculopathy—the Beaver Dam Eye Study. *Ophthalmology*. 1992;99:933–943.
8. Bressler NM, Bressler SB, Seddon JM, et al. Drusen characteristics in patients with exudative versus non-exudative age-related macular degeneration. *Retina*. 1988;8:109–114.
9. Sarks JP, Sarks SH, Killingsworth MC. Evolution of geographic atrophy of the retinal pigment epithelium. *Eye*. 1988;2:552–577.
10. Gass JDM. Drusen and disciform macular detachment and degeneration. *Arch Ophthalmol*. 1973;90:206–217.
11. Leibowitz HM, Krueger DE, Maunder LR, et al. Framingham Eye Study. VI. Macula. Degeneration. *Surv of Ophthalmol*. 1980;24:428–442.
12. Hyman LG, Lilienfeld AM, Ferris FL III, et al. Senile macular degeneration: a case-control study. *Am J Epidemiol*. 1983;118:213–227.
13. Klein R, Davis MD, Magli YL, et al. The Wisconsin age-related maculopathy grading system. *Ophthalmology*. 1991;98:1,128–1,134.
14. Bressler NM, Bressler SB, West SK, et al. The grading and prevalence of macular degeneration in Chesapeake Bay watermen. *Arch Ophthalmol*. 1989;107:847–852.
15. Age-Related Eye Disease Study Research Group. Risk factors associated with age-related macular degeneration. *Ophthalmology*. 2000;107:2,224–2,232.
16. Casswell AG, Kohen D, Bird AC. Retinal pigment epithelial detachments in the elderly: classification and outcome. *Br J Ophthalmol*. 1985;69:397–403.
17. Lewis ML. Idiopathic serous detachment of the retinal pigment epithelium. *Arch Ophthalmol*. 1978;96.620–624.
18. Meredith TA, Braley RE, Aaberg TM. Natural history of serous detachments of the retinal pigment epithelium. *Am J Ophthalmol*. 1979;88:643–651.
19. Green SN, Yarian D. Acute tear of the retinal pigment epithelium. *Retina*. 1983;3:16–20.
20. Blair CJ. Geographic atrophy of the retinal pigment epithelium. *Arch Ophthalmol*. 1975;93:19–25.
21. Hoskin A, Bird AC, Sehmi K. Tears of detached retinal pigment epithelium. *Br J Ophthalmol*. 1981;65:417–422.
22. Yanuzzi LA, Gitter KA, Schatz H. Detachment of the retinal pigment epithelium. In: *The Macula: A Comprehensive Text and Atlas*. Baltimore: Williams and Wilkins; 1979:166–179.
23. Schatz H, Yanuzzi LA, Gitter KA. Subretinal neovascularization. In: *The Macula: A Comprehensive Text and Atlas*. Baltimore: Williams and Wilkins; 1979:180–201.
24. Puliafito CA, Rogers AH, Martidis A, et al. AMD and subfoveal choroidal neovascularization. In: *Ocular Photodynamic Therapy*. Thorofare, New Jersey: Slack Incorporated; 2002:2–11.
25. Green WR, Key SN. Senile macular degeneration: a histopathologic study. *Trans Am Ophthalmol Soc*. 1977;75:180–254.
26. MPS Study Group. Subfoveal neovascular lesions in age-related macular degeneration. Guidelines for evaluation and treatment in the Macular Photocoagulation Study. *Arch Ophthalmol*. 1991;109:1,242–1,257.
27. Chamberlin JA, Bressler NM, Bressler SB, et al. The use of fundus photographs and fluorescein angiograms in the identification and treatment of choroidal neovascularization in the Macular Photocoagulation Study. *Ophthalmology*. 1989;96:1,526–1,534.

Polypoidal Choroidal Vasculopathy

6

Christina M. Klais   *Antonio P. Ciardella*   *Lawrence A. Yannuzzi*

More than two decades ago, a peculiar hemorrhagic disorder of the macula, polypoidal choroidal vasculopathy (PCV), was first described (1). This entity has also been designated as *posterior uveal bleeding syndrome* (2,3) and *multiple recurrent retinal pigment epithelium detachments in black women* (4). It has characteristic morphological features that distinguish it from other exudative maculopathies. In 1990, Yannuzzi et al. suggested the term *idiopathic PCV* because the pathogenesis was unknown, the primary abnormality involved the choroidal circulation, and the characteristic lesion was an inner choroidal vascular network of vessels ending in an aneurismal bulge or outward projection, visible clinically as a reddish-orange, spheroid, polyp-like structure (5). Clinically this entity was associated with multiple, recurrent, serosanguineous detachments of the retinal pigment epithelium (RPE) and neurosensory retina secondary to leakage and bleeding from the peculiar choroidal vascular lesion (Fig. 6.1).

The spectrum of PCV has been expanded further, thus allowing us to describe the pathogenesis, clinical manifestations, demographic profile, fluorescein and indocyanine green (ICG) angiographic findings, natural course, modalities of treatment, and visual prognosis in patients with PCV with more detail and precision (6,7).

PATHOGENESIS

The pathogenesis of PCV is not completely understood, but it is generally thought to originate in the inner choroid. A few clinicopathological studies of PCV have been reported (8–13). MacCumber et al. examined an enucleated eye with multiple recurrent serosanguineous RPE detachments and disclosed extensive fibrovascular proliferation within Bruch's membrane and in the subretinal space, reflecting that the eye had probably reached an end stage of this disease (8). They did not observe choroidal varices or aneurismal dilation of choroidal vessels except that some choroidal veins were quite large. Spraul et al. described a sub-RPE, intra-Bruch's fibrovascular membrane without subretinal component and aneurysmal vessels in an enucleated eye displaying choroidal vascular-like bulbous structures (9). Lafaut et al. reported light-microscopic findings in submacular tissue removed from an eye with PCV in age-related macular degeneration (AMD) (10). They described a sub-RPE, intra-Bruch's fibrovascular membrane containing several dilated thin-walled vessels under diffuse drusen. These abnormal vessels are lined by a thin endothelium with occasional pericytes. Some lesions were associated with islands of lymphocytic infiltration. The authors noted that the aneurysmal vessels appeared to be of venular rather than of arteriolar origin, and were probably the pathological counterpart of the lesions identified with ICG angiography. Other investigators reported grossly dilated, thin-walled vessels in surgically removed neovascular membranes suggestive of PCV (11,12). Okubo et al. found tortuous, unusually dilated venules adjacent to an arteriole with marked sclerotic changes in a surgically removed, submacular polypoidal lesion (13). The authors hypothesized that hyperpermeability and hemorrhages due to stasis of blood in the arteriole and dilated venules might cause edema and degeneration of the tissue. Further, they suggested that a venule affected by stasis may become so fragile that it forms a beaded and polypoidal configuration. The authors also observed newly formed capillaries within the wall of the degenerate arteriole and near the dilated venule. Neovascularization for recanalization and collateral circulation is known to occur in ischemic areas associated with bran retinal vein occlusion (14). Teresaki et

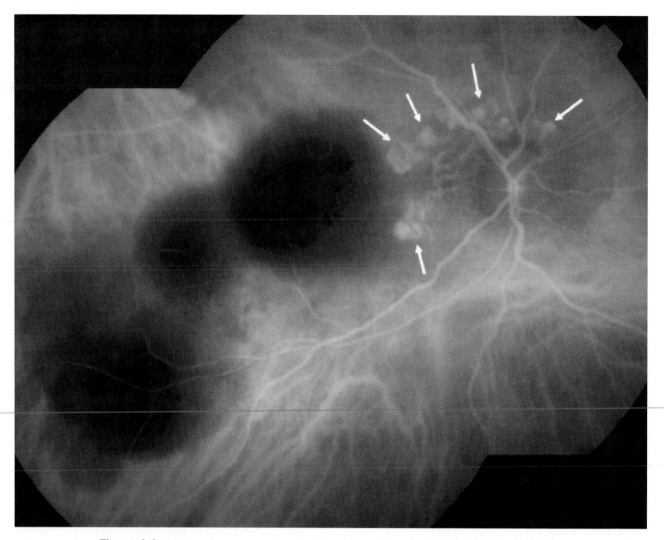

Figure 6.1 Indocyanine green angiogram of a patient with polypoidal choroidal vasculopathy shows peripapillary network of dilated choroidal lesions ending in polypoidal lesions (arrows). Note the large hemorrhagic pigment epithelium detachments blocking the background fluorescence.

al. found clusters of dilated thin-walled vessels surrounded by macrophages and fibrinous material in neovascular membranes obtained during macular translocation surgery for PCV (15).

Many questions remain unanswered regarding the pathogenesis of PCV. New information is now available to assist in our pursuit to understand the clinical nature of this disorder. Previously, this entity was reported exclusively in females of pigmented races; cases that are more recent included Caucasians of both genders (4,6,16–18) (Fig. 6.2). The predisposition for pigmented races contrasts the relative immunity to AMD and disciform scarring seen in these patients (19–21). Lafaut et al. suggested a possible coexistence of AMD and PCV, a finding certainly supported by our own clinical experience (10). Nevertheless, while associated with multiple recurrent serosanguineous macular detachments, PCV is not linked to significant fibrous proliferation commonly observed in end-stage neovascular AMD (22). Ciardella et al. reported a link between PCV and chorioretinal inflammation seen in three cases. They identified typical

clinical findings of PCV after previous inflammatory disease (7). Immunohistochemical findings in a case with PCV demonstrated both T and B lymphocytes in the choroid and fibrovacsular tissue (8).

There have been references to the association of PCV with other ocular disorders. Ross et al. reported a correlation between retinal macroaneurysms and PCV in two hypertensive black females (23). They proposed a relation between the retinal vascular changes in retinal macroaneurysms and hypertensive retinopathy, such as vascular remodeling, aneurysmal dilation, and focal vascular constriction to the characteristic choroidal lesions in PCV. A recent study confirmed, that choroidal blood flow increases significantly with increasing blood pressure (24). Untreated hypertension was found to be a risk factor in development and progression of choroidal vascular pathologies.

In spite of these observations, the association of PCV, inflammation, or other ocular disorders is still inconclusive and must be investigated further. Other potential pathogenic

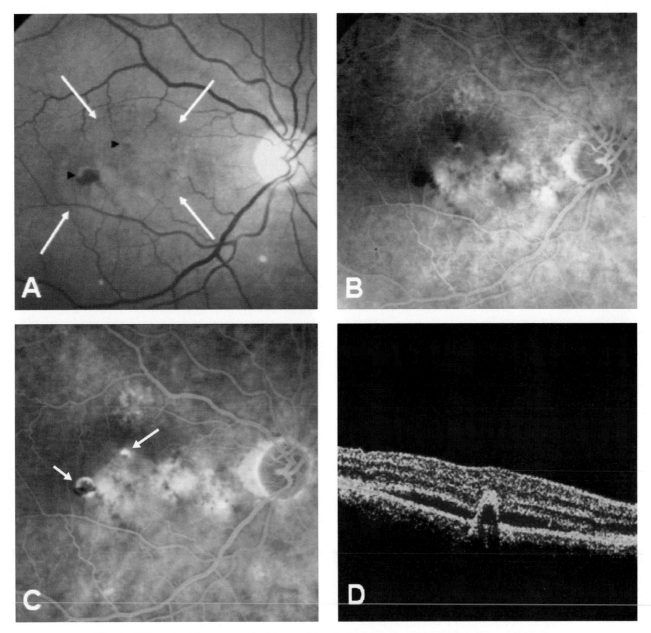

Figure 6.2 **A.** Red-free image of a 56-year-old male Caucasian reveals large detachment of the neurosensory retina (white arrows) and serosanguineous pigment epithelium detachments (black arrow heads). **B.** The early-phase fluorescein angiography shows small areas of blockage of choroidal fluorescence by the serosanguineous pigment epithelium detachments and a large area ill-defined subfoveal hyperfluorescence. **C.** There are two hot spots (white arrows) in the indocyanine green angiogram. One of these spots is partly covered by blood. **D.** The optical coherence tomography reveals a dome-shaped elevation of the retinal pigment epithelium overlying undefined hyper-reflective area characteristic of polypoidal choroidal vasculopathy. There is also a detachment of the neurosensory retina at the fovea.

factors include the possibility of a peculiar choroidal tumor, vascular malformation, or systemic hypertension. PCV may represent a variant of AMD, as is commonly recognized in a white population, or the two conditions might be distinct. Whether or not genetic or environmental factors play a role in the pathogenesis of PCV as they do in AMD remains to be determined.

When the lesion increases in size, it usually does so by three proposed mechanisms: The lesion may enlarge by simple vessel hypertrophy, by conversion of the lesion into the advancing edge of a vascular channel, and by unfolding of a cluster of aneurysmal elements and subsequent transformation into enlarging, vascular, tubular components. The third mechanism is usually apparent on clinical examination as a large, reddish-orange subretinal mass corresponding to a cluster of aneurysmal elements. The reddish-orange color can be attributed to abundant erythrocytes in the dilated vessels and in extracellular spaces. On ICG images, the subretinal mass is shown to be composed of multiple, polypoidal elements that project anteriorly from the inner choroid toward the outer retina. With time, these mass-like lesions flatten out and expand tangentially in their plane. The overlying RPE may show signs of variable atrophy.

EPIDEMIOLOGY

PCV is usually diagnosed in patients who are between the ages of 50 and 65, but age at diagnosis can range from 20 to 80 years. The average age of onset for all affected patients from the literature is 60.1 years.

Previously, it had been thought that PCV exclusively affects women. In recent studies, it has been demonstrated that female cases outnumber male ones by a ratio of approximately 4.7:1. In Asians, men seem to be more frequently affected (22).

Individuals of African American and Asian descendants are at higher risk of developing PCV (4,22), as this distinct disorder seems to preferentially affect pigmented individuals (Fig. 6.3). However, more recent reports have shown that PCV occurs in a broader range of races than it has been demonstrated in the past.

Lafaut et al. studied the prevalence of PCV in Caucasians with occult choroidal neovascularization (CNV). In a consecutive series of 374 eyes with occult CNV, 4% were diagnosed with PCV by ICG angiographic findings (17). Pauleikhoff et al. diagnosed PCV in 13.9% of 101 consecutive German patients with pigment epithelium detachment (PED) (25). Other investigators diagnosed PCV in 85% among a consecutive series of Caucasians presenting with large exudative or hemorrhagic PEDs in the absence of drusen (26). Yannuzzi et al. diagnosed PCV in 13 (7.8%) of 167 consecutive Caucasian patients with presumed neovascular AMD (27). Scassellati-Sforzolini et al. found a PCV prevalence of 9.8% in Italian patients with newly diagnosed neovascular AMD (18).

The prevalence of PCV among Chinese patients with AMD was found to be 9.3% (28). In this patient series, the most common clinical finding at presentation was subretinal hemorrhage (63.6%), followed by exudative neurosensory detachment (59.1%) and hemorrhagic PED (59.1%)—the cases were predominantly male (68.4%). Most of the polypoidal lesions were at the macula (63.6%) and unilateral (84%). In contrast, a Japanese study reported a much higher prevalence of PCV among patients with newly diagnosed neovascular AMD (29). They studied 164 eyes with PEDs and CNV, and detected PCV in 59% of the eyes. In 70%, the PED had a hemorrhagic component. Other investigators confirmed the predilection for male gender in the Japanese population, as well as unilateral involvement (22).

CLINICAL FINDINGS

Vitreous hemorrhage, relatively minimal fibrous scarring, absence of drusen, retinal vascular disease, pathologic myopia, and signs of intraocular inflammation are accepted clinical features of maculopathy caused by PCV. It is generally accepted that PCV is a bilateral disease (5). Most patients with the evidence of PCV in one eye have similar lesions in the fellow eye (Fig. 6.4); however, several patients

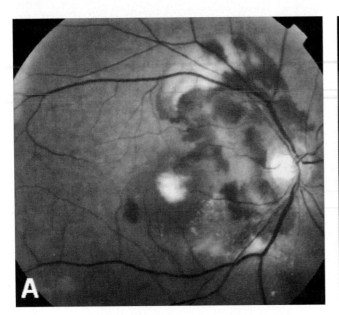
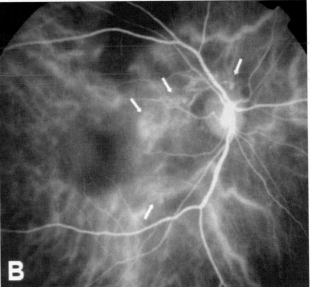

Figure 6.3   A. Red-free photograph of a 74-year-old Asian female reveals a serosanguineous pigment epithelium detachment at the macula associated with serosanguineous pigment epithelium detachments peripapillary and along the temporal superior arcade. **B.** The indocyanine green angiogram confirms the diagnosis of polypoidal choroidal vasculopathy. There is a cluster of leaking polypoidal vessels (arrows). Note the hypofluorescent areas of the pigment epithelium detachments caused by blood and exudates.

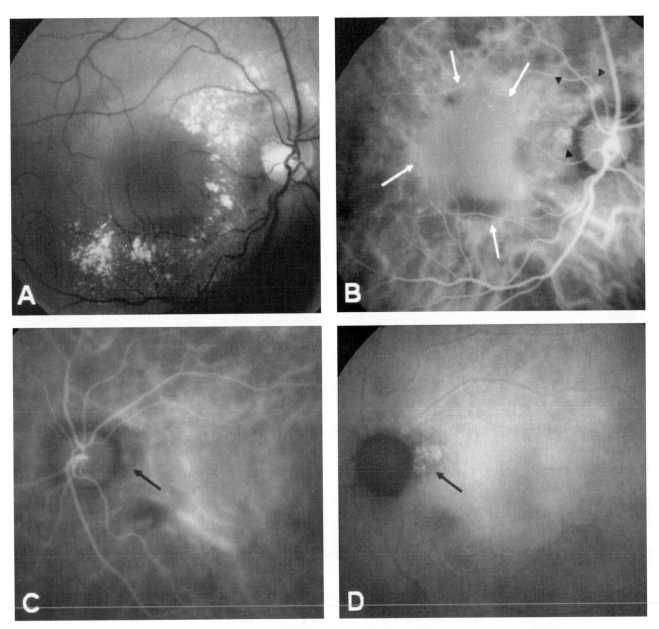

Figure 6.4 A 72-year-old Caucasian female noticed a sudden loss of vision in her right eye. **A.** The red-free photograph shows a serosanguineous retinal pigment epithelium detachment in the center of the fovea surrounded by lipid exudation. **B.** The indocyanine green angiogram reveals a cluster of actively leaking polypoidal vessels (black arrow heads) in the peripapillary area and a large hypofluorescent retinal pigment epithelium detachment (white arrows). **C.** The indocyanine green angiogram of the fellow eye, which had no symptoms, shows polypoidal vessels in the peripapillary area (arrow). **D.** The very late stage of indocyanine green angiogram demonstrates the washout phenomenon consistent with non-leaking lesion (arrow).

with PCV, who have been monitored for more than 10 years, show no evidence of the condition in the other eye so far. Iida et al. demonstrated that retinal microangiopathy may occur in a chronic macular detachment secondary to polypoidal CNV (30). They hypothesized that hypoxia from the chronic detachment, a neurotoxic effect from lipid deposition, or a biochemically-induced microvascular abnormality from secretion of vasogenic mediators as possible mechanisms.

THE POLYPOIDAL VASCULAR ABNORMALITY

Although the lesion of PCV is invariably localized to the choroidal vascular network, other characteristics of the lesion often differ. Significant variance is observed in size and location to the optic disk, fovea, and cross-section of the retina.

Size

PCV is usually categorized into small, medium, or large lesions. The width of the lesions varies depending on the affected vascular channels. With involvement of outer choroidal vessels, the polypoidal lesions appear larger. Such lesions are easily diagnosed on biomicroscopy, especially when atrophic RPE is overlying. With ICG angiography, these lesions are well detectable. Teitawa et al. reported large vascular networks expanding across the vascular arcade, which showed characteristics of CNV (31). When the middle choroidal vasculature is affected, polypoidal lesions appear smaller. In this case, it is more challenging to diagnose on clinical examination, and the preferential method for diagnosis is fluorescein angiography (5,32,33).

Location

Choroidal vascular lesions of PCV are usually located in the peripapillary area, although recent evidence suggests that lesions could also be found in the central macula and in the midperiphery (34,35) (Fig. 6.5). Lesions are found in a single location in the fundus or widespread involving more than one site.

Lafaut et al. detected polypoidal lesions in the macula in 22 of 45 eyes, which were diagnosed as PCV. They found 16 polypoidal lesions in the peripapillary area, six under the temporal vascular arcade and six in the midperiphery (17).

Due to limited reports on clinicopathologic relationship between PCV lesions and retinal layers, the precise location of the polypoidal vascular lesion in the cross-sectional structure remains unknown. Optical coherence tomography (OCT) studies were able to localize the polypoidal lesions under Bruch's membrane (36), but further studies are required to correlate the histologic finding and the results of OCT imaging.

NATURAL COURSE

The natural course of PCV is becoming better understood as the knowledge of PCV expands. This disease often follows a remitting-relapsing course, and clinically, it is associated with chronic, multiple, recurrent serosanguineous detachments of the neurosensory retina and the RPE with long-term preservation of good vision. Despite multiple recurrent serosanguineous macular detachments, fibrous proliferation resulting in typical plaque characteristics of

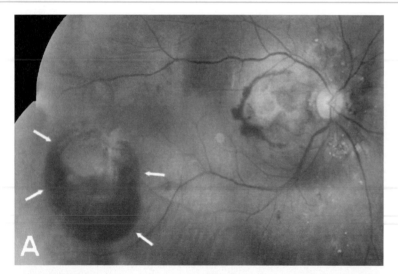

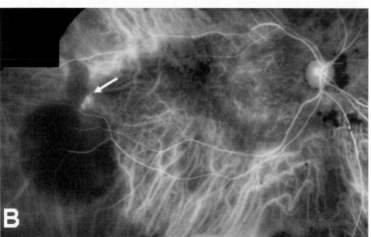

Figure 6.5   A. The red-free photograph composite of a 54-year-old African American reveals a large fibrovascular scar in the central macula. There is a large subretinal hemorrhage in the temporal periphery (arrows). **B.** Indocyanine green angiogram confirms the diagnosis of polypoidal choroidal vasculopathy showing a cluster of hyperfluorescent hot spots consistent with actively leaking polypoidal lesions (arrow). The large serosanguineous pigment epithelium detachment blocks the background fluorescence.

end-stage neovascular AMD is not seen in eyes with PCV. On the other hand, this may present difficulties with the diagnosis of PCV when the lesion is inactive. In some cases, polypoidal lesions have evolved with resolution of the serosanguineous changes, and ICG angiography reveals a non-specific plaque, which can be interpreted as CNV of the usual type. This may be due to autoinfarction, regression, or flattening of the lesion from the subpigment epithelial space into the inner portion of the choroid (Fig. 6.6). Still, some patients may develop chronic atrophy and cystic degeneration of the fovea associated with severe vision loss. Others may experience vitreous hemorrhage or secondary CNV with disciform scarring and central vision loss (1,3,8,20,37). Massive spontaneous choroidal hemorrhage is a rare but severe complication. Despite immediate drainage procedure, the visual outcome is poor (38).

Uyama et al. followed 14 eyes of 12 consecutive patients with PCV for at least 2 years without any treatment (22). They demonstrated that 50% of the eyes had favorable course. In the remaining half, the disorder persisted for a long time with occasional recurrent hemorrhages and leakage, resulting in macular degeneration and vision loss. Eyes with clusters of grape-like polypoidal dilations of the vessels had a high risk for severe visual loss.

There is an ongoing search to establish possible underlying systemic and local factors linked to the development and progression of PCV. Recent evidence suggests a possible association of PCV to hypertension and acquired macroaneurysms (23). In spite of these findings, the association between PCV and acquired retinal macroaneurysms is doubtful because retinal macroaneurysms are usually related to retinal veno-occlusive disease. They are found in

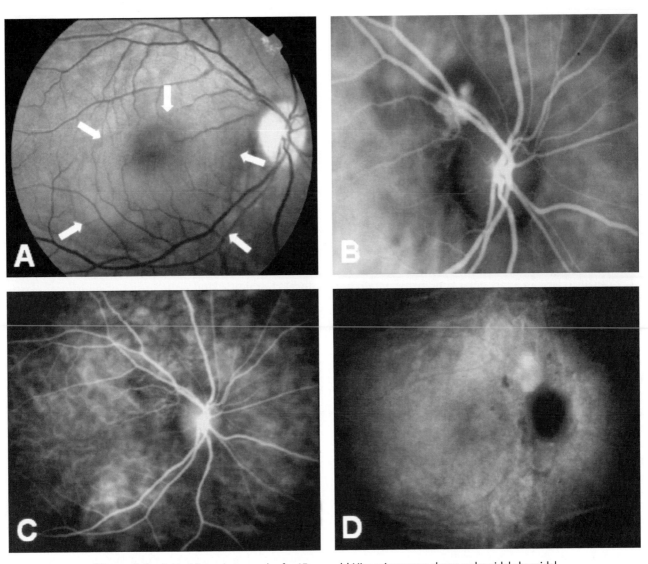

Figure 6.6 **A.** Red-free photograph of a 65-year-old Hispanic woman shows polypoidal choroidal vasculopathy with neurosensory detachment of the macula masquerading as central serous chorioretinopathy (arrows). **B.** Indocyanine green angiogram reveals leaking polypoidal vascular abnormality in the peripapillary region responsible for the neurosensory detachment. **C.** This indocyanine green angiogram was performed 5 years later, which shows resolution of the serosanguineous changes. **D.** The very late phase indocyanine green angiogram reveals a non-specific plaque, which can be mistaken as choroidal neovascularization of the usual type.

the distribution of an occluded vein, whereas polypoidal lesions predominantly occupy multiple venous watershed zones in ICG angiography (32). Smith et al. reported a patient with PCV and concurrent sickle cell disease (39). Other cases of PCV have been described in eyes with melanocytoma of the optic nerve, central retina vein occlusion (40,41). Neither of these case reports, nor our own clinical experience, demonstrates sufficient evidence finding an association between PCV and retinal vascular ischemic diseases, chorioretinal inflammation, or sickle cell disease.

DIAGNOSIS

Although fluorescein angiography can sometimes confirm the diagnosis of PCV, ICG angiography is the choice for imaging this entity. ICG angiography uses a longer wavelength, which penetrates the RPE and the surrounded exudation, allowing improved imaging of the choroidal circulation and enhanced identification of PCV lesions (32).

In early-phase ICG angiography, as larger choroidal vessels are filled with dye, a distinct network of small vessels within the choroid is visualized. With ICG imaging, the vessels of the polypoidal lesion are usually more numerous and far-reaching than is seen on clinical examination. The appearance of vessels in PCV often depends on their location in the fundus. In juxtapapillary lesions, the vascular channels may follow a radial, arching pattern and may be interconnected with smaller spanning branches more evident and numerous at the edges of the lesions. When PCV is limited to the macula, a vascular network often arises in the macula and follows oval distribution. With macular and juxtapapillary involvement, vessels in the network usually course in an irregular latticework and do not follow the lobular pattern of choroidal vasculature.

In the early-phase ICG angiograms, larger PCV vessels are filled before retinal vessels, but the area within and immediately surrounding the polypoidal lesions remains hypofluorescent compared to uninvolved choroid. When the network of vessels can be identified by ICG angiography, small hyperfluorescent polyps become visible within the choroid. These polyps seem to arise from larger choroidal vessels and do not appear on every vessel of the network. These polypoidal lesions on ICG imaging are correspondent with red-orange lesions visible on biomicroscopy. Although the network of vessels appears more extensive on ICG angiography, polypoidal lesions routinely appear smaller in earlier phases of ICG angiography. However, in mid-phase ICG angiography, lesion size approximate the choroidal excrescences have been observed clinically.

The late-phase ICG angiography is associated with reversal of the pattern of fluorescence observed in earlier studies. The area surrounding the polypoidal lesion becomes hyperfluorescent and the center shows hypofluorescence. In patients with PCV, late ICG staining associated with non-polypoidal CNV is not observed. Lesion size seems to influence the reversal pattern. Lesions smaller than half disc diameter appear to have intense uniform fluorescence, whereas internal details seem to be visible in larger polypoidal lesions (32). These findings suggest presence of an internal architecture (32).

The very late stages of ICG angiography demonstrate disappearance of the fluorescence from the lesions, thus defining the term *washout*. The washout is only seen in non-leaking lesions, whereas the leaking lesions remain hyperfluorescent. Varying degrees of hypopigmentation of the RPE overlying an involved area may enhance visualization of the abnormal vessels, yet the late ICG staining results from the intrinsic characteristics of the lesion rather than from RPE alterations (32).

OCT has also proven to be useful in the diagnosis of PCV. Recent OCT studies demonstrated dome-like elevation of the RPE and moderate reflex or nodular appearance beneath the RPE at the area of polypoidal lesions (42,43). The orange-red lesions in eyes with PCV were found to have more sharply peaked RPE detachment than observed in serous PED (36). In our experience, imaging polypoidal lesions with OCT is not always possible and requires much experience of the investigator.

DIFFERENTIAL DIAGNOSIS

The differential diagnosis of PCV lesions could be divided in three major subgroups: vascular anomaly, CNV, and peculiar type of choroidal tumor.

Inflammatory lesions that may be similar to PCV include posterior scleritis and other inflammatory diseases involving the RPE and choroid, such as panuveitis, multifocal choroiditis, and acute posterior multifocal placoid pigment epitheliopathy. Other inflammatory diseases, such as Harada disease, sympathetic uveitis, and birdshot chorioretinopathy could be ruled out due to the absence of concurrent anterior uveitis, vitritis, pain, or staining of the optic disc in fluorescein angiography (32). Other clinical characteristics of inflammatory diseases, including scleral or choroidal thickening, or fluid in the subtenon space have never been described in patients with PCV. Eyes with PCV frequently have lipid deposits, which are not commonly seen with any of the inflammatory conditions.

Other diseases, such as choroidal hemangioma, metastasis from carcinoid syndrome, and occasionally renal cell carcinoma, may also be confused with PCV.

Two decades ago, PCV was considered an entity with demographic characteristics, risk factors, a natural course, clinical interpretations, and outcomes distinct from AMD. Features such as Caucasian origin, macular location, presence of drusen, frequent recurrences, rapid rate of progression, disciform scarring, and poor visual prognosis were considered typical of AMD and used to differentiate the two entities (20). Since the definition of PCV has expanded over the past two decades, the diagnosis is no longer restricted to those specific demographic attributes or to a specific retinal location (17,35). In addition, it becomes more evident from the increasing volume of reports about PCV and from our own clinical experience that the patients may have manifestations attributable to PCV and AMD. For example, some of our patients diagnosed with AMD undergoing ICG guided-laser treatment in the past had an exceptional and unexpectedly good outcome. Later, on reviewing their records, we determined that the patients with better results were actually patients with PCV-type CNV rather than a typical form of AMD.

Presently, we believe that PCV represents a subtype of CNV in AMD. However, some characteristics distinguish PCV from other types of CNV observed in AMD. First, vascular proliferative changes associated with non-polypoidal CNV tend to produce small caliber vessels that are associated with grayish membrane and grayish discoloration of the overlying retina. These vessels are not easily detected clinically (44,45). In contrast, eyes with vascular changes typical for PCV form a network of vessels ending with saccular polypoidal lesions that have a reddish-orange color and are evident with slit lamp biomicroscopy unless they are covered by overlying blood or exudates (5,16). Second, angiographic and histopathologic characteristics tend to distinguish other types of CNV from PCV. AMD is associated with diminishing choroidal thickness and with signs of stromal fibrosis without any changes in the size of choriocapillaris or evidence of inflammatory changes (46). These findings were not observed in clinicopathological reports on PCV (8,10). Third, poorly defined CNV secondary to AMD is clinically associated with indistinct subretinal thickening and is not manifested by the detectable choroidal vascular channels terminating in polyp-like structures.

Fluorescein and ICG angiography can be used to distinguish the two types of vascular abnormalities. In both, CNV is characterized by diffuse, late-staining plaque (21). In contrast, early-phase ICG angiography reveals PCV as a prominent vascular network, which becomes washed out during the late phase. The late phase is also distinguished by a typical outline of the nonleaking large choroidal vessels. If the vessels leak, staining in the walls of aneurysmal lesions and exudation into the surrounding choroid and subretinal space are observed (32).

The natural course and clinical location of PCV are different from those of CNV. Subfoveal CNV tends to organize into a fibrotic or disciform scar, leading to severe macular damage and vision loss (45). PED seen in eyes with PCV virtually never forms a fibrotic scar (5), whereas PED associated with occult CNV in AMD usually has a poor prognosis (47).

Some eyes with PCV may present purely exudative changes masquerading chronic decompensation of the RPE, a variant of central serous chorioretinopathy (33). PCV lesions presenting with symptoms of central serous chorioretinopathy are usually small. Polypoidal lesions may resemble small PEDs clinically and on fluorescein angiography. The diagnosis becomes especially challenging in a patient with chronic central serous chorioretinopathy presenting lipid deposits in the central macula due to subfoveal polypoidal lesion. The principle of differentiating a small serous PED from a polypoidal lesion is with ICG angiography. Late staining of the PED is seen with fluorescein angiography and hypofluorescence with ICG imaging. In contrast, the polypoidal lesion is usually hyperfluorescent with ICG angiography because of its vascular nature. It is important to consider that the PCV lesion may exist under a PED. The portion of the PED overlying the polypoidal lesion will be hypofluorescent, and—if there is leakage—ICG dye may pool into the subpigment epithelial space. However, the majority of patients with PCV present with serosanguineous detachment of the RPE and neurosensory retina. These findings imply the presence of new blood vessel formation or CNV as causative factor (45).

TREATMENT

Treatment for PCV is not yet well established. If the characteristic vascular lesion of PCV is observed, a conservative approach to management is recommended unless the lesion is associated with persistent or progressive exudative change threatening central vision. In this case, conventional thermal laser treatment of the leaking polypoidal choroidal abnormality may be successful in resolution of the serosanguineous manifestation (26,48,49). Yuzawa et al. reported on visual improvement after conventional laser treatment of the entire PCV complex in nine of ten eyes (50). However, no randomized, controlled studies have been performed to prove the efficacy or safety of laser treatment. Moreover, when the CNV extends beneath the center of the fovea, thermal laser treatment is not indicated due to damage of the overlying neurosensory retina and subsequent reduction of central vision (51). It is possible that the loss of central vision due to the subfoveal treatment will exceed the damage produced by the natural course of PCV, although this is not known with any certainty. Conversely, it is not uncommon for patients with untreated subfoveal involvement with PCV to experience severe visual loss.

Due to limitations and uncertainty of the value of thermal laser coagulation and the potential devastating outcome of untreated subfoveal lesions, alternative modalities of treatment are currently being evaluated. These include vitrectomy and submacular removal of polypoidal vessels and subretinal blood. In some cases, vitrectomy is required to clear the media and recover the vision (52). Macular translocation is another surgical approach, but most patients diagnosed with PCV have relatively large vascular lesions and the surgical procedure has a number of serious complications (15,53). It has been demonstrated that radiation therapy for AMD is a possible triggering factor for the development of PCV (54).

Recent studies reported on promising results after photodynamic therapy with verteporfin in subfoveal PCV lesions (55–57). Spaide et al. reported on improvement in visual acuity in 56% of patients undergoing photodynamic therapy, while in 31% the vision was stable, and in 12% a decrease in visual acuity was noted (55). Further trials of photodynamic therapy with verteporfin for PCV are required to address long-term efficacy and safety issues.

SUMMARY

PCV seems to be a distinct clinical entity that should be differentiated from other forms of CNV associated with AMD and other known choroidal degenerative, inflammatory, and ischemic disorders. The principle abnormality in PCV, notably the branching vascular network and polypoidal structures at the borders of the lesion, seem to be unique to this entity. In patients with serosanguineous detachment of the RPE—especially in those with increased risk factors, such as pigmented race—ICG angiography should be performed to evaluate the choroidal vascular abnormality to establish a more definitive diagnosis. When ICG angiography confirms the characteristic vascular polyp-like lesion, a conservative management approach should be considered unless there is a persistent or progressive exudative change threatening the fovea and the central vision. In that event, thermal laser-coagulation of leaking aneurysmal or polypoidal components within the vascular lesion may be a rationale. Reports on photodynamic therapy for PCV demonstrate encouraging results, but randomized clinical trials are required to establish this therapeutic modality in the management of patients with PCV.

REFERENCES

1. Yannuzzi LA. Idiopathic polypoidal choroidal vasculopathy. Presented at the annual meeting of the Macular Society, Miami, 1982.
2. Kleiner RC, Brucker AJ, Johnson RL. Posterior uveal bleeding syndrome. Ophthalmology. 1984;91(Suppl 9):110.
3. Kleiner RC, Brucker AJ, Johnson RL. Posterior uveal bleeding syndrome. Retina. 1990;10:9–17.
4. Stern RM, Zakov N, Zegarra H, et al. Multiple recurrent serous sanguineous retinal pigment epithelial detachments in black women. Am J Ophthalmol. 1985;100:560–569.
5. Yannuzzi LA, Sorenson J, Spaide RF, et al. Idiopathic polypoidal choroidal vasculopathy. Retina. 1990;10:1–8.
6. Yannuzzi LA, Ciardella AP, Spaide RF, et al. The expanding clinical spectrum of idiopathic polypoidal vasculopathy. Arch Ophthalmol. 1997;115:478–485.
7. Ciardella AP, Donsoff IM, Yannuzzi LA. Polypoidal choroidal vasculopathy. Ophthalmol Clin N Am. 2002;15:537–554.
8. MacCumber MW, Dastgheib K, Bressler NM, et al. Clinicopathological correlation of the multiple recurrent serosanguineous retinal pigment epithelium detachment syndrome. Retina. 1994;14:143–152.
9. Spraul CW, Grossniklaus HE, Lang GK. Idiopathische polypöse choroidale Vaskulopathie. Klin Monatsbl Augenheilk. 1997;210:405–406.
10. Lafaut BA, Aisenbrey S, van den Broecke C, et al. Polypoidal choroidal vasculopathy pattern in age-related macular degeneration. A clinicopathologic correlation. Retina. 2000;20:650–654.
11. Reynders S, Lafaut BA, Aisenbrey S, et al. Clinicopathologic correlation in hemorrhagic age-related macular degeneration. Graefe's Arch Clin Exper Ophthalmol. 2002;240:279–285.
12. Rosa RH, Davis JL, Eifrig CW. Clinicopathologic correlation of idiopathic polypoidal choroidal vasculopathy. Arch Ophthalmol. 2002;120:502–508.
13. Okubo A; Sameshima M, Uemura A, et al. Clinicopathological correlation of polypoidal choroidal vasculopathy revealed by ultrastructural study. Br J Ophthalmol. 2002;86:1,093–1,098.
14. Frangieh GT, Green WR, Barraquer-Somers E, et al. Histopathologic study of nine branch retinal vein occlusions. Arch Ophthalmol. 1982;100:1,132–1, 140.
15. Teresaki H, Miyake Y, Suzuki T, et al. Polypoidal choroidal vasculopathy treated with macular translocation: clinical pathological correlation. Br J Ophthalmol. 2002;86:321–327.
16. Perkovich PT, Zakov N, Berlin LA, et al. An update on multiple recurrent serosanguineous retinal pigment epithelium detachments in black women. Retina. 1990;10:18–26.
17. Lafaut BA, Leyes AM, Snyders B, et al. Polypoidal choroidal vasculopathy in Caucasians. Graefe's Arcg Clin Exp Ophthalmol. 2000;238: 752–759.
18. Scassellati-Sforzolini B, Mariotti C, Bryan R, et al. Polypoidal vasculopathy in Italy. Retina. 2001;21:121–125.
19. Capone Jr A, Wallace RT, Meredith TA. Symptomatic choroidal neovascularization in blacks. Arch Ophthalmol. 1994;112:1,091–1,097.
20. Ferris III FL. Senile macular degeneration: a review of epidemiological features. Am J Epidemiol. 1983;118:213–221.
21. Yannuzzi LA, Slakter JS, Sorenson JA, et al. Digital indocyanine videoangiography and choroidal neovascularization. Retina. 1992;12:191–223.
22. Uyama M, Wada M, Nagai Y, et al. Polypoidal choroidal vasculopathy: natural history. Am J Ophthalmol. 2002;133:639–648.
23. Ross RD, Gitter GA, Cohen C, et al. Idiopathic polypoidal choroidal vasculopathy associated with retinal arterial macroaneurysm and hypertensive retinopathy. Retina. 1996;16:195–1,111.
24. Polak K, Polska E, Luksch A, et al. Choroidal blood flow and arterial blood pressure. Eye. 2003;17:84–88.
25. Pauleikhoff D, Löffert D, Spital G, et al. Pigment epithelial detachment in the elderly. Clinical differentiation, natural course, and pathogenic implications. Graefe's Arch Clin Exp Ophthalmol. 2002;240:533–538.
26. Ahuja RM, Stanga PE, Vingerling JR, et al. Polypoidal choroidal vasculopathy in exudative and hemorrhagic pigment epithelium detachments. Br J Ophthalmol. 2000;84:479–484.
27. Yannuzzi LA, Wong DW, Sforzolino MS, et al. Polypoidal choroidal vasculopathy and neovascularized age-related macular degeneration. Arch Ophthalmol. 1999;117:1,503–1,510.
28. Kwok AKH, Lai TYY, Chan CWN, et al. Polypoidal choroidal vasculopathy in Chinese patients. Br J Ophthalmol. 2002;86:892–897.
29. Imaizumi H, Takeda M. Knobby-like choroidal neovascularization accompanied with retinal pigment epithelial detachment. Nippon Ganka Gakkai Zasshi. 1999;103:527–537.
30. Iida T, Yannuzzi LA, Freund KB, et al. Retinal angiopathy and polypoidal choroidal vasculopathy. Retina. 2002;22:455–463.
31. Tateiwa H, Kuroiwa S, Gaun S, et al. Polypoidal choroidal vasculopathy with large vascular network. Graefe's Arch Clin Exp Ophthalmol. 2002;240:354–361.
32. Spaide RF, Yannuzzi LA, Slakter JS, et al. Indocyanine green videoangiography of idiopathic polypoidal choroidal vasculopathy. Retina. 1995;15: 100–110.
33. Yannuzzi LA, Freund KB, Goldbaum M, et al. Polypoidal choroidal vasculopathy masquerading as central serous chorioretinopathy. Ophthalmology. 2000;107:767–777.
34. Moorthy RS, Lyon AT, Rabb MF, et al. Idiopathic polypoidal choroidal vasculopathy of the macula. Ophthalmology. 1998;105:1,380–1,385.
35. Yannuzzi LA, Nogueira FB, Spaide RF, et al. Idiopathic polypoidal choroidal vasculopathy: a peripheral lesion. Arch Ophthalmol. 1998;116:382–383.
36. Iijima H, Iida T, Imai M, et al. Optical coherence tomography of orange-red subretinal lesions in eyes with idiopathic polypoidal vasculopathy. Am J Ophthalmol. 2000;129:105–111.
37. Spaide RF, Guyer DR, McCormick B, et al. External beam radiation therapy for choroidal neovascularization. Ophthalmology. 1998;105:24–30.
38. Yang SS, Fu AD, McDonald HR, et al. Massive spontaneous choroidal hemorrhage. Retina. 2003;23:139–144.
39. Smith RE, Wise K, Kingsley RM. Idiopathic polypoidal choroidal vasculopathy and sickle cell retinopathy. Am J Ophthalmol. 2000;129:105–111.
40. Bartlett HM, Willoughby B, Mandava N. Polypoidal choroidal vasculopathy in patients with melanocytoma of the optic nerve. Retina. 2001;21: 396–399.
41. Katsimpris JM, Petropoulas IK, Pharmakakis NM, et al. Idiopathic polypoidal choroidal vasculopathy associated with central retinal vein occlusion. J Fr Ophtalmol. 2003;26:489–492.
42. Otsuji T, Takahasi K, Fukushima I, et al. Optical coherence tomographic findings of idiopathic polypoidal choroidal vasculopathy. Ophthalmic Surg Lasers. 2000;31:210–214.
43. Giovannini A, Amato GP, D'Altobrando E, et al. Optical coherence tomography (OCT) in idiopathic polypoidal choroidal vasculopathy. Doc Ophthalmol. 1999;97:367–371.
44. Gass JDM. Stereoscopic Atlas of Macular Disease. St. Louis: CV Mosby; 1997.
45. Green WR, McDonnel PJ, Yeo JH. Pathological features of senile macular degeneration. Ophthalmology. 1985;92:615–627.
46. Arnold JJ, Sarks SH, Killingworth MC, et al. Reticular pseudodrusen. Retina. 1995;15:183–191.
47. Pauleikhoff D, Radermacher M, Spital G, et al. Visual prognosis of second eyes in patients with unilateral late exudative age-related macular degeneration. Graefe's Arch Clin Exp Ophthalmol. 2002;240:539–542.
48. Guyer DR, Yannuzzi LA, Ladas I, et al. Indocyanine green guided laser photocoagulation of focal spots at the edge of plaque of choroidal vascularization. Arch Ophthalmol. 1996;114:693–697.

49. Gomez-Ulla F, Gonzalez F, Torreiro MG. Diode laser photocoagulation in idiopathic polypoidal choroidal vasculopathy. *Retina*. 1998;18:481–483.
50. Yuzawa M, Mori R, Haruyama M. A study of laser photocoagulation for polypoidal choroidal vasculopathy. *Jpn J Ophthalmol*. 2003;47:379–384.
51. Gass JDM. Biomicroscopical and histopathologic considerations regarding the feasibility of surgical excision of subfoveal neovascular membranes. *Am J Ophthalmol*. 1994;118:285–298.
52. Shiraga F, Matsuo T, Yokoe S, et al. Surgical treatment of submacular hemorrhage associated with idiopathic polypoidal choroidal vasculopathy. *Am J Ophthalmol*. 1999;128:147–152.
53. Fujii GY, Pieramici DJ, Humayun MS, et al. Complications associated with limited macular translocation. *Am J Ophthalmol*. 2000;130:751–762.
54. Spaide RF, Leys A, Herrman-Delemazure B, et al. Radiation associated choroidal neovasculopathy. *Ophthalmology*. 1999;106:2,254–2,260.
55. Spaide RF, Donsoff I, Lam DL, et al. Treatment of polypoidal choroidal vasculopathy with photodynamic therapy. *Retina*. 2002;22:529–535.
56. Quaranta M, Mauget-Faysse M, Coscas G. Exudative idiopathic polypoidal vasculopathy and photodynamic therapy with verteporfin. *Am J Ophthalmol*. 2002;134:277–280.
57. Rogers AH, Greenberg PB, Martidis A, et al. Photodynamic therapy of polypoidal choroidal vasculopathy. *Ophthalmic Surg Lasers Imaging*. 2003;34:60–63.

Retinal Angiomatous Proliferation

Christina M. Klais   Antonio P. Ciardella   Chiara M. Eandi
Lawrence A. Yannuzzi

In patients with age-related macular degeneration (AMD), choroidal neovascularization (CNV) usually proliferates through the retinal pigment epithelium (RPE), infiltrates the retina, and communicates axonally and freely with the retinal circulation, forming a retinal-choroidal-anastomosis (RCA). Such a development is especially common in the end stage of disciform disease (1,2). Over the past decade, the spectrum of neovascular AMD has been expanded beyond the binary classic and occult CNV to include entities like polypoidal choroidal neovascularization (PCV) and retinal angiomatous proliferation (RAP) (3). The latter is a distinct subset of CNV, which is associated with proliferation of retinal capillaries and contiguous telangiectatic response, has recently been recognized and described in various stages of development (Fig. 7.1). In 1992, Harnett et al. first described retinal neovascularization as an early finding in neovascular AMD, preceding the disciform scarring stage of the disease (4). They called it a "retinal angiomatous lesion." It has also been referred to as a "deep retinal vascular anomalous complex" (5) or as "retinal choroidal anastomosis" (6,7), even though the vasogenic process is not limited to the deep retina and chorioretinal anastomoses appear to evolve only as a late and inconsistent development. These clinical findings were supported by the results of histopathological investigations of Lafaut et al. (8).

To differentiate from other forms of neovascular AMD, Yannuzzi et al. (3) proposed the term RAP for the particular characteristics of early appearance of retinal neovascularization, a contagious retinal telangiectasia, development of retinal–retinal anastomosis (RRA), progression of neovascularization in the subretinal space, as well as variable and late onset of RCA.

EPIDEMIOLOGY

The prevalence of RAP in newly diagnosed neovascular AMD is between 10 and 15% (8,9). It is found more frequently in elderly patients. In recent studies, the mean age of patients with RAP ranged between 81 and 82 years (3,10). The first clinical findings usually do not occur before the sixth decade. A marked tendency towards bilateral and symmetric neovascular disease has been found. It appears that there is a predilection for females and for Caucasians (3,11). This differentiates RAP from PCV, which has a predisposition for pigmented races (12). RAP has also been described as a rare complication in eyes with idiopathic perifoveal telangiectasis (13–15), retinal venous occlusive disease, and radiation therapy (16,17).

CLINICAL FINDINGS

Based on the presumed origin and evolution of the neovascular process, a three-stage classification was proposed to characterize clinical manifestation and progressive changes in this entity. Despite this classification, clear differentiation between the individual stages sometimes proves to be challenging.

Stage I: Intraretinal Neovascularization (IRN)

The initial lesion of RAP is by nature extrafoveolar, usually slowly growing and often asymptomatic. If the second eye becomes involved in a neovascular process, it is more noticeable to the patient and the physician. Unlike other

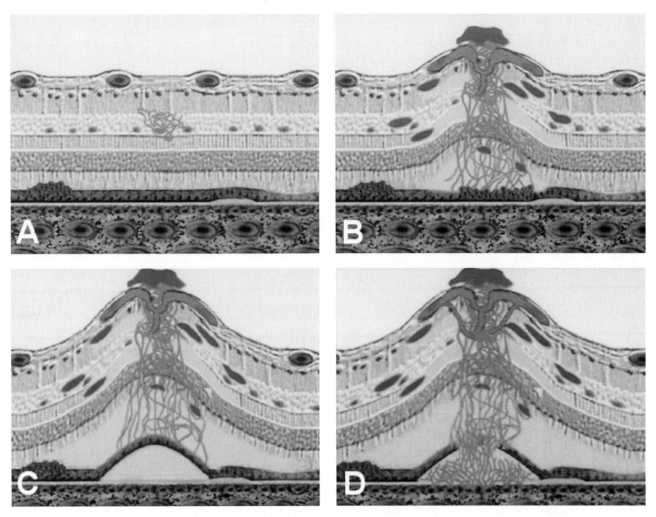

Figure 7.1   Retinal angiomatous proliferation. **A.** Stage I: intraretinal neovascularization. **B.** Stage II: subretinal neovascularization with a retinal-retinal anastomosis. **C.** Stage II: subretinal neovascularization with serous pigment epithelium detachment. **D.** Stage III: choroidal neovascularization with vascularized pigment epithelium detachment and retinal-retinal anastomosis.

forms of neovascular AMD, RAP lesions have never been described to develop from peripapillary vessels.

The earliest manifestation of RAP is IRN, a capillary proliferation within the retina originating from the deep capillary plexus in the paramacular area. The angiomatous tissue progresses predominantly vertically towards the anterior and posterior boundaries of the retina. Some lateral extension of the IRN may present as an irregular stellate figure. It is characterized by dilated retinal capillaries emanating from the focal area of the neovascularization in the shape of a sea urchin. One or more dilated compensatory retinal vessels perfuse and drain the neovascularization, sometimes forming RRA. Some intraretinal edema surrounding the core of proliferating capillaries and multiple intraretinal hemorrhages are characteristic for this stage of RAP. These hemorrhages are relatively small in nature compared to the massive hemorrhages noted in patients with well demarcated or so-called classic CNV, occult CNV, or in particular, PCV (12,18,19).

Stage II: Subretinal Neovascularization (SRN)

Stage II is diagnosed when IRN extends posteriorly beyond the photoreceptor layer of the retina into the subretinal space, forming a SRN. The SRN does not usually expand in the horizontal direction of the retina. A localized, neurosensory retinal detachment develops, and intraretinal edema increases. Compared to Stage I, more small intraretinal hemorrhages extend circumferentially to the limits of the macular detachment, but not beyond. When the RAP lesion gains access to the preretinal and subretinal space, subretinal hemorrhages are more common than preretinal hemorrhages. All hemorrhages are usually small in dimension. In 39% of Stage II lesions, Yannuzzi et al. identified a well defined retinal-retinal anastomosis, with a perfusing arteriole and draining venule, communicating in some cases in shape of a "hairpin loop" within the core of the SRN (3) (Fig. 7.2). When the SRN reaches or fuses with the RPE, a serous pigment epithelium detachment (PED) is seen in nearly all cases (Fig. 7.3).

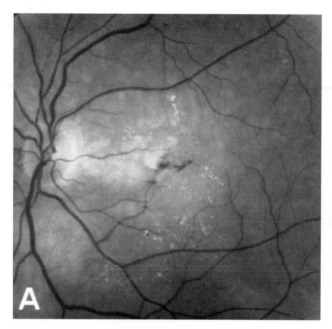
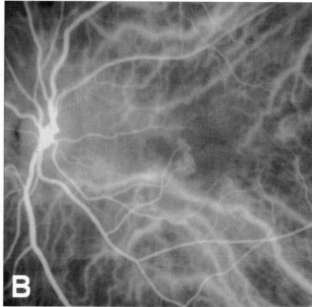

Figure 7.2 A. The red-free photograph of a 74-year-old female with retinal angiomatous proliferation Stage II shows small intraretinal and preretinal hemorrhages, detachment of the retinal pigment epithelium, and some exudates. **B.** The early-phase indocyanine green angiogram reveals a retinal-retinal anastomosis. Note the surrounding hypofluorescence caused by serous pigment epithelium detachment.

SRN connected with retinal circulation can also be observed in patients with idiopathic parafoveal telangiectasia (13–15). The major difference, however, is that these patients have a relatively healthy RPE; a choroidal component is missing as well as the development of PED.

Stage III: CNV

In Stage III, clinical and angiographic examinations clearly demonstrate the presence of CNV, sometimes associated with vascularized PED or a predisciform scar. During the evolution of this vascularized process, an axonal communication between retinal and choroidal circulation forms a RCA, while a RRA is not commonly seen in this stage (Fig. 7.4). SRN and CNV appear to be predominantly perfused by the choroidal vessels with notable drainage into the retina. Lafaut et al. reported that removing the SRN was complicated by an intimate adherence of the membrane to the overlying neurosensory retina in an area of RCA, which supports the hypothesis that the neuroretina rather than the choroid is the primary source of the new vessels (8).

PATHOGENESIS

The precise mechanism for the development of IRN as an initiating vasogenic event in RAP is not completely understood. Animal and human studies suggest that neovascularization may derive from the organization of vascular precursor cells that are already present in the tissue, by angiogenesis, or due to tissue infiltration of the angiomatous proliferation (20–31). In transgenic mice expressing vascular endothelial growth factor (VEGF) in the photoreceptors, neovascularization originates from the deep capillary plexus—the vascular bed that is closest to the photoreceptors (21). These neovascularizations can extend beneath the photoreceptors into the subretinal space (22). With time, the neovascular lesion demonstrates gradual enlargement and coalescence with other vascular complexes (20). In the subretinal space, RPE cells close to the new vessel begin to proliferate. These findings were confirmed by clinicopathological studies of submacular tissue surgically removed from patients with CNV (8). The over-expression of VEGF is sufficient to produce IRN and SRN in an animal and human model (24,25,27–29). Also clinically, increased expression of VEGF and possibly other vasogenic mediators from the vitreous, retina, or even the choroid can stimulate neovascular proliferation in the retina, particularly in the elderly eye with chronic degeneration, detachment, or ischemia (23,24,29,32,33). VEGF is up-regulated by retinal hypoxia and ischemia (34,35), which at the same time increases capillary permeability, thereby producing leakage and hemorrhage. The development of RRA appears to compensate the increase in vascular flow. Additional retinal capillaries may extend from the RAP lesion to the RRA. This component of intraretinal microangiopathy presents as tangential capillary proliferation or multiple compensatory telangiectatic capillaries or both.

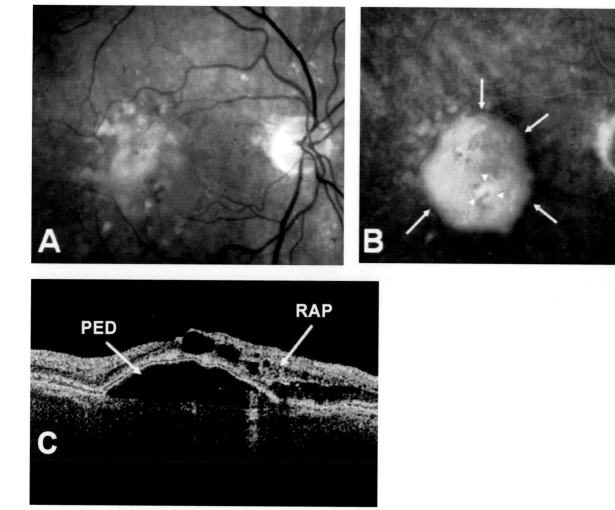

Figure 7.3 **A.** The red-free photograph of a patient with retinal angiomatous proliferation (RAP) Stage II reveals intraretinal hemorrhages, serous pigment epithelium detachment, and detachment of the neurosensory retina. **B.** Late-phase fluorescein angiogram shows complete staining of the subpigment epithelium space simulation occult choroidal neovascularization (*white arrows*). There is an area of intense hyperfluorescence at the area of the RAP lesion caused by leaking capillaries as well as intraretinal and subretinal neovascularization. **C.** Optical coherence tomography reveals a large pigment epithelium detachment (PED), detachment of the neurosensory retina, cystic spaces, and a RAP lesion.

The posterior extension of SRN infiltrates the RPE leading to reactive pigmentary changes, which are a characteristic RPE response to neovascularization in the subretinal space (36,37). It represents an attempt by the RPE to envelop new vessels and to induce an inhibitory, antivasogenic environment (36,38,39). These focal areas of hyperpigmentation were found to have high levels of autofluorescence and had absorption characteristics suggesting that the pigment seen was derived, at least in part, from lipofuscin (40). In rabbits, it has been demonstrated that injection of lipid peroxide (oxidative stress) in the subretinal space caused migration of RPE cells into the subretinal space and outer retina (41). The detached cells had phagocytized droplets of lipid peroxide. These findings suggest that after exposure to oxidative stress, RPE cells may detach and migrate into the subretinal space and outer retina and increase the VEGF secretion.

FLUORESCEIN AND INDOCYANINE GREEN (ICG) ANGIOGRAPHY FINDINGS

Although fluorescein angiography is the standard diagnostic adjunct for fundus imaging, it is often of limited value in the diagnosis, evaluation, and classification of RAP.

In Stage I, fluorescein angiography usually reveals a focal area of intraretinal staining with indistinct borders corresponding to the IRN and surrounding intraretinal edema. The surrounding capillary proliferation and leakage can also lead to misdiagnosis as non-specific microangiopathy. Early Stage I lesions can also mimic the appearance of a classic CNV. Later stages of RAP are often classified as minimally classic CNV or purely occult CNV. Yannuzzi et al. demonstrated that the majority of neovascularizations in RAP were categorized as occult CNV (61%), most with a small component of classic CNV, and only 19% were categorized as

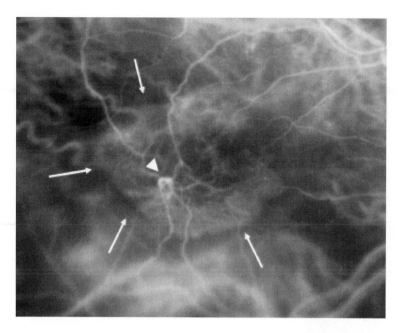

Figure 7.4 The indocyanine green angiogram in a patient with Stage III retinal angiomatous proliferation reveals intraretinal and subretinal neovascularization (*small arrow*) overlying a large area of choroidal neovascularization (*arrowhead*) with multiple retinal-choroidal anastomoses.

classic CNV (3). In 20% of the eyes, though, fluorescein angiograms were inadequate for review. In Stage III, fluorescein angiography can sometimes detect evidence of a vascularized PED. However, SRN, CNV, and vascularized PED blend into a homogenous nonspecific hyperfluorescence with fluorescein angiography, leading to an erroneous interpretation of occult CNV.

ICG angiography is useful in determining an accurate diagnosis in most cases. It reveals a focal area of intense hyperfluorescence corresponding to the neovascularization (hot spot) and some late extension of leakage within the retina from the IRN (Stage I). The late staining of intraretinal edema is quite characteristic for RAP. Intraretinal exudates surrounding the IRN contain fibrin (8) which stains with ICG dye in the mid to late stages of the angiogram (Fig. 7.5). In contrast, fibrin is invisible on fluorescein angiography. In some cases, a retinal-retinal anastomosis can be visualized by ICG angiography.

In Stage II, the ICG angiogram reveals a hot spot at the site of neovascularization within and beneath the retina. A serous PED remains hypofluorescent. The ICG dye does not leak extensively into subretinal and subpigment epithelial spaces. A precise localization of the hot spot within or within and below the retina is not possible with ICG angiography. Therefore, a hot spot in RAP must be distinguished from the two other forms of known subretinal hot spots vis-

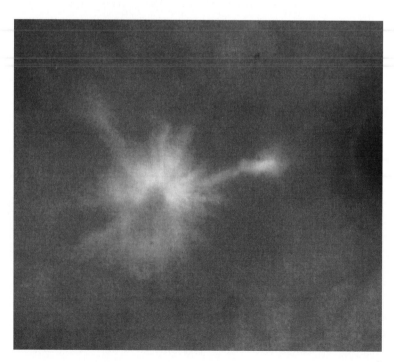

Figure 7.5. The late indocyanine green angiogram of a retinal angiomatous proliferation shows leakage into the retina, presumably from fibrin accumulation.

ible with ICG angiography: polypoidal CNV and focal occult CNV (11). These two forms of neovascularization are produced by proliferation of choroidal vessels beneath the detached macula and may be associated with serous detachment of the neurosensory retina or RPE. They do usually not show anastomotic connections between retinal and choroidal circulation and are not associated with multiple small hemorrhages as evident in RAP. An intraretinal hot spot on ICG angiography in RAP must be differentiated from small capillary hemangiomas and macroaneurysms.

As SRN progresses towards the subretinal space and the RPE, CNV becomes part of the neovascular complex. At this stage, there is often clinical and angiographic evidence of a vascularized PED. ICG angiography better images the presence of vascularized PED, because the serous component of PED remains dark during the study and the vascular component appears as hyperfluorescence. At this stage, ICG angiography may sometimes be able to image a direct communication between the retinal and choroidal component of the neovascularization thus forming a RCA.

High-speed ICG videoangiography also allows accurate identification of the RAP lesion, retinal feeding arterioles, draining venules, as well as RRA and RCA.

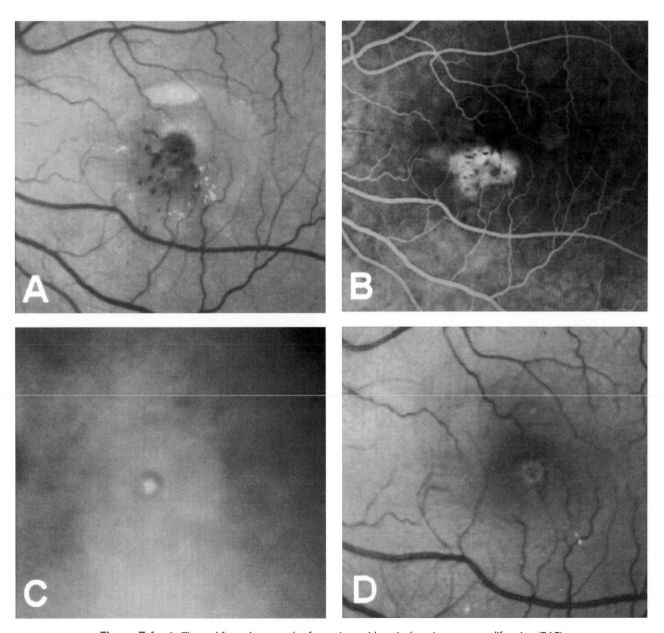

Figure 7.6   **A.** The red-free photograph of a patient with retinal angiomatous proliferation (RAP) Stage II shows intraretinal hemorrhages, lipid exudation, detachment of the neurosensory retina, and pigment epithelium. **B.** The late-phase fluorescein angiogram showing diffuse staining of the area of the RAP lesion. **C.** The late-phase indocyanine angiogram reveals a hot spot at the area of the intraretinal and subretinal neovascularization. **D.** This is a red-free photograph 2 years after successful combined therapy with an angiostatic agent and photocoagulation. There is a complete resolution of the hemorrhages, exudates, subretinal fluid, as well as the pigment epithelium detachment.

THERAPY

Although clinical manifestation and vasogenic sequence of RAP is now better appreciated, little is known about its natural course, and there is scarce evidence of successful therapy. Some investigators noted that patients with RAP have poor visual outcome after conventional laser photocoagulation even when the focal lesion is located extrafoveolar (4,5,7,42). We have found that an uncomplicated focal area of IRN may be amenable to conventional thermal laser treatment with a good result. In contrast, a stage that is more advanced involving vascularized PED and RCA is not likely to respond to any form of treatment currently available. Photodynamic therapy with verteporfin may have a different effect on RAP than on classic CNV or occult CNV (43,44). Given the tendency of ICG dye to stain the retina in eyes with RAP, there is a possibility that similar distribution may occur with the verteporfin molecule, theoretically predisposing the retina to photochemical damage when exposed to excitatory light used in photodynamic therapy. This possibility is obviously still speculation since verteporfin has not yet been imaged successfully with good spatial and temporal definition in the human. However, its fluorescein characteristics, in conjunction with its affinity to bind to protein, may produce some similarities with the ICG molecule. Since eyes with RAP in AMD are generally classified as pure occult CNV with FA, it is possible that patients with RAP were actually included in the VIP trial (44). Since ICG angiography was not used to determine eligible patients in this trial, the frequency of RAP in the subset of patients classified as occult CNV is not known. Ongoing studies on the expanded use of photodynamic therapy with verteporfin are incorporating ICG angiography, which should help to characterize the true nature and frequency of RAP and its response to this treatment.

A recent study reported on surgical ablation of retinal feeding arterioles and draining venules in Stage II lesions with serous PED (10). In all four cases, an increase in visual acuity as well as a complete resolution of the intraretinal fluid was noted. After 1 year, no recurrent lesion was observed. Preservation of underlying RPE could possibly explain the good outcome of this surgical procedure. Therefore, patients with advanced RAP may not be good surgical candidates because of the existing connection between retinal and choroidal circulation and advanced damage of the RPE.

Kuroiwa et al. reported on an unsuccessful outcome with rapid progressive scar formation after transpupillary thermotherapy in eyes with RAP (45).

In another pilot study, anecortave acetate, an angiostatic agent, was given as posterior juxtascleral injection to patients with RAP. While no major subretinal, intraretinal, or preretinal hemorrhages have been reported, loss of visual acuity could not be prevented in the majority of patients (46). Based on our experience, a combination of anecortave acetate or other antivasogenic drugs and phototherapy seems to be a promising new treatment modality (Fig. 7.6).

SUMMARY

Clinical knowledge and recognition of RAP is important since this form of neovascular AMD may be distinct from other forms of neovascular AMD concerning its natural course, visual prognosis, and response to treatment. Since RAP may simply present as IRN or it may progress to SRN (and feature with or without a serous-PED, CNV or RCA), different forms of treatment may be suitable for each stage of this complex disorder.

REFERENCES

1. Green WR, Gass JDM. Senile disciform degeneration of the macula. *Arch Ophthalmol.* 1971;100:487–494.
2. Green WR, Enger C. Age-related macular degeneration histopathologic studies: the 1992 Lorenz E. Zimmerman lecture. *Ophthalmology.* 1993;100:1,519–1,535.
3. Yannuzzi LA, Negrao S, Iida T, et al. Retinal angiomatous proliferation in age-related macular degeneration. *Retina.* 2001;21:416–434.
4. Harnett ME, Weiter JJ, Gardts A, et al. Classification of retinal pigment epithelial detachments associated with drusen. *Graefes Arch Clin Exp Ophthalmol.* 1992;230:11–19.
5. Harnett ME, Weiter JJ, Staurenghi G, et al. Deep retinal vascular anomalous complexes in advanced age-related macular degeneration. *Ophthalmology.* 1996;103:2,042–2,053.
6. Slakter JS, Yannuzzi LA, Schneider U, et al. Retinal choroidal anastomoses and occult neovascularization in age-related macular degeneration. *Ophthalmology* 1994;107:742–754.
7. Kuhn D, Meunier I, Soubrane G, et al. Imaging of chorioretinal anastomoses in vascularized retinal pigment epithelium detachments. *Arch Ophthalmol.* 1995;113:1,392–1,398.
8. Lafaut BA, Aisenbrey S, Broecke CV, et al. Clinicopathological correlation of deep retinal vascular anomalous complex in age-related macular degeneration. *Br J Ophthalmol.* 2000;84:1,269–1,274.
9. Bermig J, Tylla H, Jochmann C, et al. Angiographic findings in patients with exudative age-related macular degeneration. *Graefe`s Arch Clin Exp Ophthalmol.* 2002;240:169–175.
10. Borrillo JL, Sivalingam A, Mrtidis A, et al. Surgical ablation of retinal angiomatous proliferation. *Arch Ophthalmol.* 2003;121:558–561.
11. Fernandes LH, Freund KB, Yannuzzi LA, et al. The nature of focal areas of hyperfluorescence or hot spots imaged with indocyanine green angiography. *Retina.* 2002;22:557–568.
12. Yannuzzi LA, Wong DWK, Sforzolino BS, et al. Polypoidal choroidal vasculopathy and neovascularized age-related macular degeneration. *Arch Ophthalmol.* 1999;117:1,503–1,510.
13. Gass JDM, Blodi BA. Idiopathic juxtafoveal retinal telangiectasis. Update of classification and follow-up study. *Ophthalmology.* 1993;100:1,526–1,546.
14. Lee BL. Bilateral subretinal neovascular membrane in idiopathic juxtafoveal telangiectasis. *Retina.* 1996;16:344–346.
15. Park D, Schatz H, McDonald R, et al. Fibrovascular tissue in bilateral juxtafoveal telangiectasis. *Arch Ophthalmol.* 1986;114:1,092–1,096.
16. Boozalis GT, Schachat AP, Green WR. Subretinal neovascularization from the retina in radiation retinopathy. *Retina.* 1987;7:156–161.
17. Babek E, Green WR. Histopathological study of presumed parafoveal telangiectasia. *Retina.* 1999;19:332–335.
18. Yannuzzi LA, Slakter JS, Sorensen JA, et al. Digital indocyanine videoangiography and choroidal neovascularization. *Retina.* 1992;12:191–223.
19. Yannuzzi LA, Hope-Ross M, Slakter JS, et al. Analysis of vascularized pigment epithelium detachments using indocyanine green videoangiography. *Retina.* 1994;13:99–113
20. Okamoto N, Takao T, Hackett SF, et al. Transgenic mice with increased expression of vascular endothelial growth factor in the retina. *Am J Pathol.* 1997;151:281–291.
21. Vinores SA, Seo MS, Okamato N, et al. Experimental models of growth factor-mediated angiogenesis and blood-retinal barrier breakdown. *Gen Pharmacol.* 2000;25:233–239.
22. Tobe T, Okamoto N, Vinores MA, et al. Evolution of neovascularization in mice with overexpression of vascular endothelial growth factor in photoreceptor. *Invest Ophthalmol Vis Sci.* 1998;39:180–188.
23. Adamis AP, Miller JW, Bernal MT, et al. Increased vascular endothelial growth factor levels in the vitreous of eyes with proliferative diabetic retinopathy. *Am J Ophthalmol.* 1994;118:445–450.
24. Malecaze F, Clamens S, Simorre-Pinatel V, et al. Detection of vascular endothelial growth factor messenger RNA and vascular endothelial growth factor-like activity in proliferative diabetic retinopathy. *Arch Ophthalmol.* 1994;112:1,476–1,482.
25. Aiello LP, Avery RL, Arrigg PG, et al. Vascular endothelial growth factor in ocular fluid of patients with diabetic retinopathy and other retinal disorders. *N Engl J Med.* 1994;331:1,480–1,487.

26. Pierce AE, Avery RL, Foley ED, et al. Vascular endothelial growth factor/vascular permeability factor expression in a mouse model of retinal vascularization. *Proc Natl Acad Sci USA.* 1995;92:905–909.

27. Pe'er J, Shweiki D, Itin A, et al. Hypoxia-induced expression of vascular endothelial growth factor by retinal cells is a common factor in neovascularizing ocular diseases. *Lab Invest.* 1995;72:638–645.

28. Lopez PF, Sippy BD, Lambert HM, et al. Transdifferentiated retinal pigment cells are immunoreactive for vascular endothelial growth factor in surgically excised age-related macular degeneration-related choroidal neovascular membranes. *Invest Ophthalmol Vis Sci.* 1996;37:855–868.

29. Wells JA, Murthy R, Chibber R, et al. Levels of vascular endothelial growth factor are elevated in the vitreous of patients with subretinal neovascularization. *Br J Ophthalmol.* 1996;80:363–366.

30. Tolentino MJ, Miller JW, Gragoudas ES, et al. Intravitreous injections of vascular endothelial growth factor produce retinal ischemia and microangiopathy in an adult primate. *Ophthalmology.* 1996;103:1,820–1,828.

31. Stone J, Itin A, Alon T, et al. Development of retinal vasculature is mediated by hypoxia-induced vascular endothelial growth factor (VEGF) expression by neuroglia. *J Neurosci.* 1995;15:4,738–4,747.

32. Khiffen M, Sharma HS, Mooy CM, et al. Increased expression of angiogenic growth factors in age-related maculopathy. *Br J Ophthalmol.* 1997;81:154–162.

33. Reddy MR, Zamora RL, Kaplan HJ. Distribution of growth factors in subfoveal neovascular membranes in age-related macular degeneration and presumed ocular histoplasmosis syndrome. *Am J Ophthalmol.* 1995;120:291–301.

34. Shweiki D, Itin A, Soffer D, et al. Vascular endothelial growth factor induced by hypoxia may mediate hypoxia-initiated angiogenesis. *Nature.* 1992;359:843–845.

35. Miller JW, Adamis AP, Shima DT, et al. Vascular endothelial growth factor/vascular permeability factor is temporally and spatially correlated with ocular angiogenesis in a primate model. *Am J Pathol.* 1994;145:574–584.

36. Miller H, Miller B, Ryan SJ. The role of retinal pigment epithelium in the involution of subretinal neovascularization. *Invest Ophthalmol Vis Sci.* 1986;27:1,644–1,652.

37. Iida T, Hagimura N, Sato T, et al. Optical coherence tomographic features of idiopathic submacular choroidal neovascularization. *Am J Ophthalmol.* 2000;130:763–768.

38. Glaser BM, Campochiaro PA, Davis JL, et al. Retinal pigment epithelial cells release inhibitors of neovascularization. *Arch Ophthalmol.* 1985;103:1,870–1,875.

39. Glaser BM, Campochiaro PA, Davis JL, et al. Retinal pigment epithelial cells. *Ophthalmology.* 1987;94:780–784.

40. Spaide RF. Fundus autofluorescence and age-related macular degeneration. *Ophthalmology* 2003;110:392–399.

41. Tamai K, Spaide RF, Ellis EA, et al. Lipid hyperperoxide-stimulated subretinal choroidal neovascularization in the rabbit. *Exp Eye Res.* 2002;74:301–308.

42. Da Pozzo S, Battaglia, Parodi M, et al. A pilot study of ICG-guided laser photocoagulation for occult choroidal neovascularization presenting as a focal spot in age-related macular degeneration. *Int Ophthalmol.* 2001;24:187–194.

43. Bressler NM, Arnold J, Benchaboune M, et al. Verteporfin therapy of subfoveal choroidal neovascularization in patients with age-related macular degeneration: additional information regarding baseline lesion composition's impact on vision outcomes-TAP report no. 3. *Arch Ophthalmol.* 2002;120:1,443–1,454.

44. Verteporfin in Photodynamic Therapy Study Group. Verteporfin therapy of subfoveal choroidal neovascularization in age-related macular degeneration: two-year results of a randomized clinical trial including lesions with occult with no classic choroidal neovascularization-verteporfin in photodynamic therapy report 2. *Am J Ophthalmol.* 2001;131:541–560.

45. Kuroiwa S, Arai J, Gaun S, et al. Rapidly progressive scar formation after transpupillary thermotherapy in retinal angiomatous proliferation. *Retina.* 2003;23:417–420.

46. Yannuzzi LA, Klancnik J, Gross N, et al. Retinal angiomatous proliferation: treatment with anecortave acetate. Presented at the annual meeting of the Macula Society, Naples, Florida, 2003.

Differential Diagnosis of Age-Related Macular Degeneration

8

Mohan Iyer   William F. Mieler

INTRODUCTION

Various ophthalmic conditions can present with fundus findings similar to those seen in age-related macular degeneration (AMD). While approximately 90% of individuals with AMD develop non-neovascular changes and associated vision loss, 10% develop choroidal neovascularization (CNV) and severe vision loss. An extensive number of conditions can predispose one to CNV, and differentiation of these conditions is important because of the variability in their natural history and available treatment options. This chapter discusses the differential diagnosis of non-neovascular AMD and CNV, as well as conditions that can be associated with CNV. Because the list of conditions associated with CNV is extensive, only the more common conditions are discussed in this chapter. Discussion of the conditions is kept brief; however, the ophthalmoscopic and angiographic features that allow differentiation from AMD are emphasized in this chapter.

NON-NEOVASCULAR AMD

Non-neovascular findings in AMD include drusen and retinal pigment epithelial atrophy (1,2). Drusen are round, yellow lesions that represent deposits between the plasma membrane and basement membrane of the retinal pigment epithelium (RPE), known as basal laminar deposits, and deposits within the Bruch's membrane, known as basal linear deposits (3). Drusen are classified based on size (small: <64 μm in diameter; intermediate: 64–125 μm;

large: >125 μm) and boundary (hard: discrete boundaries; soft: amorphous boundaries; confluent: contiguous boundaries). The presence of large, soft, and/or confluent drusen increases the risk of progression to atrophy or CNV. Occasionally, drusen may appear refractile due to dystrophic calcification and are called calcified drusen. RPE atrophy may appear clinically as areas of mottled depigmentation, and when present in contiguous areas, as geographic atrophy. This is often accompanied by atrophy of underlying choriocapillaris and attenuation of overlying photoreceptors with resultant visual loss. In addition, pigment migration leading to pigment clumps or a reticulated pattern of hyperpigmentation may also be observed.

Differential Diagnosis of Non-Neovascular AMD

Conditions that can mimic non-neovascular changes of AMD are listed in Table 8.1. The differential diagnosis of non-neovascular AMD includes central serous chorioretinopathy (CSC), pattern dystrophy, basal laminar or cuticular drusen, chloroquine toxicity, dominant drusen syndrome, Type II membranoproliferative glomerulonephritis, and central areolar RPE atrophy.

Resolved CSC may present with RPE changes and mottled areas of depigmentation similar to non-neovascular AMD changes (4–9). While the typical patient is male and between 25 and 45 years of age, CSC in individuals over 50 years of age has been associated with a greater female prevalence (50%) (7). Features that help differentiate CSC from AMD in this older age group include a "gutterlike"

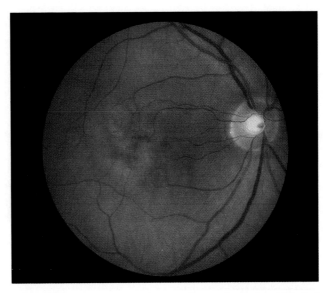

Figure 8.1 Resolved central serous chorioretinopathy with retinal pigment epithelium changes similar to non-neovascular age-related macular degeneration.

distribution of RPE atrophy, with or without multiple small serous detachments, and an absence of drusen (Fig. 8.1).

Pattern dystrophy may be seen in a younger patient with focal or reticular hyperpigmentation, and vitelliform, yellowish abnormality in the outer retina (10–16). Fluorescein angiography (FA) can help distinguish this condition from AMD with early hypopigmentation and surrounding hyperpigmentation and late staining of vitelliform areas (Fig. 8.2).

Basal laminar or cuticular drusen may be seen in patients in their third to fourth decades with numerous small drusen and a classic starry-night pattern on FA (3), often with vitelliform deposits in the macula (Fig. 8.3). Chloroquine toxicity may present as RPE mottling and nongeographic atrophy (17); the absence of drusen and a positive history of drug ingestion are essential for making the diagnosis (Fig 8.4). Patients with dominant drusen syndrome (18,18a) present with drusen in both the macula and around the vascular arcades at a younger age; a familial history and/or genetic testing may be helpful in the diagnosis (Figs. 8.5, 8.6). Sorsby's macular degeneration, an autosomal dominant disorder, has features of bilateral drusen in younger patients that may progress to CNV. Type II membranoproliferative glomerulonephritis (Fig. 8.7) may present with drusen-like deposits in the macula (19–21). Central areolar RPE atrophy (Fig. 8.8) in a

younger patient can simulate atrophic changes seen in AMD (2,23). RPE atrophy or depigmentation may occur from previous episodes of inflammatory chorioretinitis, typically in a younger patient (Fig. 8.9).

NEOVASCULAR AMD

Any pathologic process that disturbs the RPE and choroid and leads to the disruption of Bruch's membrane can be associated with CNV. The disruption in Bruch's membrane can occur from a traumatic process or by breakthrough of capillary-like new vessels from the choroid into the sub-RPE space (type I CNV) or into the sub-retinal space (type II CNV) (2,22). Although CNV was first described nearly a century ago, Gass is credited with elaborating much of our current concepts of CNV, including the recognition of

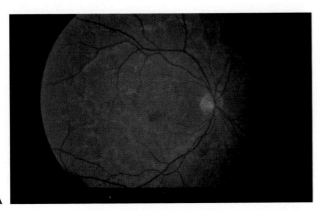
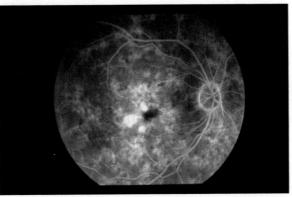

A   B

Figure 8.2 **A.** Pattern dystrophy of the retinal pigment epithelium. **B.** Fluorescein angiogram reveals central hypofluorescence surrounded by hyperfluorescence, with eventual late staining centrally.

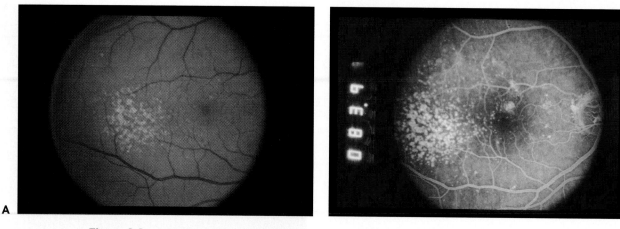

Figure 8.3 **A.** Basal laminar drusen. **B.** Fluorescein angiography showing starry-night pattern.

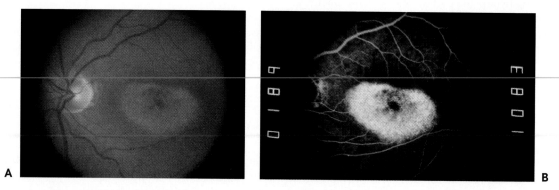

Figure 8.4 **A.** Chloroquine toxicity. Note the lack of drusen and presence of retinal pigment epithelium changes similar to non-neovascular age-related macular degeneration. **B.** Fluorescein angiography of the same fundus.

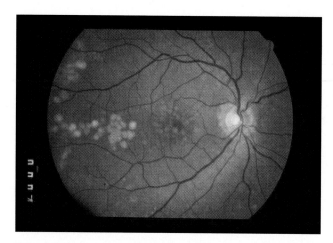

Figure 8.5 Dominant drusen syndrome.

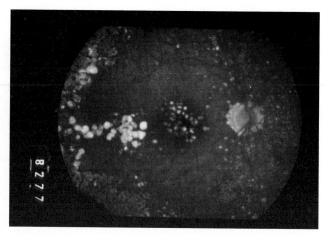

Figure 8.6 Fluorescein angiography of dominant drusen syndrome.

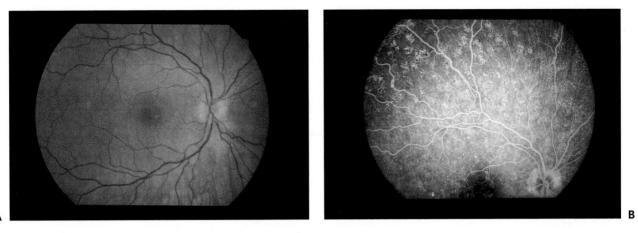

Figure 8.7 **A.** Type II membranoproliferative glomerulonephritis. **B.** Fluorescein angiography of the same fundus.

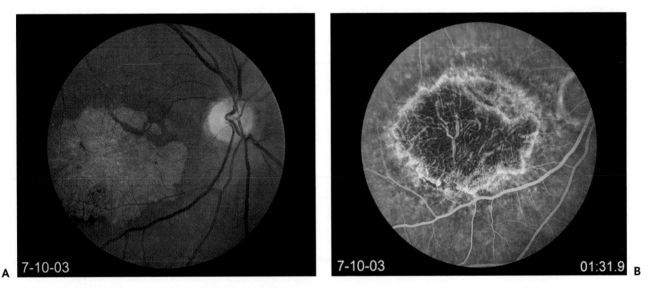

Figure 8.8 **A.** Central areolar retinal pigment epithelium atrophy. **B.** Fluorescein angiography of the same fundus.

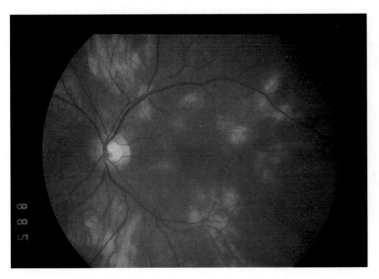

Figure 8.9 Retinal pigment epithelium changes in a young patient following inflammatory choroiditis.

AMD as the most common cause of CNV (1,2). Cellular mechanisms underlying the pathogenesis of CNV are still being elucidated and the etiology is thought to be multifactorial; thus, a number of conditions can result in CNV.

CNV primarily occurs in the macula or peripapillary area. It can rarely occur peripherally, where it may mimic a mass lesion. Clinical features include the presence of one or more of the following: retinal or subretinal hemorrhage, subretinal fluid, and lipid exudates. Associated features may include RPE detachment, subretinal plaque, or disciform scar. CNV is classified as either classic or occult based on FA findings. Classic CNV on FA has a distinct, lacy, bright hyperfluorescence in early transit phase with well-demarcated boundaries that become obscured due to leakage in late phases. Occult CNV is of two types: (a) late leakage of undetermined source or (b) fibrovascular pigment epithelial detachment (PED). In late leakage of undetermined source, FA demonstrates late punctate leakage not corresponding to RPE irregularities and a poorly demarcated lesion boundary. In fibrovascular PED, there is hyperfluorescence, best seen 1 to 2 minutes after dye injection, beneath irregular RPE with either well or poorly defined boundaries, and persistent staining or late leakage. The classification was important because photodynamic therapy (PDT), until recently, was approved only for predominantly classic lesions in the United States. Recent evaluations of PDT are focused more on lesion size rather than the above classification, and this may lead to a more consistent treatment algorithm for practicing retinal specialists, given the current variability in FA interpretation.

Neovascular AMD—Differential Diagnosis

The differential diagnosis of neovascular AMD includes macroaneurysm, vitelliform degeneration, CSC, macular hemorrhage, inflammatory conditions, and choroidal tumors (Table 8.2).

Retinal arterial macroaneurysms are typically unilateral and occur more commonly in women over 60 years of

TABLE 8.2
DIFFERENTIAL DIAGNOSIS OF NEOVASCULAR AMD
Retinal arterial macroaneurysms
Vitelliform lesions in adults
Central serous chorioretinopathy
Macular hemorrhage
Inflammatory conditions
Choroidal tumors

age (24). Preretinal, intraretinal, or subretinal hemorrhage may be present; and when the hemorrhage or associated lipid extends into the macula, it may be confused with CNV (Fig. 8.10). The epicenter of the hemorrhage can usually be identified overlying a retinal artery, and FA may aid in the diagnosis with early filling of the aneurysm, and focal narrowing of the artery proximal and distal to the aneurysm. Systemic hypertension is the most common associated condition, and work-up of a patient with macroaneurysm should include measurement of blood pressure. Vitelliform lesions in adults can have fundus features that can be mistaken for a PED (10,14). The staining of the vitelliform material on FA may also be mistaken for CNV (Fig. 8.11). However, unlike FA features of CNV, this material shows early hypofluorescence and typically a ring of irregular hyperfluorescence surrounding the hypofluorescent or nonfluorescent area.

CSC (4–9) may present with subretinal fluid that can be confused with CNV associated with AMD (Fig. 8.12). The diagnostic clues include absence of drusen, absence of hemorrhage, patches of RPE atrophy in a gutterlike distribution secondary to previous episodes of CSR, or the presence of multiple PEDs. CSC, however, can be associated with CNV (Fig. 8.13), and it is important to rule out CNV with the aid of FA.

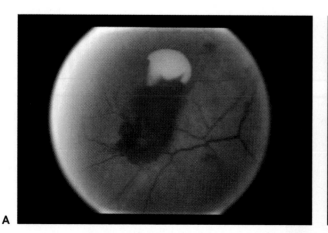
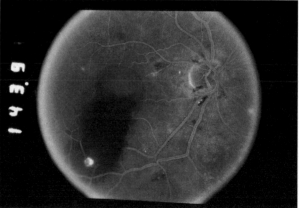

A   B

Figure 8.10 **A.** Retinal macroaneurysm. The presence of hemorrhage and exudates extending into the macula may lead to a diagnosis of choroidal neovascularization. **B.** Fluorescein angiography demonstrates the early filling of the macroaneurysm.

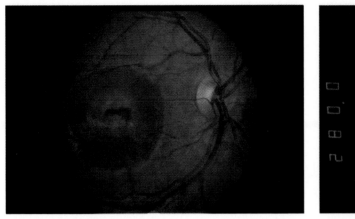
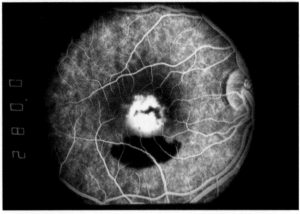

Figure 8.11 **A.** Vitelliform dystrophy. **B.** Fluorescein angiography of the same fundus. Unlike choroidal neovascularization, this material shows early hypofluorescence and typically a ring of irregular hyperfluorescence surrounding the hypo- or nonfluorescent area.

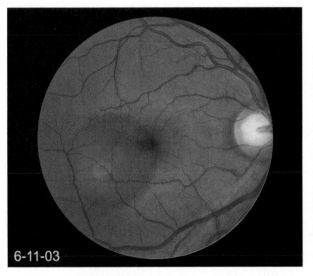
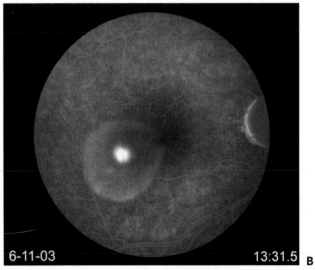

Figure 8.12 **A.** Central serous chorioretinopathy (or ICSC). Fundus photograph shows presence of subretinal fluid. Note the absence of drusen or hemorrhage. **B.** Fluorescein angiography reveals an expansile hyperfluorescent spot.

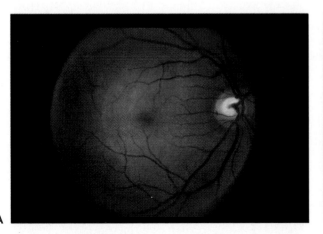
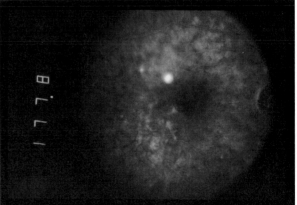

Figure 8.13 **A.** Choroidal neovascularization associated with central serous chorioretinopathy. A small amount of parafoveal hemorrhage is observed. **B.** Fluorescein angiography of the same fundus. The patient later underwent focal laser treatment with central serous chorioretinopathy resolution and recovery of visual acuity.

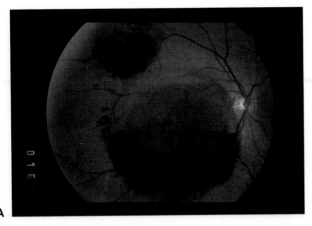
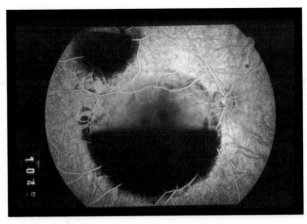

A   B

Figure 8.14 **A.** Macular hemorrhage related to Valsalva retinopathy. **B.** Fluorescein angiography of the same fundus.

Macular hemorrhage related to trauma, myopia, or Valsalva may mimic hemorrhage associated with CNV, but may be distinguished from AMD based on the lack of typical features of AMD (Fig. 8.14). Inflammatory conditions, including choroiditis, Harada's disease (25), and posterior scleritis, may have exudative changes simulating changes seen in AMD (Fig. 8.15); however, the typical features of these conditions are often sufficient for making the diagnosis. A choroidal tumor (Fig. 8.16) may present as an elevated lesion and associated CNV that may mimic CNV related to AMD (26); in such cases, ultrasonography may be employed to further delineate the lesion.

CONDITIONS ASSOCIATED WITH CNV

Many disease conditions can be associated with CNV as listed in Table 8.3. Distinguishing the correct diagnosis is important because the natural history of the CNV and the

response to therapy can be quite variable depending on the underlying condition. The more common conditions are discussed below.

Ocular Histoplasmosis Syndrome (OHS)

The most common inflammatory condition causing CNV is OHS. The fungus *Histoplasma capsulatum* is endemic to the Mississippi and Ohio River Valley areas in the United States. Over 90% of individuals from these areas with typical fundus features have positive skin testing to histoplasmin. However, there have been reports of patients with similar fundus findings from Europe and other parts of the United States where histoplasmosis is not endemic (27,28).

The triad of fundus features includes peripapillary chorioretinal atrophy, peripheral punched-out chorioretinal scars ("histo spots") or linear atrophic streaks, and macular hemorrhage or scar (2) (Fig. 8.17). Other inflam-

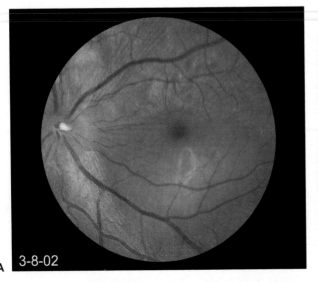
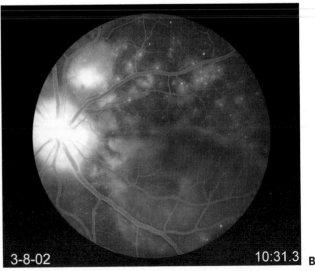

Figure 8.15 **A.** Exudative changes related to choroiditis, Harada's disease or posterior scleritis may be confused with choroidal neovascularization. **B.** Fluorescein angiography of the same fundus.

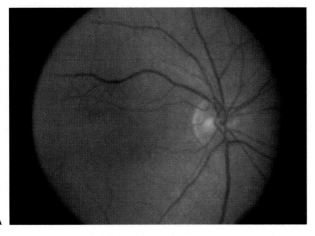
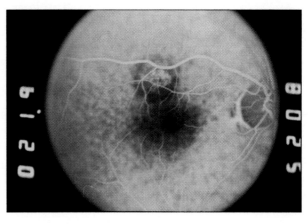

A   **B**

Figure 8.16 **A.** Choroidal melanoma with choroidal neovascularization. **B.** Fluorescein angiography of the same fundus.

matory conditions, such as multifocal choroiditis, which may predispose to CNV and have lesions similar to OHS, may be distinguished by the absence of vitreous inflammation in OHS.

The pathogenesis is thought to involve damage to the Bruch's membrane, RPE, and choriocapillaris by focal choroiditis that results in an exudative detachment of the retina or subretinal hemorrhage. Resolution of the choroiditis leaves an area of atrophy. A hemorrhagic detachment may occur that may gradually evolve into a disciform scar.

OHS tends to be associated with type II (in subneurosensory retina) CNV compared to type I (subretinal pigment epithelium) CNV seen in AMD. Natural history studies reveal a better prognosis of this form of CNV compared to CNV associated with AMD. Spontaneous regression has also been observed (2,29,30), but, as with AMD, CNV recurrence rates remain high.

The Macular Photocoagulation Study (MPS) showed a treatment benefit for juxtafoveal and extrafoveal CNV (31). After 5 years, for patients with juxtafoveal CNV, the proportion of eyes with severe visual loss (i.e., loss of at least six lines of vision) was 12% in the treated group versus 28% in the untreated group; for those patients with extrafoveal CNV, 9% in the treated group had severe visual loss, versus 44% in the untreated group. The MPS did not address subfoveal CNV. PDT and submacular surgery are the current modalities of treating subfoveal CNV (32–35).

Pathologic Myopia

Myopic degeneration occurs in 5% to 10% of myopias, especially those with greater than 6D myopia or with axial lengths greater than 26.5 mm. Fundus findings (Fig. 8.18) include tilted optic discs, peripapillary chorioretinal atrophy, lacquer cracks or linear breaks in Bruch's membrane, isolated subretinal hemorrhage not associated with CNV that may resolve spontaneously, Fuchs spots (RPE hyper-

plasia associated with small nonprogressing areas of CNV), posterior staphyloma, cystoid, cobblestone, or lattice degeneration, and thinning and hole formation in peripheral retina.

Reports of the natural history of untreated CNV in high myopia have varied: some reports describe a relatively self-limited course (36,37), while others report a poor prognosis related to untreated CNV (38–40). Older age of onset of CNV may portend a poorer prognosis (39,41). The role of laser photocoagulation for CNV related to myopia is uncertain. Progressive enlargement of the photocoagulation scar can result in decreased visual outcome despite regression of CNV (36,42,43). In addition, laser photocoagulation can be associated with elongation of pre-existing lacquer cracks or development of new ones (43). Given the concerns over laser photocoagulation related visual loss, PDT and surgical removal of subfoveal CNV have become accepted alternative treatment modalities for CNV associated with myopia (34,35,44–46).

Angioid Streaks

Angioid streaks are irregular, radiating lines emanating from the peripapillary area (Fig. 8.19). The name derives from their striking resemblance to blood vessels, although, in reality, they represent linear cracks in thickened and calcified Bruch's membrane. Loss of vision can occur from CNV through breaks in Bruch's membrane, typically in the peripapillary area, or from choroidal rupture and submacular hemorrhage following minor trauma. Associated systemic conditions found in 50% of patients with angioid streaks included pseudoxanthoma elasticum, Paget's disease, sickle cell disease, Ehlers-Danlos syndrome, and thalassemia (47). Identification of angioid streaks may thus lead to the diagnosis of a systemic condition. FA shows irregular transmission hyperfluorescence of the streaks due to overlying RPE atrophy,

TABLE 8.3
CONDITIONS ASSOCIATED WITH CNV

Degenerative and Heredodegenerative Conditions
Age-related macular degeneration
Myopic degeneration
Angioid streaks
Best's disease
Fundus flavimaticus
Optic nerve head drusen
Tilted disc syndrome
Chorioretinal coloboma
Idiopathic juxtafoveal retinal telangiectasia
Idiopathic polypoidal choroidal vasculopathy
Membranoproliferative glomerulonephritis Type II
Choroideremia

Inflammatory and Infectious Conditions
Ocular histoplasmosis syndrome
Multifocal choroiditis
Serpiginous choroiditis
Vogt-Kayanagi-Harada syndrome
Birdshot chorioretinopathy
Punctate inner choroidopathy
Acute multifocal posterior placoid pigment epitheliopathy
Multiple evanescent white-dot syndrome (MEWDS)
Behcet syndrome
Sarcoidosis
Toxoplasma retinochoroiditis
Toxocariasis
Rubella
Endogenous *Candida* endophthalmitis
Sympathetic ophthalmia

Trauma
Choroidal rupture
Intense photocoagulation
Intraocular foreign body
Retinal cryo-injury
Subretinal fluid drainage

Tumor
Choroidal nevus
Choroidal melanoma
Choroidal hemangioma
Metastatic choroidal tumors
Hamartomas of the retinal pigment epithelium
Choroidal osteoma

Miscellaneous
Idiopathic
Anterior ischemic optic neuropathy
Idiopathic central serous chorioretinopathy
Radiation retinopathy
Chronic papilledema

(52), indocyanine green (ICG) mediated feeder vessel treatment (53), submacular surgery (34,35), and limited macular translocation (54) are not well defined.

Multifocal Choroiditis and Panuveitis (MCP)

MCP (55) involves punched-out chorioretinal lesions that in their chronic stage may be similar to OHS (Fig. 8.20). A notable difference from OHS is the presence of varying degrees of vitreous inflammation in MCP. Some patients with inferior, peripheral punched-out lesions and vitritis diagnosed with MCP were later shown to have noncaseating granulomas by nondirected conjunctival biopsy leading to a diagnosis of sarcoidosis (56). The differential diagnosis of chorioretinal lesions and vitreous inflammation should include sarcoidosis, tuberculosis, and intraocular lymphoma, especially in the elderly patient.

This condition primarily occurs in mildly myopic females, with an average age at onset of 30 to 35 years, and typically, a presenting visual acuity of 20/50 or better (57). Bilateral disease is seen in 67% to 75% of patients (55). Enlargement of blind spot has been frequently associated with MCP (58,59). Recurrences may occur in one or both eyes, and present with yellowish-gray appearance of the chorioretinal scars. FA reveals hyperfluorescence of the borders of acute lesions with late staining of the centers and transmission hyperfluorescence of old punched-out scars.

Visual outcome is dependent on the number of macular lesions, development of CNV or CME. Brown et al. (57) reported on a series of 41 patients with MCP and a mean follow-up of 39 months with 95% having 20/40 or better vision in at least one eye. CNV developed in nearly one-third of the patients and was associated with visual acuity of 20/200 or worse.

Treatment with corticosteroids has occasionally led to regression of CNV while controlling the associated inflammation (57,60). The persistence of CNV despite corticosteroid treatment prompted Spaide et al. (61) to investigate the role of PDT in a series of seven patients, with stabilization or improvement of vision in all patients. Wachtlin et al. (62) also reported promising results with PDT for the treatment of CNV related to inflammatory diseases. In a study of submacular surgery in 10 eyes with MCP, Brindeau et al. (63) found that after 12 months of follow-up, 80% had visual acuity of 20/200 or worse.

Serpiginous Choroiditis

Serpiginous choroiditis is a chronic, progressive, episodic, bilateral disease that affects young-to-middle-aged otherwise healthy patients without racial or sex predilection (64–68). In the acute process, grayish-yellow areas of edema are seen at the level of the RPE extending from the optic disc in a centrifugal pattern in a pseudopodal configuration

which may be poorly visualized in eyes with darkly pigmented choroids. Treatment options for CNV, which occurs in 70% to 86% of eyes, are limited for this condition. Visual prognosis is guarded as the CNV progresses with or without laser treatment (48–51), and the roles of PDT

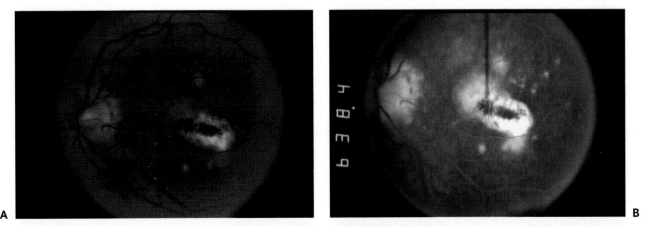

Figure 8.17 Ocular histoplasmosis syndrome. **A.** Fundus photograph showing the peripapillary atrophy, punched out lesions, and macular hemorrhage. **B.** Fluorescein angiography of the same fundus revealing choroidal neovascularization.

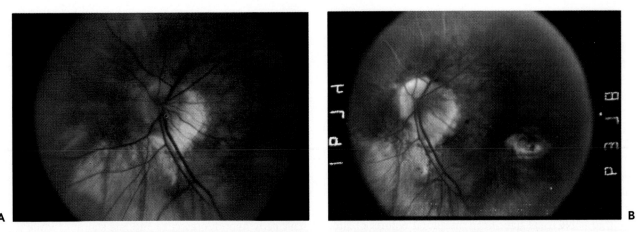

Figure 8.18 **A.** Myopic degeneration with characteristic tilted optic disc, peripapillary chorioretinal atrophy, and lacquer cracks. **B.** Fluorescein angiography of the same fundus with a Fuchs spot representing retinal pigment epithelium hyperplasia associated with a small, non-progressing area of choroidal neovascularization.

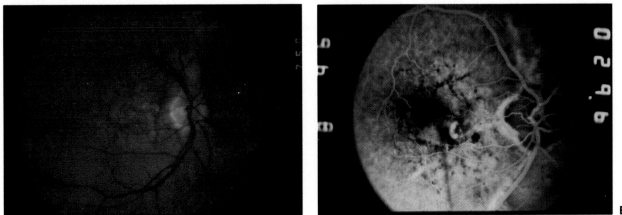

Figure 8.19 **A.** Angioid streaks with associated choroidal neovascularization. **B.** Fluorescein angiography of the same fundus.

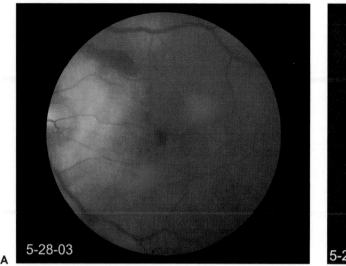

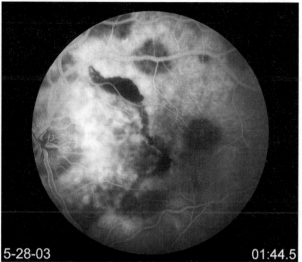

Figure 8.20 **A.** Multifocal choroiditis and choroidal neovascularization. **B.** Fluorescein angiography of the same fundus.

(Fig. 8.21). The anterior segment is usually unremarkable, and vitreous cells may be present in the acute stage. Visual loss results from chorioretinal atrophy, CME, or subretinal neovascularization (65,67–69). FA of acute lesions reveals early hypofluorescence, presumably from either nonperfusion of the underlying choriocapillaris or blockage from damaged RPE, followed by hyperfluorescence of the borders of the lesion with gradual central staining.

Treatment has primarily involved corticosteroids (69) and/or combination immunosuppressive therapy (70), particularly in patients with lesions threatening the fovea. Successful treatment with alkylating agents has been reported (71). There have been anecdotal reports of successful treatment with acyclovir, and although culture negative, VZV and HSV DNA by PCR were detected in the aqueous humor in a six of nine patients with serpiginous choroiditis (72). Laser photocoagulation to limit progression of lesions toward the fovea were unsuccessful (2,73).

Successful argon laser treatment of extrafoveal CNV has been reported (68,69). Combined ICG-mediated photothrombosis and intravitreous triamcinolone induced significant visual acuity recovery in one case of peripapillary CNV complicating serpiginous choroiditis (74).

Punctate Inner Choroidopathy (PIC)

Patients with PIC are young, myopic, healthy women who present with blurred vision, photopsia, and central or paracentral scotoma (75). The lesions are yellow and tend to smaller than those in MCP, and there is an absence of vitreous inflammation (Fig. 8.22). FA reveals acute lesions to have early hypofluorescence and late staining, while older scars show transmission defects. In one series of 30 eyes (57), visual acuity was 20/40 or better in 77% of eyes. CNV around scars developed in 27% to 40% of eyes (57,75). Small CNV may spontaneously resolve (57). Submacular surgery is complicated by recurrences (76). The role of PDT

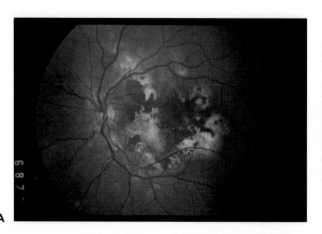

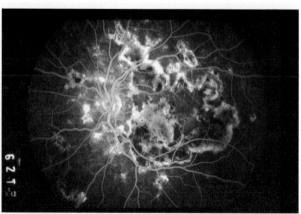

Figure 8.21 **A.** Choroidal neovascularization in a patient with serpiginous choroiditis. **B.** Fluorescein angiography of the same fundus.

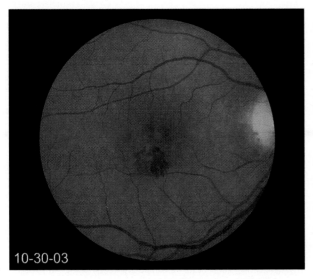
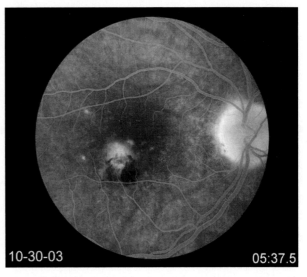

Figure 8.22 A. Choroidal neovascularization in a patient with punctate inner choroiditis. **B.** Fluorescein angiography of the same fundus.

for subfoveal CNV in patients with PIC is uncertain with few case reports published thus far (62,77).

Idiopathic CNV

CNV in the absence of any other fundus abnormality or associated condition has been termed idiopathic CNV (78). This condition should be considered a diagnosis of exclusion. In a retrospective study of 19 patients with subfoveal involvement followed for a median of 87 months, 95% of patients had stable or significantly improved visual acuity, whereas only 5% had significant visual loss (78). The MPS showed benefit from laser treatment to extrafoveal and juxtafoveal lesions (31), and benefit from PDT (52,79,80) of subfoveal idiopathic CNV has been reported. Only small case series have been reported that evaluate the role of PDT (52,79,80), subfoveal surgery (34), or limited macular translocation (54) for idiopathic CNV. In a study of seven eyes treated with PDT, the median initial acuity was 20/150; and after a mean follow up of 13.5 months, the final acuity was 20/45 (79).

OTHER CONDITIONS ASSOCIATED WITH CNV

Other conditions associated with CNV include idiopathic polypoidal choroidal vasculopathy (PCV) (81–83), hereditary dystrophies including Best's disease (84,85), idiopathic juxtafoveal retinal telangiectasia (86), optic nerve head drusen (87), sarcoidosis (88), Harada's disease (89,90), infectious causes such as toxocara and toxoplasmosis (91,92), tumors such as choroidal osteoma (93), choroidal hemangiomas (94,95), malignant melanoma (96), choroidal nevus (97), choroidal rupture (98–100),

and following focal laser photocoagulation (101)—to name just a few. A comprehensive list of conditions associated is presented in Table 8.3.

SUMMARY

The differential diagnosis of AMD is extensive. A step-wise approach would first make the distinction of whether the fundus findings appear non-neovascular or neovascular. Fundus and FA features can aid in further distinguishing the lesion. Conditions that may mimic neovascular AMD because of the presence of subretinal fluid, hemorrhage, or exudates, should be excluded, as treatment options for these conditions are considerably different. Many entities have CNV as their final pathway; an accurate diagnosis will aid in establishing systemic associations and in assessing treatment efficacy.

REFERENCES

1. Gass JDM. Drusen and disciform macular detachment and degeneration. *Arch Ophthalmol.* 1973;90:206–217.
2. Gass JD. *Stereoscopic Atlas of Macular Disease: Diagnosis and Treatment,* 4th Ed. St Louis: Mosby; 1997.
3. Russell SR, Mullins RF, et al. Location, substructure, and composition of basal laminar drusen compared with drusen associated with age-related macular degeneration. *Am J Ophthalmol.* 2000;129:205–214.
4. Gass JDM. Pathogenesis of disciform detachment of the neuroepithelium. II. Idiopathic central serous choroidopathy. *Am J Ophthalmol.* 1960;63:.587–615.
5. Yannuzzi LA, Shakin JL, Fisher YL, et al. Peripheral retinal detachments and retinal pigment epithelial atrophic tracts secondary to central serous pigment epitheliopathy. *Ophthalmology.* 1984;91:1,554–1,572.
6. Spaide RF, Campeas L, Haas A, et al. Central serous chorioretinopathy in younger and older adults. *Ophthalmology.* 1996;103:2,070–2,079; discussion 2,079–2,080.
7. Spaide RF, Hall LS, Haas A, et al. Indocyanine green videoangiography of older patients with central serous chorioretinopathy. *Retina.* 1996;16:203–213.
8. Marmor MF. New hypotheses on the pathogenesis and treatment of serous retinal detachment. *Graefes Arch Clin Exp Ophthalmol.* 1988;226:548–552.
9. Tittl MK, Spaide RF, Wong D, et al. Systemic findings associated with central serous chorioretinopathy. *Am J Ophthalmol.* 1999;128:63–68.
10. Gass JDM. A clinicopathologic study of a peculiar foveomacular dystrophy. *Trans Am Ophthalmol Soc.* 1974;72:139–156.

11. Marmor MF, Byers B. Pattern dystrophy of the pigment epithelium. *Am J Ophthalmol.* 1977;84:32–44.
12. Hsieh RC, Fine BS, Lyons JS. Patterned dystrophies of the retinal pigment epithelium. *Arch Ophthalmol.* 1977;95:429–435.
13. Patrinely JR, Lewis RA, Font RL. Foveomacular vitelliform dystrophy, adult type. A clinicopathologic study including electron microscopic observations. *Ophthalmology.* 1985;92:1,712–1,718.
14. Jaffe GJ, Schatz H. Histopathologic features of adult-onset foveomacular pigment epithelial dystrophy. *Arch Ophthalmol.* 1988;106:958–960.
15. Wells J, Wroblewski J, Keen J, et al. Mutations in the human retinal degeneration slow (RDS) gene can cause either retinitis pigmentosa or macular dystrophy. *Nat Genet.* 1993;3:213–218.
16. Battaglia Parodi M, Da Pozzo S, Ravalico G. Photodynamic therapy for choroidal neovascularization associated with pattern dystrophy. *Retina.* 2003;23(2):171–176.
17. Michael F, Marmor MD, Ronald E, et al. Recommendations on screening for chloroquine and hydroxychloroquine retinopathy: a report by the American Academy of Ophthalmology. *Ophthalmology.* 2002;109(7):1,377–1,382.
18. Deutman AF, Jansen LMAA. Dominantly inherited drusen of Bruch's membrane. *Br J Ophthalmol.* 1979;82:4.
18a. Stone EM, Lotery AJ, Munier FL, et al. A single EFEMP1 mutation associated with both Malattia Leventinese and Doyne honeycomb retinal dystrophy. *Nat Genet.* 1999 22(2):199–202.
19. Leys A, Vanrenterghem Y, Van Damme B, et al. Fundus changes in membranoproliferative glomerulonephritis type II. A fluorescein angiographic study of 23 patients. *Graefes Arch Clin Exp Ophthalmol.* 1991;229(5):406–410.
20. Kim DD, Mieler WF, Wolf MD. Posterior segment changes in membranoproliferative glomerulonephritis. *Am J Ophthalmol.* 1992;114(5):593–599.
21. Hassenstein A, Richard G. Choroidal neovascularization in type II membranoproliferative glomerulonephritis. Photodynamic therapy as a treatment option—a case report. *Klin Monatsbl Augenheilkd.* 2003;220(7):492–495. [German].
22. Gass JDM. Pathogenesis of disciform detachment of the neuroepithelium. *Am J Ophthalmol.* 1967;63:573–711.
23. Leveille AS, Morse PH, Kiernan JP. Autosomal dominant central pigment epithelial and choroidal degeneration. *Ophthalmology.* 1982;89(12):1,407–1,413.
24. Rabb MF, Gagliano DA, Teske MP. Retinal arterial macroaneurysms. *Surv Ophthalmol.* 1988;33(2):73–96.
25. Moorthy RS, Chong LS, Smith RE, et al. Subretinal neovascular membranes in Vogt-Koyanagi-Harada syndrome. *Am J Ophthalmol.* 1993;116: 164–170.
26. Annesley WH. Peripheral exudative hemorrhagic chorioretinopathy. *Trans Am Ophthalmol Soc.* 1980;78:321.
27. Suttorp-Schulten MS, Bollemeijer JG, Bos PJ, et al. Presumed ocular histoplasmosis in the Netherlands: an area without histoplasmosis? *Br J Ophthalmol.* 1997;81:7–11.
28. Watzke RC, Klein ML, Wener MH. Histoplasmosis-like choroiditis in a nonendemic area: the northwestern United States. *Retina.* 1998;18: 204–212.
29. Orlando RG, Davidorf FH. Spontaneous recovery phenomenon in the presumed ocular histoplasmosis syndrome. *Int Ophthalmol Clin.* 1983;23:137–149.
30. Kleiner RC, Ratner CM, Enger C, et al. Subfoveal neovascularization in the ocular histoplasmosis syndrome: a natural history study. *Retina.* 1988;8:225.
31. The Macular Photocoagulation Study Group. Laser photocoagulation for juxtafoveal choroidal neovascularization. Five-year results from randomized clinical trials. Macular Photocoagulation Study Group. *Arch Ophthalmol.* 1994;112(4):500–509.
32. Verteporfin in Photodynamic Therapy (VIP) Study Group. Photodynamic therapy of subfoveal choroidal neovascularization in pathologic myopia with verteporfin: 1-year results of a randomized clinical trial–VIP report no. 1. *Ophthalmology.* 2001;108:841–852.
33. Saperstein DA, Rosenfeld PJ, Bressler NM, et al. Photodynamic therapy of subfoveal choroidal neovascularization with verteporfin in the ocular histoplasmosis syndrome: one-year results of an uncontrolled, prospective case series. *Ophthalmology.* 2002;109(8):1,499–1,505.
34. Thomas MA, Dickinson JD, Melberg NS, et al. Visual results after surgical removal of subfoveal choroidal neovascular membranes. *Ophthalmology.* 1994;101:1,384–1,396.
35. Adelberg DA, Del Priore LV, Kaplan HJ. Surgery for subfoveal membranes in myopia, angioid streaks, and other disorders. *Retina.* 1995;15:198–205.
36. Avila MP, Weiter JJ, Jalkh AE, et al. Natural history of choroidal neovascularization in degenerative myopia. *Ophthalmology.* 1984;91:1,573–1,581.
37. Fried M, Siebert A, Meyer-Schwickerath G. A natural history of Fuchs' spot: a long-term follow-up study. *Doc Ophthalmol.* 1981;28:215–221.
38. Hampton GR, Kohen D, Bird AC. Visual prognosis of disciform degeneration in myopia. *Ophthalmology.* 1983;80:923–926.
39. Tabendeh H, Flynn HW Jr, Scott IU, et al. Visual acuity outcomes of patients 50 years of age and older with high myopia and untreated choroidal neovascularization. *Ophthalmology.* 1999;106:2,063–2,067
40. Yoshida T, Ohno-Matsui K, Ohtake Y, et al. Myopic choroidal neovascularization: A 10-year follow-up. *Ophthalmology.* 2003;110(7):1,297–1,305.
41. Yoshida T, Ohno-Matsui K, Ohtake Y, et al. Long-term visual prognosis of choroidal neovascularization in high myopia: A comparison between age groups. *Ophthalmology.* 2002;109(4):712–719.
42. Jalkh AE, Weiter JJ, Trempe CL, et al. Choroidal neovascularization in degenerative myopia: role of laser photocoagulation. *Ophthalmic Surg.* 1987;18:721–725.
43. Johnson DA, Yannuzzi LA, Shakin JL, et al. Lacquer cracks following laser treatment of choroidal neovascularization in pathologic myopia. *Retina.* 1998;18:118–124.
44. Verteporfin in Photodynamic Therapy (VIP) Study Group. Photodynamic therapy of subfoveal choroidal neovascularization in pathologic myopia with verteporfin: 1-year results of a randomized clinical trial—VIP report 1. *Ophthalmology.* 2001;108:841–852.
45. Verteporfin in Photodynamic Therapy (VIP) Study Group. Verteporfin therapy of subfoveal choroidal neovascularization in pathologic myopia: 2-year results of a randomized clinical trial—VIP report no. 3. *Ophthalmology.* 2003;110(4):667–673.
46. Bottoni F, Airaghi P, Perego E, et al. Surgical removal of idiopathic, myopic and age-related subfoveal neovascularization. *Graefes Arch Clin Exp Ophthalmol.* 1996;234:542–550.
47. Clarkson JG, Altman RD. Angioid streaks. *Surv Ophthalmol.* 1982;26:235–246.
48. Haruyama M, Yuzawa M. Utility of laser photocoagulation of choroidal neovascularization in angioid streaks. *Jpn J Ophthalmol.* 2003;47(6):625.
49. Gelisken O, Hendrikse F, Deutman AF. A long-term follow-up study of laser coagulation of neovascular membranes in angioid streaks. *Am J Ophthalmol.* 1988;105:299–303.
50. Lim JI, Bressler NM, Marsh MJ, et al. Laser treatment of choroidal neovascularization in patients with angioid streaks. *Am J Ophthalmol.* 1993;116:414–423.
51. Pece A, Avanza P, Galli L, et al. Laser photocoagulation of choroidal neovascularization in angioid streaks. *Retina.* 1997;17:12–16.
52. Sickenberg M, Schmidt-Erfurth U, Miller JW, et al. A preliminary study of photodynamic therapy using verteporfin for choroidal neovascularization in pathologic myopia, ocular histoplasmosis syndrome, angioid streaks, and idiopathic causes. *Arch Ophthalmol.* 2000;117:327–336.
53. Costa RA, Calucci D, Cardillo JA, et al. Selective occlusion of subfoveal choroidal neovascularization in angioid streaks by using a new technique of ingrowth site treatment. *Ophthalmology.* 2003;110(6):1,192–1,203.
54. Fujii GY, Humayun MS, Pieramici DJ, et al. Initial experience of inferior limited macular translocation for subfoveal choroidal neovascularization resulting from causes other than age-related macular degeneration. *Am J Ophthalmol.* 2001;131:90–100.
55. Dreyer RF, Gass DJ. Multifocal choroiditis and panuveitis. A syndrome that mimics ocular histoplasmosis. *Arch Ophthalmol.* 1984;102:1,776–1,784.
56. Hershey JM, Pulido LM, Rosenberg MA. Non-caseating conjunctival granulomas in patients with multifocal choroiditis and panuveitis. *Ophthalmology.* 1994;101:569–601.
57. Brown J, Reddy CV, Kimura AE, et al. Long term visual prognosis of multifocal choroiditis, punctate inner choroidopathy and the diffuse subretinal fibrosis syndrome. *Ophthalmology.* 1996;103:1,100–1,105.
58. Khorram KD, Jampol LM, Rosenberg MA. Blind spot enlargement as a manifestation of multifocal choroiditis. *Arch Ophthalmol.* 1991;109:1,403–1,407.
59. Reddy CV, Brown J, Folk JC, et al. Enlargement of the blindspot in chorioretinal inflammatory diseases. *Ophthalmology.* 1996;103:606–617.
60. Morgan CM, Schatz H. Recurrent multifocal choroiditis. *Ophthalmology.* 1986;93:1,138–1,147.
61. Spaide RF, Freund KB, Slakter J, et al. Treatment of subfoveal choroidal neovascularization associated with multifocal choroiditis and panuveitis with photodynamic therapy. *Retina.* 2002;22:545–549.
62. Wachtlin J, Heimann H, Behme T, et al. Long-term results after photodynamic therapy with verteporfin for choroidal neovascularizations secondary to inflammatory chorioretinal diseases. *Graefes Arch Clin Exp Ophthalmol.* 2003;241(11):899–906.
63. Brindeau C, Glacet-Bernard A, Coscas F, et al. Surgical removal of subfoveal choroidal neovascularization: visual outcome and prognostic value of fluorescein angiography and optical coherence tomography. *Eur J Ophthalmol.* 2001;11(3):287–95.
64. Schatz H, Maumenee AE, Patz A. Geographic helicoid peripapillary choroidopathy: clinical presentation and fluorescein angiographic findings. *Trans Am Acad Ophthalmol Otolaryngol.* 1974;78:747–761.
65. Franceschetti A. A curious affection of the fundus oculi: helicoid peripapillar chorioretinal degeneration. Its relation to pigmentary paravenous chorioretinal degeneration. *Doc Ophthalmol.* 1962;16:81–110.
66. Laatikainen L, Erkkila H. A follow-up study on serpiginous choroiditis. *Acta Opthalmol.* 1981;59:707–718.
67. Mansour AM, Jampol LM, Packo KH, et al. Macular serpiginous choroiditis. *Retina.* 1988;8:125–131.
68. Jampol LM, Orth D, Daily MJ, et al. Subretinal neovascularization with geographic (serpiginous) choroiditis. *Am J Ophthalmol.* 1979;88:683–689.
69. Wu JS, Lewis H, Fine SL, et al. Clinicopathologic findings in a patient with serpiginous choroiditis and treated choroidal neovascularization. *Retina.* 1989;9:292–301.
70. Hooper PL, Kaplan HJ. Triple agent immunosuppression in serpiginous choroiditis. *Ophthalmology.* 1990;97:109.
71. Akpek EK, Jabs DA, Tessler HH, et al. Successful treatment of serpiginous choroiditis with alkylating agents. *Ophthalmology.* 2002;109(8):1,506–1,513.

72. Priya K, Madhavan HN, Reiser BJ, et al. Association of herpesviruses in the aqueous humor of patients with serpiginous choroiditis: a polymerase chain reaction-based study. *Ocul Immunol Inflamm.* 2002;10(4):253–261.
73. Chisolm IH, Gass DJM, Hutton WL. The late stage of serpiginous (geographic) choroiditis. *Am J Ophthalmol.* 1976;82:343–351.
74. Navajas EV, Costa RA, Farah ME, et al. Indocyanine green-mediated photothrombosis combined with intravitreal triamcinolone for the treatment of choroidal neovascularization in serpiginous choroiditis. *Eye.* 2003;17(5):563–566.
75. Watzke RC, Packer AJ, Folk JC, et al. Punctate inner choroidopathy. *Am J Ophthalmol.* 1984;98:572–584.
76. Olsen TW, Capone A Jr, Sternberg P Jr, *et al.* Subfoveal choroidal neovascularization in punctate inner choroidopathy. Surgical management and pathologic findings. *Ophthalmology.* 1996;103:2,061–2,069.
77. Chatterjee S, Gibson JM. Photodynamic therapy: a treatment option in choroidal neovascularization secondary to punctate inner choroidopathy. *Br J Ophthalmol.* 2003;87(7):925–927.
78. Ho AC, Yannuzzi LA, Pisicano K, et al. The natural history of idiopathic subfoveal choroidal neovascularization. *Ophthalmology.* 1995;102:782–789.
79. Spaide RF, Martin ML, Slakter J, et al. Treatment of idiopathic subfoveal choroidal neovascular lesions using photodynamic therapy with verteporfin. *Am J Ophthalmol.* 2002;134(1):62–68.
80. Rogers AH, Duker JS, Nichols N, et al. Photodynamic therapy of idiopathic and inflammatory choroidal neovascularization in young adults. *Ophthalmology.* 2003;110(7):1,315–1,320.
81. Stern RM, Zakov ZN, Zegarra HZ, et al. Multiple recurrent serosanguinous retinal pigment epithelial detachments in Black women. *Am J Ophthalmol.* 1985;100:560–569.
82. Yannuzzi LA, Sorenson J, Spaide RF, et al. Idiopathic polypoidal choroidal vasculopathy (IPCV). *Retina.* 1990;10:1–8.
83. Ciardella AP, Donsoff IM, Huang SJ, et al. Polypoidal choroidal vasculopathy. *Surv Ophthalmol.* 2004;49(1):25–37.
84. Marano F, Deutman AF, Leys A, et al. Hereditary retinal dystrophies and choroidal neovascularization. *Graefes Arch Clin Exp Ophthalmol.* 2000;238(9):760–764.
85. Miller SA, Bresnick GH, Chandra SR. Choroidal neovascular membrane in Best's vitelliform macular dystrophy. *Am J Ophthalmol.* 1976;82(2):252–255.
86. Potter MJ, Szabo SM, Chan EY, et al. Photodynamic therapy of a subretinal neovascular membrane in type 2A idiopathic juxtafoveolar retinal telangiectasis. *Am J Ophthalmol.* 2002;133(1):149–151.
87. Harris MJ, Fine SL, Owens SL. Hemorrhagic complications of optic nerve drusen. *Am J Ophthalmol.* 1981;92:70–76.
88. Gragoudas ES, Regan CD. Peripapillary subretinal neovascularization in presumed sarcoidosis. *Arch Ophthalmol.* 1981;99:1,194–1,197.
89. Lertsumitkul S, Whitcup SM, Nussenblatt RB, et al. Subretinal fibrosis and choroidal neovascularization in Vogt-Koyanagi-Harada syndrome. *Graefes Arch Clin Exp Ophthalmol.* 1999;237(12):1,039–1,045.
90. Ober RR, Smith RE, Ryan SJ. Subretinal neovascularization in Vogt-Koyanagi-Harada syndrome. *Int Ophthalmol.* 1983;6:225–234.
91. Fine SL, Owens SL, Haller JA, et al. Choroidal neovascularization as a late complication of ocular toxoplasmosis. *Am J Ophthalmol.* 1981;91:318–322.
92. Holland GN. Ocular toxoplasmosis: a global reassessment: part II: disease manifestations and management. *Am J Ophthalmol.* 2004;137(1):1–17.
93. Gass JDM. New observations concerning choroidal osteomas. *Int Ophthalmol.* 1979;1:71–84.
94. Witschel H, Font RL. Hemangioma of the choroids. A clinicopathologic study of 71 cases and a review of the literature. *Surv Ophthalmol.* 1976;20:415–431.
95. Shields CL, Honavar SG, Shields JA, et al. Circumscribed choroidal hemangioma: Clinical manifestations and factors predictive of visual outcome in 200 consecutive cases. *Ophthalmology.* 2001;108(12):2,237–2,248.
96. Lubin JR, Gragoudas ES, Albert DM. Choroidal neovascularization associated with malignant melanoma: a case report. *Acta Ophthalmol (Copenh).* 1982;60(3):412–418.
97. Waltmann DD, Gitter KA, Yannuzzi LA, et al. Choroidal neovascularization associated with choroidal nevi. *Am J Ophthalmol.* 1978;85:704–710.
98. Gitter KA, Slusher M, Justice J Jr. Traumatic hemorrhagic detachment of retinal pigment epithelium. *Arch Ophthalmol.* 1968;79:729–732.
99. Smith RE, Kelley JS, Harbin TS. Late macular complications of choroidal ruptures. *Am J Ophthalmol.* 1974;77:650–58.
100. Higashide T, Sugiyama K. Optical coherence tomography characteristics of a hemorrhagic detachment of the retinal pigment epithelium after blunt trauma. *Am J Ophthalmol.* 2003;136(3):567–569.
101. Varley M, Frank E, Purnell EW. Subretinal neovascularization after focal argon laser for macular edema. *Ophthalmology.* 1988;95:567–573.

Fluorescein Angiography

9

J. Michael Jumper   Arthur D. Fu   H. Richard McDonald

Robert N. Johnson   Everett Ai

INTRODUCTION

Sodium fluorescein was first used as a research tool in ophthalmology soon after the molecule was synthesized by Baeyer in 1871 (1). Ninety years later, Novotny and Alvis introduced the concept of serial fundus photographs after intravenous injection of sodium fluorescein dye to study the retinal and choroidal circulation (2). Their initial observations were of diabetic and hypertensive patients, but it was not long before the utility of this novel technique was seen for age-related macular degeneration (AMD). While innovations in imaging systems and digital capture have occurred over the past four decades, the technique originally described remains largely unchanged. The true advances have been in image interpretation and clinicopathologic correlation. This chapter focuses on the application of the powerful tool of fluorescein angiography (FA) to AMD; the classification system that has developed as a result of detailed observations and the findings of clinical trials, which have used FA in directing treatment and retreatment of choroidal neovascularization (CNV).

FA PRINCIPLES AND TECHNIQUES

FA represents an application of the physical phenomenon of luminescence: light emission after atomic or molecular excitation by non-thermal radiation (3). After exposure to photic energy, free electrons in an excited state can emit energy in the form of light as they return to a lower energy state. The afterglow of luminescence represents a slower decay of an atom or molecule from its higher to lower energy state. Fluorescence represents luminescence with a near instantaneous decay rate, such that no afterglow is apparent.

Sodium fluorescein ($C_{20}H_{12}O_5Na$) is a hydrocarbon that emits green-yellow light of wavelength 520 nm to 530 nm after excitation with blue light of wavelength 465 nm to 490 nm. Because these frequencies are within the visible spectrum of light, conventional photographic devices and techniques are able to capture angiographic images. This small molecule with a weight of 376.27 Daltons—compared to 775 Daltons for indocyanine green (ICG)—readily diffuses through the fenestrated vessels of the choriocapillaris, but does not cross the intercellular tight junctions between retinal pigment epithelium (RPE) or retinal vascular endothelium (RVE). Thus, any condition that compromises the intact blood-retinal barrier, obstructs blood flow, or changes the normal pigmentation of the retina or pigment epithelium can cause abnormalities on angiography. FA has added the dimension of physiology to the clinical study of the fundus (4).

Maximal fluorescence of sodium fluorescein occurs at a pH of 7.4, ideal for human blood (3). It is relatively inert, making intravenous injection safe and severe adverse reactions rare (5). When mixed with human blood, fluorescein becomes 80% bound to plasma proteins (compared to near total binding of ICG to serum globulins). Such binding leaves fewer free electrons to fluoresce, thus requiring greater volumes of sodium fluorescein to be injected and brighter illumination necessary than if no plasma binding occurred.

The first angiography system developed by Novotny and Alvis was a modification of a Zeiss fundus camera (2). The authors note in their original article that the main limitation of this prototype was the flash apparatus causing a

12-second delay between photographs. Initial advances in the angiography system included modifications of the power pack and flash unit, dual camera backs for ease in performing color fundus photography and FA, a motor drive for rapid and motionless film advancement, and a stereo separator for stereophotography (6).

More recently, digital image capture systems have gained in popularity (7). Advantages of such systems include immediate image processing compared to the development time of film, and ease in file storage, transfer, and incorporation into electronic medical record systems. Physicians are able to make immediate treatment decisions, and the photographer is able to assess the quality of the study as it is ongoing, allowing immediate feedback and training that is more rapid. Newer digital systems are of comparable on-screen image quality to film angiography. Variability of digital print quality may not allow adequate assessment of printed digital images. While the capture of stereoscopic images is identical to film angiography, viewing of stereo pairs is more difficult, which has led to the development of devices for on-screen stereo viewing (8). Most large, multicenter treatment trials for AMD have used film angiography, and no study has directly compared the two photographic systems in determining neovascular lesion composition and size (9).

Scanning laser ophthalmoscopy has also been modified to perform FA (10). By using argon and infrared laser illumination, high temporal and spatial resolution can be achieved using low light intensity, even through a small pupil or with media opacity. In addition, dual wavelength imaging can be performed, allowing simultaneous FA and ICG angiography (11).

In the Macular Photocoagulation Study (MPS), Treatment of AMD with Photodynamic Therapy (TAP) Study, and the Verteporfin in Photodynamic Therapy (VIP) Study, similar angiographic protocols were used, including early-, mid-, and late-phase 30-degree film stereophotos centered on the macula after rapid (less than 6 seconds) injection of 5 ml of 10% of sodium fluorescein solution (9,12). Stereoscopic FA is superior to nonstereoscopic angiography in determining the presence, location, and extent of CNV (13). Similar protocols have been advocated in the office management of AMD (14). A standardized photographic plan should be used to ensure maximal capture of angiographic information and to facilitate a thorough interpretation. First, stereo color and red-free photographs are taken of the macula. After fluorescein injection, angiophotography commences in 10 to 12 seconds. Six rapid sequence photos are taken of the primary macula during the filling phase (6). This is followed by a stereo pair of the primary macula at approximately 30, 40, 60, 90, and 180 seconds post-injection. Late stereophotos are taken between 5 and 10 minutes post-injection (15).

When indicated, the angiogram should be expeditiously performed and interpreted by a physician experienced in the diagnosis and treatment of neovascular AMD (16). In the MPS, the FA used for treatment was obtained not greater than 72 to 96 hours prior to treatment (15). Based on findings of the TAP study, treatment for subfoveal CNV with verteporfin photodynamic therapy (PDT) should be performed within a week. In grading the FA, the distance of the neovascular lesion to the center of the fovea, the membrane size, and leakage characteristics are noted using a stereo viewer. For film angiography, a reticule measurement divided by the camera magnification factor is used to measure the lesion dimensions. Many digital angiography systems contain measurement software for exact measurements and automatic conversion for different camera settings. An enlarged early- or mid-frame FA image is invaluable during thermal laser treatment to ensure adequate coverage of the CNV. This can be achieved using a microfilm reader, angiogram projector, or a digital display in the laser treatment suite.

The patient should be properly informed of the rare but potentially serious risks of FA (5,17). Any facility that performs FA should be equipped with a proper resuscitation kit and have in place a care plan and adequately trained personnel in the event of an adverse reaction (6).

FA INTERPRETATION

AMD represents a retinal disease in which all of the various abnormal FA patterns can be observed (Fig. 9.1). These angiographic abnormalities are broadly classified as those leading to abnormally increased fluorescence (hyperfluorescence) or decreased fluorescence (hypofluorescence) (18). Hypofluorescence either represents blocked fluorescence or a vascular filling defect. As it pertains to AMD, blocked fluorescence is typically due to intraretinal/subretinal/sub-pigment epithelial hemorrhage or pigment proliferation/clumping. In advanced non-neovascular AMD, hypofluorescence can develop from choroidal vascular atrophy and retinal vascular occlusion can occur after thermal laser or verteporfin PDT.

Hyperfluorescence in AMD can be the result of loss of the normal barrier to background choroidal fluorescence known as transmitted fluorescence. Examples include hard drusen, nongeographic atrophy (non-GA) of the RPE in which abnormal background fluorescence fades during the course of the study (window defect), and geographic atrophy (GA) of the RPE in which atrophy of the choriocapillaris reveals the staining of the underlying sclera (19). Leakage of dye into a confined space is characterized by progressive, uniform hyperfluorescence known as pooling, which can be seen with soft drusen and serous RPE detachment. Abnormal blood vessels are noteworthy for their lack of intercellular tight junctions allowing permeability to fluorescein. CNV and intraretinal neovascularization in AMD lead to early and progressive hyperfluorescence with late leakage.

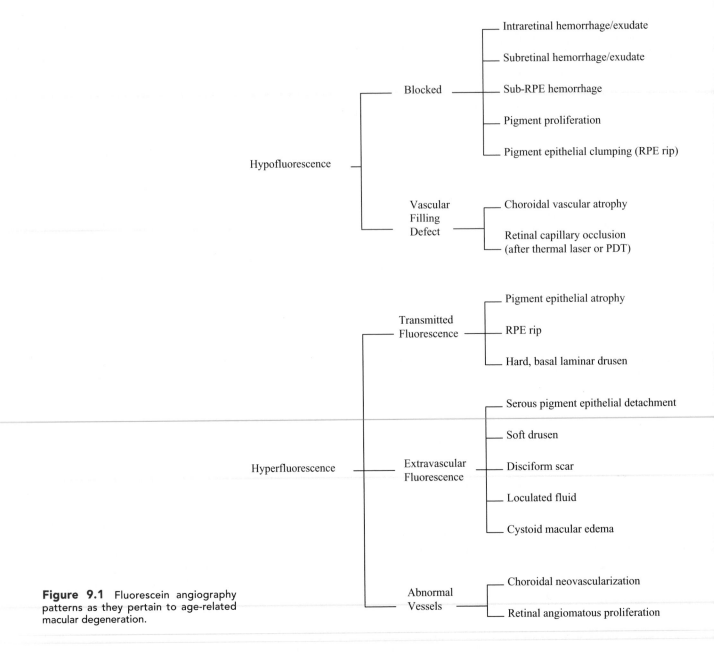

Figure 9.1 Fluorescein angiography patterns as they pertain to age-related macular degeneration.

INDICATIONS FOR FA IN AMD

While FA is an integral part in the care process of AMD, it does not replace history and careful ophthalmic examination in assessing a patient, and it is not indicated in all patients or at each visit (16). FA is indicated for any patient with AMD and vision loss, metamorphopsia, or new scotoma in which CNV is suspected (20–22). Because not all patients with neovascular AMD are symptomatic, those at high risk for developing CNV should be carefully examined for signs of such changes (23). While stereoscopic slit lamp ophthalmoscopy can usually detect evidence of CNV (including subretinal fluid, hard exudate, blood, pigment epithelial elevation, or a gray-green membrane), angiography is needed to detect the size, exact location, and leakage characteristics of the lesion (24). CNV may be unde-

tectable by clinical examination alone. In patients with clinical signs of advanced non-neovascular AMD, FA may be helpful to assess for progression of pigment epithelial atrophy, particularly if vision changes are reported.

Because of the increasing incidence of AMD with age, elderly patients with media opacity that may limit careful macular examination, such as cataract or keratopathy, may benefit from FA (19). Angiography may reveal neovascular or non-neovascular changes that might alter the treatment recommendations or pre-operative counseling regarding cataract extraction or corneal transplantation.

FA is a crucial part of the postoperative assessment in patients with CNV who have undergone thermal laser photocoagulation or verteporfin PDT. FA has a greater sensitivity in detecting CNV and will reveal a significant percentage of recurrent lesions not suspected on clinical examination (25). With thermal laser, the initial postoperative FA is indicated between 2 and 4 weeks to confirm that the entire CNV lesion has been treated and is obliterated. If adequate treatment is present, repeat FA should be performed in 4 to 6 weeks followed by intervals at the discretion of the treating physician (16). Following verteporfin PDT, the best evidence suggests repeat FA should be performed at 3-month intervals with retreatment as indicated (26).

Over the past two decades, a great deal of effort and expense has gone into the study of new treatments for neovascular AMD. These studies could not be carried out without the ability of FA to objectively document treatment response. Ongoing trials with injected antiangiogenic drugs, non-verteporfin PDT, prophylactic laser to high risk non-neovascular AMD, transpupillary thermotherapy, radiation therapy, selective feeder vessel laser therapy, serum apheresis, submacular surgery, and macular translocation all include FA in their pretreatment and post-treatment protocol. At this time, there is insufficient data to direct the use of FA after these unproven treatments (16).

ANGIOGRAPHIC PATTERNS IN AMD

Non-Neovascular AMD

The majority of patients with AMD have the non-neovascular form, which consists of drusen and RPE abnormalities. Several types of drusen exist that differ histopathologically and angiographically. Hard drusen are small ($= 63\ \mu m$), round discrete deposits on ophthalmoscopy that correspond to lipidized RPE or accumulation of

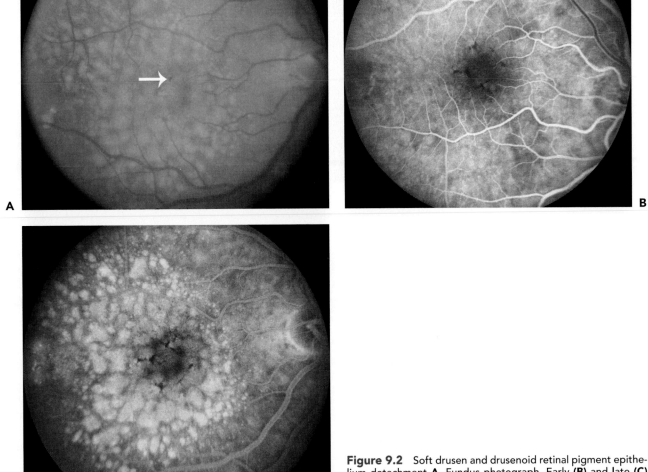

Figure 9.2 Soft drusen and drusenoid retinal pigment epithelium detachment **A.** Fundus photograph. Early **(B)** and late **(C)** angiogram demonstrating progressive hyperfluorescence from dye pooling. Arrow indicates an area of focal hyperpigmentation.

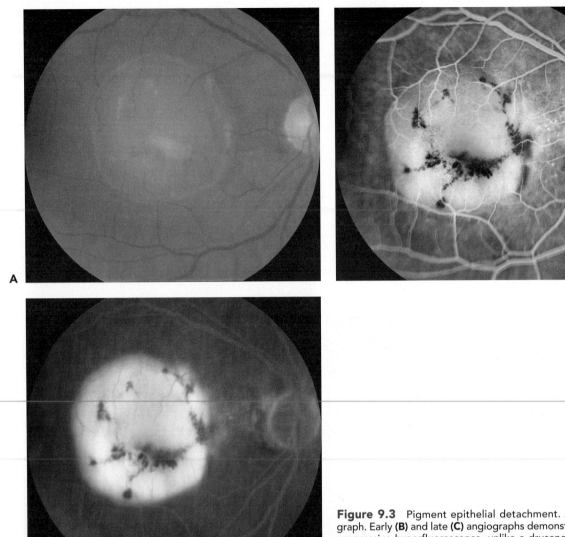

Figure 9.3 Pigment epithelial detachment. **A.** Fundus photograph. Early **(B)** and late **(C)** angiographs demonstrating the uniform progressive hyperfluorescence, unlike a drusenoid retinal pigment epithelial detachment, which is less fluorescent and stains faintly in the late phases of the study (see Figure 9.2).

hyaline material in the inner and outer collagenous zones of Bruch's membrane (27). With FA, hard drusen typically appear as transmission defects due to overlying RPE thinning or depigmentation (28). Angiography often reveals a greater number of hard drusen than can be seen clinically (13).

Soft drusen are larger (>63 μm) with irregular, poorly defined borders and the propensity to coalesce and become confluent. FA of soft drusen shows progressive hyperfluorescence and dye pooling without leakage beyond its margin (Fig. 9.2). Histopathologically, soft drusen are localized detachment between the RPE and 1) basal laminar deposit in an eye with diffuse basal laminar deposit, 2) basal linear deposit in an eye with diffuse basal linear deposit, or 3) localized accumulation of basal linear deposit in an eye without diffuse basal linear deposit (27,29,30). Studies have also identified vascularization of soft drusen, which may account for a component of the hyperfluorescence (28). When soft drusen coalesce, the

resulting irregular, shallow elevation of the RPE is referred to as drusenoid RPE detachment (29). Unlike a serous RPE detachment, where FA staining uniformly increases during the study and remains bright in the late phases, drusenoid RPE detachment is less fluorescent and either stain faintly or fade in the late phases of the study (19) (Figs. 9.2 and 9.3).

Basal laminar drusen represent angiographically and histologically distinct deposits, which appear as innumerable, small, round, semi-translucent, yellow lesions on fundus biomicroscopy. FA reveals early, discrete hyperfluorescence and late fading that has been described as "stars-in-the-sky"(31) (Fig. 9.4). Histopathology reveals basal laminar drusen to be nodularity of a diffusely thickened inner Bruch's membrane (31).

In addition to drusen, non-neovascular AMD is defined by the presence of RPE abnormalities, including hyperpigmentation, non-GA, and GA. All forms of RPE change may be present in the same eye over time or

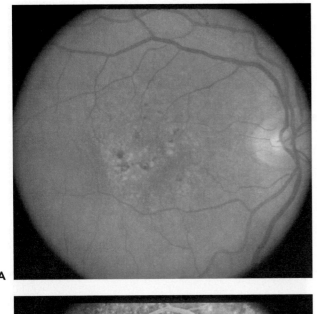

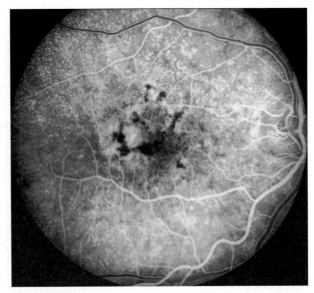

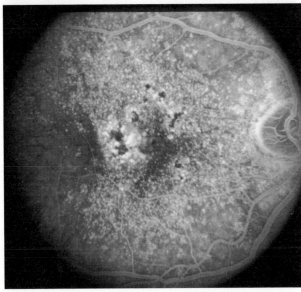

Figure 9.4 Basal laminar drusen. **A.** Fundus photograph shows innumerable, small, round, semitranslucent, yellow lesions. **B.** Fluorescein angiography reveals early, discrete hyperfluorescence. **C.** Late fading that has been described as "stars-in-the-sky."

simultaneously. Focal hyperpigmentation appears as a blocked fluorescence on FA and is characterized histopathologically by focal RPE hypertrophy and pigment migration into the subretinal space and outer retina (28). Focal hyperpigmentation is often associated with soft drusen, geographic atrophy, or neovascular AMD, but may appear alone (Fig. 9.2).

RPE atrophy is a common feature in AMD and has been documented to replace regressed drusen or follow collapse of a serous RPE detachment (27,32). Non-GA and GA share the common histopathologic feature of RPE loss. However, in GA, this loss is more extensive and there is associated atrophy of the overlying retina and underlying choriocapillaris leading to the difference in fluorescein appearance (Fig. 9.5). Non-GA typically appears as mottled early hyperfluorescence, which fades late consistent with window defect. Conversely, GA does not hyperfluoresce early because of the loss of underlying choriocapil-

laris; only larger choroidal vessels are apparent. Late in the FA, well-defined hyperfluorescence from staining of the exposed deep choroid and sclera is apparent (19).

NEOVASCULAR AMD

The term neovascular AMD refers to the presence of abnormal blood vessels, serous or hemorrhagic detachment of the pigment epithelium, lipid exudation, subretinal fibrosis, or disciform scar formation. The growth of abnormal blood vessels from the choroid into Bruch's membrane, as well as under and into the neurosensory retina, is known as CNV and accounts for the majority of severe vision loss in AMD. Angiographic classification by the MPS of CNV into classic and occult patterns has formed the basis of our understanding of the natural history and defined our treatment of AMD. The interpretation of CNV evolved during

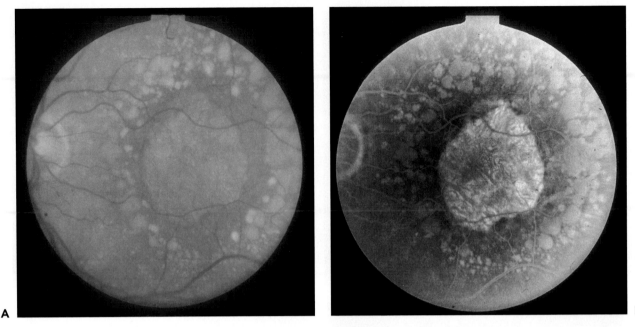

Figure 9.5 Geographic atrophy of the retinal pigment epithelium (RPE). **A.** Fundus photograph demonstrating loss of RPE with sharp borders and surrounding large drusen. **B.** Angiograph reveals well-defined hyperfluorescence from staining of the exposed deep choroid and sclera.

the course of the MPS and later investigations into the system described below. The MPS has defined the term lesion component as the area of the retina containing CNV or interfering with the ability to define the boundaries of CNV. A neovascular lesion represents the entire complex of lesion components and may include the CNV and the features that block the view of the boundaries (33).

Classic CNV is typically brightly hyperfluorescent in the early phase of the angiogram, corresponding to choroidal filling. Initially, the boundaries are well demarcated, allowing the clinician to accurately determine the location of the lesion and the distance from the lesion border to the center of the foveal avascular zone. Occasionally, the capillaries of the CNV are apparent as a lacy cartwheel network in the early phase. Because the new vessels leak, progressive hyperfluorescence and blurring of the lesion edge continues during the course of the FA (Fig. 9.6). This leakage may pool in the subretinal

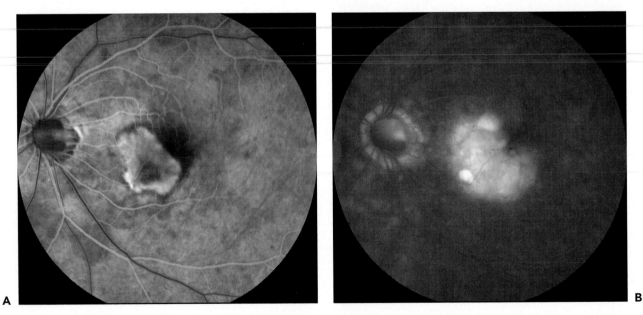

Figure 9.6 Classic choroidal neovascularization. Early **(A)** and late **(B)** angiographs showing early well-demarcated hyperfluorescence with late leakage.

space if a neurosensory retinal detachment is present, or may collect in the outer plexiform layer in the form of cystic retinal edema. When dye pooling is well demarcated in a confined space of a localized sensory retinal detachment or within intraretinal cystic spaces, it has been termed loculated fluid (34). Loculated fluid was a common finding in patients with new subfoveal CNV in the MPS and may confuse the treating physician as to the boundary of the lesion. A variant of classic CNV has been described in which new vessel filling is slower and the boundaries are not distinguished until approximately 2 minutes after dye injection. Despite a slow fill, the boundaries present initially correspond to the area of leakage in the late frames (15). Classic CNV has been further categorized based on location with respect to the fovea: 1) extrafoveal CNV is greater than 200 μm from the foveal center, 2) juxtafoveal CNV is located between 1 and 199 μm from the foveal center, and 3) subfoveal CNV is located under the center of the fovea. In the TAP and VIP studies, lesion component proportions were further delineated. A neovascular lesion in which the classic CNV component is greater than 50% of the total lesion size is defined as predominately classic. Lesions in which the classic CNV component comprises less than 50% of the total area are referred to as minimally classic (9).

Occult CNV is that which is not classic and has been categorized as fibrovascular pigment epithelial detachment (FVPED) or late leakage of undetermined source (33). FVPED is defined as an irregular elevation of the RPE detected on stereoangiography associated with stippled hyperfluorescence apparent 1 to 2 minutes after fluorescein injection and ill-defined staining or leakage in the late frames (Fig. 9.7). FVPED differs from classic CNV in

that the early hyperfluorescence is not as discreet or as bright and the boundaries usually remain indeterminate. In addition, the smooth RPE elevation, uniform progressive hyperfluorescence, and late, well-demarcated pooling of a classic, serous PED should not be confused with FVPED. Occult CNV with late leakage of undetermined source lacks a discernible, well-demarcated area of leakage in the early frames of the FA. Speckled hyperfluorescence with no visible source becomes apparent 2 to 5 minutes after dye injection and later pools in the overlying subretinal space (Fig. 9.8). This differs from the slow-filling variant of classic CNV in that the leakage source is never apparent.

Aside from drusenoid PED and the FVPED form of occult CNV discussed previously, other forms of PED exist in AMD, including serous and hemorrhagic PED. Serous PED may or may not be associated with CNV. Typically, serous PED is easily seen on fundus biomicroscopy as a round or oval translucent elevation of the RPE. Early arteriovenous phase of the angiogram reveals progressive, uniform hyperfluorescence with late, intense pooling of fluorescein. The progression of hyperfluorescence (often described as "turning up a rheostat") reflects the rapid movement of fluorescein across Bruch's membrane into the sub-RPE space (6) (Fig. 9.3). A notch in the otherwise smooth border of a serous PED may be an indication of CNV. A hemorrhagic PED is easily differentiated from serous PED on clinical examination. The translucence of serous fluid is replaced by a dark, reddish-brown mass. While hemorrhagic PED can appear clinically similar to uveal melanoma, the blood blocks normal choroidal and CNV-associated fluorescence unlike the punctate hyperfluorescence of the intrinsic circulation of melanoma.

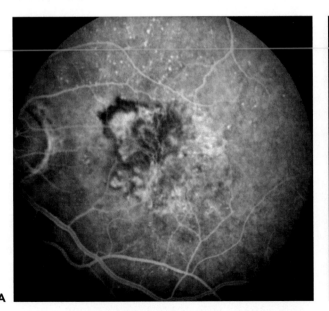

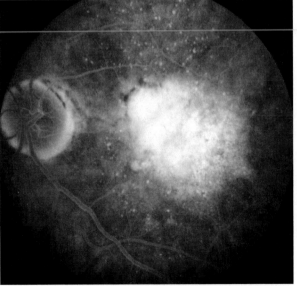

A   B

Figure 9.7 Mid **(A)** and late **(B)** angiogram of occult choroidal neovascularization in the form of fibrovascular pigment epithelial detachment. There is stippled hyperfluorescence apparent 1 to 2 minutes after fluorescein injection with ill-defined leakage in the late frames.

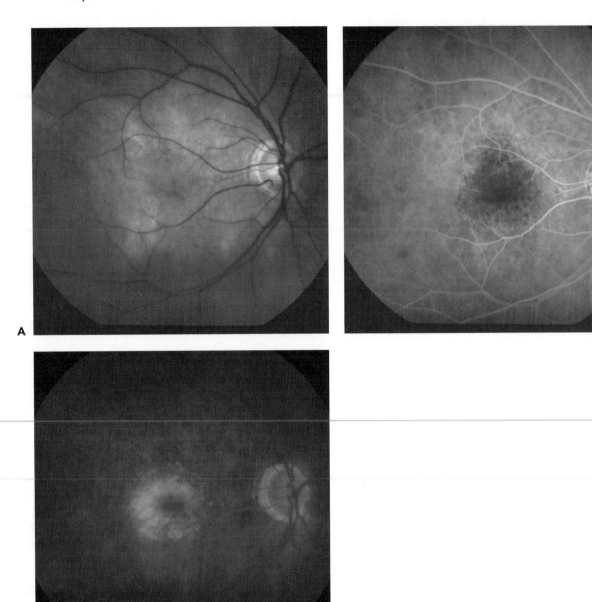

Figure 9.8 Occult choroidal neovascularization in the pattern of late leakage of undetermined source. **A.** Fundus photograph. **B.** Early frame angiograph demonstrating no apparent leakage source. **C.** Late frames reveal leakage into the subretinal space.

Furthermore, the standardized ultrasonographic patterns of the two lesions differ.

Lesion components associated with neovascular AMD that can obscure the boundaries of CNV include changes that block fluorescence, such as blood, fibrous tissue, RPE hyperplasia, or RPE redundancy (from an RPE tear). Alternatively, CNV can be obscured by greater fluorescence from staining fibrous tissue or a serous PED. When contiguous with CNV, such lesions can make it impossible to determine the exact boundary of the CNV and are referred to as components of the lesion. As such, they are included in the laser treatment plan unless otherwise indicated.

OTHER CNV PATTERNS IN AMD

Disciform scar represents the evolution of CNV and is comprised of variable amounts of active CNV as well as fibrovascular and cellular proliferation. The color varies from white to yellow to brown depending on the amount of fibrous tissue, RPE hyperplasia, blood, and lipid exudate present. Variable amounts of serous retinal detachment may be associated with disciform scar. Angiography, while not typically indicated at this stage of the disease, reveals blockage from RPE hyperplasia and blood, staining of the fibrous component and leakage of the active CNV component, if present (Fig. 9.9).

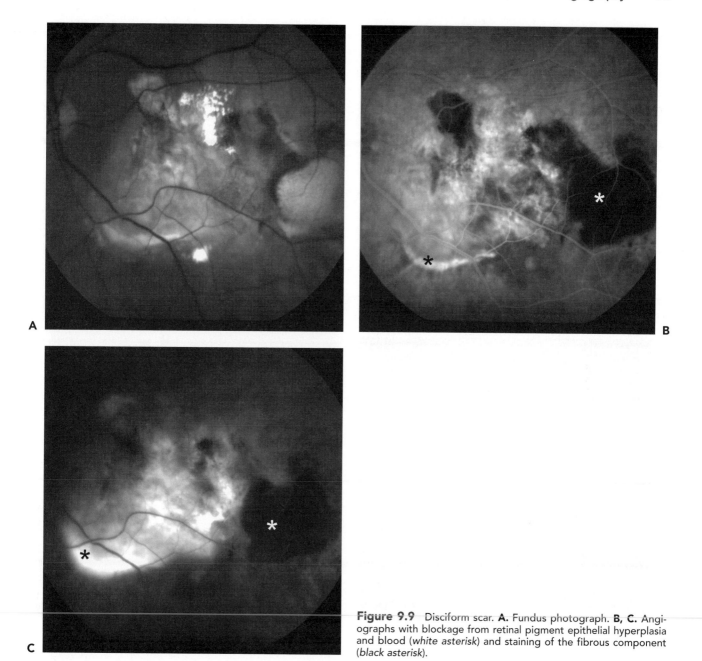

Figure 9.9 Disciform scar. **A.** Fundus photograph. **B, C.** Angiographs with blockage from retinal pigment epithelial hyperplasia and blood (*white asterisk*) and staining of the fibrous component (*black asterisk*).

Like hemorrhagic PED, FA is helpful in differentiating an atypical, dark disciform scar from an uveal melanoma. A common vascular change that occurs during the disciform scar process is a retinal-choroidal anastomosis, in which CNV communicates with the retinal circulation (30).

Recently, a distinct form of neovascular AMD referred to as retinal angiomatous proliferation (RAP) has been described in which the vasogenic process originates in the retina (35,36). Yannuzzi et al. have proposed that formation of RAP begins as intraretinal neovascularization, which progresses to subretinal neovascularization and finally an anastomosis to CNV (Fig 9.10). They describe

the formation of a retinal-retinal anastomosis in some cases. Stereo FA of early RAP lesions revealed intraretinal hyperfluorescence most commonly defined as occult. As the neovascularization process involves the subretinal space, a serous PED commonly developed which finally becomes vascularized. In their series, the authors state that this form of neovascular AMD was found almost exclusively in whites, with a female to male ratio of 3:1. While the different stages they describe were difficult to differentiate by examination and angiography, ICG was helpful in making the diagnosis.

With neovascular AMD, a tear in the RPE can occur spontaneously, as a result of thermal laser photocoagulation or

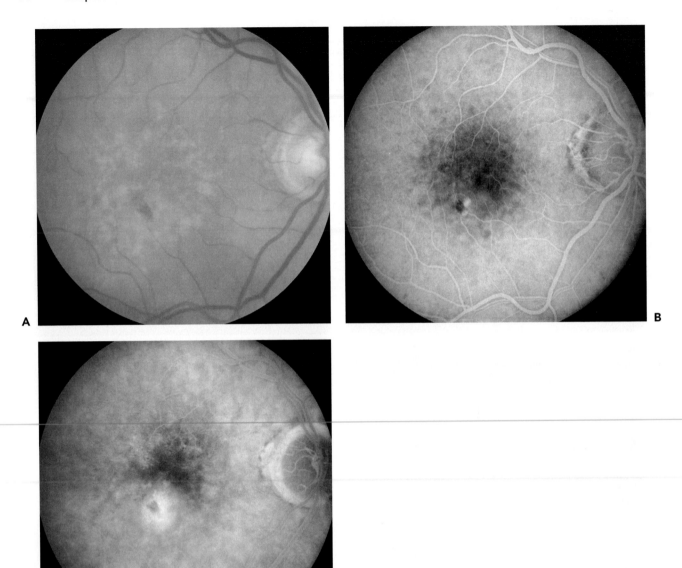

Figure 9.10   Retinal angiomatous proliferation. **A.** Fundus photograph reveals intraretinal hemorrhage and new vessels. Early **(B)** and late **(C)** angiography reveals progressive intraretinal hyperfluorescence.

after verteporfin PDT (37–39). Gass has hypothesized that serous PED adjacent to FVPED tears at a point opposite the fibrovascular change and retracts toward the fibrovascular mound (40). His theory explains the uneven hyperfluorescence and distribution of drusen (not evident in the serous PED portion of the lesion) noted prior to RPE rip. The unique angiographic appearance after RPE rip includes early hyperfluorescence with late staining in the area of absent pigmented RPE and hypofluorescence with stippled hyperfluorescent staining in the area of redundant RPE and fibrovascular tissue (Fig. 9.11). Gass explains that the reason the denuded Bruch's membrane does not leak fluorescein into the subretinal space is due to the growth of hypopigmented metaplastic RPE shortly after the tear occurs (40).

FA AFTER LASER TREATMENT

Thermal Laser Photocoagulation

Immediate effects of laser photocoagulation of CNV may include changes leading to hypofluorescence (retinal edema, temporary closure of retinal capillaries and choroidal vessels) and/or hyperfluorescence (thermal vasculitis of retinal and choroidal vessels). These immediate and variable changes usually stabilize by 2 to 4 weeks when the first postoperative FA is indicated. Features at the initial FA of a well-treated CNV membrane include early hypofluorescence in the area of treatment. Later frames may show areas of staining or leakage within the area of treatment and uniform staining at the periphery of the

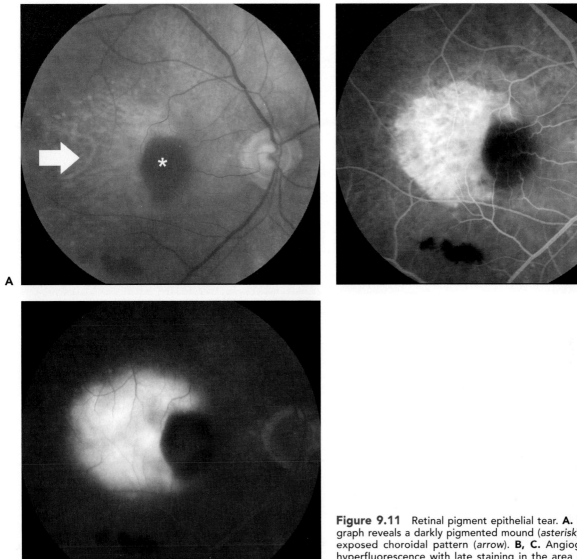

Figure 9.11 Retinal pigment epithelial tear. **A.** Fundus photograph reveals a darkly pigmented mound (*asterisk*) with adjacent exposed choroidal pattern (*arrow*). **B, C.** Angiography reveals hyperfluorescence with late staining in the area of absent pigmented retinal pigment epithelium (RPE) and hypofluorescence in the area of redundant RPE and fibrovascular tissue.

lesion (41). Persistence of CNV is defined by the MPS as leakage at the periphery of the laser treated area in the early (<6 weeks) postoperative FA and is considered inadequately treated original CNV tissue. CNV recurrence implies new fluorescein leakage contiguous to a previously treated lesion after (>6 weeks) initial FA showed no evidence of persistence. The leakage is present in the late frames of the study and is usually preceded by moderate hyperfluorescence in earlier frames (41) (Fig. 9.12).

In the MPS, a significant number of post-treatment angiograms could not be clearly interpreted as having recurrence or not (42). A category of questionable recurrence was defined as one of three angiographic patterns shown to carry a risk for developing recurrent CNV: 1) focal staining along the laser lesion edge, 2) new blocked fluorescence from hemorrhage, and 3) speckled hyperfluorescence beyond the edge of the laser lesion (42). Close

follow-up is warranted if any of these patterns are present in the postoperative period.

A large choroidal vessel leading to the CNV may be visible on FA. Such feeder vessels may be seen in untreated neovascular AMD, but are most commonly seen in recurrent CNV after thermal laser treatment. Feeder vessels are considered lesion components, which should be considered in the treatment plan (33).

Verteporfin PDT

In the TAP and VIP studies, follow-up angiograms were graded for evidence of leakage as: 1) progression of leakage—CNV beyond the area of baseline CNV, 2) moderate leakage—area of active CNV occupying = 50% of baseline CNV without progression, 3) minimal leakage—area of active CNV occupying <50% of baseline CNV, and 4)

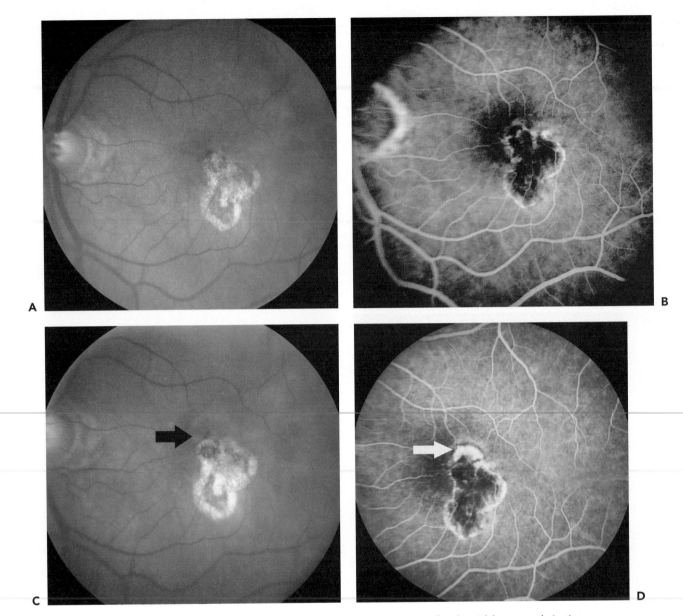

Figure 9.12 Angiographic patterns after thermal laser treatment for choroidal neovascularization (CNV). Photograph **(A)** and midphase angiograph **(B)** of well-treated CNV. There is uniform staining at the periphery of the lesion. Two months later **(C)**, new subretinal fluid is present (*arrow*) with midphase angiograph **(D)** demonstrating progressive hyperfluorescence at the margin of CNV recurrence (*arrow*).

absence of leakage—no active CNV within baseline CNV and no progression (43). Lesions with leakage at follow-up visits were considered for retreatment at 3-month intervals (9). After treatment, the ability to differentiate classic from occult CNV becomes increasingly difficult (Fig. 9.13). Regardless, lesions with any leakage were considered for treatment. More importantly, the ability to differentiate leakage from staining of various lesion components becomes increasingly difficult after treatment (9,44).

CONCLUSIONS

AMD remains a challenging disease to evaluate and treat. The ideal imaging study for this disease would be: (1) non-

invasive, (2) rapid, (3) safe, (4) inexpensive, (5) able to detect neovascular changes under pigmented lesions or serous PED, (6) able to differentiate neovascular from non-neovascular disease, and (7) able to differentiate active from inactive CNV. FA falls short of ideal because it requires an intravenous injection, has known (albeit minimal) risks, is limited in its ability to differentiate neovascular from other lesions, and to detect CNV margins due to obscuring lesions. Regardless, FA remains the gold standard in the diagnosis and treatment of neovascular AMD. More importantly, FA has been crucial in our understanding the pathophysiology of AMD.

Digital FA is replacing film angiography in clinical trials just as it largely has in practice. All new retinal imaging technologies must be compared to FA in efficacy and cost

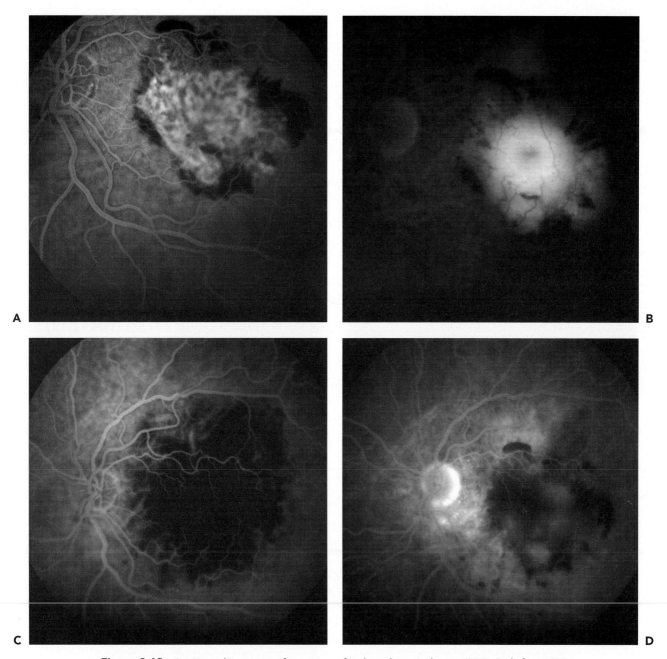

Figure 9.13 Angiographic pattern after verteporfin photodynamic therapy (PDT). Early-frame **(A)** and late-frame **(B)** angiographs of classic choroidal neovascularization before verteporfin PDT. One month after PDT, there is closure of the vessels in the early frames **(C)** with only mild staining within the original borders of the lesion in the late frames **(D)**.

(45). A combination of FA with ICG, optical coherence tomography, retinal thickness analysis, and/or confocal microscopy may, one day, be proven to improve the management of AMD. Yet-unpublished clinical trials may answer this question in the near future.

REFERENCES

1. Ehrlich P. Uber provicierte Fluoreszenzerscheinungen am Auge. *Dtsch Med Wschr.* 1882;8:8–21.
2. Novotny HR, Alvis DL. A method of photographing fluorescence in circulating blood in the human retina. *Circulation.* 1961;24:82–86.
3. Wolfe DR. Fluorescein angiography: basic science and engineering. *Ophthalmology.* 1986;93:1,617–1,620.
4. Norton EW. Doyne memorial lecture, 1981. Fluorescein angiography. Twenty years later. *Trans Ophthalmol Soc UK.* 1981;101(Pt2):229–233.
5. Yannuzzi LA, Rohrer KT, Tindel LJ, et al. Fluorescein angiography complication survey. *Ophthalmology.* 1986;93:611–617.
6. Johnson RN, Schatz H, McDonald HR, et al. Fluorescein angiography: basic principles and interpretation. In: Ryan SJ, Schachat AP, Eds. *Retina.* St. Louis: Mosby;875–942.
7. Friberg TR, Rehkopf PG, Warnicki JW, et al. Use of directly acquired digital fundus and fluorescein angiographic images in the diagnosis of retinal disease. *Retina.* 1987;7:246–251.
8. Klein ML, Steinkamp PN. Stereoscopic digital fluorescein and indocyanine green videoangiography. *Retina.* 1997;17:359–360.
9. Barbazetto I, Burdan A, Bressler NM, et al. Photodynamic therapy of subfoveal choroidal neovascularization with verteporfin: fluorescein angiographic guidelines for evaluation and treatment—TAP and VIP report No. 2. *Arch Ophthalmol.* 2003;121:1,253–1,268.
10. Gabel VP, Birngruber R, Nasemann J. [The scanning laser ophthalmoscope and its use as a fluorescein angiography instrument]. *Fortschr Ophthalmol.* 1988;85:569–573.
11. Bischoff PM, Niederberger HJ, Torok B, et al. Simultaneous indocyanine green and fluorescein angiography. *Retina.* 1995;15:91–99.

12. Macular Photocoagulation Study Group. *Manual of Procedures.* Baltimore: MPS Coordinating Center. US Dept of Commerce; 1991.

13. Bressler NM, Bressler SB, Fine SL. Age-related macular degeneration. *Surv Ophthalmol.* 1988;32:375–413.

14. Singerman LJ. Fluorescein angiography. Practical role in the office management of macular diseases. *Ophthalmology.* 1986;93:1,209–1,215.

15. Chamberlin JA, Bressler NM, Bressler SB, et al. The use of fundus photographs and fluorescein angiograms in the identification and treatment of choroidal neovascularization in the Macular Photocoagulation Study. The Macular Photocoagulation Study Group. *Ophthalmology.* 1989;96:1,526–1,534.

16. Chew EY, Benson WE, Boldt HC, et al. *Preferred Practice Patterns: Age-Related Macular Degeneration.* San Francisco: American Academy of Ophthalmology; 2003.

17. Kwiterovich KA, Maguire MG, Murphy RP, et al. Frequency of adverse systemic reactions after fluorescein angiography. Results of a prospective study. *Ophthalmology.* 1991;98:1,139–1,142.

18. Rabb MF, Burton TC, Schatz H, et al. Fluorescein angiography of the fundus: a schematic approach to interpretation. *Surv Ophthalmol.* 1978;22:387–403.

19. Pieramici DJ, Bressler SB. Fluorescein angiography. In: Berger JW, Fine SL, Maguire MG, ed. *Age-Related Macular Degeneration.* St. Louis: Mosby; 219–236.

20. Macular Photocoagulation Study Group. Laser photocoagulation of subfoveal neovascular lesions in age-related macular degeneration. Results of a randomized clinical trial. *Arch Ophthalmol.* 1991;109:1,220–1,231.

21. Macular Photocoagulation Study Group. Argon laser photocoagulation for neovascular maculopathy. Five-year results from randomized clinical trials. *Arch Ophthalmol.* 1991;109:1,109–1,114.

22. Macular Photocoagulation Study Group. Laser photocoagulation for juxtafoveal choroidal neovascularization. Five-year results from randomized clinical trials. *Arch Ophthalmol.* 1994;112:500–509.

23. Pieramici DJ, Bressler SB. Age-related macular degeneration and risk factors for the development of choroidal neovascularization in the fellow eye. *Curr Opin Ophthalmol.* 1998;9:38–46.

24. Wilkinson CP. The clinical examination. Limitation and over-utilization of angiographic services. *Ophthalmology.* 1986;93:401–404.

25. Sykes SO, Bressler NM, Maguire MG, et al. Detecting recurrent choroidal neovascularization. Comparison of clinical examination with and without fluorescein angiography. *Arch Ophthalmol.* 1994;112:1,561–1,566.

26. Bressler NM. Verteporfin therapy of subfoveal choroidal neovascularization in age-related macular degeneration: two-year results of a randomized clinical trial including lesions with occult with no classic choroidal neovascularization—verteporfin in photodynamic therapy report 2. *Am J Ophthalmol.* 2002;133:168–169.

27. Sarks SH. Council Lecture. Drusen and their relationship to senile macular degeneration. *Aust J Ophthalmol.* 1980;8:117–130.

28. Green WR, Key SN, III. Senile macular degeneration: a histopathologic study. *Trans Am Ophthalmol Soc.* 1977;75:180–254.

29. Bressler NM, Silva JC, Bressler SB, et al. Clinicopathologic correlation of drusen and retinal pigment epithelial abnormalities in age-related macular degeneration. *Retina.* 1994;14:130–142.

30. Green WR, McDonnell PJ, Yeo JH. Pathologic features of senile macular degeneration. *Ophthalmology.* 1985;92:615–627.

31. Gass JD, Jallow S, Davis B. Adult vitelliform macular detachment occurring in patients with basal laminar drusen. *Am J Ophthalmol.* 1985;99:445–459.

32. Meredith TA, Braley RE, Aaberg TM. Natural history of serous detachments of the retinal pigment epithelium. *Am J Ophthalmol.* 1979;88:643–651.

33. Macular Photocoagulation Study Group. Subfoveal neovascular lesions in age-related macular degeneration. Guidelines for evaluation and treatment in the macular photocoagulation study. *Arch Ophthalmol.* 1991;109:1,242–1,257.

34. Bressler NM, Bressler SB, Alexander J, et al. Loculated fluid. A previously undescribed fluorescein angiographic finding in choroidal neovascularization associated with macular degeneration. Macular Photocoagulation Study Reading Center. *Arch Ophthalmol.* 1991;109:211–215.

35. Hartnett ME, Weiter JJ, Staurenghi G, et al. Deep retinal vascular anomalous complexes in advanced age-related macular degeneration. *Ophthalmology.* 1996;103:2,042–2,053.

36. Yannuzzi LA, Negrao S, Iida T, et al. Retinal angiomatous proliferation in age-related macular degeneration. *Retina.* 2001;21:416–434.

37. Cantrill HL, Ramsay RC, Knobloch WH. Rips in the pigment epithelium. *Arch Ophthalmol.* 1983;101:1,074–1,079.

38. Decker WL, Sanborn GE, Ridley M, et al. Retinal pigment epithelial tears. *Ophthalmology.* 1983;90:507–512.

39. Gelisken F, Inhoffen W, Partsch M, et al. Retinal pigment epithelial tear after photodynamic therapy for choroidal neovascularization. *Am J Ophthalmol.* 2001;131:518–520.

40. Gass JD. Pathogenesis of tears of the retinal pigment epithelium. *Br J Ophthalmol.* 1984;68:513–519.

41. Macular Photocoagulation Study Group. Recurrent choroidal neovascularization after argon laser photocoagulation for neovascular maculopathy. *Arch Ophthalmol.* 1986;104:503–512.

42. Dyer DS, Brant AM, Schachat AP, et al. Angiographic features and outcome of questionable recurrent choroidal neovascularization. *Am J Ophthalmol.* 1995;120:497–505.

43. Treatment of Age-Related Macular Degeneration with Photodynamic Therapy (TAP) Study Group. Photodynamic therapy of subfoveal choroidal neovascularization in age-related macular degeneration with verteporfin: one-year results of 2 randomized clinical trials—TAP report 1. *Arch Ophthalmol.* 1999;117:1,329–1,345.

44. Kaiser RS, Berger JW, Williams GA, et al. Variability in fluorescein angiography interpretation for photodynamic therapy in age-related macular degeneration. *Retina.* 2002;22:683–690.

45. Bressler NM. Evaluating new retinal imaging techniques. *Arch Ophthalmol.* 1998;116:521–522.

Indocyanine Green Angiography

10

Lindsay M. Smithen   *Christina M. Klais*   *Chiara M. Eandi*
Michael D. Ober   *Antonio P. Ciardella*   *Jason S. Slakter*

Indocyanine green (ICG) angiography has rapidly emerged as an invaluable tool in the arsenal of ophthalmologists worldwide. It allows for visualization of choroidal pathology resulting in a diagnosis that is more accurate and a better characterization of chorioretinal disease. The applications of ICG angiography continue to grow in number; the full extent of its capabilities is not yet known.

HISTORY

Initially used in the photographic industry, ICG was introduced into medicine in 1957 (1). Its first applications in medicine were in the field of cardiology, specifically in measuring cardiac output. ICG was soon utilized as a method of measuring hepatic blood flow and function (2,3). The first angiogram from ICG was performed on the carotids (4).

In 1972, Flower and Hochheimer applied ICG angiography to ophthalmology (5,6). They performed intravenous absorption ICG angiography to view the choroidal circulation. However, the film and associated technology at the time were not sensitive enough to allow for adequate capture of the low-intensity ICG fluorescence. In 1976, Orth et al. used a movie camera to record the angiographic images, but the camera did not permit visualization of the fundus during the exam (7).

Improvements in technology in the ensuing years contributed to acceptance of ICG as an important diagnostic tool. Hayashi et al. improved the quality of filter combinations that screen out all but the desired wavelengths of light. Videoangiography, a technique that employs an infrared-sensitive camera to record images on a videocassette, was introduced (8–10). Angiography was better than the infrared film at the time, but it was still limited by resolution. Scheider and Schroedel later utilized a scanning laser ophthalmoscope (SLO) in ICG videoangiography (11), further enhancing the diagnostic capabilities of the exam. In 1992, Guyer et al. (12) and Yannuzzi et al. (13) introduced a new more affordable and marketable digital imaging system based upon high-resolution ICG images. This new system allowed ICG angiography to achieve clinical practicality (14).

ICG

Chemical Properties

ICG is a sterile, water-soluble tricarbocyanine dye with the empirical formula $C_{43}H_{47}N_2NaO_6S_2$ and a molecular weight of 775 Daltons. Chemically, it is known as an anhydro-3,3,3′,3′-tetramethyl–1-1′-di-(4-sulfobutyl)-4,5,4′,5′-dibenzoindotricarbocyanine hydroxy sodium salt (15) with both lipophilic and hydrophilic characteristics.

ICG is the product of a complex, synthetic process. Sodium iodine is incorporated to create an ICG lyophilisate that can then be dissolved in solvent. Once dissolved, ICG has a tendency toward aggregation at high concentration. It also aggregates when mixed in physiologic saline. Accordingly, ICG is supplied with prepared, sterile water at pH between 5.5 and 6.5. The aqueous ICG dye solution can decay at a rate of approximately 10% in 10 hours and should be used within this time period (16).

Optical Properties

When in solution with blood, ICG absorbs light from 650 nm to 850 nm, with peak absorption at 805 nm. Its emission spectrum ranges from 770 nm to 880 nm, peaking at 835 nm. Both the absorption and emission spectra are shifted towards shorter wavelengths when ICG is in an aqueous solution, while the overall intensity of the fluorescence is diminished.

Whereas fundus photography and fluorescein angiography (FA) do not provide images of the choroidal circulation, the physical characteristics of ICG allow for visualization of the choroid and associated abnormalities (17). ICG effectively penetrates normal ocular pigments, such as melanin and xanthophylls; the retinal pigment epithelium (RPE) and choroid absorb 21% to 38% of near-infrared light as compared with 59% to 75% of the blue-green light (500 nm) associated with fluorescein dye. Near-infrared light emission also allows visualization of the choroidal circulation and associated pathology through overlying hemorrhage, serous fluid, lipid, and pigment that may block the blue-green light used to excite fluorescein. Enhanced imaging of conditions, such as choroidal neovascularization (CNV) and pigment epithelial detachment (PED), is the result (2,18).

Pharmacokinetics

ICG is both lipophilic and hydrophilic, allowing it to bind to a number of molecules. In vivo, ICG is 98% protein bound. Although it was previously thought to bind strictly to serum albumin (19), it is now known that 80% of ICG molecules actually bind to globulins, such as A1-lipoprotein. Relatively small sodium fluorescein molecules remain mostly unbound from protein and easily leak out of the choriocapillaris vessels. ICG molecules, on the other hand, bind to serum proteins forming complexes that are too large to pass through the fenestrated capillary walls in the choroid. It is this property that gives ICG angiography an advantage over FA in highlighting choroidal vasculature (20).

Originally, it was thought that the protein-binding capacity of ICG limited it to travel within choroidal vessel walls. It has, however, been demonstrated that ICG dye diffuses through the choroidal stroma during angiography, accumulating within RPE cells. It diffuses slowly, however, staining the choroid within 12 minutes of injection.

ICG is excreted entirely by the liver (3). It is taken up by hepatic parenchymal cells and secreted, unchanged, into bile (21,22). As a result of strong binding to plasma proteins, ICG is not taken up by the kidney, lungs, or cerebrospinal fluid. It does not cross the placenta (23–25). The half-life of ICG is approximately 2 to 4 minutes.

Toxicity

ICG is a relatively safe dye; adverse reactions are rare, and are less common than with sodium fluorescein (26–30). Mild reactions, such as nausea, vomiting, and pruritus, occur in 0.15% of patients. There have been isolated reports of hypotensive shock, anaphylactic shock, and vasovagal-type reactions. There are two reported deaths from ICG administration during cardiac catheterization (16).

Sterile ICG manufactured in the United States contains small amounts of iodine and therefore should be used with caution in patients with iodine allergy. ICG should also be avoided in uremic patients and in those with hepatic disease. ICG is classified in pregnancy category C which means that it has not been shown to be harmful to the human fetus, but that there still exists reason for concern (31). Emergency equipment should always be on hand when ICG is administered.

Injection Technique

ICG should be dissolved in the aqueous solvent provided and should be used within 10 hours of preparation (16) (IC Green; Akorn, Inc., Buffalo Grove, Illinois). The standard concentration is 25 mg of ICG in 5 mL solvent (32). In patients with a poorly dilated pupil or those with a heavily pigmented fundus, the dose of ICG must be increased to 50 mg. For wide-angle angiography, the dose of ICG is 75 mg, but for SLO angiography, the dose remains 25 mg. It is imperative not to administer too much ICG, as higher ICG concentrations in the bloodstream decrease the effectiveness of the test.

The solution is injected intravenously and allowed to circulate within the systemic vasculature. Rapid injection is essential. The injection may be followed with an immediate 5 mL saline flush. Early-phase photographs are taken almost immediately after injection, mid-phase photographs occur at both 5 and 10 minutes post-injection, and late-phase photographs are taken at 20 and 40 minutes post-injection (32). A red-free fundus photograph is often taken before injection to aid in interpretation of test results (33).

DIGITAL IMAGING SYSTEMS

A filter, called an excitation filter, is placed over the light source, which allows only the passage of near-infrared light (34). This light is absorbed by the ICG molecules in the eye, which in turn emit slightly lower energy light. A barrier filter is used to capture only this light emitted from the ICG into the camera by blocking wavelengths shorter than 825 nm.

The images produced by ICG allow for visualization of choroidal circulation, but ICG's application in this realm was only accepted when appropriate mechanisms of image capture were developed. Methods of image acquisition include the fundus camera, the video camera, or the scanning laser ophthalmoscope.

A video fundus camera is connected to a digital imaging system. Flash synchronization allows high-resolution image capture. These images are recorded on computer hard-drive, CD-ROM, or DVD and can be edited. The development of high-resolution digital imaging systems has increased the use of ICG angiography dramatically.

Recent advances in the technology associated with ICG angiography include real-time angiography, wide-angle angiography (35), digital subtraction angiography (36), and high-speed ICG videoangiography (11,37,38).

Real-time ICG angiography utilizes a modified camera with a diode laser illumination system that has an 805 nm output (Topcon 501AL camera). It can capture images at 30 frames per second and thus allows for continuous recording. The images are recorded as a continuous film or as single images at a frequency of 30 per second. Single frames can be digitalized to make a printed copy, but the resolution of these prints is limited to 640 × 480 pixels.

Wide-angle ICG angiography (WAICGA) is achieved with the use of a wide-angle contact lens. The lens produces an image that lies about 1 cm in front of the lens. Accordingly, the fundus camera must be set on A or + in order to focus on the image plane. WAICGA allows for instantaneous imaging of a large area of the fundus. When the contact lens is combined with the laser illumination system, real-time imaging of up to 160 degrees of the fundus is possible (Fig. 10.1).

Digital subtraction ICG angiography (DS-ICGA) is a technique that involves digital subtraction of sequentially acquired ICG angiographic frames to image the progression of the dye front within the choroidal circulation. With a digital image, it is possible to "subtract" the pre-contrast image (or just the previous image) to visualize the vascular structures by following the progression of dye as it moves through the vascular network. The purpose of subtraction is to eliminate everything but the choroidal vasculature. Pseudo-color imaging of the choroid allows for differentiation and identification of choroidal arteries and veins. DS-ICGA allows imaging of occult CNV in greater detail and in a shorter period of time than with conventional ICG angiography (39).

The development of the confocal SLO was instrumental in eliminating a fundamental problem in fundus imaging.

Reflection from interfaces of the ocular optical media can obscure any picture of the retina; these reflections must be minimized. The SLO utilizes a low-power, infrared laser diode (795 nm) to "scan" the fundus. A laser beam is transmitted through the pupil, centrally, and scans the surface of the retina point by point. The reflected light is captured, transduced, and amplified. The varying reflectance of the retina to the laser beam creates an image of the fundus. The SLO captures 20 to 30 images per second, but the resolution is limited to 256 × 256 pixels or 512 × 512 pixels.

The result is a clearer picture with fewer reflective obscurations and distortions. Confocal SLO also allows for simultaneous ICG and FA. This system is also used in high-speed ICG angiography. Generally, scanning laser systems record the filling phases with greater temporal resolution than do fundus camera systems. Nonetheless, late phase photographs are better imaged with video cameras.

Recently, Teschner and co-workers reported that three-dimensional confocal angiography produces reliable quantitative and qualitative analysis of defects, exudation, and proliferative vascular lesions (40).

INTERPRETATION

The phases of an indocyanine green angiogram are analogous to those of a FA. The early phases of the ICG angiogram show both choroidal and retinal vascular filling, which occur in parallel, but not exactly in phase. Within seconds of dye injection, the larger choroidal vessels start to fluoresce slightly before the retinal arterioles. While the retina usually fills from one central artery, the choroid fills from a number of separate vessels simultaneously causing rapid movement of the dye into the choroid. The dye progresses to the smaller arterioles and on to the choriocapillaris. The dye front reaches the post-capillary venules and then the larger veins. This trip occurs within a few seconds in a healthy individual, but in an elderly person, the artery to vein time may be increased. The transition to the venous phase happens more quickly in the choroid than in the retina.

Interpretation of ICG angiography is quite complex. A wide spectrum of "normal" exists when referring to choroidal circulation, making it difficult to assign a standard for the basis of comparison. It is necessary to approach ICG interpretation with an algorithm in mind. Similarly to FA interpretation, the first step involves identifying areas of hypofluorescence or hyperfluorescence. In the presence of hypofluorescence, it is necessary to make a determination as to whether the fluorescence is blocked or whether there is a vascular filling defect. Blockage can be produced by pigment, hemorrhage, exudation, myelination, and scarring. Vascular filling defects reflect either a vascular occlusion or a response to tissue atrophy.

With hyperfluorescence, the possible causes include transmitted fluorescence, abnormal vessels, leakage, or artifact from misalignment of barrier and excitatory filters.

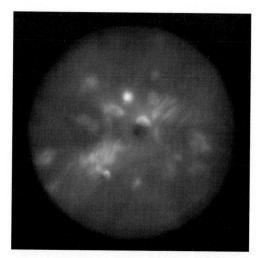

Figure 10.1 The wide-angle indocyanine green angiogram of a patient with central serous chorioretinopathy illustrates multifocal hyperpermeable areas of presumed occult pigment epithelial detachments that extend far beyond the posterior pole.

Transmitted fluorescence is most often seen with atrophy of the RPE, although scleral thinning is another identified cause.

APPLICATIONS

ICG angiography was originally used in the diagnoses and interpretation of CNV in age-related macular degeneration (AMD). Although this remains the primary application of the procedure, there are a growing number of uses for ICG angiography, extending into the anterior segment. In the following section, the current applications of ICG angiography will be detailed, including definitions, expected angiogram results, and clinical significance.

AMD

ICG angiography has advanced our understanding of the pathologic process and the appropriate management of AMD. Although AMD can be suspected from clinical exam, angiography is necessary for accurate diagnosis, characterization, and monitoring. ICG angiography does not replace FA in AMD; instead, it serves in conjunction with FA to enhance appreciable knowledge of a particular patient's condition.

Definitions

The terminology used to describe the angiographic manifestations of AMD was established by the Macular Photocoagulation Study Group (MPS) (41). The most relevant definitions from this study have been described extensively, but the information made available through ICG has added to our understanding of these conditions and have led to slight modifications of prior definitions (2,5,6,8–12,14,42).

Serous PED

A serous PED is an ovoid or circular detachment of the RPE that appears on ICG angiography as variable, minimal blockage of normal choroidal vessels most evident in the mid-phases of the study. In comparison to its appearance on FA, a serous PED is hypofluorescent on ICG study. ICG molecules are large and protein bound and are thus prevented from free passage through the fenestrated choriocapillaris into the sub-RPE space. Approximately 1.5% of newly diagnosed neovascular AMD patients present with this form of pure serous PED (8,11,12).

CNV

CNV is defined as choroidal capillary proliferation through a break in the outer aspect of Bruch's membrane, under the RPE and the neurosensory retina. CNV can be classified into many categories based on its presenting characteristics (Fig.10.2).

Classic CNV

Classic CNV, representing only 12% of newly diagnosed neovascular AMD, presents as a well-demarcated area of early hyperfluorescence with progressive leakage on FA (2,5,9,35,42). The findings are similar on ICG, but do not present as clearly as they do on FA.

Occult CNV

Occult CNV is seen in more than 85% of newly diagnosed neovascular AMD patients. The characteristics of occult CNV can vary immensely; the FA findings in occult CNV lack the clear delineation seen in cases of classic CNV. Occult CNV is characterized as either fibrovascular PED with irregular elevation of the RPE or as late leakage of undetermined origin. There are two major classifications of occult CNV as recognized by ICG angiography: with and without serous PED. Occult CNV can also be subclassified as hot spot (focal) or plaque. Polypoidal choroidal vasculopathy (PCV) and retinal angiomatous proliferation (RAP) represent subtypes of CNV, which often present with a hot spot.

Without Serous PED

This type of occult CNV, which represents two-thirds of newly diagnosed cases of occult CNV, is characterized by increasing subretinal hyperfluorescence and irregular staining caused by sub-RPE CNV. ICG angiography reveals early vascular hyperfluorescence and late-staining of abnormal vessels. Any image with distinct margins on ICG angiography is considered well-defined CNV.

With Serous PED

This type of occult CNV, representing the remaining one-third of newly diagnosed patients with occult CNV patients, is associated with a serous PED. The combination of CNV and serous PED has been termed vascularized PED (V-PED) and results from sub-RPE neovascularization associated with a serous PED. In these patients, ICG angiography reveals early vascular hyperfluorescence and late staining of the CNV. The serous PED, as previously noted, is comparatively hypofluorescent because only minimal leakage occurs beneath the serous detachment. ICG is more helpful in differentiating between a serous PED and a V-PED as FA in both cases presents as hyperfluorescence. ICG is also superior for identifying the vascularized and serous component of V-PEDs, as the serous component of a PED is hypofluorescent while the vascular component is hyperfluorescent (8,36–38).

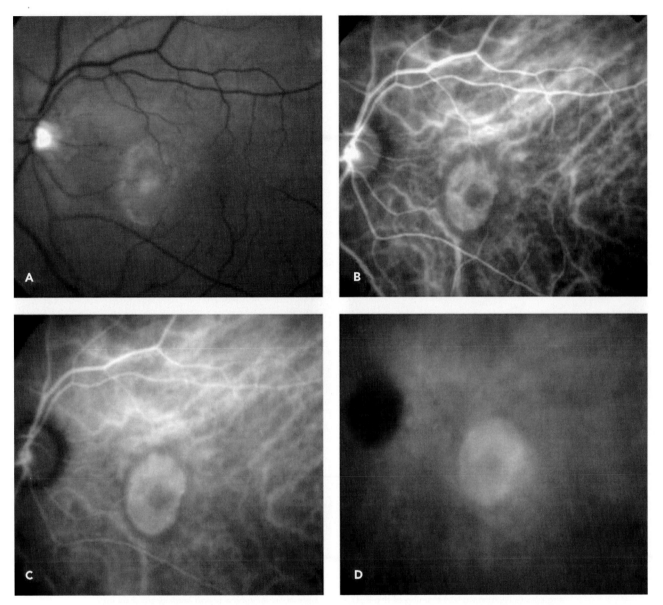

Figure 10.2 A. This is the red-free photograph of a patient with classic choroidal neovascularization (CNV). **B.** The early-phase indocyanine green (ICG) angiogram reveals hyperfluorescence of the CNV. Mid-phase **(C)** and late-phase ICG angiograms **(D)** show staining of the hyperfluorescent CNV.

Hot spots

Hot spots, or focal CNV, (Fig. 10.3) appear on ICG angiography as a well-delineated area of CNV no more than one disc diameter in size. Hot spots represent an area of active occult CNV, an area of neovascularization that exhibits active proliferation and a high level of permeability. RAP, focal occult CNV, and polypoidal-type CNV are subgroups of hot spots that will be discussed later in this chapter.

Plaque

A plaque is an area of occult CNV larger than one disc diameter in size. Plaques can be either well-defined or ill-

defined depending on the presence or absence of distinct margins throughout the study or the presence or absence of blockage. Approximately 60% of plaques are characterized as ill-defined, meaning there are either indistinct margins or blockage of blood flow at some point in the ICG study. They are often formed by late-staining vessels that are more likely to be quiescent areas of neovascularization and are not associated with appreciable leakage. Plaques of occult CNV seem to grow slowly in dimension.

Occult CNV can also appear as a combination lesion with both hot spot(s) and plaque(s). A recent review of 1,000 patients with occult CNV revealed the following relative frequencies: 61% plaques alone, 29% hot spots alone, 8% combination lesions (43). The combination lesions

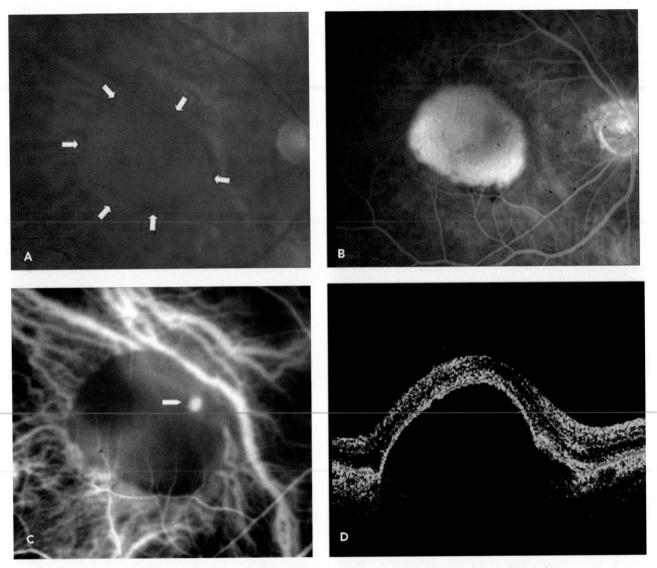

Figure 10.3 **A.** Clinical photograph showing a large pigment epithelial detachment (PED) (*white arrows*) in a patient with focal occult choroidal neovascularization. **B.** Late-phase fluorescein angiogram illustrating late staining of the PED. **C.** Mid-phase indocyanine green angiogram showing a focal area of abnormal hyperfluorescence (hot spot). **D.** The OCT scan confirms a large PED.

were then further subclassified as marginal spots, overlying spots, and remote spots, depending on the location of hot spots in relation to plaques (38). Marginal spots are lesions in which hot spots occur at the edge of the plaques of neovascularization. Overlying spots are lesions in which hot spots reside on top of plaques. Remote spots are lesions in which hot spots are not contiguous with plaques.

While FA remains the standard for diagnosis and management of classic CNV, ICG plays an important role in cases of occult CNV. Even when clinical and fluorescein findings suggest occult CNV, ICG angiography can often clearly document, delineate, and localize the lesion as areas of CNV that appear poorly defined during FA (8–10,15,26,43–50).

It is common for both classic and occult neovascularization to be present in the same patient. In these cases, the

area of the each type in relation is used to characterize a lesion. Lesions with greater than 50% classic CNV (i.e., 80% classic and 20% occult) are termed *predominantly classic*. Lesions with less than 50 percent classic CNV are termed *minimally classic* lesions.

Characterization of CNV lesions is important as only a small percentage of patients with CNV are eligible for treatment. One study revealed that approximately 40% of patients diagnosed with occult CNV actually presented with early, well-defined focal areas of fluorescence on ICG videoangiography (2).

It is clear that ICG does not replace FA in characterizing CNV, but it is an important adjunctive study. FA is superior for imaging well-defined CNV. ICG angiography, however, is indispensable in cases of occult CNV as it can identify well-defined, treatable lesions in approximately

30% of occult CNV cases (45,51). Accordingly, it is advisable to perform ICG angiography as an adjunct to FA for occult lesions in order to diagnose and manage accurately.

POLYPOIDAL CHOROIDAL VASCULOPATHY (PCV)

PCV is characterized by the presence of an inner choroidal vascular network ending in an aneurismal bulge clinically seen as a reddish-orange, spheroid, polyp-like structure. It was initially reported exclusively in middle-aged, Black females, but has since been recognized as a variant of CNV that can be found in all patients with AMD. In PCV, leakage and bleeding from the peculiar choroidal vascular abnormality result in multiple, recurrent, serosanguinous detachments of the RPE and the neurosensory retina (39,41,46). ICG can be used to identify and to characterize the vascular abnormality with high sensitivity and specificity (41,43–45,50,52–74). The early-phase of ICG angiogram shows a distinct network of vessels within the choroid. Patients with juxtapapillary involvement show a radial, arching pattern as vascular channels extend and connect with smaller, spanning branches that are more numerous and thus have increased prominence at the edge of the PCV lesion. Larger choroidal vessels in the PCV lesion begin to fill before retinal vessels. The area within and surrounding the network is relatively hypofluorescent compared to the involved choroid. The vessels of the network seem to fill at a slower rate than retinal vessels.

Shortly after the network is first visualized on ICG angiogram, small, hyperfluorescent polyps are seen within the choroid (Fig. 10.4). These polypoidal structures correspond to the reddish-orange choroidal excrescence seen clinically. They leak slowly creating increasing hyperfluorescence. In the late-phases of ICG angiography, a uniform washout is seen as the dye disappears from the polypoidal vascular structure; the late staining that is characteristic of occult CNV is not seen in PCV.

PCV may also be localized to the macular area without any peripapillary component. In addition, it may present as a network of small branching vessels ending in polypoidal dilation. ICG angiography is necessary to image the latter presentation (Fig. 10.5).

Many studies suggest the importance of ICG angiography in the diagnosis of PCV (65,75,76). In these studies, ICG angiography has established the presence of PCV in patients with occult CNV in 4% to 8% of patients. The prevalence of PCV in patients with large hemorrhagic and exudative neurosensory detachments but no drusen was 85% (Fig. 10.6) (52).

ICG has also revealed the presence of early polyps in the peripapillary, macular, and peripheral areas (Fig.10.7) (72). The identification of these polyps has lead to several investigations into potential treatment. In this regard, ICG angiography has helped our understanding of PCV and will likely lead to improvements in treatment strategies that, in turn, will improve visual outcomes.

RETINAL ANGIOMATOUS PROLIFERATION (RAP)

RAP is a distinct subgroup of neovascular AMD in which the first manifestation of angiomatous proliferation occurs within the retina. As the condition progresses through the

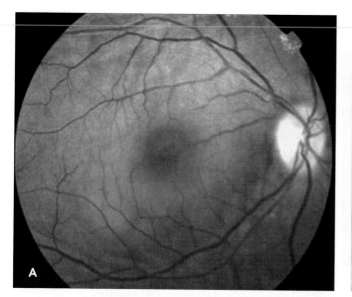

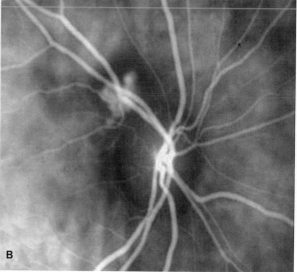

Figure 10.4 **A.** Red-free photograph of a 62-year-old female illustrating a neurosensory retinal detachment in the central macula. **B.** Indocyanine green angiogram reveals the presence of a polypoidal choroidal vascular abnormality in the superior temporal juxtapapillary region.

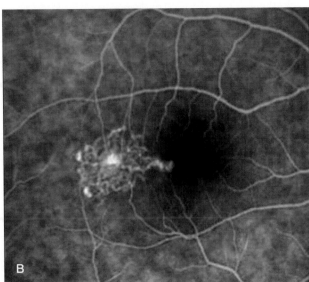

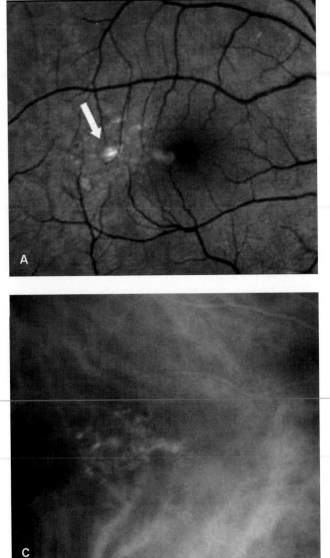

Figure 10.5 This is a 56-year-old Caucasian male who had three transient episodes of visual disturbance, who was diagnosed with central serous chorioretinopathy. **A.** Red-free photograph reveals a flat macula overlying multiple, nummular elevations suggestive of small serous pigment epithelial detachments. There is a patch of fibrous metaplasia (*arrow*) at the center of the lesion. **B.** Fluorescein angiogram reveals a net of subretinal inner choroidal vessels terminating in aneurismal or polypoidal lesions. **C.** Late-phase indocyanine green angiogram confirms the presence of polypoidal vascular abnormality.

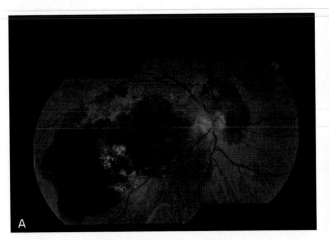

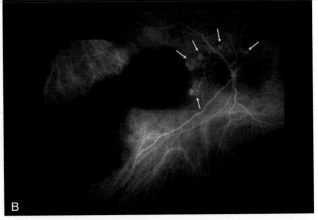

Figure 10.6 This is a 66-year-old Caucasian male with sudden deterioration vision in his right eye. **A.** Color photograph composite shows large subretinal and intraretinal hemorrhages at the posterior pole and surrounding the optic nerve. There are areas with dense lipid exudation. **B.** Mid-phase indocyanine green angiogram illustrates a large hyperfluorescent area. In the peripapillary area, there is a net of subretinal inner choroidal vessels that terminates in polypoidal lesions (*white arrows*).

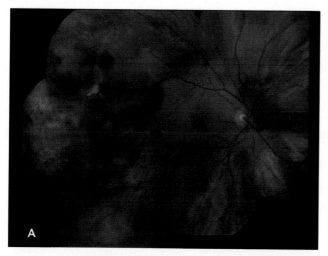 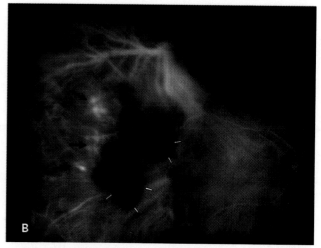

Figure 10.7 **A.** Color photograph composite of the fundus of a patient with polypoidal choroidal vasculopathy demonstrates hemorrhagic pigment epithelial detachment (PED) in the temporal periphery and subretinal hemorrhages. Note the subretinal fluid exudation involving the macula. **B.** Indocyanine green angiography composite of the right fundus reveals a cluster of actively leaking polypoidal vessels in the retinal periphery (*black arrows*). Note the two hemorrhagic PEDs blocking the background fluorescence (*white arrows*).

retina and into the subretinal space, dilated retinal vessels, hemorrhages, and exudates develop. One or more of the enlarged, compensatory retinal vessels perfuse and drain the neovascularization, occasionally forming a retinal-retinal anastomosis (RRA). In these patients, the same indistinct staining seen in occult CNV is present on a FA, and ICG angiography is useful in making an accurate diagnosis (Fig. 10.8) (77).

ICG angiograms of RAP lesions reveal a focal area of intense hyperfluorescence (hot spot) with some late extension of the leakage within the retina due to intraretinal neovascularization (IRN) and subretinal neovascularization (SRN). As the IRN progresses through the subretinal space, it may anastomose with the underlying choroidal circulation. At this stage, clinical and angiographic evidence of a V-PED is often present. As stated previously, ICG is the preferred method of imaging a V-PED because the serous component of the PED remains hypofluorescent while the vascular component displays hyperfluorescence (Fig. 10.9). ICG angiography may be able to capture direct communication between the retinal and the choroidal component of the neovascular complex as they meet to form a retinal-choroidal anastomosis (RCA) (78).

Through the use of ICG, Kuhn et al. were the first to identify RCA as a potential manifestation of RAP (79). They found ICG angiographic evidence of RCA in 28% of patients with AMD associated with V-PED. A second report revealed that in patients with neovascular AMD, the neovascularization is associated with RAP in 16% of cases (80). Again, ICG angiography is necessary to make this determination; it has demonstrated use in making an accurate diagnosis when IRN progresses beneath the neurosensory retina (Fig. 10.10).

ICG-GUIDED LASER TREATMENT OF CNV

Laser photocoagulation therapy, guided either by FA or by ICG, is a proven treatment strategy against CNV in AMD. Unfortunately, only a small percentage of patients with CNV are eligible for treatment.

Eligibility for treatment includes either classic, well-defined, extrafoveal CNV demonstrated on FA or an ICG-angiographically identified focal lesion in occult CNV. Approximately 13% of patients fall into the first category, classic CNV, and can thus receive FA-guided laser treatment (81). Recurrence occurs in up to 50% of these cases; accordingly, only 6.5% of all CNV patients benefit from FA-guided treatment.

ICG angiography has increased immensely the population eligible for treatment. The vast majority (approximately 85%) of patients with CNV have the occult type of CNV that has traditionally remained untreatable (81). ICG angiography can identify treatable, focal lesions (hot spots) in close to 30% of these cases (45,51). The hot spots represent areas of actively leaking neovascularization that can be obliterated by laser photocoagulation; plaques, by contrast, appear to represent a thin layer of neovascularization that is not actively leaking and thus does not appear to be affected by laser treatment.

In the case of a combined lesion (both plaque and hot spot), treatment eligibility depends on the relative location of the lesions. Laser treatment has been successful in treating lesions in which the hot spot is at the margin of the plaque (46). Poor results are seen in attempts to treat hot spots that lay directly over a plaque.

The success of laser treatment on RCA lesions is dependent on the presence of an associated serous PED. When

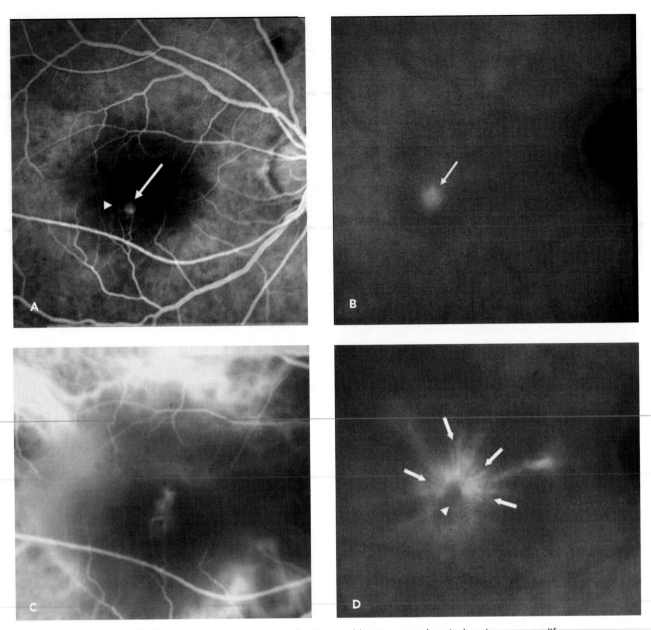

Figure 10.8 **A.** Fluorescein angiogram of a 73-year-old patient reveals retinal angiomatous prolif-eration stage I (*arrow*). Note the telangiectasia surrounding this area (*arrowhead*). **B.** Indocyanine green (ICG) angiogram showing a focal area of intense hyperfluorescence (*arrow*) or so-called "hot spot." **C.** The ICG angiogram 1 year later illustrates a retinal-retinal anastomosis and subretinal neo-vascularization. **D.** The late-phase ICG angiogram shows intraretinal leakage (*arrows*) surrounding the fading angiomatous proliferation (*arrowhead*).

serous PED is present, laser treatment has achieved little success at treating RCA (82). Slakter et al. found that laser treatment is effective in 66% of patients with occult CNV associated with an elevation of the neurosensory retina; this success dropped to 43% when the occult CNV was associated with a PED (79,83).

Overall, 26% of all eyes with exudative maculopathy are eligible for ICG-guided laser photocoagulation. A success rate of 35% with ICG-guided treatment translates to an additional 9% of the overall patient population affected with CNV that can be treated effectively. With only 6.5% of patients helped with FA-guided laser treatment and 9%

aided by ICG-guided treatment, the majority of patients are still either untreatable or are refractory to treatment (84).

Feeder vessels (FVs) identified by dynamic ICG angiography, but not by FA, can be treated with argon green laser (85). ICG angiography is then performed at regular inter-vals following treatment to determine response. A second laser treatment is administered if ICG angiography reveals a patent FV. A 40% success rate was found, initially, with a more recent report of 75% success. It appears that dynamic ICG angiography detects smaller FVs and could thus be used in treatment of these vessels (86).

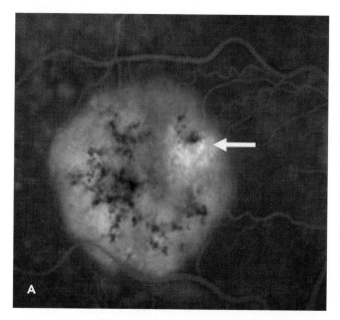

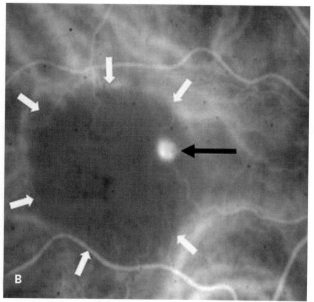

Figure 10.9 **A.** The fluorescein angiogram of a patient with stage II retinal angiomatous proliferation (RAP) reveals late staining of a pigment epithelial detachment (PED). There is an increase in the intensity of fluorescence in the area of the RAP lesion (*arrow*). **B.** The indocyanine green angiogram shows hypofluorescence in the area of the PED (*white arrows*) and a "hot spot" corresponding to the RAP (*black arrow*).

CENTRAL SEROUS CHORIORETINOPATHY (CSC)

CSC is a relatively common condition characterized by an idiopathic recurrent serous detachment of the macula.

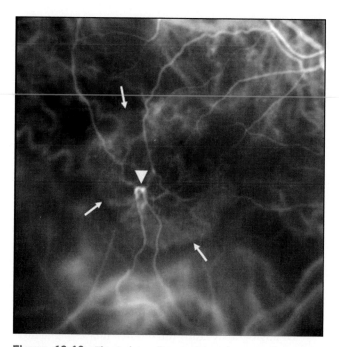

Figure 10.10 The indocyanine green angiogram of a patient with stage III retinal angiomatous proliferation shows intraretinal and subretinal neovascularization (*arrowhead*) overlying a large area of choroidal neovascularization (*arrows*) with multiple retinal-choroidal anastomoses.

Traditionally, there has been great debate regarding the pathogenesis of CSC, but ICG angiography has expanded our knowledge of the disease (2,18,73,76,86–100).

In CSC, ICG angiography reveals multiple areas of hyperfluorescence in the early- and mid-phases of the study that tend to fade in the late-phases (Fig. 10.11). These areas of hyperfluorescence correspond with areas that display leakage on FA, but also appear in areas that appear clinically and angiographically normal, as well as in the seemingly normal, fellow eye. The hyperfluorescence is thought to represent diffuse choroidal hyperpermeability and can be seen on WAICGA far beyond the posterior pole (87). They are presumed to be occult PEDs.

Although further pathologic correlation is necessary, the sheer number of PEDs seen with ICG suggests that PEDs may be much more common in CSC than previously identified. In addition, the presence of PEDs on ICG angiograms in eyes that appear inactive by both clinical exam and FA suggests that CSC may be more diffuse and widespread than originally believed. It has been suggested that the persistence of abnormal findings in cases of inactive disease is a reflection of chronic and not recurrent disease (Fig. 10.12).

In addition to identifying PEDs, ICG is able to delineate a serous PED associated with AMD from a serous PED in CSC. In CSC, there is increased permeability of the choriocapillaris that allows leakage of the ICG molecules under the PED. As a result, a serous PED in CSC is bright (hyperfluorescent), while a serous PED in AMD is hypofluorescent.

ICG-guided photodynamic therapy has a role in the treatment of CSC. Yannuzzi et al. reported rapid resolution of subretinal fluid in patients with chronic CSC treated with ICG-guided photodynamic therapy (73).

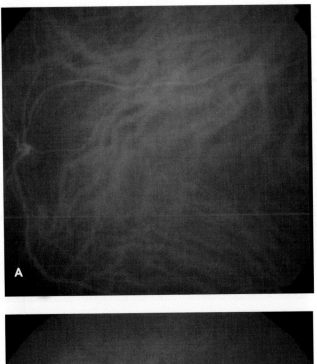

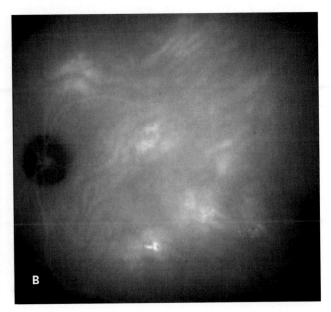

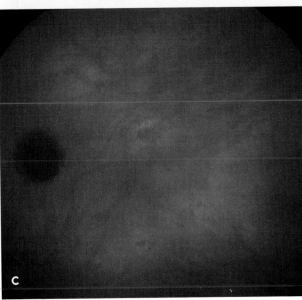

Figure 10.11 This is a 43-year-old Caucasian female with chronic central serous chorioretinopathy in the left eye. Indocyanine green angiography is essentially normal in the early-phase **(A)**, but reveals multiple patchy areas of hyperfluorescence in the mid-phase **(B)** that fade in the last phase of the study **(C)**.

Occasionally, CSC is indistinguishable from PCV both clinically and on FA. In these cases, ICG angiography is helpful in determining the true diagnosis (1,97).

INTRAOCULAR TUMORS

ICG angiography is an important tool in the diagnosis and evaluation of intraocular tumors. Guyer et al. reported that certain tumors have characteristic ICG videoangiographic patterns (100,101).

Choroidal Melanoma

Pigmented choroidal melanomas contain large amounts of melanin that, in high density, absorb the near-infrared light. Fluorescence is blocked; the tumor and underlying choroidal vasculature cannot be visualized through the dense tumor pigmentation. The hypofluorescence caused by tumor blockage is often larger than clinically suspected, thus yielding a better understanding of the severity of the tumor. When a pigmented choroidal melanoma thickens or develops prominent intrinsic vasculature, ICG angiography reflects this change with an increase in fluorescence in the late-phase (Fig. 10.13) (102).

ICG angiography can thus differentiate pigmented choroidal melanomas from non-pigmented tumors, such as hemangiomas and osteomas. It is, however, difficult to distinguish melanomas from other pigmented lesions, such as nevi or metastatic cutaneous melanoma.

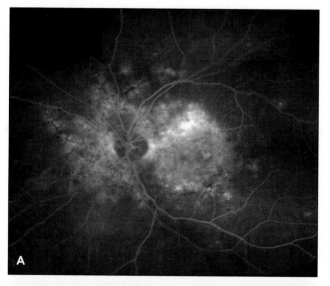

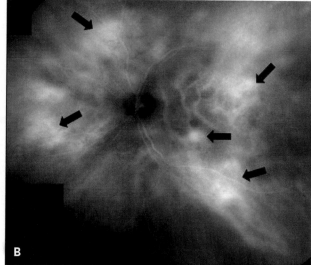

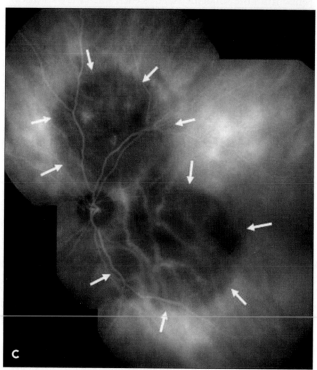

Figure 10.12   A. Fluorescein angiogram of the left eye of a 53-year-old patient with central serous chorioretinopathy shows diffuse decompensation of the retinal pigment epithelium. **B.** The mid-phase indocyanine green (ICG) angiogram reveals multifocal areas of hyperfluorescence (*black arrows*) that do not always correspond with the leaking points seen on FA. **C.** ICG angiography 3 weeks after photodynamic therapy. Leaking choroidal areas show resolution of the inner choroidal staining.

Choroidal Hemangioma

The vascularity of choroidal hemangiomas results in a marked, progressive hyperfluorescence on ICG angiography (102). In the early phases, a network of small-caliber vessels is visible in a web-like configuration that tends to obscure the normal choroidal pattern. Choroidal hemangiomas completely fill with dye within 1 minute. ICG is also helpful in evaluating vascular lesions underlying hemorrhage. ICG, unlike FA, may allow visualization of the tumor through an overlying hemorrhage.

Piccolino developed a technique for studying the vasculature of choroidal hemangiomas that involves performing ICG angiography with artificially increased intraocular pressure (99). The increased intraocular pressure serves to slow choroidal circulation allowing better delineation of the feeding and draining vessels and of the inner circulation of the tumor.

Choroidal Metastases

Choroidal metastases display different patterns on ICG angiography depending on vascularity, pigmentation, and primary location of the lesion (101). In the early-phase, choroidal metastases show diffuse, homogeneous

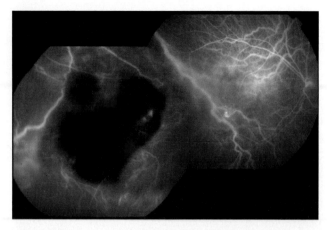

Figure 10.13 In this indocyanine green (ICG) angiogram composite, the fluorescence is blocked by the large amount of melanin, which characterizes pigmented choroidal melanomas. ICG angiography shows intrinsic vasculature (*arrows*), which develops when pigmented choroidal melanoma thickens.

hypofluorescence that often allows for visualization of the normal choroidal perfusion pattern that lies below.

The origin of the tumor is often reflected on ICG angiography. Breast metastases show moderate blockage. Metastatic thyroid carcinoma and metastatic bronchial carcinoid tumors show hyperfluorescence. Metastatic skin melanoma displays marked blockage and is often indistinguishable from primary choroidal melanoma (101).

ICG angiography can usually distinguish a metastatic choroidal lesion from a choroidal hemangioma. A case has been reported in which a metastatic lesion with heavy vascularization was confused with a choroidal hemangioma (87). This case emphasized the need to place ICG findings in the context of clinical examination, ultrasound, and FA.

Choroidal Osteomas and Others

A choroidal osteoma is a tumor that contains bone at various stages of calcification. Early-phase ICG angiography shows characteristic small vessels that often leak too fast to be detected by FA (103). Variable hypofluorescence is observed in the bony areas. They may show hyperfluorescence in the mid-to-late-phases of the ICG angiogram.

ICG can be used to identify varices of vortex veins that appear similar to choroidal tumors. If a diagnosis cannot be made clinically, ICG angiography of these varices shows marked dilation of the vortex veins (104).

The introduction of SLO in ICG has allowed for in vivo imaging of histologically demonstrated microcirculatory patterns (MCP) (104). In some cases, the MCP is tied to the behavior of uveal melanoma; in these cases, visualization of the MCP allows for better characterization of tumor activity (105). It has been demonstrated that the presence of complex MCPs on angiogram in eyes with melanocytic lesions is associated with clinical evidence of lesion growth (98).

INFLAMMATORY DISEASES

ICG angiography assists in the evaluation and management of inflammatory diseases. It has also contributed immensely to our knowledge of these disease processes (106). In cases of retinal vasculitis, ICG contributes little information that is not provided by FA; it does, however, help establish diagnosis, management, and treatment effectiveness in a variety of inflammatory disorders.

Serpiginous Choroidopathy

Serpiginous choroidopathy is a rare disorder that affects primarily the inner choroid and RPE and, secondarily, the outer retinal layers. A progressive condition, it begins at the optic nerve and advances centrifugally. In cases of serpiginous choroidopathy, ICG can be used to delineate the acute phase from the subacute stage as each stage shows a distinct pattern on the angiogram. The acute stage of serpiginous choroidopathy is characterized by generalized hypofluorescence in all phases of the study. In the subacute stage, midsized and large choroidal vessels can be visualized within the lesion. Delay in or lack of filling in the smaller choroidal vessels, including the choriocapillaris, yields a generalized hypofluorescence in all phases of the study. The subacute phase produces a more detailed picture than the acute stage as there is resolution of acute inflammatory changes and associated edema. The late-phase in subacute serpiginous chorioretinopathy reveals well-demarcated lesions that represent choroidal perfusion abnormalities and blockage by inflammatory exudates, along with edema of the RPE and of the outer retina. When serpiginous choroidopathy becomes inactive, atrophy of the RPE and choriocapillaris allows for visualization of the deep choroidal vessels (107).

A recent report by Giovannini et al. suggests the presence of occult satellite lesions in the choroid seen on ICG angiography without clinical or angiographic (fluorescein) evidence (107). It has been suggested that these quiescent lesions represent occult manifestations of the disease.

ICG angiography is particularly useful to distinguish between serpiginous choroidopathy and other choroidal vascular inflammatory diseases, such as Vogt-Koyanagi-Harada Syndrome (VKH), ocular sarcoidosis, ocular tuberculosis, and birdshot choroidopathy (108). In these conditions, there is diffuse choroidal hyperfluorescence in the late-phases of angiography due to involvement in the large choroidal vessels.

Acute Multifocal Posterior Placoid Pigment Epitheliopathy (AMPPPE)

AMPPPE occurs in young adults and consists of multifocal, yellow-white, flat, placoid lesions in the RPE at the posterior pole and mid-peripheral fundus (109). These lesions are hypofluorescent throughout the ICG study that may be due to occlusive vasculitis that results in a partial occlusion in the choroidal circulation (110). This hypofluorescence remains even once lesions have healed; ICG angiograms in these cases show early hypofluorescence that becomes more clearly delineated in the late-phases.

Multiple Evanescent White Dot Syndrome (MEWDS)

MEWDS is a syndrome of unknown etiology that presents acutely with unilateral visual loss in healthy young women. The RPE-photoreceptor complex is the primary site of involvement (111). Clinical exam reveals subtle white dots; FA displays an indistinct pattern of punctate hyperfluorescence. ICG, on the other hand, elucidates a pattern of hypofluorescent spots throughout the posterior pole and peripheral retina that appear approximately 10 minutes after dye injection, and remain through the late-phases. When compared to clinical exam, the dots appear larger with ICG angiography. Additionally, a greater number of lesions are detected on ICG angiography than with FA.

MEWDS occasionally presents with enlargement of the blind spot on visual field examination. In these cases, a ring of hypofluorescence is visualized around the optic disc. It has been shown that resolution of the enlarged blind spot and return of vision does not correlate completely with the disappearance of hypofluorescent areas on ICG angiography; these lesions often remain visible on ICG study. These findings suggest that MEWDS may result in persistent abnormalities in choroidal circulation, even after vision has been restored (Fig. 10.14) (112,113).

Hypofluorescent spots are also present in adjacent vessels. Ikeda et al. suggest that inflammatory lesions extend to the inner layers of the retina when MEWDS is complicated by periphlebitis (112). The inflammatory changes involve the choroid and all layers of the retina and thus block weak background fluorescence. The result is hypofluorescence in the late-phase of ICG angiography.

Birdshot Chorioretinopathy

Birdshot chorioretinopathy is a disorder of bilateral, painless decrease in vision and floaters in otherwise healthy adults. The disease acquired its name from its hallmark "birdshot" appearance of scattered, creamy lesions. Birdshot chorioretinopathy is an uncommon, but potentially serious inflammatory disorder of both the choroid and the retina with no known associations to systemic disease. There is a strong correlation with the HLA-A29 class I antigen, suggesting a genetic predisposition to disease.

Although ICG angiography is not usually necessary to make the diagnosis of birdshot chorioretinopathy, it does allow for differentiation from other inflammatory disorders. In birdshot chorioretinopathy, the angiogram reveals multiple hypofluorescent lesions that follow the larger choroidal vessels, appearing early in the study and persisting throughout the later phases. The dots visualized with ICG are similar in size to, but are more numerous than those seen clinically. A study by Howe et al. established that ICG detects birdshot lesions more rapidly than does FA, making it potentially more valuable in assessing disease activity (Fig. 10.15) (114).

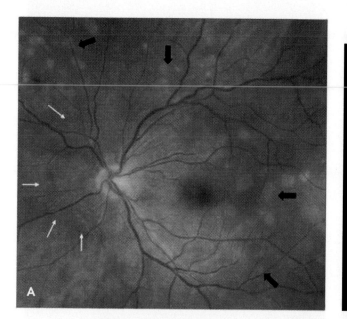
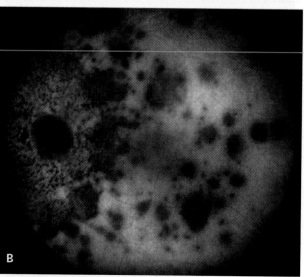

Figure 10.14 This is a 29-year-old female with unilateral visual disturbance caused by multiple evanescent white dot syndrome. **A.** The clinical photograph shows multiple round, white to yellow-white spots (*black arrows*) distributed over the posterior fundus. In the peripapillary region, there are multiple small yellow dots (*white arrows*). **B.** The mid-phase indocyanine green reveals multiple large and small hypofluorescent spots in the posterior pole. Note the ring of hypofluorescence surrounding the optic disc.

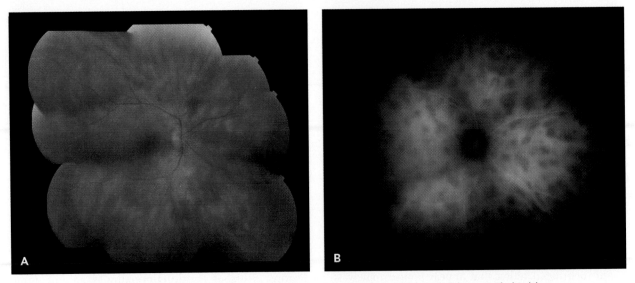

Figure 10.15 This is a 46-year-old Caucasian female with newly diagnosed birdshot retinochoroidopathy. **A.** Clinical photograph composite reveals multiple creamy round lesions. **B.** Mid-phase indocyanine green illustrates multiple hypofluorescent lesions resembling "holes" in the fluorescence of the choriocapillaris.

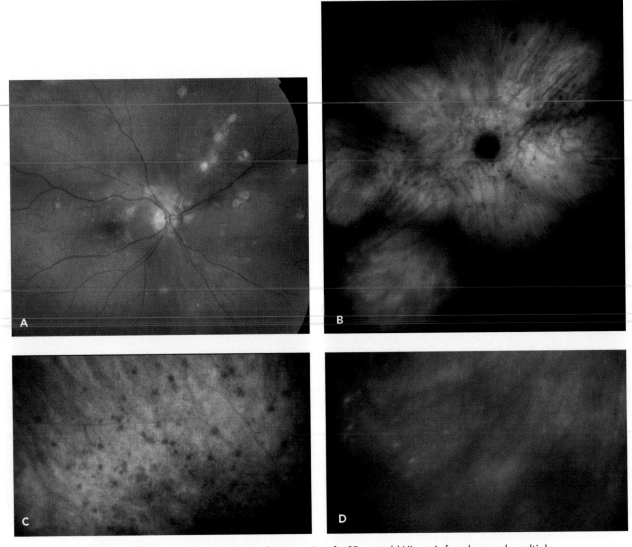

Figure 10.16 **A.** Clinical photograph composite of a 35-year-old Hispanic female reveals multiple flat, yellow, round lesions at the level of the retinal pigment epithelium and the inner choroid distributed over the posterior pole consistent with the diagnosis of multifocal choroiditis. Indocyanine green angiogram composite **(B)** shows multiple hypofluorescent spots **(C)**, as well as hyperfluorescent foci **(D)**. Note the confluent hypofluorescence surrounding the optic nerve.

Multifocal Choroiditis (MFC)

MFC is an idiopathic inflammatory disorder of the choroid with varied presentation and clinical course, but with classic findings on clinical exam: punched out chorioretinal spots, peripapillary atrophy, peripheral chorioretinal curvilinear lesions, and neovascularized macular degeneration or disciform scar.

ICG angiography of MFC shows multiple areas of hypofluorescence, best seen in the late-phases of angiography that result from blockage of fluorescence by MFC lesions. Hyperfluorescent foci that do not correlate with lesions seen clinically or by FA can also be observed (115). These areas may represent subclinical foci of choroiditis.

Slakter et al. report that in a series of 14 patients with MFC, 50% of eyes that were found to have large hypofluorescent spots in the posterior pole do not correspond to lesions seen on clinical exam or by FA. Twenty five percent of eyes exhibited enlargement of the blind spot on visual field exam, ICG angiography revealed confluent hypofluorescence surrounding the optic nerve (Fig. 10.16). It has also been reported that ICG angiography is useful in following the natural course of MFC and in evaluating the response to oral prednisone. In 29% of cases, ICG angiography displayed changes that correlate with the clinical course. After administration of prednisone, there was a decrease in symptoms experienced by patients, less inflammation on clinical exam, and a corresponding reduction in the size and number of hypofluorescent spots seen with ICG angiography. One patient was noted to have complete resolution of angiographic lesions following treatment with prednisone.

SUMMARY

ICG angiography was introduced into ophthalmology in the 1970s and has since become an important tool for imaging the retinal and choroidal vasculature. The physical properties of the dye allow for visualization of choroidal circulation that is not possible with sodium fluorescein. Interpretation of ICG angiography is quite complex, but, once mastered, can contribute immensely to the diagnosis, characterization, and management of chorioretinal pathology.

Although its predominant use resides in CNV secondary to AMD, ICG angiography has a growing number of applications. It has become increasingly clear that ICG is an important tool that should be utilized in conjunction with both clinical examination and FA. As technology improves and advances, it is likely that our knowledge and use of ICG angiography will continue to expand beyond its current scope.

REFERENCES

1. Fox JJ, Brooker L, Heselstine D, et al. A tricarbocyanine dye for continuous recording of dilution curves in whole blood independent of variations in blood oxygen saturation. *Proc Staff Meeting Mayo Clinic.* 1957;32: 478–484.
2. Yannuzzi LA, Slakter JS, Sorenson JS, et al. Digital indocyanine green videoangiography and choroidal neovascularization. *Retina.* 1992;12: 191–223.
3. Caesar J, Shaldon S, Chianduss L, et al. The use of indocyanine green in the measurement of hepatic blood flow and as a test of hepatic function. *Clin Sci.* 1961;21:43–57.
4. David NJ. Infrared absorption fundus angiography. In: *Proceedings of International Symposium on Fluorescein Angiography, Albi, France, 1969.* Basel: Karger; 1971.
5. Flower RW, Hochheimer BF. Clinical infrared absorption angiography of the choroid. *Am J Ophthalmol.* 1972;73:458–459.
6. Flower RW. Infrared absorption angiography of the choroid and some observations on the effects of high intraocular pressure. *Am J Ophthalmol.* 1972;74:600–614.
7. Orth DH, Patz A, Flower RW. Potential clinical applications of indocyanine green angiography—preliminary report. *Eye, Ear, Nose, Throat Monthly.* 1976;55:15–28.
8. Hayashi K, DeLaey JJ. Indocyanine green angiography of neovascular membranes. *Ophthalmologica.* 1985;190:30–39.
9. Hayashi K, Hasegawa Y, Tazawa Y, et al. Clinical application of indocyanine green angiography to choroidal neovascularization. *Jpn J Clin Ophthalmol.* 1989;33:57–68.
10. Hayashi K, Hasegawa Y, Tokoro T, et al. Value of indocyanine green angiography in the diagnosis of occult choroidal neovascular membrane. *Jpn J Clin Ophthalmol.* 1988;42:827–829.
11. Scheider A, Schroedel C. High resolution indocyanine green angiography with scanning laser ophthalmoscope. *Am J Ophthalmol.* 1989;108: 458–459.
12. Guyer DR, Duker J, Puliafito CA. Indocyanine green angiography and dye-enhanced diode laser photocoagulation. *Semin Ophthalmol.* 1992;7: 172–176.
13. Yannuzzi LA, Slakter JS, Gross NE, et al. Indocyanine green angiography guided photodynamic therapy for treatment of chronic central serous chorioretinopathy: a pilot study. *Retina.* 2003.
14. Guyer DR, Yannuzzi LA, Slakter JS, et al. The status of indocyanine green videoangiography. *Curr Opin Ophthalmol.*
15. Patz A, Flower RW, Klein ML, et al. Clinical applications of indocyanine green angiography. *Doc Ophthalmol Proc Series.* 1976;9:245–251.
16. Indocyanine Green. Mosby's Drug Consult. Available at MDConsult.
17. Geeraets WJ, Berry ER. Ocular spectral characteristics as related to hazards from lasers and other light sources. *Am J Ophthalmol.* 1968;66: 15–20.
18. Fox IJ, Wood EH. Application of dilution curves recorded from the right side of the heart or venous circulation with the aid of a new indicator dye. *Proc Mayo Clin.* 1957;32:541.
19. Cherrick GR, Stein SW, Leevy CM, et al. Indocyanine green: observations on its physical properties, plasma decay, and hepatic extraction. *J Clin Invest.* 1960;39:592–596.
20. Baker KJ. Binding of sulfobromophthalein (BSP) sodium and indocyanine green (ICG) by plasma a1-lipoproteins. *Proc Soc Exp Biol Med.* 1966;122: 957–963.
21. Goresky CA. Initial distribution and rate of uptake of sulfobromophthalein in the liver. *Am J Physiol.* 1964;207:13–17.
22. Levy CM, Bender J, Silverberg M, et al. Physiology of dye extraction by the liver: comparative studies of sulfobromophthalein and indocyanine green. *Ann N Y Acad Sci.* 1963;111:161–163.
23. Ketterer SG, Wiengand BD. Hepatic clearance of indocyanine green. *Clin Res.* 1959;7:289–292.
24. Ketterer SG, Wiengand BD. The excretion of indocyanine green and its use in the estimation of hepatic blood flow. *Clin Res.* 1959;7:71–75.
25. Prunte C, Flammer J. Choroidal capillary and venous congestion in central serous chorioretinopathy. *Am J Ophthalmol.* 1996;121:26–34.
26. Bischoff PR, Flower RW. Ten years experience with choroidal angiography using indocyanine green dye: a new routine examination or an epilogue? *Doc Ophthalmol.* 1985;60:235–291.
27. Fox IJ, Wood EH. Indocyanine green: physical and physiological properties. *Mayo Clinic Proc.* 1960;35:372–376.
28. Hochheimer BF. Angiography of the retina with indocyanine green. *Arch Ophthalmol.* 1971;86:564–565.
29. Levy CM, Smith F, Kiesman T. Live function test. In: Bockus HL, ed. *Gastroenterology*, vol 3, 3rd Ed. Philadelphia: WB Saunders; 1976.
30. Shabetai R, Adolph RJ. Principles of cardiac catheterization. In: Fowler NO, ed. *Cardiac Diagnosis and Treatment*, 3rd Ed. Hagerstown, MD; 1980.
31. Fineman MS, Maguire JI, Benson WE, et al. Safety of indocyanine green angiography during pregnancy. *Arch Ophthalmol.* 2001;119:353–355.

32. Stango PE, Lim JI, Hamilton P. Indocyanine green angiography in chorioretinal diseases: indications. an evidence-based update. *Ophthalmol.* 2003;110(1):15–24.
33. Piccolino FC, Borgin L, Zinicola E, et al. Pre-injection fluorescence in indocyanine green angiography. *Ophthalmol.* 1996;103:1,837–1,845.
34. Uyama M, Matsubara T, Fukushima I, et al. Idiopathic polypoidal choroidal vasculopathy in Japanese patients. *Arch Ophthalmol.* 1999;117: 1,035–1,042.
35. Spaide RF, Orlock DA, Herrmann-Delamazure B, et al. Wide-angle indocyanine green angiography. *Retina.* 1998;18:44–49.
36. Spaide RF, Orlock DA, Yannuzzi LA, et al. Digital subtraction indocyanine green angiography of occult choroidal neovascularization. *Ophthalmology.* 1998;105:680–688.
37. Giovannini A, Scassellati-Sforzolini B, D'Altobrando E. Choroidal findings in the course of idiopathic serous pigment epithelium detachment detected by indocyanine green videoangiography. *Retina.* 1997;17:286–293.
38. Flower RW. Extraction of choriocapillaris hemodynamic data from ICG fluorescence angiograms. *Invest Ophthalmol Vis Sci.* 1993;34:2,720–2,729.
39. Webb RH, Hughes GW, Delori FC. Confocal scanning laser ophthalmoscope. *Applied Optics.* 1987;26:1,492–1,499.
40. Teschner S, Noack J, Birngruber R, et al. Characterization of leakage activity in exudative chorioretinal disease with three-dimensional confocal angiography. *Ophthalmology.* 2003;110:687–697.
41. Macular Photocoagulation Study Group. Occult choroidal neovascularization. Influence on visual outcome in patients with age-related macular degeneration. *Arch Ophthalmol.* 1996;114:400–412.
42. Hayashi K, Hasegawa Y, Tokoro T. Indocyanine green angiography of central serous chorioretinopathy. *Int Ophthalmol.* 1986;9:37–41.
43. Guyer DR, Yannuzzi LA, Slakter JS, et al. Classification of choroidal neovascularization by digital indocyanine green videoangiography. *Ophthalmology.* 1996;103:2,054–2,060.
44. Chang B, Yannuzzi LA, Ladas ID, et al. Choroidal neovascularization in second eyes of patients with unilateral exudative age-related macular degeneration. *Ophthalmology.* 1995;102:1,380–1,386.
45. Destro M, Puliafito CA. Indocyanine green videoangiography of choroidal neovascularization. *Ophthalmology.* 1988;95:846–853.
46. Guyer DR, Yannuzzi LA, Ladas I, et al. Indocyanine green guided laser photocoagulation of focal spots at the edge of plaques of choroidal neovascularization: a pilot study. *Arch Ophthalmol.* 1996;114:693–697.
47. Guyer DR, Puliafito CP, Mones JM, et al. Digital indocyanine green angiography in chorioretinal disorders. *Ophthalmology.* 1992;99:287–290.
48. Lee BL, Lim JI, Grossniklaus HE. Clinicopathologic features of indocyanine green angiography-imaged, surgically excised choroidal neovascular membranes. *Retina.* 1996;16:64–69.
49. Scheider A, Kaboth A, Neuhauser L. Detection of subretinal neovascularization membranes with indocyanine green and infrared scanning laser ophthalmoscope. *Am J Ophthalmol.* 1992;113:45–51.
50. Yannuzzi LA, Hope-Ross M, Slakter JS, et al. Analysis of vascularized pigment epithelium detachments using indocyanine green videoangiography. *Retina.* 1994;14:99–113.
51. Schwartz S, Guyer DR, Yannuzzi LA, et al. Indocyanine green videoangiography guided laser photocoagulation of primary occult choroidal neovascularization in age-related macular degeneration. *Invest Ophthalmol Vis Sci.* 1995;36:186.
52. Ahuja RM, Stanga PE, Vingerling JR, et al. Polypoidal choroidal vasculopathy in exudative and hemorrhagic pigment epithelial detachments. *Br J Ophthalmol.* 2000;84:479–484.
53. Capone A Jr, Wallace RT, Meredith TA. Symptomatic choroidal neovascularization in Blacks. *Arch Ophthalmol.* 1994;112:1,091–1,097.
54. Kwok AKH, Lai TYY, Chan CWN, et al. Polypoidal choroidal vasculopathy in Chinese patients. *Br J Ophthalmol.* 2002;86:892–897.
55. Schneider U, Gelisken F, Inhoffen W. Clinical characteristics of idiopathic polypoidal choroid vasculopathy. *Ophthalmologe.* 2001;98:1,186–1,191.
56. Shiraga F, Matsuo T, Yokoe S, et al. Surgical treatment of submacular hemorrhage associated with idiopathic polypoidal choroidal vasculopathy. *Am J Ophthalmol.* 1999;128:147–154.
57. Smith RE, Wise K, Kingsley RM. Idiopathic polypoidal choroidal vasculopathy and sickle cell retinopathy. *Am J Ophthalmol.* 2000;129:544–546.
58. Scassellati-Sforzolini B, Mariotti C, Bryan R, et al. Polypoidal choroidal vasculopathy in Italy. *Retina.* 2001;21:121–125.
59. Tateiwa H, Kuroiwa S, Gaun S, et al. Polypoidal choroidal vasculopathy with large vascular network. *Graefe's Arch Clin Exp Ophthalmol.* 2002;240: 354–361.
60. Tateiwa H, Kuroiwa S, Gaun S, et al. Polypoidal choroidal vasculopathy with large vascular network. *Graefe's Arch Clin Exp Ophthalmol.* 2002;240: 354–361.
61. Iida T, Yannuzzi LA, Freund KB, et al. Retinal angiopathy and polypoidal choroidal vasculopathy. *Retina.* 2002;22:455–463.
62. Kleiner RC, Brucker AJ, Johnston RL. The posterior uveal bleeding syndrome. *Retina.* 1990;10:9–17.
63. Kleiner RC, Brucker AJ, Johnston RL. The posterior uveal bleeding syndrome. *Ophthalmol.* 1984;91(Suppl 9):110.
64. Lafaut BA, Aisenbrey S, van den Broecke C, et al. Polypoidal choroidal vasculopathy pattern in age-related macular degeneration. *Retina.* 2000;20: 650–654.
65. Lafaut BA, Leyes AM, Snyers B, et al. Polypoidal choroidal vasculopathy in Caucasians. *Graefes Arch Clin Exp Ophthalmol.* 2000;238:752–759.
66. Lip PL, Hope-Ross MW, Gibson JM. Idiopathic polypoidal choroidal vasculopathy: a disease with diverse clinical spectrum and systemic associations. *Eye.* 2000;5:695–700.
67. Lois N. Idiopathic polypoidal choroidal vasculopathy in a patient with atrophic age-related macular degeneration. *Br J Ophthalmol.* 2001;85: 1,011–1,012.
68. Macular Photocoagulation Study Group. Argon laser photocoagulation for neovascular maculopathy: five year results from randomized clinical trials. *Arch Ophthalmol.* 1991;109:1,109–1,114.
69. Mohand-Said M, Nodarian M, Salvanet-Bouccara A. Idiopathic polypoidal choroidal vasculopathy: 2 case report. *J Franc Ophtal.* 2002;25: 517–521.
70. Ross RD, Gitter KA, Cohen G, et al. Idiopathic polypoidal choroidal vasculopathy associated with retinal arterial macroaneurysm and hypertensive retinopathy. *Retina.* 1996;16:105–111.
71. Spaide RF, Yannuzzi LA, Slakter JS, et al. Indocyanine green videoangiography of idiopathic polypoidal choroidal vasculopathy. *Retina.* 1995;15: 100–110.
72. Yannuzzi LA, Ciardella AP, Spaide RF, et al. The expanding clinical spectrum of idiopathic polypoidal choroidal vasculopathy. *Arch Ophthalmol.* 1999;115:478–485.
73. Yannuzzi LA, Freund KB, Goldbaum M, et al. Polypoidal choroidal vasculopathy masquerading as central serous chorioretinopathy. *Ophthalmology.* 2000;107:767–777.
74. Yannuzzi LA, Sorenson JS, Spaide RF, et al. Idiopathic polypoidal choroidal vasculopathy. *Retina.* 1990;10:1–8.
75. Yannuzzi LA, Wong DW, Sforzolini SB, et al. Polypoidal choroidal vasculopathy and neovascularized age-related macular degeneration. *Arch Ophthalmol.* 1999;17:1,503–1,510.
76. Pauleikhoff D, Loffert D, Spital G, et al. Pigment epithelial detachment in the elderly. Clinical differentiation, natural course and pathogenetic implications. *Graefe's Arch Clin Exp Ophthalmol.* 2002;240:533–538.
77. Yannuzzi LA, Negrao S, Iida T, et al. Retinal angiomatous proliferation in age-related macular degeneration. *Retina.* 2001;21:416–434.
78. Moorthy RS, Lyon AT, Rabb MF, et al. Idiopathic polypoidal choroidal vasculopathy of the macula. *Ophthalmology.* 1998;105:1,380–1,385.
79. Kuhn D, Meunier I, Soubrane G, Coca G. Imaging of chorioretinal anastomoses in vascularized retinal pigment epithelium detachments. *Arch Ophthalmol.* 1995;113:1,392–1,396.
80. Fernandes LHS, Freund BK, Yannuzzi LA, et al. The nature of focal areas of hyperfluorescence or hot spots imaged with indocyanine green angiography. *Retina.* 2002;22:557–568.
81. Freund KB, Yannuzzi LA, Sorenson JA, et al. Age-related macular degeneration and choroidal neovascularization. *Am J Ophthalmol.* 1993;115: 786–791.
82. Slakter JS, Yannuzzi LA, Scheider U, et al. Retinal choroidal anastomosis and occult choroidal neovascularization. *Ophthalmology.* 2000;107: 742–753.
83. Slakter, JS, Yannuzzi, LA, Sorenson, JA, et al. A pilot study of indocyanine green videoangiography-guided laser photocoagulation of occult choroidal neovascularization in age-related macular degeneration. *Arch Ophthalmol.* 1994;112:465–472.
84. Mandava N, Guyer DR, Yannuzzi LA, et al. Indocyanine green videoangiography-guided laser photocoagulation of occult choroidal neovascularization. *Ophthalmic Surgery and Lasers.* 1997;28:844–852.
85. Flower RW. Optimizing treatment of choroidal neovascularization feeder vessels associated with age-related macular degeneration. *Am J Ophthalmol.* 2002;134:228–239.
86. Staurenghi G, Orzalesi N, La Capria A, et al. Laser treatment of feeder vessels in subfoveal choroidal neovascular membranes: a revisitation using dynamic indocyanine green angiography. *Ophthalmology.* 1998;105: 2,297–2,305.
87. Bacin F, Buffet JM, Mutel N. Angiographie par absorption, en infrarouge, au vert d'inocyanine, aspects chez le sujet normal et dans les tumeurs choridenned. *Bull Soc Ophthalmol Fr.* 1981;81:315.
88. Escano MF, Fujii S, Ishibashi K, et al. Indocyanine green videoangiography in macular variant of idiopathic polypoidal choroidal vasculopathy. *Jap J Ophthalmol.* 2000;44:313–316.
89. Guyer DR. Central serous chorioretinopathy. In: Yannuzzi LA, Flower RW, Slakter JS eds. *Indocyanine Green Angiography.* St. Louis: Mosby Year Book; 1997:297–304.
90. Guyer DR, Yannuzzi LA, Slakter JS, et al. Digital indocyanine green videoangiography of central serous chorioretinopathy. *Arch Ophthalmol.* 1994;112:1,057–1,062.
91. Lafaut BA, De Laey JJ. Indocyanine green angiography in central serous chorioretinopathy. *Bull Soc Belge Ophthalmol.* 1996:262:55–61.
92. Okushiba U, Takeda M. Study of choroidal vascular lesions in central serous chorioretinopathy using indocyanine green angiography. *Nippon Ganka Gakkai Zasshi.* 1997;101:74–82.
93. Piccolino FC, Borgia L, Zinicola E, et al. Indocyanine green angiographic findings in central serous chorioretinopathy. *Eye.* 1995;9: 324–332.
94. Prunte C, Flammer J. Choroidal capillary and venous congestion in central serous chorioretinopathy. *Am J Ophthalmol.* 1996;121:26–34.

95. Scheider A, Hintschich C, Dimitriou S. Central serous chorioretinopathy. Studies of the site of the lesion with indocyanine green. *Ophthalmologe.* 1994;91:745–751.

96. Spaide RF, Campeas L, Haas A, et al. Central serous chorioretinopathy in younger and older adults. *Ophthalmology.* 1996;103:2,070–2,080.

97. Katsimpris J, Donati G, Kapetanios A, et al. The value of indocyanine green angiography in detection of central serous chorioretinopathy. *Klin Monatsbl Augenheilkd.* 2001;218:335–337.

98. Mueller AJ, Freeman WR, Schaller UC, et al. Complex microcirculation patterns detected by confocal indocyanine green angiography predict time to growth of small choroidal melanocytic tumors. *Ophthalmology.* 2002;109:2,207–2,214.

99. Piccolino FC, Borgia L, Zinicola E. Indocyanine green angiography of circumscribed choroidal hemangiomas. *Retina.* 1996;16:19–28.

100. Sallet S, Amoakn WM, Lafaut BA, et al. Indocyanine green angiography of choroidal tumors. *Graefes Arch Clin Exp Ophthalmol.* 1995;223:677–689.

101. Guyer DR, Yannuzzi LA, Krupsky S, et al. Digital indocyanine green angiography of intraocular tumors. *Semin Ophthalmol.* 1993;8:224–229.

102. Shields CL, Shields JA, De Potter P. Patterns of indocyanine green videoangiography of choroidal tumors. *Br J Ophthalmol.* 1995;79:237–245.

103. Kardmas EF, Weiter JJ. Choroidal osteoma. *Int Ophthalmol.* 1997;37:171–182.

104. Singh AD, De Potter P, Shields CL, et al. Indocyanine green angiography and ultrasonography of a varix of the vortex vein. *Arch Ophthalmol.* 1993;100:1,283–1,284.

105. Seregard S, Spanberg B, Juul C. et al. Prognostic accuracy of the mean of the largest nucleoli, vascular pattens, and PC-10 in posterior uveal melanoma. *Ophthalmology.* 1998;105:485–491.

106. Krupsky S, Foster S, Guyer DR, et al. Digital indocyanine green angiography of choroidal inflammatory disorders. *Invest Ophthalmol.* 1992;33(Suppl).

107. Giovannini A, Ripa E, Scassellati-Sforzolini B, et al. Indocyanine green angiography in serpiginous choroidopathy. *Eur J Ophthalmol.* 1996;6:299–306.

108. Bouchenaki N, Cimino L, Auer C, et al. Assessment and classification of choroidal vasculitis in posterior uveitis using indocyanine green angiography. *Klin Monatsbl Augenheilkd.* 2002;219:243–249.

109. Howe LJ, Woon H, Graham EM, et al. Choroidal hypoperfusion in acute multifocal posterior placoid pigment epitheliopathy: an indocyanine green angiography study. *Ophthalmology.* 1995;102:790–798.

110. Park D, Schatz H, McDonald HR, et al. Indocyanine green angiography of acute multifocal posterior placoid pigment epitheliopathy. *Ophthalmology.* 1995;102:1,877–1,883.

111. Ie D, Glaser BM, Murphy RP, et al. Indocyanine green angiography in multiple evanescent white-dot syndrome. *Am J Ophthalmol.* 1994;117:7–12.

112. Ikeda N, Ikeda T, Nagata M, et al. Location of lesions in multiple evanescent white dot syndrome and the cause of the hypofluorescent spots observed by indocyanine green angiography. *Graefes Arch Clin Exp Ophthalmol.* 2001;239:242–247.

113. Yen MT, Rosenfeld PJ. Persistent indocyanine green angiographic findings in multiple evanescent white dot syndrome. *Ophthalmic Surg Lasers.* 2001;32:156–158.

114. Howe LJ, Stanford MR, Graham EM, et al. Choroidal abnormalities in birdshot chorioretinopathy: an indocyanine green angiography study. *Eye.* 1997;11:554–559.

115. Slakter JS, Giovannini A, Yannuzzi LA, et al. Indocyanine green angiography of multifocal choroiditis. *Ophthalmology.* 1997;104:1,813–1,819.

The Use of Optical Coherence Tomography in the Diagnosis and Assessment of AMD

Robin Singh   Rama D. Jager   D. Virgil Alfaro, III   Carmen Puliafito

BACKGROUND

Diagnosis of age-related macular degeneration (AMD) has typically been achieved using direct optical analysis from indirect ophthalmoscopy, fundus photography, and scanning laser ophthalmoscopy. These images can be enhanced by the use of contrast agents such as fluorescein (FA) for the improved depiction of vascular lesions. Such techniques, in addition to concerns surrounding the use of contrast agents, provide little information about certain key aspects of age-related macular degeneration, including retinal thickness.

Biomedical image analysis has been rapidly developing over the past few years to the point where a range of alternative imaging modalities is available. These include differential electro-magnetic absorption (CT), differential proton density and excitation states (MRI), differential position emission tomography (PET), and differential sound wave reflection through the use of ultrasound (U/S). All of the above modalities enable the acquisition of anatomical, tissue characterizing and functional images of human tissue, in vivo. When applied to imaging of the posterior segment of the eye, all exhibit often-preclusive limitations. In particular, the frequently employed posterior segment conventional U/S typically achieves spatial resolutions only in the range of 120 to 150 μm. (1)

Partial coherence imaging, also known as optical coherence tomography (OCT) when applied to cross-sectional imaging, is a rapidly emerging biomedical technology. It has demonstrated a wide range of biological and medical applications. It offers non-invasive, real-time high spatial resolution (μm) imaging of cell and tissue microstructure to a depth of a few millimeters in biological tissue. Such properties offer an exciting prospect for ophthalmic imaging, particularly of the posterior segment structures, including the individual layers of the retina.

EVOLUTION OF OCT

Developed by a collaboration of ophthalmologists and bioengineers at the Massachusetts Institute of Technology, OCT imaging was first applied to the anterior segment and retinal tissues of the eye in the early nineties (2,3). Following the release of the first commercial series of machines in 1995 (OCT1, Zeiss Humphrey Instruments) through 2002 (OCT3), the technique has been applied to a very wide range of medical scenarios. In vitro and in vivo diagnostic OCT imaging has now been performed in urology, dermatology, cardiology, gastroenterology, and other general tumor diagnostics (4–8). Furthermore, the technique has been expanded to provide a role in surgical intervention (e.g., image-guided identification of breast carcinoma [9]) and molecular research (e.g., tracking the in vivo migration of neural crest cells or visualization of mitotic activity within a cell [10]). In a demonstration of its versatility, OCT has even been used to read data from multi-layer optical discs (11).

In retinal disease, the use of OCT has now been validated in a range of pathologies, including diabetic retinopathy, macular edema, macular holes and diseases causing alterations in retinal thickness (12). The changes are often detected before the onset of physical symptoms. It has also been used to guide retinal photocoagulation. As we subsequently detail, OCT is emerging as a useful technique for the detection of the range of pathologies that comprise AMD.

PRINCIPLES IN OCT

OCT essentially performs optical ranging in biological tissue. Typically, a 200-μW beam of near infrared light (between 800 nm and 1500 nm) from a superluminescent diode is projected via a slit lamp and through a +78 D biomicroscopy lens onto biological tissue (the retina). Each interface between different types of tissue (where the optical index of refraction changes) reflects a portion of the incident beam. The relative position of such interfaces can then be determined by using interferometric calculations (see below). This produces simple ranging information along a single longitudinal axis, analogous to an A-Scan of ultrasonography. When the axis of ranging is moved in a horizontal direction, the composite of several such projections produces a cross-sectional image (analogous to B-scan of ultrasonography). A typical OCT3 B-Scan is comprised of 512 A-scans, with the OCT3 machine capable of simultaneous acquisition of up to six A-scans in approximately 1 s. Alignment of scans is performed relative to the very high reflectivity of the retinal pigment epithelium. Modified scanning patterns may be used, including radial scans centered at a given point and annular scans of varying diameters. Fixed scan patterns may be used for comparison in follow-up examinations.

Rather then simply calculating the time difference of reflections, as in ultrasound, OCT utilizes the principle of white light interference, originally described by Sir Isaac Newton. When two light beams cross each other's paths, an interference pattern is produced. With low-coherence light the pattern is only detectable when the path lengths of the two beams are equal (or within a small distance known as the *coherence length* of the beam, related to the wavelength in the center of the spectrum of the incident light). This principle is utilized in an OCT machine (Fig. 11.1) by splitting the original low-coherent light into two beams by use of a partially reflective mirror (splitter). The reflected (or reference beam) is directed onto an adjustable mirror, while the transmitted beam (or optical beam) is directed

onto the tissue. The optical beam (now known as the measurement beam) is reflected from various tissue interfaces back to the splitter, where it is redirected onto the photo detector. By adjusting the position of the reference mirror, patterns will appear at the photodetector that correspond to the path lengths set by various tissue interfaces, whose relative positions can then be plotted.

The resolution of this axial ranging is related to coherence length, which itself is dependent upon spectral bandwidth (the difference in wavelengths between the shortest and longest wavelengths in the originally produced light) and wavelength in the center of that spectrum. Broad spectrums and low-center wavelengths produce high axial resolutions, but the latter is rapidly attenuated in biological tissue, limiting the range of penetration. An OCT3 system is capable of an axial resolution less than 10 μm (13).

The transverse resolution in an OCT system is independent of the axial resolution and is primarily dependent upon the focus area of the transmitted beam (known as spot size). Smaller spot sizes produce higher transverse resolutions, but also limit the depth to which the beam can be focused. The field of view of an OCT image is limited to about 30 degrees. It is possible to image through media opacities, including cataract or vitreous hemorrhage, though the resolutions falls.

The magnitude (or intensity) of the interference pattern depends on the optical properties of the tissue from which the beam is reflected and can be converted to a logarithmic grey scale image or, for more intuitive viewing, to a standardized false color rainbow image. Blue is used to represent areas of low reflectivity, with green, yellow, red and white representing progressively higher reflectivity. A typical false color image of the posterior segment is shown in Figure 11.2.

An OCT image is actually an image map of the different optical properties of tissue, rather than the real differences in histology *per se*. However, particularly with the newer OCT3 system, different colors on an OCT image have been shown to correlate well with the traditional histological stains that differentiate tissue types (13).

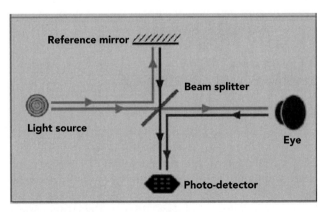

Figure 11.1 Stylized representation of the OCT system showing elements involved in interferometry.

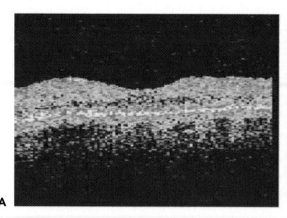 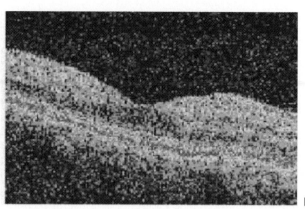

Figure 11.2 OCT and OCT3 representations of a normal posterior pole.

The quality of an OCT image can be quantitatively measured by the signal-to-noise ratio (SNR) of the image, a measure of the actual amount of information (signal) in the image relative to all other sources of error (noise). The SNR decreases with greater beam penetration and with increased number of imaged elements (resolution). A more powerful incident beam increases the SNR. The maximum power is limited by safety standards designed to prevent harmful biological effects. In practice, such safety limits currently correspond to a maximum imaging depth of 1 to 3 mm in highly scattering tissue, while maintaining images in the 10 to 15 μm range. In more transparent structures, such as the eye (anterior to the retinal layer), up to 10 to 20 mm imaging depth is possible. Additionally, as newer OCT systems employee narrow fiber-optic cable probes (125 μm) for beam guidance, the fiber itself can easily be advanced to the surface of the tissue to be examined, even when this is deep within the body. The SNR will also fall as the frame rate (the rate of repeat capture of the same image) increases due to the allocation of the available signal between the frames. Thus, acquisition rates are also limited by available power (or bandwidth).

After the image is captured at the photo-detector, digital image processing may be employed to enable algorithmic enhancement of the incoming signal in particular ways, including edge detection or contrast enhancement, or preferential imaging of one tissue type.

THE NORMAL OCT IMAGE

Figure 11.2 shows an OCT2 (2a) and corresponding OCT3 (2b) image of a normal posterior segment. The retinal pigment epithelium (RPE) and choriocapillaris appear as a high reflectivity (red) line. They are used as a central reference, with an area of lower reflectivity (yellow-green) above representing the retina. The internal limiting membrane (vitreoretinal interface) is then the demarcation between the retina and the non-reflective posterior vitreous. Retinal thickness is defined as the distance between

this demarcation and the anterior surface of the RPE. If any degree of vitreoretinal detachment is present, the posterior hyaloid face may be visible as a thin hyper-reflective (red-white) line against the vitreous. The foveal depression is clearly visible. Foveal thickness, as measured by OCT3, is approximately 160 μm (14).

The area deep to the red reference line shows a poorer SNR due to attenuation. This hyporeflective (green) layer is the choroid, with the choroidal bloods vessels appearing as even more hyporeflective structures within.

OCT IN AMD

The range of pathologies in AMD may broadly be split into three groups. The earliest signs are non-exudative changes: pigment abnormalities known as drusen and geographic atrophy. Later, changes of serous and hemorrhagic detachment of the retina and RPE, and tears of the RPE can develop. Finally neovascular lesions (fibrovascular pigment epithelial detachments (FVPED), well-defined choroidal neovascularization (CNV), and poorly defined CNV) and fibrous scarring can appear.

GROUP 1—EARLY NON-EXUDATIVE CHANGES

Soft, non-calcified, drusen in non-exudative AMD (Fig. 11.3) appear as elevations of the highly reflective (red) RPE layers. This is consistent with accumulation of amorphous material within or adjacent to Bruch's membrane. The lack of optical shadowing in the choroid below these contours differentiates it from serous detachment of RPE.

With geographic atrophy, OCT demonstrates a well-defined region of increased reflectivity in the normally hyporeflective choroid due to increased incident (and reflected) light reaching the choroid via the atrophic pigment layer. The contour of the fovea may be altered and the hyporeflective photoreceptor layer absent (Fig. 11.4).

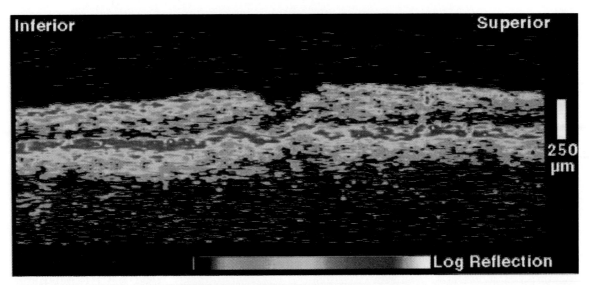

Figure 11.3   Soft drusen of non-exudative AMD.

GROUP 2—DETACHMENT OF THE RETINA

Retinal detachments appear as elevation of the central hyper-reflective (red) layer, corresponding to the RPE. Serous detachment of RPE appears as elevation of this central (red) line over a serous, fluid filled, optically clear (black) cavity, with optical shadowing of the choroidal reflections beneath (Fig. 11.5). Areas of adjacent sub-retinal fluid accumulation may be noted in more advanced cases.

Detachment of the neurosensory layer alone, without the RPE, would not show elevation of the central red line. Hemorrhagic detachment shows the same elevation of the RPE but with moderate (green) reflectivity beneath the detachment instead of an optically clear space, corresponding to the region of hemorrhage. Again, optical shadowing occurs and adjacent serous (black) areas may be present. When a tear is present, the normal dome shaped profile of the RPE is lost, often replaced by a double red reflective layer representing folded RPE (Fig. 11.6). Adjacent to this, an area of hyper-reflective choroid appears allowing greater penetration of light due to the loss of the RPE.

GROUP 3—NEOVASCULARIZATION OF AMD

Of the neovascular lesions, FVPED presents very similarly to hemorrhagic detachment with elevation of the red line over an area of moderate reflectivity. However, this elevation

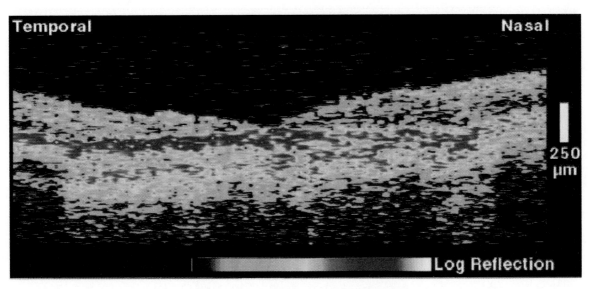

Figure 11.4   Geographic atrophy of AMD.

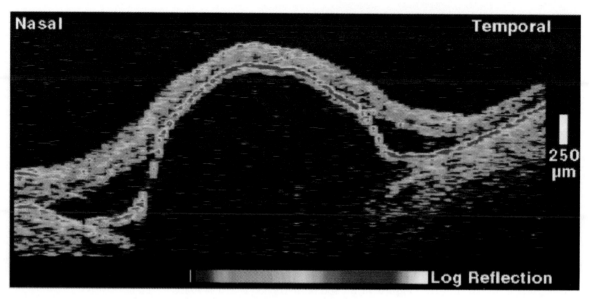

Figure 11.5 Serous detachment of the retinal pigment epithelium.

represents new vessel formation and does not cause significant optical shadowing or attenuation (Fig. 11.7). Consistent with all neovascularization, the RPE is thickened and fragmented, initially, along the inferior border.

When such thickening and fragmentation of the RPE has well defined borders, often with fusiform morphology, it is known as well defined CNV (analogous to classical CNV on angiography, and thought to be new vessels penetrating via breaks in the RPE) (Fig. 11.8). In poorly defined CNV, the RPE changes are more irregular and variable on cross-sectional appearance. Disciform scars are often difficult to distinguish from CNV on OCT, but the former is usually associated with thinning or atrophy of the RPE.

OCT AFTER PHOTODYNAMIC THERAPY

OCT appears to be a useful tool for monitoring the response of the RPE and retina after photodynamic therapy (PDT) performed for CNV in AMD (Fig. 11.9). In one study (15), OCT identified specific signs for monitoring the response in the period after treatment with PDT with Visudyne™ for predominantly classical subfoveal CNV. One of these signs included measurement of the fluid to fibrosis ratio, providing a more accurate indication of the distinction between cystic macular edema and the return of neovascular activity, both of which may have been misinterpreted as new leakage on a corresponding FA. While not replacing angiography for post-therapy evaluation, this

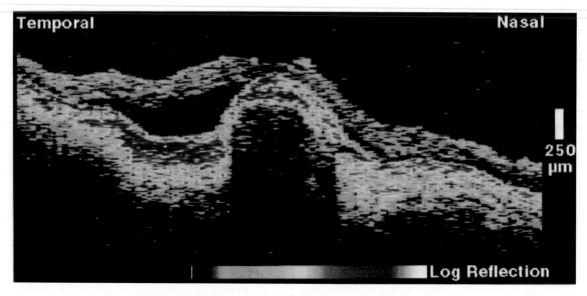

Figure 11.6 Spontaneous tear of the retinal pigment epithelium.

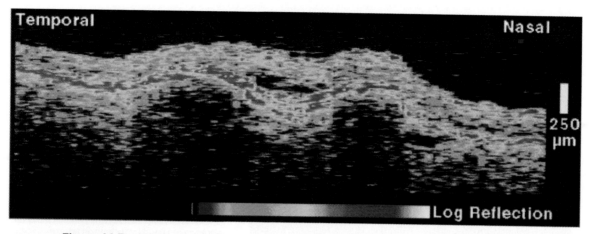

Figure 11.7   OCT showing fibrovascular pigment epithelial detachments at two sites in the retina.

staging system for OCT appearance was found to be a useful adjunct to determine whether repeat therapy was likely to be beneficial rather than detrimental.

LIMITATIONS AND COMPARATIVE ADVANTAGE

OCT is a technique that picks up where ultrasound left off, providing a new range of high resolution cross sectional images of posterior segment structures, including the vitreous, retina and choroid. In AMD, drusen, geographic atrophy, sub-retinal and intra-retinal fluid accumulation, hemorrhage, RPE detachments, RPE tears and neovascularization all show distinct patterns, enabling accurate identification and differentiation.

Of these, the importance of the early detection of neovascular membranes in CNV cannot be understated. AMD is the leading cause of blindness in the elderly population of the developed world. Though CNV only makes up 20% of visual loss in AMD (16), it is most likely to lead to blindness. Early and appropriate treatment may lead to

measurably and significantly improved visual acuity and an increase in quality of life.

A key feature CNV is RPE thickening. The Retinal Thickness Analyzer (RTA, Talia Technology Inc, Tampa, Florida, USA) and the Heidelberg Retinal Tomograph (HRT, Heidelberg Engineering, Heidelberg, Germany) can both produce cross sectional and surface tomographic retinal images with quantitative thickness data. Retinal thickness measured by OCT and RTA correlate very well and in certain situations (early diabetic retinopathy, but not AMD) the RTA may have an increased sensitivity to the onset of retinal thickening (17–19). However, RTA produces more false positive measurements of retinal thickening (19) and is more adversely affected by media opacities (18). HRT is more effective than either OCT or RTA when imaging the outer layers of the retina in the presence of hemorrhage and hard exudates (20), but is slower to acquire an image, requiring patients to maintain fixation for extended periods of time.

Classical angiography uses FA, captured by fundus photography or SLO. A portion of FA occult CNV has been shown to be well defined (and thus amenable to intervention) by both the newer technique of digital high-speed (<1 image/second) indocyanine green (ICG) angiography (which also has a near-infrared spectrum similar to OCT) and OCT (Fig. 11.10) (21).

Furthermore the high temporal resolutions of both of these techniques (though now high-speed FA is also available) have enabled the accurate identification of so-called feeder vessels that supply blood to new vessels in CNV (22). This high temporal resolution is needed to capture flow information in the choroid, which has the highest blood flow to tissue weight ratio of any tissue in the body (being approximately 20 to 30 times greater than that of retinal blood flow [23]). Furthermore the fluorescent lesion size on ICG correlates much better with the actual CNV membrane size than FA (which often overestimates the true lesion size [24]) and correlates well with the membrane size as measured by OCT (21).

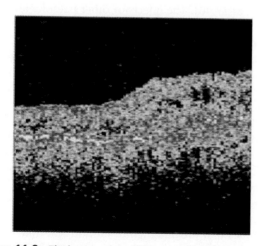

Figure 11.8   Thickening of the RPE consistent with CNV.

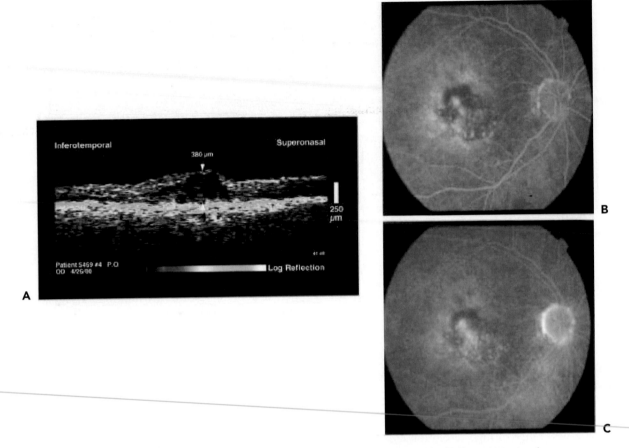

Figure 11.9 OCT clarifies the nature of leakage detected by angiography (**B,C**) as cystic macular edema (**A**) and not recurrence of CNV activity.

There are several advantages of OCT over ICG or FA. It is non-invasive and does not use dye and thus may be used in those allergic to FA or ICG dyes or those with other contraindications to such dyes. It does not require a needle-stick and is often well tolerated in children, who do not readily tolerate dye angiography. Furthermore it provides clear intuitive analysis of retinal thickness, easily understood by both patients and more junior levels of the medical staff (25). In certain pathologies, in particular RPE detachments, one study found that OCT often showed lesion sizes greater than that of ICG (or the older FA) which to correlate with altered histology that was not observable by ICG (or FA) (21).

Conversely, the OCT is relatively expensive and thus not widely available, requires a reasonable degree of patient cooperation, and is degraded in the presence of opacity within the media. Furthermore, severe hemorrhagic or exudative RPE detachments reduce light penetration to the choroid and may cause CNV lesions to go undetected. Certain lesions may be better detected in the *en-face* view of angiography (or even of simple stereoscopic fundoscopy) because of the nature of OCT's cross-sectional imaging.

OCT, like ultrasound, is also operator dependent, with a clear learning curve. Attention to detail is required to create a useful OCT image. However, most centers have little diffi-culty in training technicians to achieve high quality OCT images. After such training, studies have found excellent reproducibility both between technicians for the same patient and for repeated OCT measurements on the same patient (26–28). For retinal thickness, intersession variability and repeatability coefficients were found to be <2% and correlation coefficients were >0.89 (27). Measurement of retinal thickness appears not to be affected by the presence of nuclear cataracts (29) or the state of dilation of the pupil (26–27,30). The effects of other pathologies on reproducibility, such as miosis or changes in refractive index, remain to be determined.

Most studies conclude that OCT and newer angiographic techniques are complementary in the diagnosis and assessment of posterior segment pathology. Another optical imaging technique that also provides non-invasive pictures is field of diffusion optical imaging. This modality collects multiply scattered diffusing photons that have traveled relatively large distances through tissue, rather than the backscattered photons used in OCT (31–32). Though it affords greater tissue penetration, it has a very poor spatial resolution, typically on the order of a few millimeters.

As mentioned earlier, alternative functional neuro-imaging techniques that provide high-resolution real-time (16–32 frames per second) imaging include MRI, CT, PET and U/S.

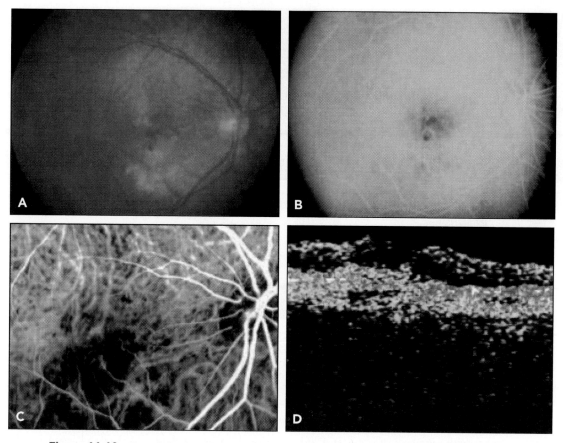

Figure 11.10   Though fundus photography **(A)**, FA angiography **(B)**, ICG angiography **(C)** all show leakage of obscure origin, OCT **(D)** is able to pinpoint the site of disruption (defined CNV).

OCT has a resolution about two orders of magnitude above that of U/S, eliminates the need for contact and thus optical index matching gels, and can employ tiny, remote fiber-optic probes. Advances in U/S technology providing 23 μm axial and 13 μm transverse resolution, in one case, have come at the expense of imaging depth ($<$1 mm) (33). OCT can also be extended with techniques utilized by U/S, such as Doppler, and with spectroscopic analysis which U/S cannot employ (see below). Disadvantages of other modalities involve the use of ionizing radiation (CT) and the cost of large expensive systems (CT, MRI, PET). However, similar to the situation with angiography, co-registration of such modalities with OCT may, in the future, provide higher levels of imaging performance.

THE FUTURE OF OCT IN AMD

The majority of current OCT systems use commercially available superluminescent diodes at wavelengths common in the telecommunications industry, typically 800 nm, 1300 nm, and 1500 nm. Such sources are reliable, cheap, compact, and produce low levels of noise. However, they also have low power output, which limits their acquisition rates, and narrow spectral bandwidth, which limits the SNR.

High-power lasers, with higher SNR, could be employed to produce higher spatial resolution and higher acquisitions speeds (which would, incidentally, reduce the biological effects on tissue and help to keep within safety limits). A wider bandwidth would provide better axial resolution, by decreasing the coherence length. Both of these have been achieved by use of very short-pulse (femtosecond) solid state lasers, such as the Ti:sapphire laser coupled with non-linear processes, providing wavelengths in a continuum from 400 to 1600 nm (34). These lasers are currently of very large size and require additional pump lasers, water-cooling and special training to maintain alignment. However, they have produced sub-micro resolution images ex vivo and, while imaging the retina, axial resolutions in the region of 1 to 3 μm (35). At this unprecedented level of detail, seven to eight distinct layers of the retina become visible (Fig. 11.11). If such high resolutions are not required, the use of longer wavelengths such as 1300 nm may be used to produce a two-to-three-fold increase in depth of imaging or to reduce imaging time and thus patient sensation.

Such detailed information allows detection of pathology at a very early stage, when intervention may be more successful and irreversible damage delayed or prevented. These high-resolution images have demonstrated two distinct

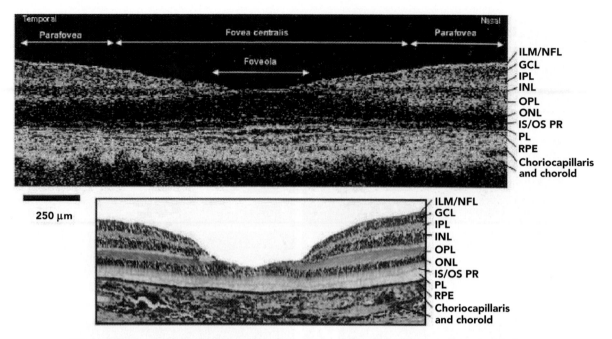

Figure 11.11 Ultra-high-resolution OCT of a normal macula with histological comparison below. GCL, ganglion cell layer; ILM/NFL, internal limiting membrane/nerve fiber layer; INL, inner nuclear layer; IPL, inner plexiform layer; IS/OS PR, photoreceptor inner segments/outer segments; ONL, outer nuclear layer; OPL, outer plexiform layer; photoreceptor; PL, plexiform layer; RPE, retinal pigment epithelium.

layers of photoreceptors with segments of cones and rods. These are thought to represent functional visual units, being concentrated in distinct shapes (cylindrical, conical, or paraboloid) in between the surrounding matrix (36). This is in excellent agreement with traditional histologic images. For the first time in vivo, the external limiting membrane and outer lamella of Bruch's membrane were clearly identified and the exact location of CNV relative to the RPE, a long standing source of controversy, was clearly delineated (36). In addition, quantitative measurements of choroidal thickness were possible. Undoubtedly the availability of such information will advance the understanding of the pathogenesis of AMD and have a significant impact on investigation and evaluation of therapy.

Coupled with advances such as rotating mirrors to change the phase of the reference beam in place of tradi-tional linear translation (37), such lasers have also enabled real-time image acquisition (up to 32 frames per second in an animal model [38]). This rapid data acquisition is use-ful in parts of the body with intrinsic motion, such as the heart. In AMD it has provided the ability to guide laser ablation in real time (5).

Motion correction technologies include algorithmic and optical compensation for the inherent motion of the eye (Fig. 11.12). This motion is produced by pulsatile changes in intra-ocular pressure, microsaccades, tremor (and changes in fixation point that cannot be compensated for). Simple, highly refined computer algorithms (39) or adaptive optics, which use a secondary sensing beam to control a deformable membrane mirror, optimize images to within the transverse pixel width and significantly increase the signal-to-noise ratio (40). Recent dispersion correction algorithms can now

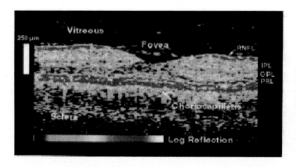
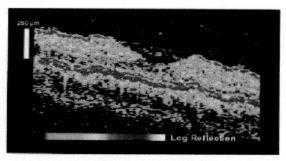

Figure 11.12 Algorithmic motion correction applied to raw false-color OCT image (right) produces clearer delineation of retinal structures (left). IPL, inner plexiform layer; OPL, outer plexiform layer.

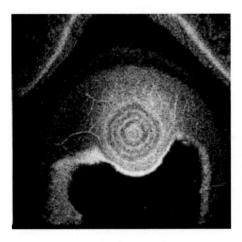
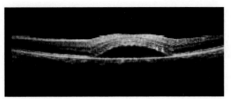

Figure 11.13   OCT C-Scan (*right*) of serous elevation of the fovea with corresponding conventional B-scan (*left*) for comparison.

automatically determine the differing levels of dispersion at different tissue depths and correct for detrimental effects (41–42). Previously, this required relatively slow digital or optical analysis, one depth at a time.

Though OCT data manipulation is still in its infancy, when compared to the sophisticated processing seen in established modalities such as CT and MRI, rapid developments are now occurring. Real-time Doppler processing is now possible (43) with applications such as the identification of feeder vessels in AMD-related CNV. Spectroscopic analysis, using Fourier or wavelet analysis of differential pattern of absorption across the several wavelengths afforded by high-bandwidth sources, promises even more resolution (44–45). Functional information such as oxygenation states or metabolic activity at the individual cell levels becomes possible. The contrast available may be enhanced with the use of near-infrared dyes, with absorption spectra features within the OCT source (46). Dyes may also potentially be used for other applications, such as enhancing contrast of specific tissues. Further investigation is required to elucidate how such information may be used in diagnostic retinal imaging.

Novel image acquisition has now been achieved by stacking several B-scans to produce a three-dimensional (3D) data set and the production of so-called C-scan (47–48) or *en-face* images familiar to ophthalmologists (Fig. 11.13). This enables co-registration of other data also captured in this orientation, such as ICG, confocal imaging or multifocal electroretinograms. A prototype machine, called the optical coherence ophthalmoscope, that uses a single illumination source to capture both 3D OCT and SLO images simultaneously, is under evaluation. As suggested by other studies where two modalities were separately captured, simultaneous dual modality images are likely to improve retinal diagnosis. Of course, 3D acquisition also makes possible *en-face* imaging of deeper planes, traditionally invisible or partially visible to optical microscopy and the use of novel oblique imaging planes unfamiliar to ophthalmology. Additionally, 3D rendering of familiar lesions such as CNV becomes possible, helping

to more accurately delineate their boundaries. Image correction may potentially be applied in all dimensions. Much investigation and education will be required before such information can be used to advantage.

CONCLUSION

Since its inception, the surge of interest in OCT has seen its use validated in a wide range of retinal pathology including that of AMD. It offers very high-resolution non-contact non-invasive imaging that is helping to redefine our understanding of many retinal disease processes. OCT remains in its infancy, with significant technical improvements expected in the next few years. More widespread availability and constructions of standard reference data sets for different age groups, racial types and sex will certainly improve interpretation. It is likely that OCT will become a readily available standard alternative imaging modality to add to U/S, CT, MRI, and PET.

REFERENCES

1. Bamber JC, Tstram M. Diagnostic ultrasound. In: Webb S, ed. *The Physics of Medical Imaging*. Philadelphia: Adam Hilger; 1988:319–388.
2. Bouma BE, Tearney GJ, eds. *Handbook of Optical Coherence Tomography*. New York: Marcel Dekker, Inc; 2001.
3. Puliafito CA, Hee MR, Lin CP, et al. Imaging of macular diseases with optical coherence tomography. *Ophthalmology*. 1995;102(2):217–29.
4. Brezinski ME, Tearney GJ, Weissman NJ, et al. Assessing atherosclerotic plaque morphology: comparison of optical coherence tomography and high frequency intravascular ultrasound. *Heart*. 1997;77:397–403.
5. Li XD, Boppart SA, Van Dam J, et al. Optical coherence tomography: advanced technology for the endoscopic imaging of Barrett's esophagus. *Endoscopy*. 2000;32(12):921–930.
6. Boppart SA, Herrmann JM, Pitris C, et al. Real-time optical coherence tomography for minimally invasive imaging of prostate ablation. *Comput Aided Surg*. 2001;6(2):94–103.
7. Schmitt JM, Yadlowsky MJ, Bonner RF. Subsurface imaging of living skin with optical coherence microscopy. *Dermatology*. 1995;191(2):93–98.
8. Boppart SA, Brezinski ME, Pitris C, et al. Optical coherence tomography for neurosurgical imaging of human intracortical melanoma. *Neurosurgery*. 1998;43(4):834–841.
9. Boppart SA, Luo W, Marks DL, et al. Optical coherence tomography: feasibility for basic research and image-guided surgery of breast cancer. *Breast Cancer Res Treat*. 2004;84(2):85–97.
10. Boppart S, Bouma B, Pitris C, et al. In vivo optical coherence tomography imaging. *Nature Med*. 1998;4:861–865.
11. Chinn S, Swanson E. Multilayer optical storage by low-coherence reflectometry. *Optic Lett*. 1996;21:899–901.

12. Williams ZY, Schuman JS, Gamell L, et al. Optical coherence tomography measurement of nerve fiber layer thickness and the likelihood of a visual field defect. *Am J Ophthalmol.* 2002;134(4):538–546.

13. Drexler W, Morgner U, Ghanta RK, et al. Ultrahigh-resolution ophthalmic optical coherence tomography. *Nat Med.* 2001;7(4):502–507. Erratum In: *Nat Med.* 2001;7(5):636.

14. Hee MR, Puliafito CA, Wong C, et al. Quantitative assessment of macular edema with optical coherence tomography. *Arch Ophthalmol.* 1995;113(8): 1,019–1,029.

15. Rogers AH, Martidis A, Greenberg PB, et al. Optical coherence tomography findings following photodynamic therapy of choroidal neovascularization. *Am J Ophthalmol.* 2002;134(4):566–576.

16. Klein R, Klein BE, Linton KL. Prevalence of age-related maculopathy. The Beaver Dam Eye Study. *Ophthalmology.* 1992;99(6):933–943.

17. Pires I, Bernardes RC, Lobo CL, et al. Retinal thickness in eyes with mild nonproliferative retinopathy in patients with type 2 diabetes mellitus: comparison of measurements obtained by retinal thickness analysis and optical coherence tomography. *Arch Ophthalmol.* 2002; 120(10):1,301–1,306.

18. Polito A, Shah SM, Haller JA, et al. Comparison between retinal thickness analyzer and optical coherence tomography for assessment of foveal thickness in eyes with macular disease. *Am J Ophthalmol.* 2002;134(2):240–251.

19. Neubauer AS, Priglinger S, Ullrich S, et al. Comparison of foveal thickness measured with the retinal thickness analyzer and optical coherence tomography. *Retina.* 2001;21(6):596–601.

20. Yoshida A. New examination methods for macular disorders—application of diagnosis and treatment. *Nippon Ganka Gakkai Zasshi.* 2000;104(12): 899–942.

21. Kim SG, Lee SC, Seong YS, et al. Choroidal neovascularization characteristics and its size in optical coherence tomography. *Yonsei Med J.* 2003;44(5):821–827.

22. Shiraga F, Ojima Y, Matsuo T, et al. Feeder vessel photocoagulation of subfoveal choroidal neovascularization secondary to age-related macular degeneration. *Ophthalmology.* 1998;105(4):662–669.

23. Alm A. Physiology of the choroidal circulation. In: Yannuzzi LA, Flower RW, Slakter JS, eds. *ICG Angiography.* New York: C V Mosby, 1987.

24. Lambert HM, Lopez PF. Surgical excision of subfoveal choroidal neovascular membranes. *Curr Opin Ophthalmol.* 1993;4(3):19–24.

25. Jaffe GJ, Caprioli J. Optical coherence tomography to detect and manage retinal disease and glaucoma. *Am J Ophthalmol.* 2004;137(1):156–169.

26. Koozekanani D, Roberts C, Katz SE, et al. Intersession repeatability of macular thickness measurements with the Humphrey 2000 OCT. *Invest Ophthalmol Vis Sci.* 2000;41(6):1,486–1,491.

27. Massin P, Vicaut E, Haouchine B, et al. Reproducibility of retinal mapping using optical coherence tomography. *Arch Ophthalmol.* 2001;119(8): 1,135–1,142.

28. Muscat S, Parks S, Kemp E, et al. Repeatability and reproducibility of macular thickness measurements with the Humphrey OCT system. *Invest Opthalmol Vis Sci.* 2002;43:490–495.

29. Schuman J, Pedut-Kloizman T, Hertzmark E, et al. Reproducibility of nerve fiber layer thickness measurements using optical coherence tomography. *Ophthalmology.* 1996;103:1,889–1,898.

30. Baumann M, Gentile RC, Liebmann JM, et al. Reproducibility of retinal thickness measurements in normal eyes using optical coherence tomography. *Ophthalmic Surg Lasers.* 1998;29:280–285.

31. Strangman G, Boas DA, Sutton JP. Non-invasive neuroimaging using near-infrared light. *Biol Psychiatry.* 2002;52(7):679–693.

32. Villringer A, Chance B. Non-invasive optical spectroscopy and imaging of human brain function. *Trends Neurosci.* 1997;20(10):435–442.

33. Yokosawa K, Sasaki K, Umemura S, et al. Intracorporeal imaging and differentiation of living tissue with an ultra-high-frequency ultrasound probe. *Ultrasound Med Biol.* 2000;26(4):503–507.

34. Unterhuber A, Povazay B, Bizheva K, et al. Advances in broad bandwidth light sources for ultrahigh resolution optical coherence tomography. *Phys Med Biol.* 2004;49(7):1,235–1,246.

35. Unterhuber A, Povazay B, Hermann B, et al. Compact, low-cost Ti:Al2O3 laser for in vivo ultrahigh-resolution optical coherence tomography. *Opt Lett.* 2003;28(11):905–907.

36. Drexler W, Sattmann H, Hermann B, et al. Enhanced visualization of macular pathology with the use of ultrahigh-resolution optical coherence tomography. *Arch Ophthalmol.* 2003;121(5):695–706.

37. Tearney GJ, Brezinski ME, Bouma BE, et al. In vivo endoscopic optical biopsy with optical coherence tomography. *Science.* 1997;276:2,037–2,039.

38. Boppart SA, Tearney GJ, Bouma BE, et al. Noninvasive assessment of the developing Xenopus cardiovascular system using optical coherence tomography. *Proc Natl Acad Sci USA.* 1997;94(9):4,256–4,261.

39. Ferguson RD, Hammer DX, Paunescu LA, et al. Tracking optical coherence tomography. *Opt Lett.* 2004;29(18):2,139–2,141.

40. Hermann B, Fernandez EJ, Unterhuber A, et al. Adaptive-optics ultra-high-resolution optical coherence tomography. *Opt Lett.* 2004;29:2,142–2,144.

41. Marks DL, Oldenburg AL, Reynolds JJ, et al. Digital algorithm for dispersion correction in optical coherence tomography for homogeneous and stratified media. *Appl Opt.* 2003;42(2):204–217.

42. Marks DL, Oldenburg AL, Reynolds JJ, et al. Autofocus algorithm for dispersion correction in optical coherence tomography. *Appl Opt.* 2003;42(16): 3,038–3,046.

43. Schaefer AW, Reynolds JJ, Marks DL, et al. Real-time digital signal processing-based optical coherence tomography and Doppler optical coherence tomography. *IEEE Trans Biomed Eng.* 2004;51(1):186–190.

44. Lietgeb R, Wojtkowski M, Kowalczyk A, et al. Spectal measurement of absorption by spectroscopic frequency-domain optical coherence tomography. *Optic Lett.* 2000;25:820–822.

45. Morgner U, Drexler W, Kartner FX, et al. Spectroscopic optical coherence tomography. *Optic Lett.* 2000;25:111–113.

46. Xu C, Ye J, Marks DL, et al. Near-infrared dyes as contrast-enhancing agents for spectroscopic optical coherence tomography. *Optics Lett.* 2004;29: 1,647–1,649.

47. Rosen RB, Podoleanu AG, Dunne S, et al. Optical coherence tomography ophthalmoscopy: In: Ciulla TA, Regillo CD, Harris A, eds. *Retina and Optic Nerve Imaging.* Lippincott: Williams and Wilkins; 2003.

48. Podoleanu AG, Dobre GM, Cucu RG, et al. Combined multiplanar optical coherence tomography and confocal scanning ophthalmoscopy. *J Biomed Opt.* 2004;9(1):86–93.

Optical Coherence Tomography Ophthalmoscope

12

Richard Rosen   *Daniel Will*   *Patricia M. C. Garcia*   *Shane Dunne*
Yale L. Fisher   *Akitoshi Yoshida*   *Adrian G. H. Podoleanu*

INTRODUCTION

Imaging eyes with macular degeneration has reached new levels of sophistication in recent years with the advent of digital technology. While original descriptions and hand drawings of the disease were recorded as far back at 1875, it was not until the mid-1960s with the development of fluorescein angiography that opthalmologists such as Gass were able to begin to unravel the complex pathophysiology (33,36). Fundus photography infused with the capability of real-time perfusion studies provided an optical means of segmenting vascular structures as a tool for in vivo dissection.

The confocal scanning laser ophthalmoscope (SLO), introduced by Webb, Pomeranzeff, and colleagues at the Schepens Eye Research Institute in the early 1980s, moved fundus imaging beyond the confines of classical optics into the realm of digital acquisition (6,7). High-resolution images composed of linear streams of reflected points captured the surface of the retina in exquisite detail, with the capability of working through small pupils and around cataracts or other media opacities. The discrete illumination and image-construction technique of the method also allowed the introduction of complex stimuli for acuity testing and microperimetry providing additional functional-testing capabilities. Despite these advances, the method is limited by the physiologic optics of the eye, which sets the maximum resolution attainable at about 300 μm—more than the normal thickness of the retina.

Optical coherence tomography (OCT), introduced by Fujimoto, Huang, Puliafito, and associates at the Massachusetts Institute of Technology in the early 1990s, gave clinicians the first cross-sectional images of the macula at near-histologic resolution in a living eye (1,2). Adapting the method of low-coherence interferometry, resolutions in the 10-to-20-μm range could be achieved, dependent solely on the bandwidth of the light source (3,4). This technology has been commercialized by Carl Zeiss, Inc., and has added a new dimension to retinal imaging and management of macular disease. As these fascinating cross-sectional images have become more important in clinical decision-making it has become evident that their precise localization and correlation with standard fundus views is very difficult to achieve.

The OCT ophthalmoscope (SLO/OCT), developed by Podoleanu, Jackson, and associates at the University of Kent at Canterbury (UKC) in 1995, provided the next step multidimensional retinal imaging with the fusion of SLO and OCT technologies (8,13–16). It combines the transverse raster-scanning approach of SLO and the optical-processing method of OCT to generate stacks of simultaneous image pairs, which document both surface anatomy and subsurface detail. A single illuminating source produces both images ensuring point-to-point correspondence, enabling precise registration of overlays, and accurate location of B-scan OCT cross-sections with respect to the SLO fundus image. Commercial development of this instrument is currently underway by Ophthalmic Technologies,

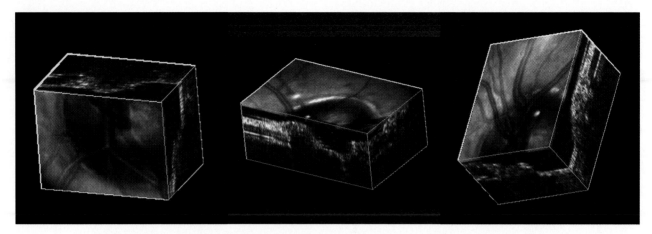

Figure 12.1 OCT ophthalmoscope imaging: a block of tissue is imaged with OCT for subsurface structure, and a simultaneously acquired SLO image provides an accurate surface positional reference. Cutting into the block reveals OCT cross-sections. True three-dimensional OCT ophthalmoscopy as shown here is not always practical in the clinic, but the principle of SLO-based landmarking can be usefully applied to individual B-scan and C-scan OCT images as well.

Inc. (Toronto, Canada). Its unique features and potential value in unraveling the complex presentation of macular degenerative lesions are the subject this chapter.

TECHNICAL PRINCIPLES

The fundamental aspects of the OCT technique are presented in a separate chapter in this book. We will focus on the distinctive features and integrated technologies of the OCT ophthalmoscope instrument.

Concept

The basic concept of imaging with the OCT ophthalmoscope is illustrated in Figure 12.1. Internal structures, imaged by OCT, are related (ideally in three dimensions) to surface landmarks on an accompanying SLO image.

ABCs of Scanning

In OCT, as in ultrasound, an *A-scan* is a one-dimensional scan along the depth axis (usually close to the optical axis of the eye). In ultrasound, A-scan data are sometimes presented individually as graphs of signal strength versus depth, but in OCT imaging, A-scans are usually captured in groups and assembled to form B-scans. A *B-scan* is a cross-sectional image in which signal strength is translated to brightness. In OCT, a B-scan is also called a *longitudinal* image (9).

A C-scan, also called a coronal, transverse, or en-face scan, is a cross-sectional image acquired on a plane at a fixed distance (depth) from the scanning apparatus. C-scans share the same orientation as conventional ophthalmoscopy and are in fact the basis of SLO scanning as found in the Heidelberg and Rodenstock systems. Their use in radiology has become more common due their availability

from computed tomography (CT) or magnetic resonance imaging (MRI). In ophthalmic ultrasound they can only be obtained as reconstructions of sets of B-scan images from three-dimensional ultrasound systems.

The C-scan orientation is particularly attractive as an acquisition strategy since the arrangement of detail in the image corresponds to standard fundus photography, offering the potential for overlaying multiple registered images (Fig. 12.2).

Scan Acquisition Strategies

OCT images, whether B-scan or C-scan in orientation, are constructed from a matrix of pixels, acquired either one

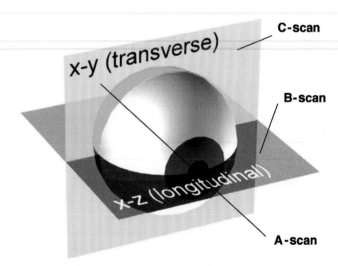

Figure 12.2 A-scan, B-scan, and C-scan orientations defined relative to the eye. An *A-scan* is a one-dimensional scan along the depth axis. A *B-scan* is any two-dimensional cross section where one axis is the depth axis. A C-scan is a two-dimensional cross section in which all points have the same depth. Three-dimensional scans can be assembled as stacks of parallel B-scans or C-scans.

Optical Coherence Tomography Ophthalmoscope   **133**

column or one row at a time. The Zeiss/Meditec OCT system employs a fast-moving reference mirror within its interferometry optics, and a slower-moving scanning mirror for transverse (lateral) scanning. As a result it captures B-scans one pixel-*column* at a time, as a sequence of A-scans. This is similar to the way ultrasound B-scans are assembled, as a series of A-scan lines captured rapidly as the transducer sweeps laterally across the target at a much slower rate.

The principle employed in the ultrasound imaging (where time-of-flight events are registered) is difficult to extend to the optical waves because of the huge difference between the speed of light and that of sound. To obtain images based on the time of flight from organs a few centimeters deep would require electronic devices to respond to femtosecond temporal events. No such devices exist. Therefore, OCT has found a way around, where low-speed electronics are used to track matching of temporal events happening on a femtosecond scale (10). In OCT, all dimensions are scanned mechanically, and so the question of which dimension is scanned most rapidly and which less rapidly is one of engineering. The research group at UKC, whose work is described in detail in the next section, designed their OCT apparatus using a fast-moving scanning mirror and a much slower interferometry reference mirror; hence, their B-scan and C-scan images are assembled one pixel-*row* at a time (11).

The order of scan acquisition is unimportant in theory, but very important in practice when the target is a living eye. During the time period required to assemble a single image, the eye will exhibit saccadic, microsaccadic, and drift motions laterally, and there will also be motion along the Z-axis or depth-axis due to head motion and pulsatile blood flow in the retina (12). The column-at-a-time strategy used in the Zeiss OCT and the row-at-a-time strategy used in the UKC design have different strengths and weaknesses, of which diagnosticians should be keenly aware (18).

In the Zeiss/Meditec column-at-a-time approach, the target area is repeatedly probed with fast A-scans. This allows for accurate detection of Z-axis motions, which manifest as imperfect alignment of adjacent pixel columns. Using suitable image processing techniques, this effect can be compensated entirely automatically; this is a major strength of the Zeiss/Meditec technique. It is not possible, however, to detect or compensate for lateral eye motion during the scan. This effectively means there is no guarantee that the B-scan image actually contains backscattering events all from the same vertical position if the lateral movement was horizontal or all from the same horizontal position if the lateral movement was vertical and implies that any lateral measurements are suspect.

In the UKC row-at-a-time approach, the target is repeatedly imaged in lateral stripes at different depths. This ensures that lateral measurements are accurate (because each line scan is fast enough to freeze even rapid eye movements), but provides no assurance that the pixels in each en-face scan originate from the same, or that the image has not been compromised by Z-axis motion of the eye or

head. In opposition to the Zeiss/Meditec principle, where the corrections for the movement along the fast-scanning direction are performed in software using information in the same OCT image, movements along the fast-scanning direction (lateral) in the UKC system can be corrected by information acquired from the SLO image. This is illustrated in Figures 12.3 and 12.4.

Three-Dimensional Scanning

Digital imaging systems make it practical to consider scanning in three dimensions rather than just two. A three-dimensional OCT scan, for example, could be built up from a series of closely spaced, parallel B-scans or C-scans. Scanning in three dimensions takes much longer than scanning in only two dimensions, because many more data points (voxels) are required. When scanning the living eye, the question of which dimension is scanned least frequently becomes important, because the eye is likely to move as the scan progresses. Hence, with current scanning technology, three-dimensional OCT is not yet practical for most patients in the clinic. That said, a modified slightly lower-resolution version of three-dimensional reconstruction of C-scan series has been implemented to generate topographic macular and optic nerve mapping (Fig. 12.5A).

The C-Scan Advantage

C-scan OCT images are somewhat novel and unfamiliar in appearance, but as with other innovations in diagnostic imaging, understanding comes with experience. The most compelling aspect of C-scan OCT is that the format layout matches standard fundus photographs; every C-scan OCT image comes with a companion SLO fundus image that provides orientation. Since the images result from parallel detector systems attached to a single illumination source, there is precise point-to-point correspondence between the paired images. The utility of this association has been exploited by software that allows marking or encircling specific features on either image and finding it on the other. There is also an adjustable transparency feature on the SLO image, which invites a view of the underlying C-scan OCT slice through the window of the SLO surface features. This feature allows the observer to easily explore the relationship between surface landmarks and the underlying internal anatomy (Figs. 12.5B-D).

C-scan OCT images can, however, be difficult to interpret in isolation, because what is imaged is a slab of tissue less than 15 μm thick. There is a tendency for individual slices to appear patchy because of the way the scanning plane intersects with curved layers of the retina. Tilting of the macular plane due to normal saccadic shifts even under the influence of controlled fixation often splays overlying retinal layers from their vertical orientation to reveal multiple depth structures within a single slice. Interpretation therefore depends upon understanding of this unique orientation and recognition of these

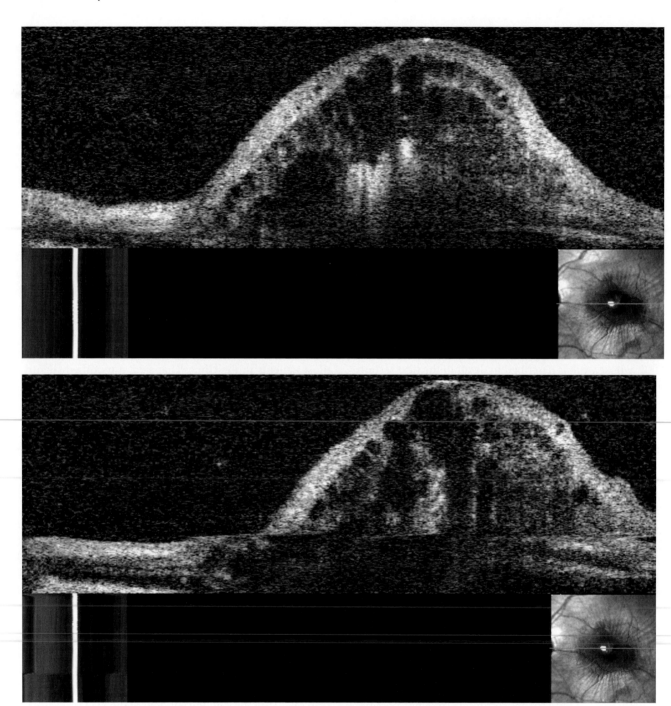

Figure 12.3   Detecting lateral motion in B-scans. Each pair of images features an OCT B-scan above and the corresponding vertical stripes *(lower left)*, and image obtained on the SLO channel *(lower right)*. The stripes on the top show a highly regular structure, indicating little or no lateral motion of the eye during scan. We can thus confidently assume that the corresponding B-scan OCT image *(above)* represents a true planar cross section of the fundus. The stripes on the image below shows variation from top to bottom, indicating that the scanned area of the fundus has changed between the beginning and the end of the scan (i.e., the eye has moved). The corresponding OCT image *(bottom right)* should be considered suspect.

movement-induced artifacts. Simulations of C-scanning has been developed using histopathologic specimens cut in the same orientation and animated computer models to help familiarize and orient clinicians to the images.

Currently, C-scan OCT finds it greatest utility integrated with B-scan OCT to insure the accurate localization of specific structures of interest. As a wide-angle sweeping tool,

the C-scan OCT can often be used as a scout for detecting subtle subsurface lesions that might otherwise be missed by single B-scan OCT slices. Because of the accurate registration that exists between different views, subtle findings on one view can quickly be explored along other axes. The ability to rapidly switch between C and B modes additionally insures the accuracy of combining views. As scanners

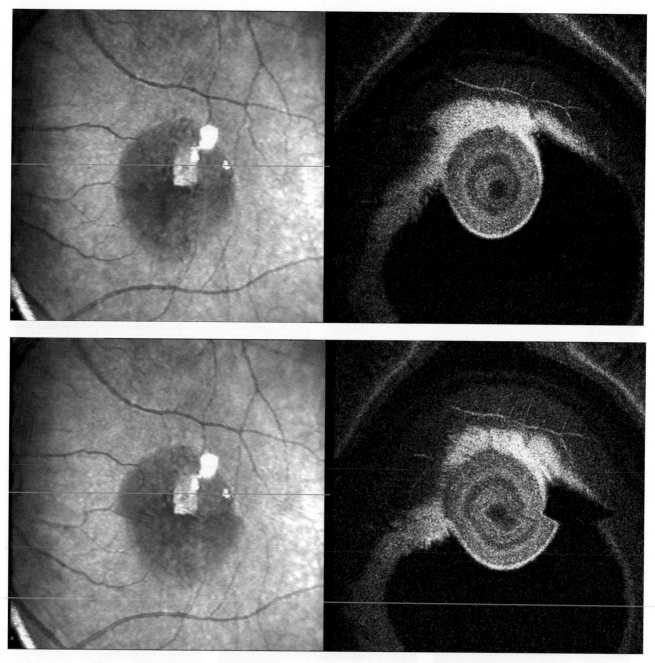

Figure 12.4 Detecting saccadic motions in C-scans. These two SLO/OCT image pairs were captured in the course of a three-dimensional scan sequence. The top SLO image *(upper left)* shows a clean view of the fundus of a patient with central serous retinopathy. The lower SLO image *(bottom left)* shows a characteristic lateral tearing appearance in the middle of the macular pigment, because the eye moved rapidly about one-half of the way through the scan from top to bottom of the frame. This effect is exaggerated in the C-scan OCT *(right)*, which shows the characteristic target appearance of small serous retinal detachments.

continue to increase in speed and versatility near real-time, high-resolution volumetric reconstructions will become more clinically relevant (Figs. 12.5E-G).

Considerations in Age-Related Macular Degeneration (AMD)

Interpretation of multiplanar images of patients with age-related macular degeneration can be quite challenging. These lesions tend to contain a mixture of components involving multiple layers of the posterior pole. Drusen, retinal pigment epithelium (RPE) detachments, serous retinal detachments, intraretinal fluid, hemorrhage, exudates, and choroidal neovascularization may be present. Although certain lesion features occur at predictable locations in the retina, other features such as neovascularization, serous fluid, and hemorrhage may be found at particular levels or extend through multiple layers simultaneously. Accurately localizing the lesion components in their entirety is extremely difficult. Multiplanar OCT imaging enhances the

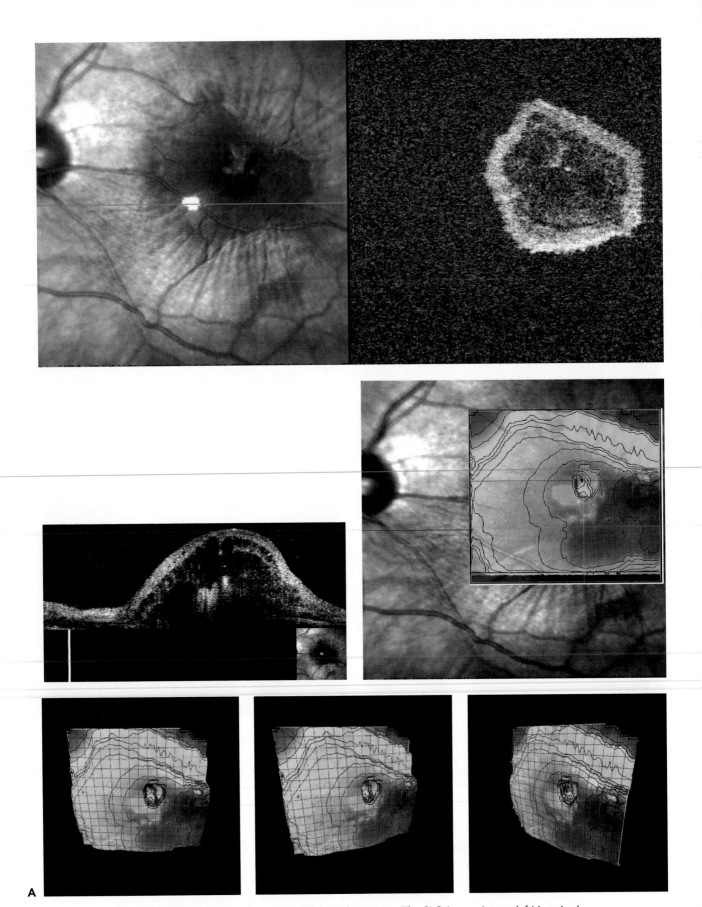

Figure 12.5 A. Imaging formats available in the system. The SLO image *(upper left)* is paired with a cut from the C-scan OCT *(upper right)* through the mound of a cicatrizing CNV. The B-scan OCT *(middle left)* shows the lesion in profile. A topographic contour map derived from a three-dimensional reconstruction of the lesion is superimposed on the SLO image *(middle right)*. Three slightly different views of the three-dimensional topographic rendering of the lesion are seen on the lower row.

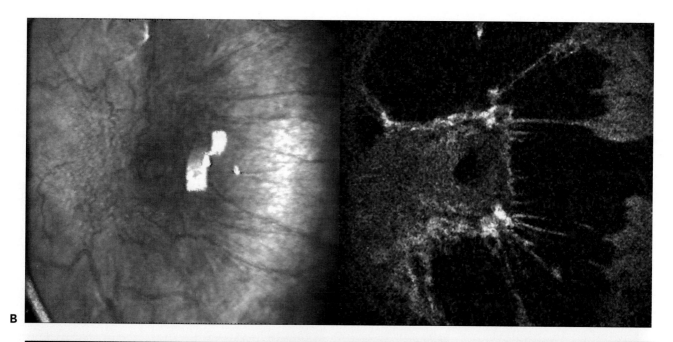

B

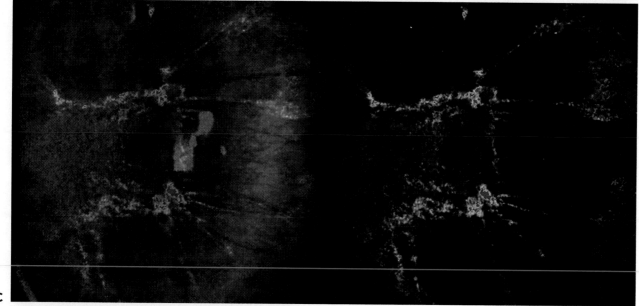

C

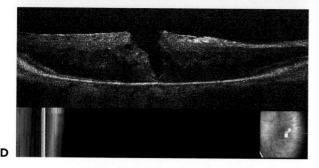

D

Figure 12.5 (*continued*)   **B–D.** The overlay facility of C-scan OCT for integrating the surface and subsurface detail. The upper pair of images shows the SLO surface image *(left)* and corresponding C-scan OCT, revealing the stellate configuration of an epiretinal membrane that has produced a pseudomacular-hole appearance. The pair below shows the use of threshold color in the same C-scan OCT *(right)* overlaid on the grayscale SLO. The B-scan OCT profile of the macular pucker is seen at the bottom.

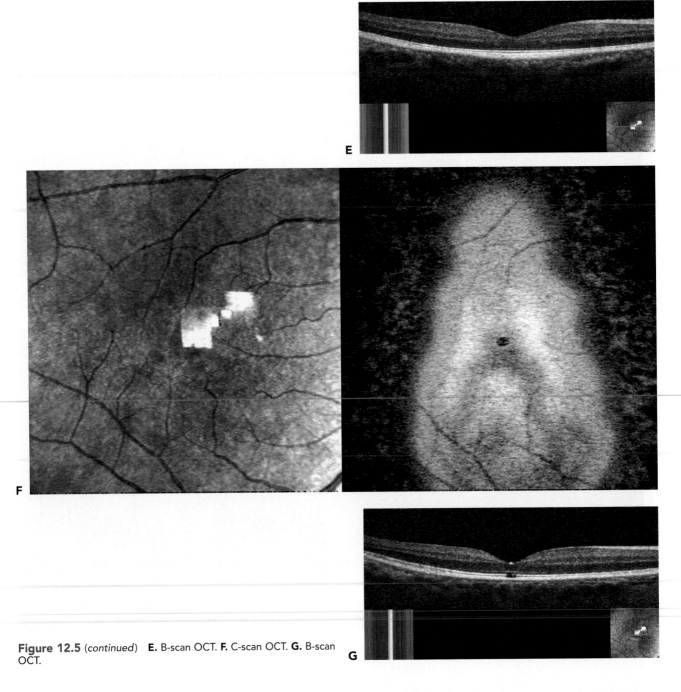

Figure 12.5 (*continued*) **E.** B-scan OCT. **F.** C-scan OCT. **G.** B-scan OCT.

clinician's ability to do this. While these complex images are the most difficult to interpret, they are among the most useful clinically.

CLINICAL EXAMPLES

Presented here are some cases of AMD seen at the New York Eye and Ear Infirmary, which have been imaged using several prototype versions of the OTI/UKC OCT ophthalmoscope.

The image examples in this chapter are presented for the most part in their native grayscale without the addition of threshold-colored representation that is standard in the Zeiss/Humphrey instrument. Grayscale images, as argued by Ishikawa and colleagues, provide better contrast and more detail than threshold-colored versions of the same images (21). When combined with a semi-transparent grayscale SLO, threshold coloring of a C-scan OCT may be useful for helping to distinguish the black-and-white surface features from the deeper-colored structures. However, colorization of images is distracting and frequently masks fine features of the anatomy, thus sacrificing some of the advantages of the technology.

To fully appreciate C-scan OCT imaging, it is important to review each study as a set of slices like a CT or MRI sequence, and avoid the tendency to accept the first B-scan

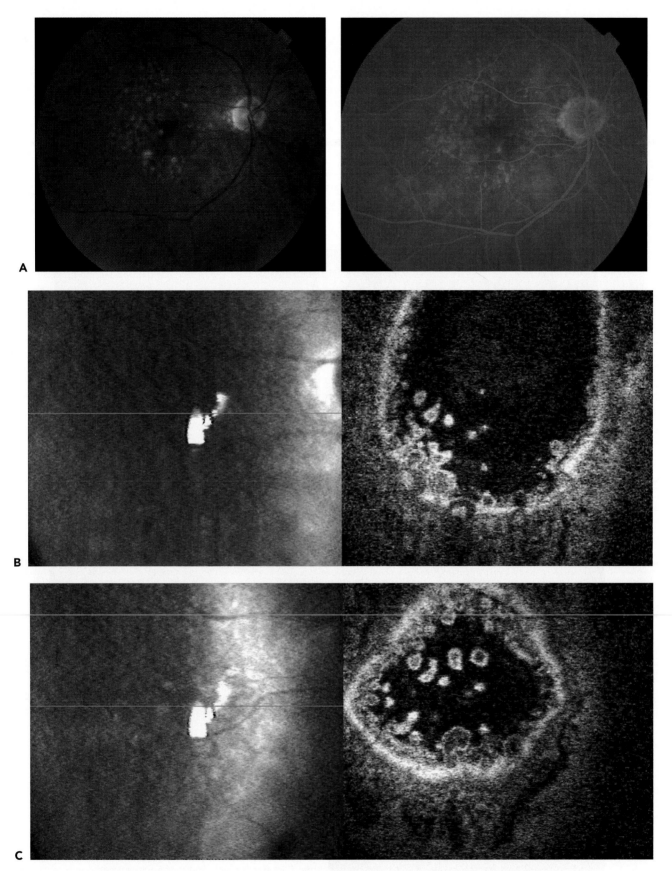

Figure 12.6   A. The color fundus photo *(left)* and corresponding fluorescein frame *(right)* of a patient with dry AMD. **B.** B-scan OCT demonstrating the cross-sectional profile of the drusen. **C.** C-scan OCT.

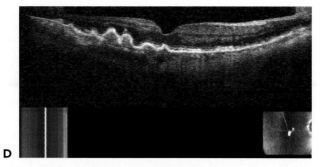

Figure 12.6 (*continued*) **D.** B-scan OCT.

OCT seen as representing an accurate portrayal of the pathology. By noting features at different depths in conjunction with related B-scan OCT images it is possible to envision a more comprehensive picture of a lesion's internal three-dimensional anatomy.

Non-Exudative AMD

Drusen are easily recognizable on clinical exam (35). Multiplanar OCT imaging in patients with drusen demonstrates thickened hyperreflective lesions that correspond to clinically observed drusen. Serial coronal images of larger, soft drusen typically demonstrate internal hyporeflectivity

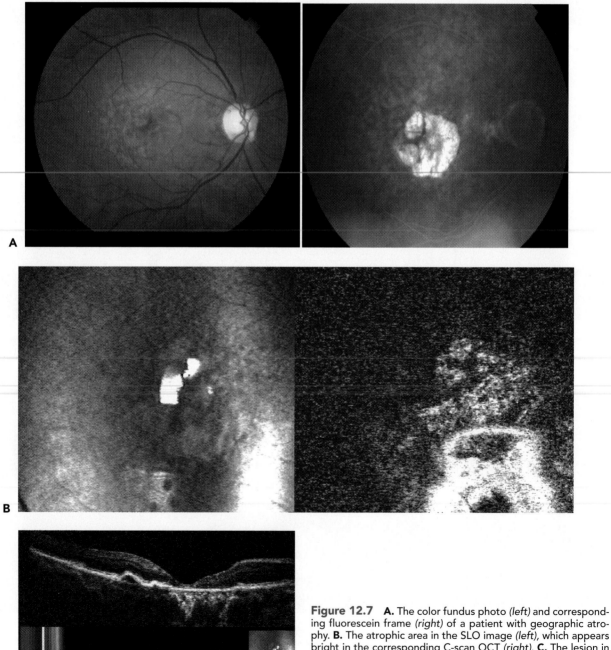

Figure 12.7 A. The color fundus photo (*left*) and corresponding fluorescein frame (*right*) of a patient with geographic atrophy. **B.** The atrophic area in the SLO image (*left*), which appears bright in the corresponding C-scan OCT (*right*). **C.** The lesion in cross section in the B-scan OCT. Note the thinning in the foveal region overlying the region of increased transmission.

consistent with what we understand of their heterogeneous composition and their similarity to small RPE detachments (Fig. 12.6).

Geographic Atrophy

Areas of geographic atrophy histologically localize to the RPE (34). Overlying photoreceptors exhibit dropout and thinning as well. Multiplanar OCT imaging demonstrates hyper-reflectivity extending into the choroidal layer. The normal masking of choroidal reflectivity by the retinal pigment epithelium is replaced by bright areas that can be described as *bright shadowing*. In Figure 12.7, the cross-sectional image shown demonstrates these features. A soft drusen is evident temporal to the area of atrophy. The coronal image demonstrates the intense signal noted in areas of

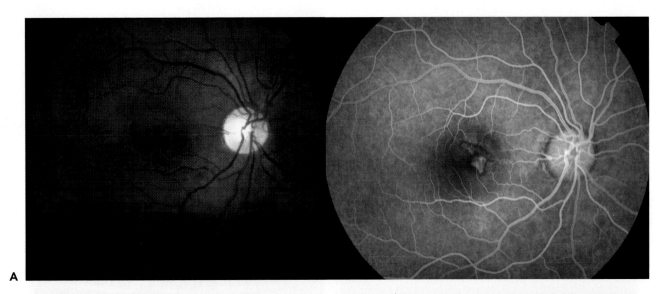

A

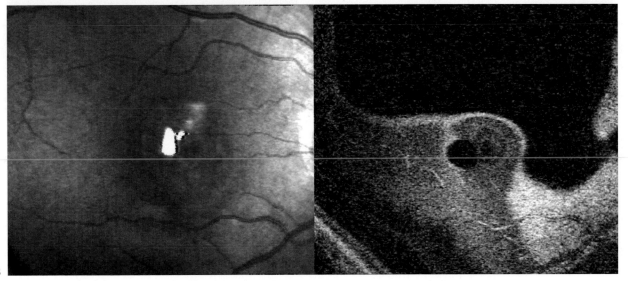

B

Figure 12.8   A. A color fundus photo *(left)* demonstrating a slightly decentered paracentral dark bleb-like lesion and corresponding fluorescein *(right)* reveals a smaller well-demarcated hyperfluorescent vascular lesion. **B–C.** Image pairs showing the SLO surface images on the left, and C-scan OCT of internal detail at two different levels on the right. The C-scan OCT in the upper pair shows the relation of the center of the lesion to a cut through the foveal depression, which is seen as a dark circle. The concentric circles of the lesion are produced as the scan slices across the alternating dark and light bands of internal retinal structure. The C-scan OCT in the lower pair appears as a slightly splayed cross section. The bright layer represents the outer retina-RPE-choriocapillaris complex, which shows evidence of disruption at the site of the lesion. There is evidence of thickening and some shadowing of the underlying bright band. Retinal vessels can be seen above and shadows of choroidal vessels can be seen below. **D.** *(left)* Negative image of the ICG angiogram that demonstrates a remarkable similarity to the shape of the lesion captured in **C. E.** *(right)* B-scan OCT of the lesion that has produced an asymmetric elevation of the retina on the nasal side of the fovea. There is clear delineation of internal retinal bands with some fluid over the thickened hyperreflective lesion and shadowing beneath obscuring the choroidal details.

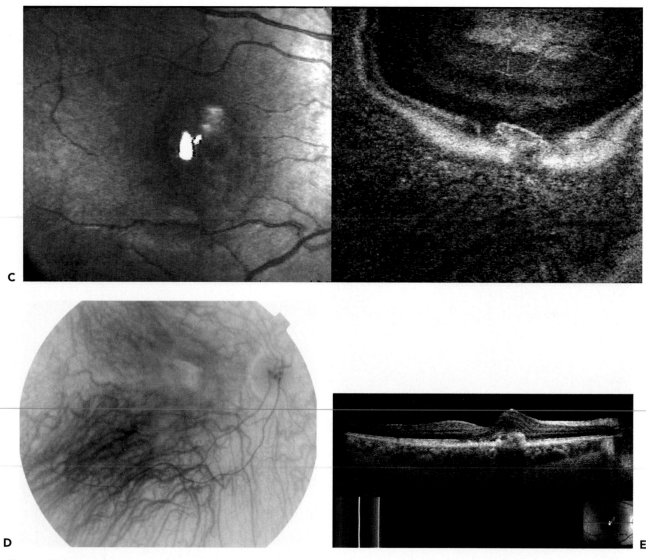

Figure 12.8 (continued)

RPE atrophy. The islands of spared RPE seen on the fundus photograph are also demonstrated in the coronal image.

The atrophy of the highly reflective RPE layer results in enhanced imaging of the deeper retinal layers. There is greater illumination of the choroid noted in both coronal and cross-sectional imaging that outlines more details of the vascular structures of the underlying choroid.

Exudative AMD

Active exudative lesions are characterized by disruption of the normal retinal architecture by blood vessels, serous fluid, hemorrhage, and lipoproteinaceous debris. Familiarity with the OCT appearance of the normal retinal architecture and the relative reflectivity of various layers is helpful in interpreting these complicated lesions. Examples of each are shown below.

Idiopathic Choroidal Neovascularization

The patient is a 29-year-old female who presented with complaints of distortion in her right eye. The fluorescein

angiogram demonstrates a classic choroidal neovascular membrane. The coronal C-scan OCT demonstrates a *bull's-eye lesion* adjacent to the foveal depression (Fig. 12.8). This is a common finding in small-to-medium-size lesions that elevate the retina, especially if a sensory retinal detachment is present. Here it corresponds to the dome of retinal elevation above the membrane. The second coronal OCT scan is an oblique cut that spreads the details of the superficial retina across the upper portion of the image, the outer retina and RPE in a curved central bright band, and the choroidal blood vessels across the lower part of the image. The choroidal neovascular membrane is seen as a thickening adjacent to hyporeflective spaces, which are contiguous between the choroid, through the RPE, and into the lesion.

Serous Retinal Pigment Epithelium Detachment

Eyes with occult choroidal neovascular membranes tend to have lesions that are very heterogeneous. Fluorescein angiography often demonstrates variable leakage and staining usually in the late phases of the study. Histopathologic studies have demonstrated these membranes within

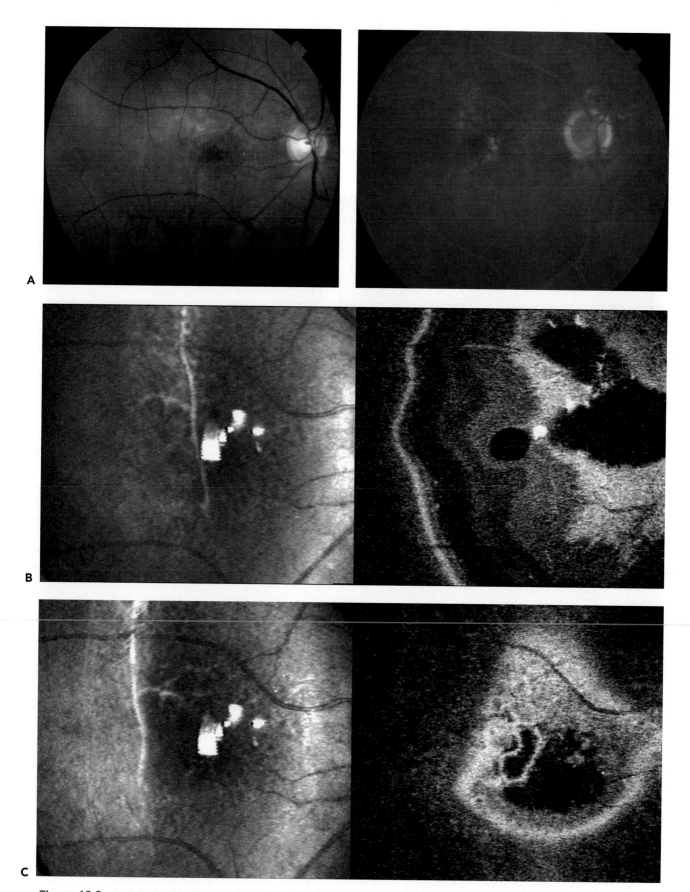

Figure 12.9   A. Color fundus photos *(left)* of the right eye demonstrate punctate areas of hypopigmentation and some pigment clumping. **B.** A late fluorescein image *(right)* reveals discreet round areas of staining. **C.** C-scan OCT images of the right eye. The upper right C-scan OCT is an oblique cut revealing the choroid on the left, the RPE line extending vertically, and the foveal cup represented by a dark oval. The dark areas in the middle to upper right show where the nasal bulge of the retina meets the vitreous. The cut is superficial to the actual RPE detachment, which can be seen as a bright, irregularly encircled area in the C-scan OCT below.

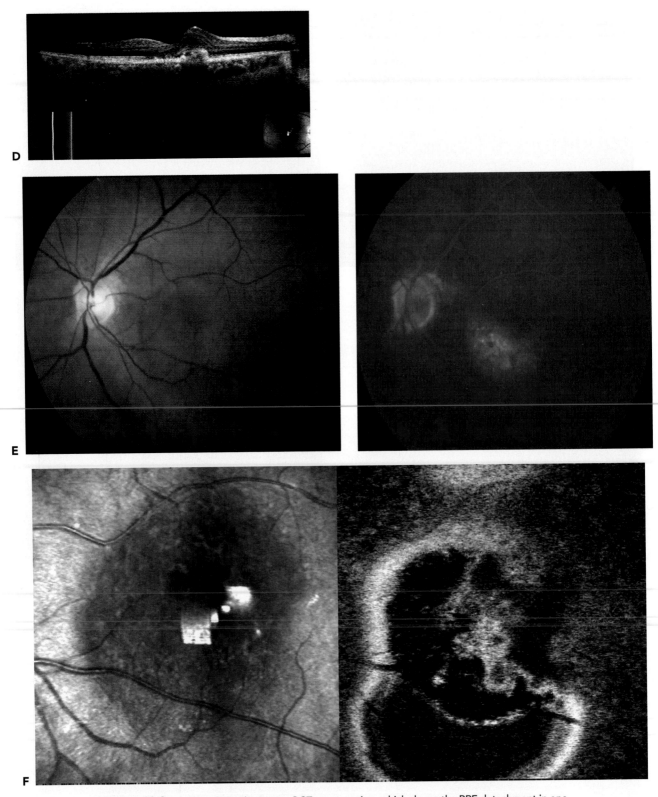

Figure 12.9 (*continued*) **D.** The B-scan OCT cross section, which shows the RPE detachment in one profile that inaccurately portrays it as having a regular dome shape. **E.** The color fundus photo (*left*) showing a circular area of blurred retinal details. A late-fluorescein image (*right*) shows a diffuse oval area of leakage. **F.** Paired SLO (*left*) and C-scan OCT (*right*) of a complex serous macular detachment. While the SLO image shows the elevation as a darkened region, the C-scan OCT, which is tilted slightly, reveals hyperreflective condensations on the internal wall of the elevation. There are also irregular confluent drusen at the edge of the detachment. The upper right quadrant of the elevation shows shadowing and some discontinuity of the RPE region, which may represent choroidal vascular invasion.

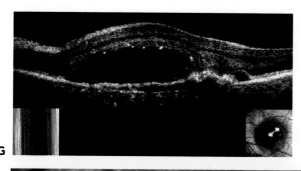

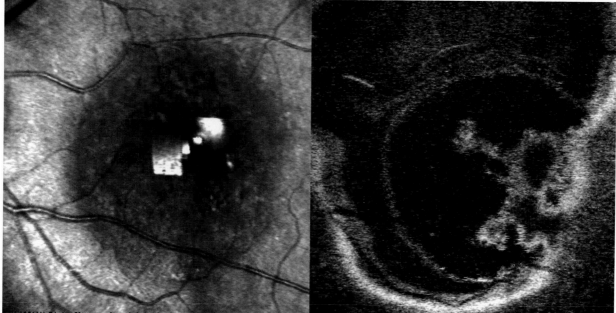

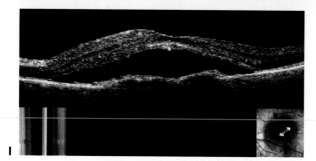

Figure 12.9 *(continued)* **G.** A B-scan OCT cross section of the same lesion. Note the split in the bright layer and the inner portion with focal condensations adherent to the elevated retina. On the right side of the lesion there is a loss of definition near the base and some elevation and nodularity of the outer portion of the bright layer. **H.** Appears more on axis than the previous image pair. The C-scan OCT shows a less distorted outline of the serous detachment, with the underlying RPE elevation appearing slightly eccentric to the left. The irregular nodularity at the RPE-retinal juncture appears more cystic in this image. **I.** A B-scan OCT cross section cut through the fovea. The fact that this cut misses the nodular lesion seen in the C-scans illustrates the limitation of relying exclusively on B-scan OCT imaging. OCT, optical coherence tomography; RPE, retinal pigment epithelium; SLO, scanning laser ophthalmoscope.

Bruch's membrane, between the RPE and Bruch's membrane, and between the retina and RPE (34). Localization of membranes clinically is close to impossible, relying upon fluorescein and indocyanine angiography alone. Multiplanar OCT imaging appears promising for noninvasively distinguishing the actual layers involved.

The next example is a 76-year-old female who presented with complaints of distortion in her left eye. Fundus photographs, fluorescein angiography, and indocyanine angiography were performed (Fig. 12.9A–D). The right eye demonstrates mottling of the retinal pigment epithelium, multiple hard drusen, and perifoveal pigmentation. The angiography

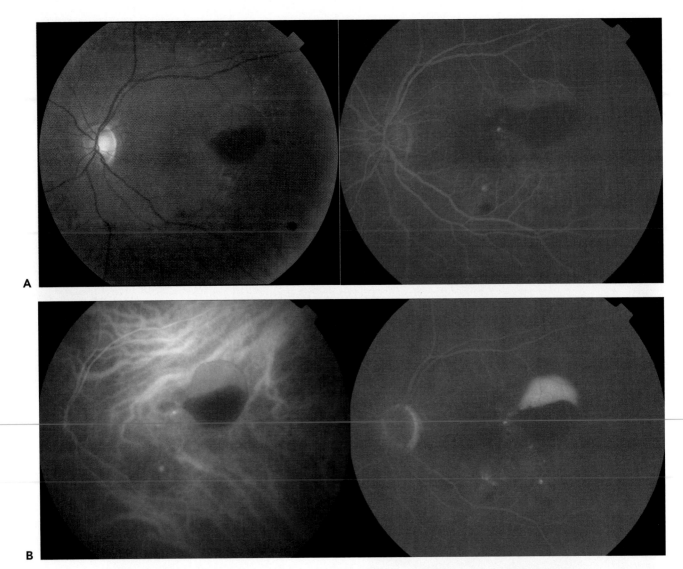

Figure 12.10 A. A color fundus image *(left)* that demonstrates soft drusen and RPE detachment that has an internal level of hemorrhage. Fluorescein angiogram *(right)* reveals additional RPE detachments and diffuse areas of leakage. **B.** Indocyanine green angiography *(left)*, which shows the bright lesions as dilated extensions of choroidal vessels. Late fluorescein *(right)* of the same lesions shows progressive filling of the hyperfluorescent lesions. **C.** SLO *(left)* that depicts the dark outline of the RPE elevations. The diagonal bowtie shaped reflex is an artifact of the lens. The long bright streak is an artifact of the tear film on the cornea. The C-scan OCT *(right)* outlines the RPE elevations that interrupt the bright double-lined circular cross section of the RPE-retina interface. The choroidal vasculature is seen is the corners of the image. **D.** A single B-scan OCT cut through the largest hemorrhagic RPE detachment and some smaller adjacent serous RPE detachments. OCT, optical coherence tomography; RPE, retinal pigment epithelium; SLO, scanning laser ophthalmoscope.

demonstrates areas of mid-phase hyperfluorescence that did not leak in the late phases. Based on the fundus pigmentation and fluorescein angiography a chronic RPE detachment might be suspected. An RPE detachment is clearly evident on cross-sectional imaging. The extent of this is best appreciated on coronal imaging, which shows a bean shaped detachment adjacent to the fovea.

Fibrovascular RPE Detachment
Eyes with fibrovascular RPE detachment show evidence of asymmetry of the elevation with disturbance of the under-

lying layers. The fellow eye of the patient in the previous example demonstrates this type of configuration. The fundus photograph shows a slightly irregular blister of fluid, while fluorescein angiography demonstrates a diffusely hyperfluorescent area inferior to the foveal region. The complexity of the lesion is further unfolded in the multiplanar OCT imaging.

There is a sensory retinal detachment that takes the form of concentric lines similar to the central serous case presented earlier in the chapter (Fig. 12.9). Abnormalities of the Bruch's/RPE complex are displayed in both coronal

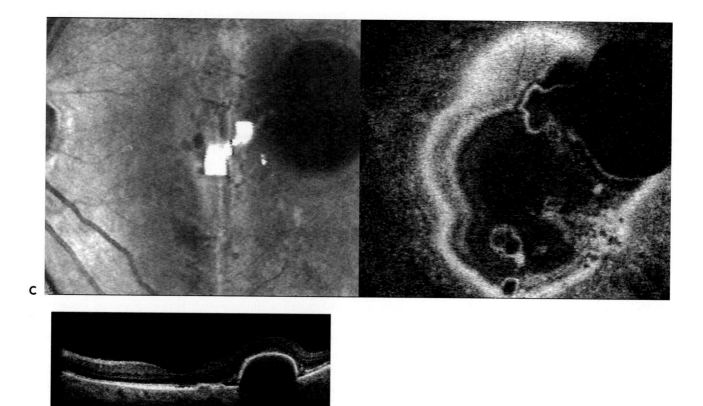

C

D

Figure 12.10 *(continued)*

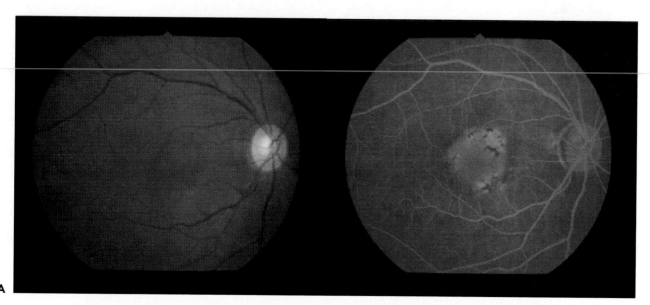

A

Figure 12.11 **A.** Color fundus photo *(left)* with a central discoid lesion containing central pigmentary changes. Fluorescein angiogram *(right)* reveals the hyperfluorescence of an RPE elevation with irregular blockage features. **B.** A B-scan OCT *(left)*, which demonstrates a large RPE elevation with an overlying interretinal hyperreflective component and some subretinal fluid. The C-scan OCT *(right)* displays the *bull's-eye* pattern recognized as indicating serous elevation with a central hyperreflective lesion. OCT, optical coherence tomography; RPE, retinal pigment epithelium.

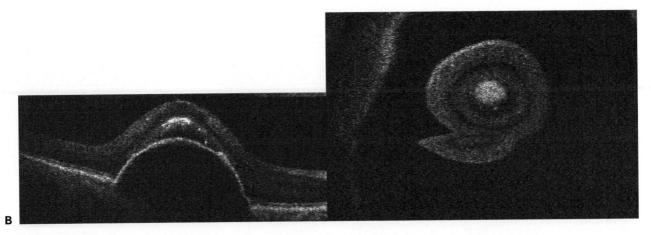

B

Figure 12.11 *(continued)*

and cross-sectional imaging. The hyperreflective band, which corresponds to the retina-RPE complex, is separated from the underlying faint hyperreflective band, which corresponds to Bruch's membrane region. These features are corroborated in the late frames of the angiogram, but are more clearly demonstrated on these images.

A single B-scan image cannot do justice to the lesion. However, the series of coronal images demonstrates how the RPE is elevated by syncytium-like mass extending from the occult membrane that appeared on the fluorescein below the fovea. A second cross-sectional image is shown from the area beneath to the fovea. A sensory retinal detachment is visible in this image as well. The RPE is separated from the underlying thin reflective band. A smaller area of sensory retinal detachment appears near the edge of the B-scan OCT separate from the larger area of sensory retinal detachment (Fig. 12.9E–I).

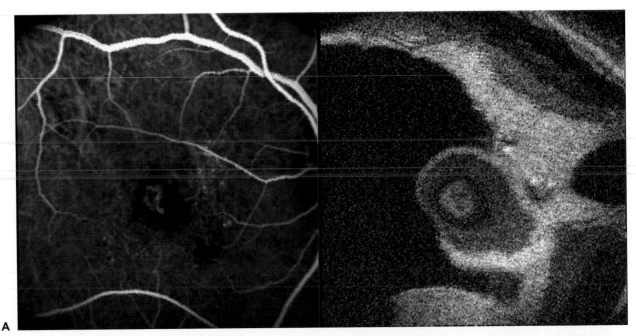

A

Figure 12.12   **A.** ICG fluorescence *(left)* of a classic well-defined choroidal neovascular membrane involving the fovea. Corresponding C-scan OCT *(right)* reveals a surrounding serous envelope subretinal fluid. **B.** The same frames with the addition of threshold color to the C-scan OCT *(right).* The overlay feature is used to show the precise relationship between the classic component of the lesion and the surrounding detachment *(left).* **C.** A B-scan OCT of the same lesion that shows the fluid pockets from the sagittal perspective. **D–F.** Progressively deeper views of the same lesion, which reveal a conduit-like feature that may be the source of the classic component of the neovascular complex. The tubular portion of the lesion originates outside of the central lesion and appears to extend through the RPE to the choroidal origin. ICG, Indocyanine green; OCT, optical coherence tomography; RPE, retinal pigment epithelium; SLO, scanning laser ophthalmoscope.

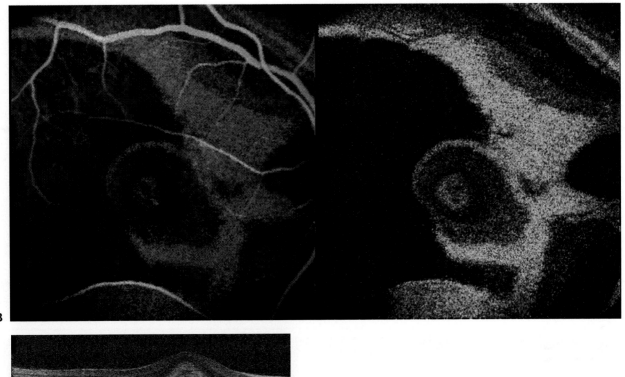

B

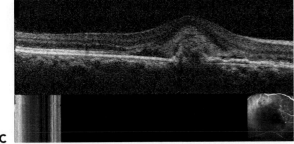

C

Figure 12.12 (continued)

Polypoidal Choroidal Vasculopathy

Polypoidal choroidal vasculopathy often presents with hemorrhagic events, and is reported more commonly in pigmented populations that typically do not develop choroidal neovascular membranes (32). Characteristic lesions include poorly defined collections of hemorrhagic RPE detachments, dilated choroidal vessels, and subretinal hemorrhage that lack any neovascular focus. C-scan OCT is able to capture the complexity of these fundi and complement the selective cross-sectional imaging of B-scan OCT.

Figure 12.10 is of a 79-year-old female who complained of progressive visual distortion in her left eye. Fundus examination revealed a partially hemorrhagic RPE detachment with multiple adjacent drusen and pigmentary alterations (Fig. 12.10A–D).

Retinal Angiomatous Proliferation (RAP)

RAP, also referred to as retinochoroidal anastomosis or deep retinal vascular anastomosis, is an unusual form of neovascular AMD, which clinicians have become increasingly aware of in recent years. The focus of the neovascular vessels appears within the neurosensory retina, but whether its origin is retinal or choroidal remains a topic of continuing controversy. Some estimate that this phenomenon may be found in as many as 20% to 30% of occult CNV, which demonstrate focal hot spots with ICG.

This example is courtesy of Dr. Akitoshi Yoshida of Asahikawa Medical College, Asahikawa, Japan who has a similar prototype SLO/OCT system (Fig. 12.11A, B).

INTEGRATED CONFOCAL INDOCYANINE GREEN ANGIOGRAPHY AND OCT IMAGING

Currently there is still no clinically viable contrast agent that can be visualized in OCT images, however, the combined SLO-OCT system opens the possibility of adding angiographic capabilities to the SLO channel. The similarity of operating spectra between OCT and ICG imaging allowed construction of a system that could utilize the same illumination source for the two functions, maintaining the precise registration between paired images. The result is a spatial sequence of C-scan OCT images at

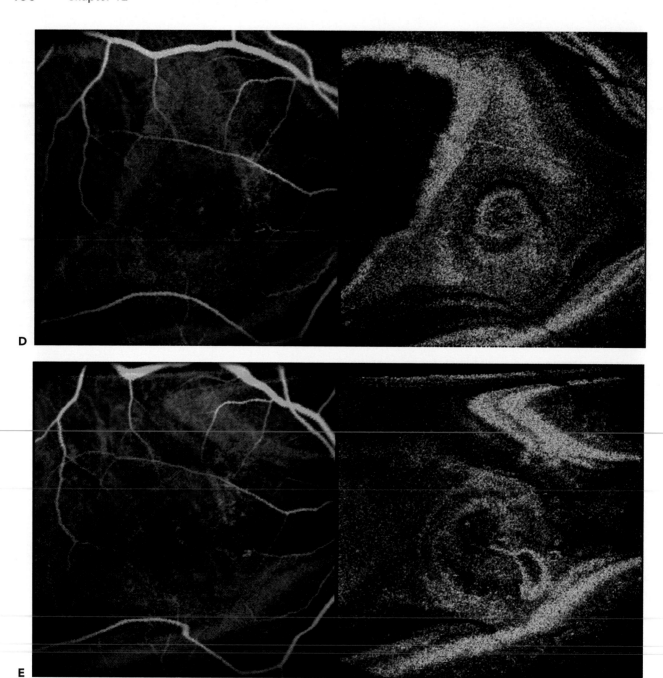

Figure 12.12 (continued)

increasing depths that parallel the temporal filling sequence of the ICG angiogram. Since the B-scan and C-scan OCT images are also precisely related, it becomes feasible to use fluorescent features in the SLO channel to precisely guide acquisition of B-scan OCT cross-sections (Fig. 12.12A–F).

The combination of angiographic and anatomic studies adds an additional dimension to multiplanar OCT imaging, which, like other combined functional imaging systems (e.g., PET-CT scanning and functional MRI), promises to help further unravel the complexity that veils our understanding of clinical disease.

LIMITATIONS

The clinical examples included here are but a small sampling of the thousands of patients scanned with this emerging technology. Currently, the challenges to refinement of the instrument involve increasing scanning speeds, minimizing artifacts, improving resolution through better light sources, and optimizing the computer interface to provide the clinician with the capability to extract the most useful information in each particular case. Parallel to these efforts are initiatives to enhance the understanding and interpretation of the

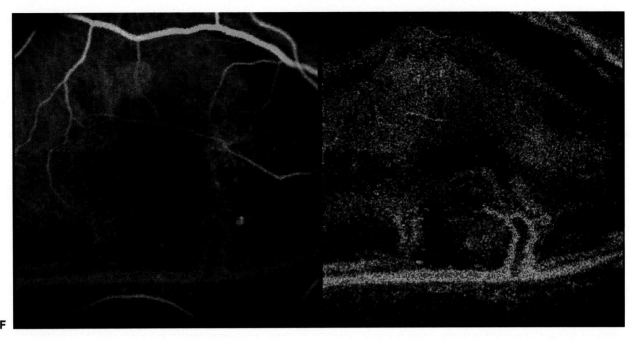

Figure 12.12 (*continued*)

enormous flood of new information harvested by this technology.

There are several important hurdles in interpreting multiplanar OCT imaging. Currently, there is no capability within the hardware that can simultaneously determine the precise location of a particular cross-sectional image at the moment it is being acquired. A close approximation may be made if particular landmarks, such as the foveal depression or some particularly identifiable lesion, are present. Coronal imaging avoids this dilemma to some extent, but may have to skip areas in the Z-plane due to patient movements. There is also the inherent phenomenon of reflective imaging that produces shadowing, an effect by which anterior reflective substances diminish the relative signal of those tissues beneath it. This introduces an additional complexity when attempting to interpret lesions found in macular degeneration, in which important details may be obscured by overlying normal pigmented or vascular tissue, fibrovascular material, blood, or exudates.

FUTURE DIRECTIONS

The Macular Photocoagulation Study used visible lesion characteristics to guide treatment. As is illustrated in these cases, there are significant microscopic details that are better appreciated using multiplanar OCT imaging than with fluorescein or indocyanine green angiography alone. The combination of anatomic and functional studies is a powerful technique for understanding the pathologies encountered. This technology may have the potential to advance treatment modalities based on

microscopic anatomic details to a greater extent than previous modality.

Gradually, as fully automated three-dimensional imaging, higher resolution, fluorescein angiography, Doppler blood flow, and spectral analysis are incorporated into the current system, it promises to evolve into "multi-functional, multi-dimensional OCT" (22–30). As it becomes available to more investigators and clinicians as a commercial device, a blossoming of experience and observations is anticipated, which should further the understanding of the information available within its images (31).

REFERENCES

1. Huang D, Swanson EA, Lin CP, et al. Optical coherence tomography. *Science*. 1991;254:1,178–1,181.
2. Puliafito CA, Hee MR, Schuman JS, et al. *Optical Coherence Tomography of Ocular Diseases*. Thorofare, NJ: SLACK; 1996.
3. Youngquist RC, Carr S, Davies DEN. Optical coherence-domain reflectometry: a new optical evaluation technique. *Optics Letters*. 1987;12: 158–160.
4. Gilgen HH, Novak RP, Salathe RP, et al. Submillimeter optical reflectometry. *J Lightwave Technol*. 1989;7:1,225–1,233.
5. Wojtkowski M, Leitgeb R, Kowalczyk A, et al. In vivo human retinal imaging by Fourier domain optical coherence tomography. *J Biomed Optics*. 2002;7(3):457–463.
6. Webb RH, Hughes GW, Pomeranzeff O. Flying spot TV ophthalmoscope. *Appl Opt*. 1980;19:2,991–2,997.
7. Elsner AE, Burns SA, Weiter JJ, et al. Infrared imaging of subretinal structures in the human ocular fundus. *Vision Res*. 1996;36:191–205.
8. Seeger M, Podoleanu AG, Jackson DA. Preliminary results of retinal tissue imaging using coherence radar technique. Applied Optics Div. Conference, Reading (UK), 16–19 September 1996. Bristol, United Kingdoms: IOP Publishing; 1996.
9. Hecht E, Zajac A. *Optics. 4th Ed*. Reading, MA: Addison-Wesley; 2001.
10. Saleh BEA, Teich MC. *Fundamentals of Photonics*. New York: John Wiley & Sons; 1991. 10/Optical Coherence Tomography Ophthalmoscopy 135
11. Henney K, ed. *Radio Eengineering Handbook. 5th Ed*. New York: McGraw-Hill; 1959.
12. Carpenter RHS. *Movements of the Eyes. 2nd Ed*. London: Pion; 1988.
13. Podoleanu AG, Dobre GM, Webb DJ, et al. Fiberised set-up for retinal imaging of the living eye using low coherence interferometry. IEE Colloquium on Biomedical Applications of Photonics. Savoy Place, London, 2 April 1997. IEE Seminar Digest ref no. 1997/124. London: Institution of Electrical Engineers; 1997.

14. Podoleanu AG, Dobre GM, Webb DJ, et al. Coherence imaging by use of a Newton rings sampling function. *Optics Letters.* 1996;121:1,789–1,791.

15. Podoleanu AG, Dobre GM, Jackson DA. En-face coherence imaging using galvanometer scanner modulation. *Optics Letters.* 1998;23:147–149.

16. Podoleanu AG, Rogers JA, Webb DJ, et al. Compatibility of transversal OCT imaging with confocal imaging of the retina in vivo. SPIE Conference on Coherence Domain Optical Methods in Biomedical Science and Clinical Applications III, San Jose, California, 27–29 January 1999. Bellingham, WA: SPIE, vol. 3598, 1999:61–67.

17. Podoleanu AG, Rogers JA, Webb DJ, et al. Criteria in the simultaneous presentation of the images provided by a stand alone OCT/SLO system. EUROPTO Conference on Lasers in Ophthalmology, Stockholm, Sweden, 11–12 September 1998. Bellingham, WA: SPIE vol. 3564, 1998: 163–168.

18. Podoleanu AG, Seeger M, Dobre GM, et al. Transversal and longitudinal images from the retina of the living eye using low coherence reflectometry. *J Biomed Optics.* 1998;3:12–20.

19. Podoleanu AG, Rogers JA, Jackson DA. OCT En-face images from the retina with adjustable depth resolution in real time. *IEEE Journal of Selected Topics in Quantum Electronics.* 1999;5:1,176–1,184.

20. Podoleanu AG, Rogers JA, Jackson DA, et al. Three-dimensional OCT images from retina and skin. *Optics Express.* 2000;7:202–298.

21. Ishikawa H, Gurses-Ozden R, Hoh ST, et al. Grayscale and proportion-corrected optical coherence tomography images. *Ophthalmic Surg Lasers.* 2000;31:223–228.

22. Podoleanu AG, Rogers JA, Jackson DA. Dynamic focus applied for correct determination of flow speed of a biological liquid using OCT. Proceedings of SPIE, vol. 3746. Kim BY, Hotate K, eds. OFS-13, International Conference on Optical Fiber Sensors, April 12–16, 1999, Kyongju, Korea. Bellingham, WA: SPIE, 1999:288–291.

23. Bouma B, Tearney GJ, Boppart SA, et al. High-resolution optical coherence tomographic imaging using a mode-locked Ti:Al2O3 laser source. *Optics Letters.* 1995;29:1,486–1,488.

24. Bouma BE, Tearney GJ, Bilinsky IP, et al. Self-phase-modulated Kerr-lens mode-locked Cr:forsterite laser source for optical coherence tomography. *Optics Letters.* 1996;21:1,839–1,841.

25. Drexler W, Morgner U, Kärtner FX, et al. In vivo ultrahigh-resolution optical coherence tomography. *Optics Letters.* 1999;24:1,221–1,223.

26. Drexler W, Morgner U, Ghanta RK, et al. Ultrahigh-resolution ophthalmic optical coherence tomography. *Nat Med.* 2001;7: 502–507.

27. Podoleanu AG, Dobre GM, Webb DJ, et al. Simultaneous enface imaging of two layers in the human retina by low coherence reflectometry. *Optics Letters.* 1997;22:1,039–1,041.

28. Podoleanu AG, Rogers JA, Dobre GM, et al. Multi-planar OCT/confocal ophthalmoscope in the clinic. *Ophthalmic Research.* 2002;(Suppl):112.

29. Podoleanu AG, Dobre GM, Cucu RG, et al. Combined multiplanar optical coherence tomography and confocal scanning ophthalmoscopy. *Journal Biomedical Optics.* 2002;9(1), 86–93.

30. Podoleanu AG, Dobre GM, Cucu RG, et al. Sequential OCT and confocal imaging. *Opt Letters.* 2001;29:364–366.

31. Podoleanu AG, Charalambous I, Plesea L, et al. Correction of distortions in OCT imaging of the eye. *Physics in Medicine and Biology.* 2004;49(7):1,277–1,294.

32. Yannuzzi LA, Flower RW, Slatker JS, eds. *Indocyanine Green Angiography.* St. Louis:Mosby; 1997.

33. Verhoeff FH, Grossman HP: Pathogenesis of disciform degeneration of the macula. *Arch Ophthalmol.* 1937;18:561–585.

34. Ambati J, Ambati BK, Yoo SH, et al. Age-related macular degeneration: etiology, pathogenesis, and therapeutic strategies. *Surv Opthalmol.* 2003;48: 257–293.

35. Abdelsalam A, Del Priore L, Zarbin MA. Drusen in age-related macular degeneration: pathogenesis, natural course, and laser photocoagulation-induced regression. *Surv Ophthalmol.* 1999;44:1–29.

36. Yannuzzi LA, Ober MD, Slakter JS, et al. Ophthalmic fundus imaging: today and beyond. *Am J Ophthalmol.* 2004;137:511–524.

37. Slakter JS, Yannuzzi LA, Schneider U, et al. Retinal choroidal anastomoses and occult choroidal neovascularization in age related macular degeneration. *Ophthalmology.* 2000;107:742–753.

38. Yannuzzi LA, Negrao S, Iida T, et al. Retinal angiomatous proliferation in age-related macular degeneration. *Retina.* 2001;21:416–434.

39. Kuhn D, Meunier I, Soubrane G, et al, Imaging of chorioretinal anastomoses in vascularized retinal pigment epithelium detachments. *Arch Ophthalmol.* 1995;113:1,392–1,398.

New Imaging Modalities

Dirk-Uwe Bartsch   Ursula Schmidt-Erfurth   William R. Freeman

INTRODUCTION

Recent developments in ophthalmic imaging have developed several new tools for visualizing the posterior pole of the human retina. These tools include the scanning laser ophthalmoscope, optical coherence tomography, retinal thickness analyzer, and scanning laser polarimetry. Along with the device development, a series of new applications has been developed, such as scanning laser tomography, scanning laser-Doppler flowmetry, scanning laser fluorescein angiography, scanning laser indocyanine green angiography, scanning laser corneal microscopy, and scanning laser microperimetry. A brief review of each technology along with limitations and some examples of the technologies are given.

BASICS

The first ophthalmoscope was invented by Hermann von Helmholtz in 1850 and it revolutionized ophthalmology. The instrument allowed the physician to look at the inside of the patient's eye and allowed to diagnose eye diseases and prevent blindness. For many years the basic concept of the ophthalmoscope remained unchanged. In the last 25 years it appears that ophthalmology has made significant improvements to all aspects of ophthalmic imaging yielding a plethora of new devices and imaging methods.

Scanning laser ophthalmoscopy was first introduced in the early 1980s by Robert Webb and colleagues from Boston (1,2). Since the first publication, this area of ophthalmic imaging has seen an explosion of applications, instruments, and research papers published in the field. Up to today, at least five different commercial companies have sold, are selling, or are planning to sell instruments that can be classified as scanning laser ophthalmoscopes (SLOs). These companies, listed alphabetically, are: Canon, Heidelberg Engineering, Laser Diagnostic Technologies, Ophthalmic Technologies, and Optos.

Before we review the applications of SLO technology, let us explore the three words that make up the instrument name. *Scanning* refers to the illumination system and the method of illuminating the retina. The main difference between a traditional fundus camera and an SLO is that the retina is sampled point by point instead of capturing an image as a whole. This property is described by the term scanning. During the acquisition of a single image, the laser beam scans at high speed across the retina one line at a time in a raster-like fashion. Thus, each point of the retina is illuminated for only a very brief fraction of a second. Typically, an SLO captures between 20 and 30 frames per second. Each frame consists of 256 to 1,536 lines, depending on the instrument and manufacturer. Each line contains 256 to 1,536 points. Therefore, a single point on the retina is illuminated for less than 1 microsecond. This is in contrast to conventional fundus cameras that illuminate the entire eye for several milliseconds during flash exposure. This high-speed scanning ensures that the images look very sharp and detailed. Essentially, the scanning mechanism acts as an ultra-short flash lamp. Even though only 30 frames are captured per second, a single point on the retina is illuminated for less than 1,000,000th of a second.

The disadvantage of the temporal scanning is that the entire image is not captured simultaneously, but over 1/30 to 1/12 of a second. Therefore, there is a difference between the time exposure per point and the time needed to complete the entire illumination sequence of a whole frame. Thus, eye motion may have an unusual effect on the image in SLOs. The upper and lower portion of a single image may not be aligned with each other due to eye motion during the acquisition of that image. This artifact is not commonly observed in traditional fundus photography, since the entire image is recorded at one time. Although this artifact is not very common in SLO imaging, the frequency of motion artifacts within a frame was reported at about 5% in serial angiographic imaging (3). Another way to look at the recording sequence of SLOs is to consider that fundus cameras capture a spatial image, while SLOs capture a temporal image. This means that in a fundus camera, the image of the retina is present in space. In contrast, SLOs code the image in the temporal domain.

The second term that is being described in scanning laser ophthalmoscope is the term laser. The principal difference between fundus cameras and SLOs is that the light source is always a laser. A laser (**L**ight **A**mplification by **S**timulated **E**mission of **R**adiation) emits light of typically one wavelength, in a collimated beam. The term *collimated* means that the light travels as a parallel beam. What is the difference between laser light and incandescent light? The use of the laser means that SLOs cannot achieve white-light imaging comparable to conventional white-light fundus photography. Some groups have developed three-color SLOs for reflectance imaging (4). Their system uses three separate lasers with three wavelengths (red, green, and blue) to offer multichromatic illumination. Similarly, Optos has recently announced that they have developed a three-color wide-field SLO system. However, one has to consider the continuous light spectrum. Therefore, it becomes evident that three lines corresponding to the three laser wavelengths do not equal the continuous spectrum of a white-light illumination source (Fig. 13.1) (5). Furthermore, the advantage of using a laser for illumination is that all the light energy can be delivered at a specific wavelength without the use of narrow bandwidth filters. Thus, red-free photography can easily be achieved with the help of the green laser light of an argon gas laser (Fig. 13.2). The appearance of this photographic imaging mode is very similar to the fundus camera setting using red-free filters. With the widespread availability of diode lasers for red and infrared wavelengths, it has been easy to achieve small compact SLOs using these wavelengths. However, until recently, blue and green wavelengths were not obtainable with diode or other solid-state compact lasers. While some blue and green diode lasers had been developed, they did not offer high temporal light output stability making them

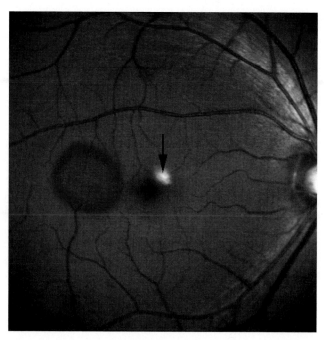

Figure 13.2   Red-free photograph in the right eye of a 37-year-old male with central serous retinopathy. The central white spot in the image (*black arrow*) is an artifact due to internal lens reflection.

unsuitable for imaging applications. Therefore, large, air-cooled gas lasers such as argon gas lasers were required for the operation of blue and green wavelengths in SLOs. However, the recent introduction of novel solid-state blue lasers has allowed some companies to replace the large gas lasers with smaller, more energy-efficient solid-state lasers. Additionally, the use of a single wavelength allows maximizing quantum efficiency in angiographic imaging. By matching the laser wavelength to the maximum excitation wavelength of the fluorescent dye, a brighter image with lower light exposure to the patient's retina can be achieved (Fig. 13.3) (6,7). The initial applications of scanning laser imaging were limited to monochromatic imaging at different

Figure 13.1   Spectrum comparison between white light and laser lines. The top shows the spectrum of white light. The bottom graph shows the spectrum that a three-wavelength laser light system exhibits.

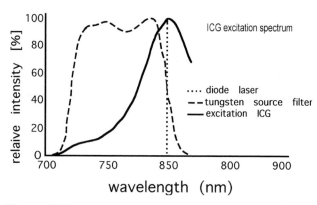

Figure 13.3   Comparison of dye excitation curve, conventional spectrum, and laser line. The vertical line represents the indocyanine green (ICG) laser excitation at 795 nm. The solid line is the excitation spectrum of ICG. The dashed line is the emission spectrum of a tungsten light source. It can be seen that a laser light delivery system is much more efficient than any continuous-spectrum light source.

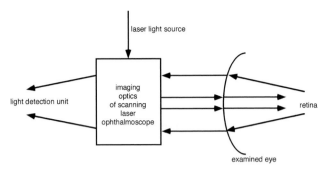

Figure 13.4 Schematic of scanning laser ophthalmoscope as inverted indirect ophthalmoscope. The light enters the eye through a small illumination aperture and the returned light is collected over a large viewing aperture.

wavelengths, fluorescein angiography, and perimetry. The first researchers quickly realized the advantages of this imaging mode as low-light level, highly light-efficient, continuous imaging, large depth of field, instantaneous image availability, and the possibility of dynamic image studies (8,9).

The SLO operates essentially as an inverted, indirect ophthalmoscope (10). This means that a small illumination aperture is used to illuminate the eye, while a large viewing aperture collects all the light emitted by the eye (Fig. 13.4). This illumination arrangement ensures that SLOs can image in undilated or dilated pupils. While dilated pupils are necessary for conventional fundus cameras to ensure proper illumination of the fundus, dilated pupils are not needed for SLO imaging. However, dilating the eye will make it easier for the operator to center the SLO's illumination within the eye's pupil and achieve even illumination of the fundus. In general, SLOs allow excellent imaging even in the presence of media opacities.

One of the additional benefits of SLOs is the higher light efficiency of the typical photo detector used in these devices. SLOs use point detectors such as avalanche photodiodes or high-efficiency photomultiplier tubes. These devices can reach a quantum efficiency of up to 70%. This offers a significant advantage over two-dimensional light detectors used in fundus cameras. Furthermore, scanning the light beam across the posterior pole of the eye allows the instrument to image the eye with a much larger depth of field compared to a traditional fundus camera. Two other advantages of scanning laser technology compared to film-based fundus photography are also shared with digital photography. The images are instantaneously available for review, and the high-capture speed allows studying dynamic processes, such as blood flow.

CONFOCAL IMAGING

By modifying the light return path of the optics in the SLO, a new imaging modality was developed. The confocal imaging mode was introduced in 1987 by Webb and associates (11). The term confocal is a contraction of the optical terms

conjugate and focal. These terms describe that the locations of the focal plane in the retina and the focal plane in the image sensor are located in conjugate positions. That means that their locations are equivalent or coinciding. The confocal imaging mode ensures that light from the retinal plane comes to a focus on the image sensor. Consequently, light from retinal locations outside of the focal plane does not come to a focus on the image sensor, but instead in front or behind the image sensor. Thus, confocal imaging allows optical sectioning of the posterior pole of the human eye. Therefore, two imaging modes are now available—nonconfocal and confocal imaging. Nonconfocal imaging has the advantage of a very large depth of field as described above. Confocal imaging typically has a depth of field of 300 μm or more depending on the wavelength and the optics of the eye, among other factors. By combining a rapid axial focus movement with the confocal imaging mode, three-dimensional imaging of the posterior pole becomes possible (Fig. 13.5). Furthermore, the confocal imaging mode allows a better discrimination between retinal and choroidal layers in angiographic imaging, as described later in this chapter. Quickly after the introduction

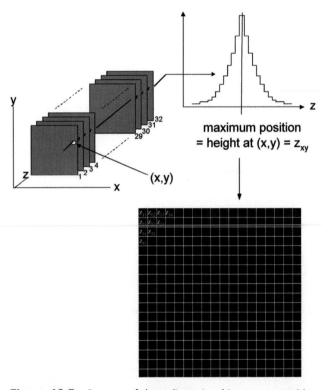

Figure 13.5 Concept of three-dimensional image composition based on 32 confocal slices. Light from the focal plane in the retina is imaged through the pinhole. The light originating from out-of-focus planes is blocked by the confocal pinhole. Therefore, each point along an axial line experiences a change in recorded light intensity. The top left diagram shows the stack of 32 confocal slices with a single axial line demonstrating the change in intensity. The axial intensity distribution for each pixel is plotted in the diagram top right. Computer curve fitting detects the centerline of the axial intensity distribution and this value is coded into a 2D image with 256 by 256 pixels (or 384 by 384 pixels for the Heidelberg Retina Tomograph II). The axial location of the maximum is color coded according to a false color scale to yield a color-coded height image.

of the confocal imaging mode, the instrument was commercialized by three different companies. There are three different instruments in clinical use that take advantage of the confocal-imaging mode to achieve three-dimensional imaging: the Heidelberg Retina Tomograph (HRT) the Heidelberg Retina Tomograph II (HRT II) (Heidelberg Engineering, Heidelberg, Germany), and the TopSS from Laser Diagnostic Technologies. The type of instrument has been used since 1989 (12–14) for imaging of the optic nerve head and the macula. The first instrument, HRT, uses 32 overlapping axial scans with 256 by 256 pixels per image. The HRT II uses a variable number of axial scans ranging from 16 to 64 slices with 384 by 384 pixels per image (Fig. 13.6). The third instrument, TopSS, has a pixilation of 256 by 256, using 32 axial scans. Confocal scanning laser ophthalmology is also known as scanning laser tomography (SLT). The initial studies of this technology focused on establishing the parameters for reproducibility and accuracy (12,15–20). However, researchers quickly realized the potential of this technology for applications in glaucoma (12,19,21–28) and retinal imaging (14,29–33).

The potential use of confocal scanning laser tomography in glaucoma is twofold. The first application is to allow discrimination between normal eyes (Fig. 13.7), eyes that may be glaucoma suspect, and glaucomatous eyes (Fig. 13.8). The second application is to allow follow-up of changes over time (Fig. 13.9). The hypothesis of the former application is that glaucomatous damage causes structural changes of the posterior pole that can be detected earlier than the appearance of functional change as recorded with perimetry. The impetus for the latter application is that follow-up with a very sensitive device allows better monitoring of treatment efficacy and to determine the need for more intervention. With the help of the three-dimensional image series, it becomes possible to calculate a number of three-dimensional descriptive parameters called stereometric

parameters. The reproducibility of these stereometric parameters has been evaluated by a number of groups (20,23,34–36). The standard deviation for the cup and rim areas was 0.04 mm^2 for normal eyes, and 0.06 mm^2 for glaucomatous eyes. The standard deviation for the cup volume was 0.01 mm^3 for normal eyes, and 0.03 mm^3 for glaucomatous eyes. The coefficient of variation ranged from 3.4% to 8% for normal eyes, and 2.9% to 9.4% for glaucomatous eyes.

In order to calculate the stereometric parameters, a contour line has to be drawn around the optic nerve head (26,37). The contour line is drawn interactively by the user at the disc border (38–40). One of the disadvantages of this instrument is the need to draw this contour line for each baseline examination. However, in a recent study, it was shown that the interobserver agreement for contour lines drawn by five different observers was almost perfect for mean height of contour (interclass correlation coefficient [ICC] = 0.94), cup shape (ICC = 0.92), and volume above curved surface (ICC = 0.83) (37). Moreover, recent software changes have improved the interactive placement of the contour line, and thus have made it easier for the novice user to accomplish proper placement of the contour line. Furthermore, Chauhan and colleagues have developed an analysis method that does not require the use of contour lines (41). This analysis method thus offers more objective assessment of optic nerve head in glaucoma.

In classification studies, researchers have been trying for years to determine which of these stereometric parameters allows the best early detection of glaucomatous damage. Mikelberg and colleagues (42,43) found that the following parameters were most useful: height variation of the contour, cup shape measure, and rim volume. Their results showed a sensitivity of up to 87%, and a specificity of 84.4% (42). When the eyes were grouped by disc area, the sensitivities were 65%, 79%, and 83%, for eyes with a disc area of less than 2 mm^2, between 2 to 3 mm^2, and more than 3 mm^2, respectively. The corresponding specificities were 83%, 90%, and 89%, respectively (43). Bathija and colleagues studied the height variation of the contour, the retinal nerve fiber layer thickness, the cup shape measure, and the rim area. Their results for eyes between 2 to 3 mm^2 in disc area showed a sensitivity of 94%, and a specificity of 82% (44); while eyes with less than 2 mm^2 had a sensitivity of 71%, and a specificity of 92%. Wollstein and colleagues analyzed the log of the rim area and the cup-to-disc area ratio. They reported a sensitivity of 84%, and a specificity of 96% for the log of the rim area, and a sensitivity of 75%, and a specificity of 98% for the cup-to-disc area ratio (45). Uchida and colleagues used a neural network classification for analyzing cup area, cup/disc area ratio, rim area, height variation of the contour, cup volume, rim volume, cup shape measure, retinal nerve fiber layer thickness, and retinal nerve fiber layer cross sectional area. They reported a sensitivity of 92%, and a specificity of 91% (46).

Other studies have focused on the correlation of stereometric parameters with visual field indices. Several groups

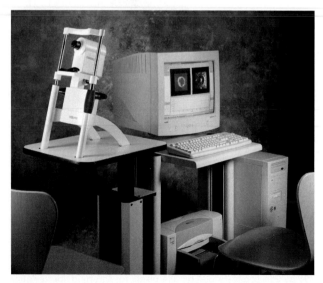

Figure 13.6 Photo of Heidelberg Retina Tomograph II. (Image courtesy of John Hawley, Heidelberg Engineering, Vista, CA.)

Heidelberg Retina Tomograph II
Initial Report

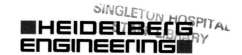

Patient:

Sex: male   DOB: Pat-ID: ---

Examination: **Date:**

Scan: Focus: -1.00 dpt   Depth: 2.25 mm   Operator: ---   IOP: ---

OD

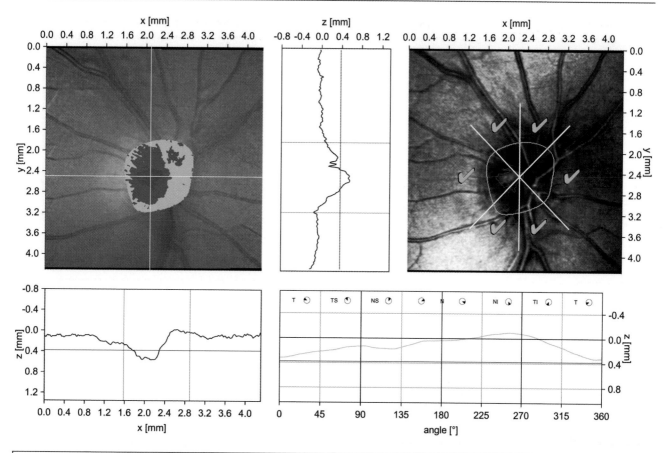

Stereometric Analysis ONH		Normal Range
Disk Area	1.569 mm²	1.69 - 2.82
Cup Area	0.140 mm²	0.26 - 1.27
Rim Area	1.429 mm²	1.20 - 1.78
Cup Volume	0.015 cmm	-0.01 - 0.49
Rim Volume	0.373 cmm	0.24 - 0.49
Cup/Disk Area Ratio	0.089	0.16 - 0.47
Linear Cup/Disk Ratio	0.299	0.36 - 0.80
Mean Cup Depth	0.129 mm	0.14 - 0.38
Maximum Cup Depth	0.420 mm	0.46 - 0.90
Cup Shape Measure	-0.247	-0.27 - -0.09
Height Variation Contour	0.421 mm	0.30 - 0.47
Mean RNFL Thickness	0.265 mm	0.18 - 0.31
RNFL Cross Sectional Area	1.177 mm²	0.95 - 1.61
Reference Height	0.376 mm	
Topography Std Dev.	17 μm	

Moorfields Classification: Within normal limits (*)

(*) Moorfields regression classification (Ophthalmology 1998;105:1557-1563). Classification based on statistics. Diagnosis is physician's responsibility.

Comments:

Date: **Signature:**

Software: IR1-V1.7/552

Figure 13.7   Printout of the baseline examination with the Heidelberg Retina Tomograph II in the right eye of a 37-year-old normal male.

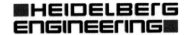
Patient:

Sex: female

Examination: Time elapsed: 25 months

Scan: Focus: 0.00 dpt   Depth: 2.75 mm

OS

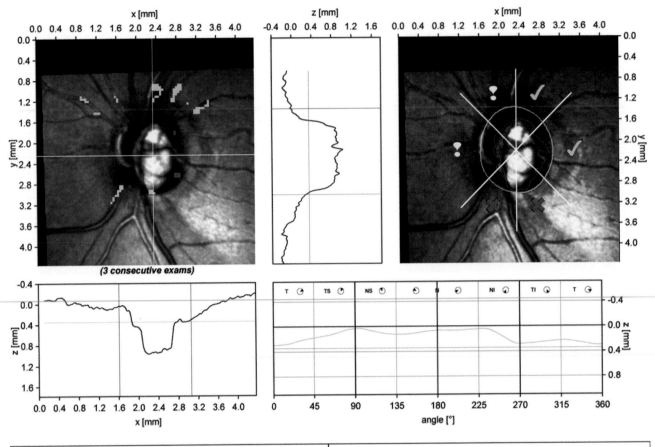

(3 consecutive exams)

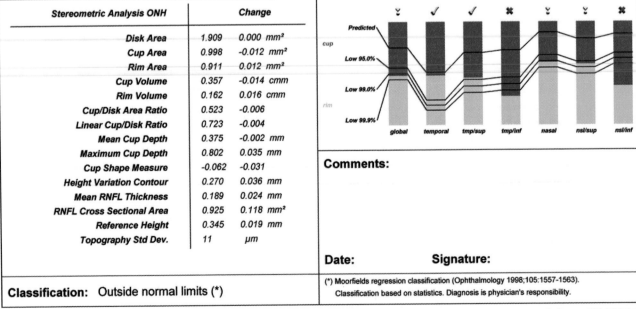

Stereometric Analysis ONH		Change
Disk Area	1.909	0.000 mm²
Cup Area	0.998	-0.012 mm²
Rim Area	0.911	0.012 mm²
Cup Volume	0.357	-0.014 cmm
Rim Volume	0.162	0.016 cmm
Cup/Disk Area Ratio	0.523	-0.006
Linear Cup/Disk Ratio	0.723	-0.004
Mean Cup Depth	0.375	-0.002 mm
Maximum Cup Depth	0.802	0.035 mm
Cup Shape Measure	-0.062	-0.031
Height Variation Contour	0.270	0.036 mm
Mean RNFL Thickness	0.189	0.024 mm
RNFL Cross Sectional Area	0.925	0.118 mm²
Reference Height	0.345	0.019 mm
Topography Std Dev.	11	µm

Comments:

Date: **Signature:**

Classification: Outside normal limits (*)

(*) Moorfields regression classification (Ophthalmology 1998;105:1557-1563).
Classification based on statistics. Diagnosis is physician's responsibility.

Software: IR1-V1.6.2.1

Figure 13.8   Printout of the baseline examination with the Heidelberg Retina Tomograph II in the left eye of a 50-year-old male with glaucoma. (Image courtesy of Dr. Robert N. Weinreb, UCSD Shiley Eye Center, University of California San Diego, CA.)

Heidelberg Retina Tomograph II
Initial Report

■HEIDELBERG
ENGINEERING■

Patient:

Sex: male

Examination:

OS

Scan: Focus: -3.00 dpt   Depth: 4.00 mm

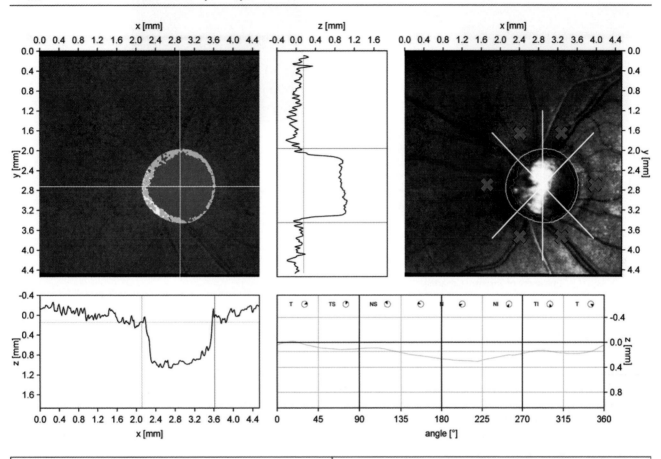

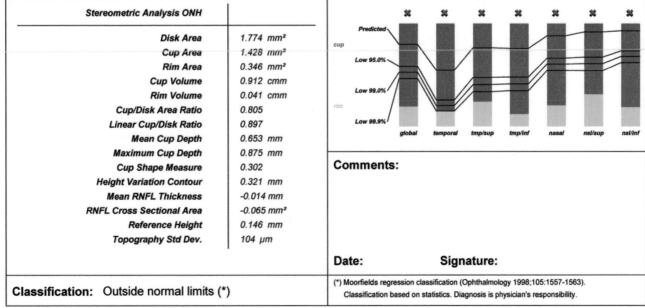

Stereometric Analysis ONH	
Disk Area	1.774 mm²
Cup Area	1.428 mm²
Rim Area	0.346 mm²
Cup Volume	0.912 cmm
Rim Volume	0.041 cmm
Cup/Disk Area Ratio	0.805
Linear Cup/Disk Ratio	0.897
Mean Cup Depth	0.653 mm
Maximum Cup Depth	0.875 mm
Cup Shape Measure	0.302
Height Variation Contour	0.321 mm
Mean RNFL Thickness	-0.014 mm
RNFL Cross Sectional Area	-0.065 mm²
Reference Height	0.146 mm
Topography Std Dev.	104 µm

Comments:

Date: **Signature:**

Classification: Outside normal limits (*)

(*) Moorfields regression classification (Ophthalmology 1998;105:1557-1563).
Classification based on statistics. Diagnosis is physician's responsibility.

Software: IR1-V1.6.2.1

Figure 13.9 Printout of the follow-up exam with the Heidelberg Retina Tomograph II in the left eye of a 63-year-old female. (Image courtesy of Dr. Robert N. Weinreb, UCSD Shiley Eye Center, University of California San Diego, CA.)

159

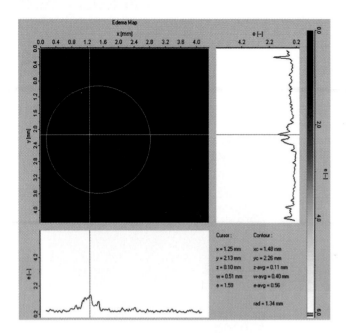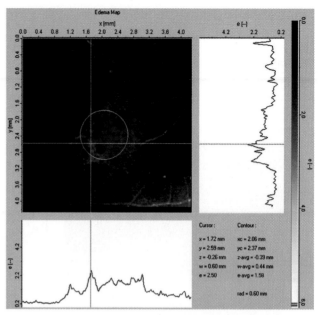

Figure 13.10 Macular edema maps in a 50-year-old male with a 12-year history of diabetic macular edema and a visual acuity of 20/140 (0.14) in the right eye and 20/250 (0.08) in the left eye. (Image courtesy of Drs. K. Guan, C. Hudson, M. Mendelcorn, J. Flanagan, Department of Ophthalmology, University of Toronto, Canada.)

associated the cup shape measure with visual field mean defect (47–50). They reported correlation coefficients ranging between −0.43 and −0.65. Other groups correlated the retinal nerve fiber layer thickness with visual field mean defect (48,51,52). These groups reported correlation coefficients ranging between 0.49 and 0.67. The rim area was also correlated to visual field mean defect by some groups (50,51,53). These groups reported correlation coefficients ranging between 0.44 and 0.62.

The reproducibility of local height measurements was also determined by a number of groups (16,20,21,35,44, 54–57). The standard deviation for normal eyes ranged from 25 to 33 μm in early software versions, and improved to 18 μm with version 2.01 (HRT). Correspondingly, the standard deviation for glaucomatous eyes ranged from 30 to 36 μm in early software versions, and improved to 21 μm with version 2.01 (HRT).

It has to be remembered that macular pathologies such as macular edema or cysts might affect the axial light reflection function and cause misinterpretations in topographic evaluations (18,58). In detail, macular cysts or areas of macular edema might cause two distinct peaks in the axial intensity distribution, while the topographic software evaluation assumes a single peak. The conventional topography algorithm above only considers the axial location of the Gaussian profile fitted to the signal width data curve. However, the data curve or axial intensity distribution (or simply Z-profile) contains information about the thickness of the retina (58). By analyzing the axial spreading or full width at half maximum of the data curve, the thickness can be extracted. The research group of Flanagan and colleagues has developed a software algorithm that analyzes the axial intensity distribution, and computes a thickness-equivalent map of the retina (59). Thus, macular edema mapping becomes possible. The software package first normalizes the axial intensity distribution by expressing the signal width as a function of the minimum and maximum signal width value within a given image. After this normalization, a Gaussian profile is fitted to the left and right portion of the axial intensity distribution, and the resulting width data expressed in arbitrary units. The main focus of this software has been to study macular edema (Figs. 13.10, 13.11). They concluded that this analysis offers non-invasive, objective, topographic, and reproducible index of macular retinal thickening. The differences between this type of scanning-laser thickness analysis (SLTA) and optical coherence tomography (OCT) (60) are in axial resolution and transverse pixel resolution. While the OCT has a better axial resolution of about 15 μm (compared to between 80 to 300 μm for SLTA), the OCT offers only a very poor coverage in the retinal plane. Depending on the type of OCT examination protocol, only 600 to 768 points are used for the calculation of a retinal thickness map compared to 147,456 points in SLTA (HRTII).

SCANNING LASER-DOPPLER FLOWMETRY

A different type of instrument is the scanning laser Doppler flowmeter (SLDF). This instrument was developed by the research group of Michelson (61–63). This instrument relies on the Doppler effect to measure particle flow. The Doppler

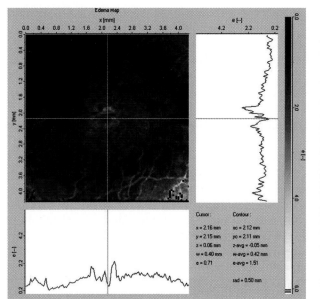 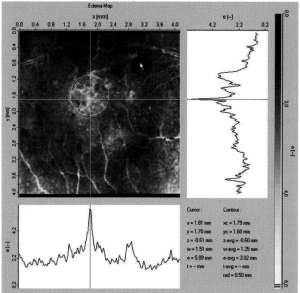

Figure 13.11 On the left side, the macular edema map in the left eye of a 56-year-old female with central retinal vein occlusion is shown. (Image courtesy of Drs. M. Rawji, W-C Lam, J. Flanagan, Department of Ophthalmology, University of Toronto, Canada.) On the right side, the macular edema map in the right eye of a 53-year-old male with a 9-year history of diabetes and cystoid diabetic macular edema is shown. The visual acuity was 20/48 (0.42). (Image courtesy of M. Rawji, C. Hudson, M. Mendelcorn, J. Flanagan, Department of Ophthalmology, University of Toronto, Canada.)

shift occurs when light interacts with moving particles within the retinal vessels. These particles are assumed to be red blood cells (RBCs). The reflection of the light from the RBCs causes a slight change in the light's frequency. By mixing the Doppler shifted light with unaltered reflected light, an interaction of these two components occurs. This interaction is called oscillation and is characterized by a flickering in intensity that is proportional to the particle velocity. By performing a fast Fourier transform, the temporal signal can be transferred to the frequency domain. The power spectrum analysis allows one to extract two independent variables and one derived variable. The independent variables are volume and flow, while the derived variable is velocity. Volume is correlated with the total number of moving particles, while flow is correlated to the overall blood flow. By dividing these parameters, velocity is calculated.

Unlike the previously described SLOs, the SLDF instrument (HRF, Heidelberg Engineering, Heidelberg, Germany) uses a different scanning algorithm. It scans each line 128 times before moving to the next line. It records a total of 64 lines with 256 points each (Fig. 13.12). Thus, the computer can analyze a temporal intensity fluctuation for each point of the scan line over 128 points in time. The reproducibility of the instrument was determined in a model eye (64). The variability of the SLDF measurements was between 3.57% and 4.05%, and was independent of flow rate. Chauhan and colleagues concluded that the instrument measures reliably and linearly within a given operating range. The use

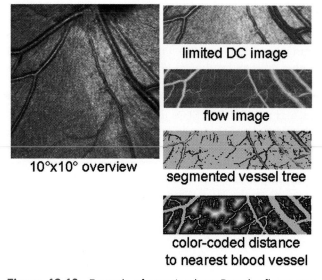

10°x10° overview

limited DC image

flow image

segmented vessel tree

color-coded distance to nearest blood vessel

Figure 13.12 Example of scanning laser-Doppler flowmeter image. The top left image shows the 10-by-10-degrees overview image for orientation. The top right image (limited DC image) shows the fundus-equivalent view of the measurement area. The blue highlighted areas are the areas that were excluded from the analysis due to underexposure or overexposure. The second image on the right (flow image) shows the blood flow image as analyzed with the automated full field analysis program described in the text. The program allows to segment blood vessels as seen in the third image on the right (segmented vessel tree). The bottom right image shows the color coded perfusion map. The color code indicates distance to nearest blood vessel. The brighter the region, the further away it is from the nearest blood vessel.

of the SLDF has been evaluated in clinical studies in glaucoma (65–68) and other pathologies (69–72). The instrument allows measuring blood flow only in arbitrary units due to the interindividual variation in retinal reflectance, hematocrit, and other parameters. The lack of calibration in this instrument requires baseline measurements at the same eye or the contralateral eye. Furthermore, there have been a number of reports concerning the factors influencing flow measurements (73–76). The studies have helped to establish a set of examination guidelines for clinical imaging and postacquisition image analysis.

To overcome some of the above limitations that were related to the small size of the measurement square, and aliasing from blood flow measurements in large blood vessels, the group of Michelson has developed an automated full-field analysis program (62,63). This software has been extensively used since its inception and provides blood flow values for the entire image after automatically excluding large blood vessels and regions of overexposure or underexposure (77–80).

ANGIOGRAPHY

Soon after the initial development of scanning laser technology, the use of fluorescein angiography (FA) was advocated (9). Scheider and colleagues subsequently suggested the use of indocyanine green (ICG) angiography with a SLO (81–85). The excitation and emission diagrams of sodium fluorescein and ICG are shown in Figure 13.13. Subsequently, Bischoff and colleagues suggested to combine both dye modalities into one instrument (86). Other groups quickly followed with a different instrument (7,87). It has to be stressed that the light sources in fundus cameras and SLOs are different. While most fundus cameras use a broadband light source such as a flash lamp, SLOs use a narrow-bandwidth laser. Therefore, the SLO can deliver all of the energy at the peak excitation wavelength of each dye. This means that in angiography, SLOs use more efficient light sources than fundus cameras. There have been five different commercial instruments for angiography. However, not all devices are still available at press time, and their features vary. These devices are the Heidelberg Retina Angiograph (HRA, Heidelberg Engineering, Heidelberg, Germany) and the Heidelberg Retina Angiograph 2 (HRA2, Heidelberg Engineering,

Heidelberg, Germany), the AngioScan (Laser Diagnostic Technologies, San Diego, CA), the Rodenstock SLO (Rodenstock, Ottobrunn, Germany; also was distributed by Canon USA), and the Optos Panoramic200 (Optos North America, Marlborough, MA). In principle, the HRA uses three lasers (argon gas with 488 nm and 514 nm wavelength, laser diode with 795 nm wavelength, and another laser diode with 835 nm wavelength), and records either 256 × 256 pixels or 512 × 512 pixels for each image. The HRA2 uses the same two laser diodes and a solid-state laser for 488 nm wavelength FA excitation. The HRA2 can record up to 1,536 × 1,536 pixels per image. The field size in both instruments can be varied between 10 by 10, 20 by 20, or 30 by 30 degrees. In combination with an automated software alignment algorithm (88), the system is capable of performing software-assisted image montages with field sizes well beyond 120 degrees, and pixel resolutions of over 3,000 by 3,000 pixels (Fig. 13.14). The AngioScan uses one infrared laser diode (795 nm wavelength), and offers a 256-by-256-pixel resolution for ICG angiography (ICGA) only. However, it simultaneously records a reflectance image alongside the fluorescence image with a separate detector. The Rodenstock SLO has a modular design and can house different laser light sources. Most commonly it uses an Argon gas with 488 nm and 514 nm wavelength and different laser diodes or a Helium-Neon laser. The device has a pixelation of either 512 by 512 (European version) or 640 by 480 (U.S. version), at video frame rates of 50 and 60 Hz, respectively.

Scanning laser angiography has a clear advantage over fundus cameras in ICGA. Flower and colleagues showed that fundus cameras are subject to a false fluorescence artifact at low-light levels in the late phase of ICG angiograms, due to diffuse scattering of infrared light (89). The scanning nature of the SLO illumination prevents this artifact.

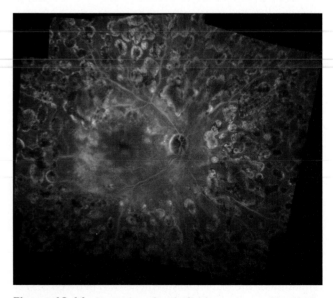

Figure 13.14 Examples of wide-field capture mode with the help of automatic montage software. On the left side you can see a fluorescein angiogram in a 52-year-old male with diabetic retinopathy and panretinal photocoagulation. The size of the image is 82 degrees tall by 70 degrees wide.

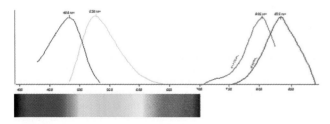

Figure 13.13 Excitation and emission spectrum of sodium fluorescein and indocyanine green in comparison. The color spectrum is for illustration only.

This artifact is not observed in fluorescein angiography, since the pigment will absorb all scattered excitation light in the visible part of the spectrum.

The high light efficiency of the SLO makes technology very suitable to the application of oral FA (90,91). While intravenous (IV) FA is the examination method of choice for many retinal diseases, it has been shown that some patients are allergic to the IV administration of the drug. It has been reported that mild allergic reactions can occur in 1% to 5% of all cases, while fatal reactions are reported in 1 in 222,000 cases (92,93). Oral FA has previously been proposed as an alternative to IV angiography and to avoid its complications (94–96). A mild skin reaction has been reported with an oral dose in a patient with personal and familial history of atopic eczema (97). However, it is generally assumed that the adverse reaction rate and severity is less with oral than with IV FA. The phenomenon of lower incidence of adverse reactions to orally-administered agent versus IV route, is well documented in the case of penicillin (97). In a recent study, Bartsch and colleagues found that oral FA with the confocal HRA allows detection of choroidal neovascularization (CNV) in all patients (91). Visualization of extent and type of CNV was possible in most eyes. Thus, oral angiography may be an excellent screening tool for CNV, and allows guidance of treatment in the majority of cases (Fig. 13.15).

Another area of application of scanning laser angiography is the imaging of malignant choroidal melanoma. This type of melanoma is the most common primary ocular tumor in adults and has a high incidence of metastasis formation, even after successful treatment of the primary tumor. Although the overall incidence of uveal melanoma is seven per million per year (98), the incidence in patients >70 years old is much higher: 16 to 17 per million per year for women, and 23 to 24 per million per year for men (99). Mueller, Freeman, and colleagues (100–103) have shown in an animal model and in a study of two patients scheduled for enucleation, that the vascularization patterns visible in ICGA with a confocal SLO are identical to the histological microvascularization patterns described by Folberg and colleagues (104–108) (Fig. 13.16). Subsequent

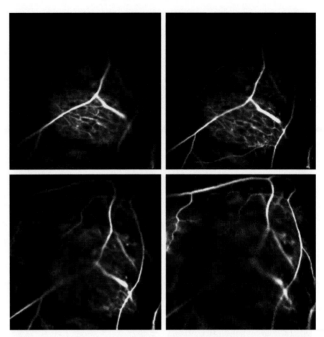

Figure 13.16 Four confocal indocyanine green angiographic image in a patient with ocular melanoma. Each image was recorded with 30-by-30-degrees field of view. The images are in consecutive order from anterior (*top left*) to posterior (*bottom right*). The blood vessels inside the tumor are clearly visible in the top two images, and partially visible in the bottom left. Due to the confocal aperture and the large size of the tumor out-of-focus regions are not visible.

prospective clinical trials have shown that microvascular patterns are capable of predicting tumor growth better than other indicators such as histologic evaluation (109–112). Thus, ICGA offers a new method of increasing prognostic accuracy for ocular melanoma.

CONFOCAL CORNEAL IMAGING

Recently, Guthoff and Stave have made a modification to an existing SLO by attaching a microscope objective lens to allow confocal corneal imaging at microscopic resolution (113). This approach effectively turns the device into a confocal scanning laser microscope (Fig. 13.17). Currently, available confocal tandem scanning laser microscopes with halogen or mercury lamp illumination offer insufficient image quality and irregular corneal illumination. These problems are of particular concern for automatic quantitative evaluation of keratocyte density before and after laser in-situ keratomileusis (LASIK) or photorefractive keratectomy (PRK).

MICROPERIMETRY

One of the first applications of scanning laser ophthalmoscopy has been orphaned by the demise of the Rodenstock SLO. This application is microperimetry. Microperimetry was proposed to allow an observer to see in real

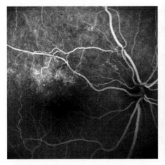 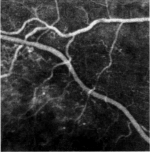

Figure 13.15 Example of oral fluorescein angiography in a patient with diabetes. The image on the left shows the 30-by-30-degrees field of view, while the right image shows with details of retinal microcirculation in a 10-by-10-degrees field of view. Areas of capillary dropout, microaneurysms, and vascular tortuosity are seen along retinal vein superotemporal to macula.

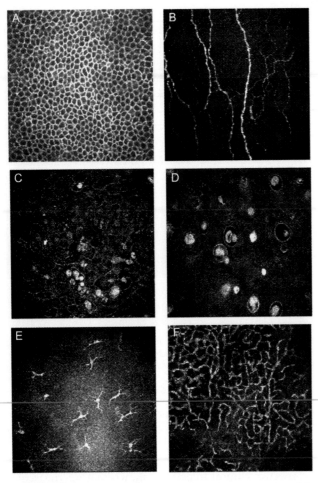

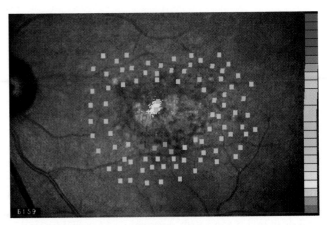

Figure 13.18 Static threshold fundus perimetry (microperimetry) examination in a 59-year-old female patient with geographic atrophy following age-related macular degeneration. The visual acuity was 20/60. The absolute central scotoma (*open blue rectangles*) and the relative scotoma surrounding the pathologic area can be seen. The scale on the right gives threshold values in 1 dB steps beginning with 0 dB at the top (*blue*) to 23 dB (*red*) at the bottom. There is a movement of the point of fixation towards the top of the scotoma, while sometimes the patient still fixated central (*yellow points* represent all single fixations during stimulus presentation). The small red cross at the vessel crossing is needed for manual fundus tracking. (Images courtesy of Prof. Dr. Klaus Rohrschneider, Heidelberg, Germany.)

Figure 13.17 Confocal scanning laser microscopic image of the cornea. Each image shows a section of the cornea of 250 μm by 250 μm. **A.** Intermediate cells (wing cells) of the epithelium in a healthy cornea (N = 5,000 cells per mm², depth = 20 μm). **B.** A subepithelial nerve plexus with thick, often parallel strands and cross-linking as well as fine bifurcations near Bowman's membrane (depth = 62 μm). **C.** A cornea with acanthamoeba keratitis in the early stages of infection with epithelial and microcystic changes. **D.** Meesmann's dystrophy of the corneal epithelium. The image shows epithelial changes similar to findings reported in histological light and electron microscopy. **E.** Langerhans cells of medium density near the basal membrane after 2 years of wearing soft contact lenses in a patient with contact lens induced corneal changes. **F.** Epidemic keratoconjunctivitis with intraepithelial lesions and highly reflective cell borders in the basal plane. (Images courtesy of Prof. Dr. med. Rudolf Guthoff and Prof. Dr. rer. nat. Joachim Stave, Rostock, Germany).

time on a television monitor the precise retinal location of the exciting stimulus and the fixation target. Typically, infrared illumination is used to view the fundus while a visible fixation target is presented along with a variable intensity test stimulus (114–117). The size of the stimulus can be varied, as well as the length of presentation time (Fig. 13.18). Microperimetry with an SLO has the advantage of correcting fixation instabilities due to the unique ability to view the fundus with both fixation and stimulus in one image. Furthermore, the high resolution allows to study foveal and excentric fixation (118–120). The method has found clinical utility with the establishment of standardized testing methods (121–125). There have been over 50 papers published in

the last 15 years on the topic of microperimetry. However, the limitation to the widespread use of this technique has been the labor-intensive examination and evaluation method.

MULTIFOCAL ELECTRORETINOGRAPHY

Sutter and Tran introduced multifocal electroretinography (mfERG) into clinical ophthalmology in 1992 (126). Since then it has proved to be a valuable addition to clinical diagnosis, follow-up, and basic research. While the initial stimulus was provided via a computer monitor, other groups have adapted the technology to incorporate the SLO as stimulator (123,127–135). An example of the results is shown in Figure 13.19. The use of the SLO allows the simultaneous visualization of the fundus during the recording of the mfERG. This procedure allows to directly monitor fixation, and may be useful in patients with unstable fixation.

NEW TECHNOLOGY

Recent advances in the laboratory have introduced new technologies to scanning laser ophthalmoscopy. These advances include the application of adaptive optics, eye tracking, and the combination of SLO-imaging with OCT-imaging mode. Adaptive optics has been used in astronomy for decades to compensate for the aberrations of the turbulent atmosphere. In 1953, Babcock originally proposed that adaptive optics could dynamically compensate for the wavefront error

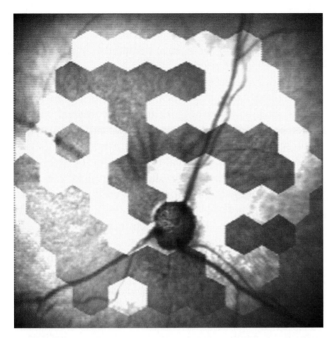

Figure 13.19 Multifocal electroretinogram (mfERG) in an abyssinian cat showing the stimulating pattern superimposed onto the retinal background. The animal was imaged with the Heidelberg Retina Angiograph, and the stimulus was provided by the Retiscan system (Roland Consult, Wiesbaden, Germany). (Image courtesy of Prof. Dr. med. Mathias Seeliger, Tübingen, Germany, and Kristina Narfström PhD, Columbia, MO.)

caused by atmospheric turbulence in ground-based telescopes (136). Recently, adaptive optics have been applied to compensate for aberrations of the human eye. Several adaptive optics systems have been reported for aberration compensation of the eye. Dreher and colleagues first used a deformable mirror in conjunction with the human eye and successfully corrected the astigmatism in one subject's eye by

using the prescription provided by a conventional refraction test (137). Liang and colleagues have built an adaptive optical system based on the astronomical, piezo-driven deformable mirror technology (138,139). They have successfully demonstrated the capability of adaptive optics to correct the eye's optical aberrations and obtained high-resolution retinal image with a conventional CCD camera. Roorda and colleagues have recently built a tabletop adaptive-optics SLO (140). The research instrument has a variable field of view ranging between 1 by 1 and 3 by 3 degrees (Fig. 13.20). They were able to resolve cone photoreceptors at retinal locations from 0.5 to 4 degrees from the fovea. Due to the high price of the adaptive optical components and the requirement for optimal eye-instrument alignment with a bite bar, these types of instruments will probably not find immediate clinical utility. However, adaptive optics will allow research institutions to achieve unprecedented resolution to improve understanding of anatomy, physiology, and for the diagnosis of pathological conditions. In particular, diseases such as diabetic retinopathy and age-related macular degeneration (AMD) will benefit from improved resolution since smaller changes in appearance can be detected.

Hammer and colleagues have recently added retinal eye tracking to imaging with an SLO (141). Their system uses a confocal reflectometer with a closed-loop optical servo system to lock onto retinal features. They were able to achieve tracking with a bandwidth of larger than 1 kHz, with an accuracy of 0.05 degrees, and image series of up to 1,000 frames. Eye tracking will allow improved imaging in patients with fixation problems (e.g., central scotoma, diabetic retinopathy, and AMD), and it may allow conducting hemodynamic studies over long observation periods.

The third area of innovation is in combining SLO imaging with OCT. The research group of Podoleanu has built a

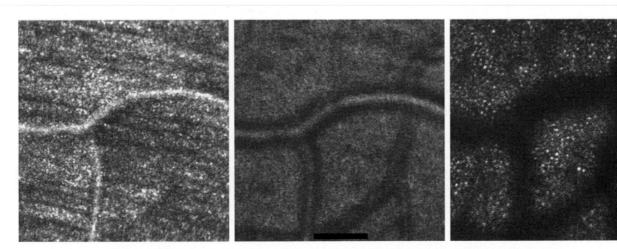

Figure 13.20 These images were taken with the Houston adaptive optics scanning laser ophthalmoscope, or AOSLO. The three panels show three optical sections of human retina. The first panel shows the nerve fibers, which run along the surface of the retina. The second section reveals more blood vessels that run beneath the nerve fiber layer. The third panel shows the photoreceptor layer, which lies deeper in the retina. The three sections span a depth of about 300 μm. The scale bar is 100 μm. (Courtesy of Austin Roorda.)

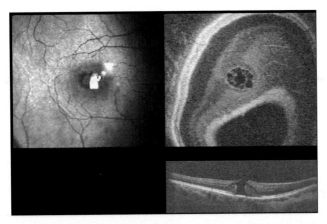

Figure 13.21 Clinical examination in a patient with macular hole with the combination optical coherence tomography-scanning laser ophthalmoscope (OCT/SLO) instrument. The top left image shows the confocal SLO view and the top right image the coronal OCT scan (*en-face view*), while the bottom right image shows the familiar OCT B-scan image. The images illustrate that a single OCT B-scan image may not cover a sufficient retinal area to appreciate the complexity of a certain pathology. (Image courtesy of Dr. Richard Rosen, New York, NY.)

device that uses a short-coherence length light source and three-dimensional scanning to achieve simultaneous confocal and OCT imaging (142–144). The advantage of this approach is that the exact location of the OCT scan line can be seen in the confocal SLO image, unlike the conventional OCT where the fundus photograph is recorded immediately after completing the OCT B-scan. An example of the combined SLO-OCT image is shown in Figure 13.21. The combination SLO/OCT has great potential for the study of glaucomatous optic nerve head and macular pathologies such as macular hole formation, diabetic retinopathy, and AMD.

Topographic Angiography

Macular disease, such as AMD, diabetic maculopathy (DMP), and others, is characterized by vascular pathologies including extravasation from retinal or choroidal vessels, retinal or choroidal perfusion changes, or leakage from neovascular proliferation. Conventional angiography allows identifying the diagnostic entity, but is limited in the evaluation of the activity of lesions and the detection of deep vascular changes. FA is compromised by masking phenomena through hemorrhage or serous fluid, and often unable to differentiate staining from residual leakage. ICGA offers improved transmission with detection of occult processes, but presents features that are often difficult to interpret and not yet classified. Confocal scanning laser ophthalmoscopy with point-source illumination and optimized excitation offers optimal contrast, high sensitivity, and depth resolution. With the option to scan through multiple tomographic sections, confocal scanning laser ophthalmoscopy can be used to identify the spatial location of the fluorescent marker and to provide a realistic three-dimensional

angiographic image. The vascular pattern of retina and choroid as well as extravasate is documented so that structural and perfusion- or leakage-related dynamic processes can be captured effectively.

The principle of topographic angiography is the use of a series of consecutive confocal series of fluorescence, and by introducing a smart algorithm, to reconstruct a three-dimensional profile of the intravascular and extravascular fluorescence distribution (145,146). Data acquisition is performed using a confocal SLO preferably with a 30-degree field. For FA, an argon laser emitting at 488 nm is used for excitation and blocking filters for wavelengths below 510 nm are used for detection. For ICGA, excitation is performed using a diode laser emitting at 795 nm, and blocking filters for wavelengths below 835 nm are used for detection. A refractive correction of +3 diopters is added to create a preretinal initial focus for complete sectioning. A series of 32 tomographic sections is usually taken over a depth of 4 mm with a distance of 125 μm between sections. All 32 lateral images are aligned and corrected for translational eye movements. An additional averaging over 3 by 3 neighboring pixels accounts for rotational artifacts. A two-dimensional intensity profile is generated based on the maximum fluorescence intensity for each image point. Subsequently, an axial depth profile is extracted from the stack of the 32 aligned angiograms for each image point in the x/y plane. The topographic software program identifies the position of the threshold fluorescence and generates a topographic relief. Superficial fluorescence appears as prominence, and deep fluorescence is represented as a defect within the background level. In contrast to conventional two-dimensional angiography, SLO topography delineates physiologic and pathologic vasculature with its precise location and configuration, and also identifies related exudation. Masking by hemorrhage or absorbing fluid does not preclude the detection of the underlying processes. Superimposed fluorescence features seen in conventional FA/ICGA appear as distinct lesions with characteristic anatomy (147–149).

SLO topography offers a three-dimensional image of the choriocapillary surface and the overlying retinal vasculature. Changes in the choroidal perfusion are seen as defects in the choroidal surface. In geographic atrophy, absence of the RPE layer produces a bright window defect without insight into the vascular pathology (Fig. 13.22A). Topography, however, is able to detect the absence of a normal choriocapillary layer: size and depth of choroidal non-perfusion is documented as precisely as the configuration of the retinal vascular arcades and the avascular cavity of the optic nerve (Fig. 13.22B). Drusen as a characteristic sign of early-stage AMD are associated with RPE dysfunction leading to choroidal leakage or atrophy. An inhomogeneous pattern of staining and nonstaining areas is seen by conventional ICGA (Fig. 13.23A). Topography identifies the different stages of the drusen pathology: while dark areas are consistent with focal prominence

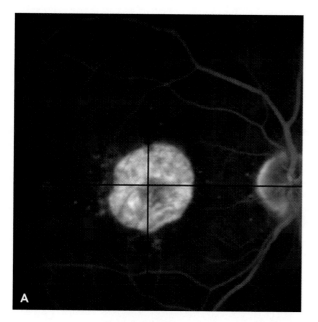

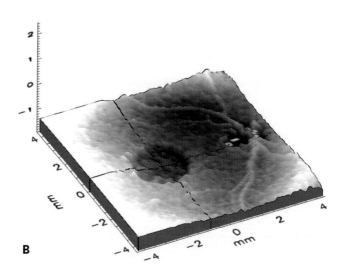

Figure 13.22   **A.** On the left side the indocyanine green angiogram shows intensive hyperfluorescence indicating a window defect in geographic atrophy. **B.** On the right side the topographic angiography identifies absence of choriocapillary perfusion in the area of hyperfluorescence.

reflecting localized fluid pooling, bright drusen cover areas with perfusion defects (Fig. 13.23B).

CNV, a feature of exudative AMD, is diagnosed by angiography and differentiated into classic and occult subtypes. Hemorrhage and serous fluid often obscure the neovascular features in conventional angiography. Hemorrhagic CNV appears as an area of blocked fluorescence by FA as well as ICGA (Fig. 13.24A). Topography demonstrates the typical prominent configuration of a classic lesion type with steep borders and central crater (Fig. 13.24B). The sharp elevation of classic CNV is often surrounded by a halo of choroidal depression that might reflect choroidal perfusion changes. Occult CNV types are by definition ill defined with fuzzy borders and absence of a neovascular pattern (Fig. 13.25A).

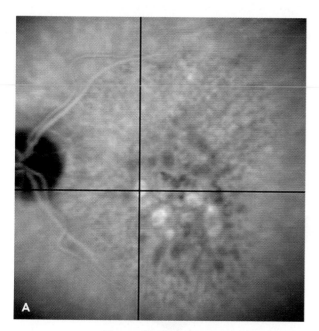

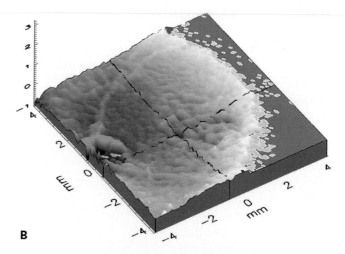

Figure 13.23   **A.** The left shows the indocyanine green angiography in a patient with large drusen demonstrating a variable pattern with areas of hypofluorescence seen in the upper and lower macular area and hyperfluorescent staining in the central portion. **B.** The right side shows the three-dimensional topographic angiography view of hypofluorescent drusen harboring focal prominent lesions consistent with fluid pooling underneath the RPE, the hyperfluorescent drusen in the center are associated with choriocapillary defects.

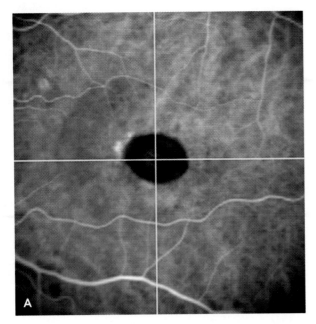

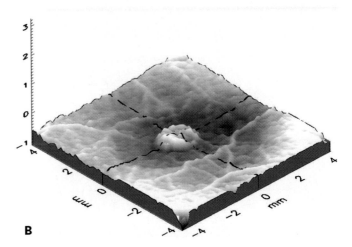

Figure 13.24 **A.** The left side shows the indocyanine green angiogram of a patient with subretinal hemorrhage masking choroidal neovascularization. **B.** On the right the neovascular structures are well delineated by topographic imaging without any masking by overlying blood.

This lesion type appears as irregular prominence with a flat convex shape (Fig. 13.25B). Steep borders and the central crater formation of classic lesions are missing. Even highly prominent lesions can be precisely imaged by SLO topography. In large choroidal hemangioma, conventional angiography is unrevealing with a flat pattern of spotty hyperfluorescence (Fig. 13.26A). By topography, the vascular mass is shown with substantial prominence. RPE destruction and leakage in the central portion of the lesion as well as the

intact retinal vasculature overlying the tumor are represented (Fig. 13.26B).

Retinal vascular pathology is another entity typically identified by angiography. In branch retinal vein occlusion (BRVO) capillary dropout is seen during early FA (Fig. 13.27A), and leakage due to ischemia is observed during late ICGA (Fig. 13.27B). Extravasation of fluid into the retina with consecutive retinal thickening is detected by topographic angiography only (Fig. 13.27C). The

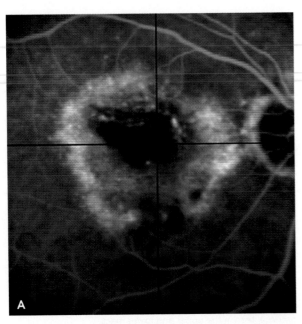

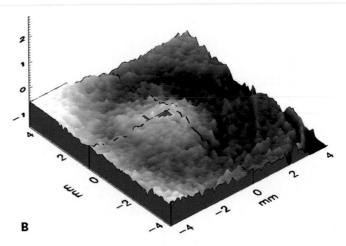

Figure 13.25 **A.** The left side shows the indocyanine green angiogram of a patient with occult choroidal neovascularization (CNV) demonstrating inhomogeneous leakage from the choroidal background. **B.** The topographic angiography shows that the flat convexity of occult CNV differs substantially from the distinct prominence of classic lesion types.

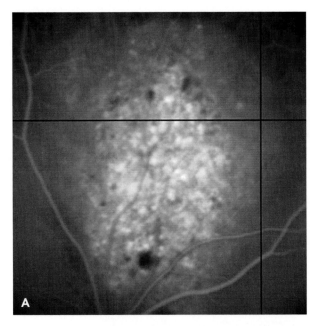
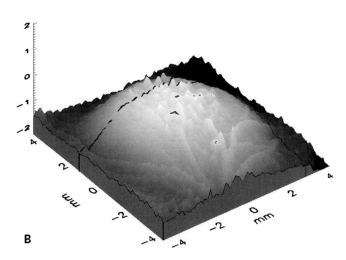

Figure 13.26 A. The conventional indocyanine green angiogram (*left*) shows that angiographic features of choroidal hemangioma are limited to a flat pattern of spotty hyperfluorescence in the center of the lesion. **B.** The topographic angiography shows that the tumor height and shape is clearly represented by topographic imaging.

quadrant affected by BRVO appears elevated, consistent with intraretinal fluid accumulation. Extension and degree of thickening are well-delineated.

Confocal topographic angiography offers high-resolution, three-dimensional imaging of chorioretinal vascular disease. Structural changes such as neovascular proliferation or vascular atrophy are identified in respect to localization, size, and prominence/depth. Dynamic phenomena (i.e., perfusion, extravasation, or barrier dysfunction) are identified and may be quantified more precisely than by conventional angiography. SLO topography is a useful technique in the diagnosis of chorioretinal disease, allows a precise

evaluation of therapeutic interventions, and may improve the understanding of the pathophysiology of macular disease.

In conclusion, SLO offers a wide variety of clinical applications covering diseases such as glaucoma, AMD, diabetic retinopathy, corneal dysfunctions, and ocular melanoma. The type of disease and application dictates which instrument should be used. However, the user should be aware of the underlying physical principles and become familiar with the theory of the devices to avoid misinterpretation of data. History and the marketplace have shown that this technology is here to stay.

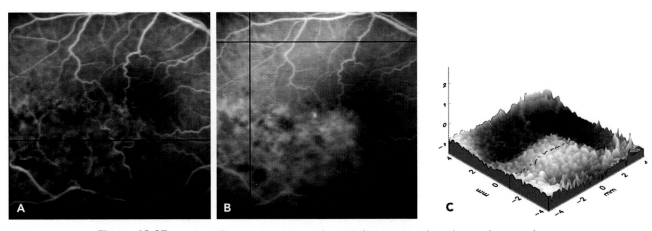

Figure 13.27 A. Early fluorescein angiography (FA) demonstrates branch retinal vein occlusion with venous tortuosity and avascular areas is seen in the left image. **B.** The middle image shows diffuse leakage with macular edema in late phase FA. **C.** Retinal thickening following intraretinal extravasation of fluid in the temporal inferior portion of the retina is well demarcated by topographic angiography (*right*).

ACKNOWLEDGMENTS

This study was sponsored in part by a grant from the National Eye Institute (NIH-NEI grant EY13304 [DUB], NIH grant EY07366 [WRF]), and Research to Prevent Blindness (UCSD).

The authors would like to thank John Hawley (Heidelberg Engineering, Vista, CA); Dr. John Flanagan (Waterloo, Canada); Prof. Dr. med. Rudolf Guthoff (Rostock, Germany); Dr. Austin Roorda (Houston, TX); Prof. Dr. rer. nat. Joachim Stave (Rostock, Germany); and Dr. Robert N. Weinreb (La Jolla, CA) for contributing photos for this chapter.

REFERENCES

1. Webb R, Hughes G, Pomerantzeff O. Flying spot TV ophthalmoscope. *Appl Opt.* 1980;19:2,991–2,997.
2. Webb R, Hughes G. Scanning laser ophthalmoscope. *IEEE Trans Biomed Eng.* 1981;28:488–492.
3. Bartsch DU, Mueller AJ, Freeman WR. Motion artifacts in confocal infrared scanning laser ophthalmoscopy using indocyanine green. Presented at the 5th International Meeting on Scanning Laser Ophthalmoscopy, Tomography and Microscopy. San Antonio, TX, 1995.
4. Manivannan A, Vander Hoek J, Vieira P, et al. Clinical investigation of a true color scanning laser ophthalmoscope. *Arch Ophthalmol.* 2001;119(6): 819–824.
5. Bartsch DU, Freeman WR, Lopez AM. A false use of "true color." *Arch Ophthalmol.* 2002;120(5):675–676; author reply 676.
6. Bartsch DU, Weinreb RN, Zinser G, et al. Confocal scanning infrared laser ophthalmoscopy for indocyanine green angiography. *Am J Ophthalmol.* 1995;120(5):642–651.
7. Freeman WR, Bartsch DU, Mueller AJ, et al. Simultaneous indocyanine green and fluorescein angiography using a confocal scanning laser ophthalmoscope [see comments]. *Arch Ophthalmol.* 1998;116(4):455–463.
8. Timberlake G, Mainster MA, Webb RH, et al. Retinal localization of scotomata by scanning laser ophthalmoscopy. *Invest Ophthalmol Vis Sci.* 1982;22:91–97.
9. Mainster M, Timberlake GT, Webb RH, et al. Scanning laser ophthalmoscopy. Clinical applications. *Ophthalmology.* 1982;89:852–857.
10. Webb RH, Dorey CK. The pixelated image. In: Pawley JB, ed. *Handbook of Biological Confocal Microscopy.* New York: Plenum; 1990:41–51.
11. Webb R, Hughes G, Delori F. Confocal scanning laser ophthalmoscope. *Appl Opt.* 1987;26:1,492–1,499.
12. Kruse FE, Burk RO, Völcker HE, et al. Reproducibility of topographic measurements of the optic nerve head with laser tomographic scanning. *Ophthalmology.* 1989;96(9):1,320–1,324.
13. Kruse FE, Burke RO, Völker HE, et al. [3-dimensional biomorphometry of the papilla using a laser tomography scanning procedure—initial experiences with pathologic papillar findings]. *Fortschr Ophthalmol.* 1989;86(6): 710–713.
14. Bartsch DU, Intaglietta M, Bille JF, et al. Confocal laser tomographic analysis of the retina in eyes with macular hole formation and other focal macular diseases. *Am J Ophthalmol.* 1989;108(3):277–287.
15. Janknecht P, Funk J. Optic nerve head analyser and Heidelberg retina tomograph: accuracy and reproducibility of topographic measurements in a model eye and in volunteers. *Br J Ophthalmol.* 1994;78(10):760–768.
16. Chauhan BC, Le Blanc RP, McCormick TA, et al. Test-retest variability of topographic measurements with confocal scanning laser tomography in patients with glaucoma and control subjects. *Am J Ophthalmol.* 1994; 118(1):9–15.
17. Dreher AW, Weinreb RN. Accuracy of topographic measurements in a model eye with the laser tomographic scanner. *Invest Ophthalmol Vis Sci.* 1991;32(11):2,992–2,996.
18. Bartsch DU, Freeman WR. Laser-tissue interaction and artifacts in confocal scanning laser ophthalmoscopy and tomography. *Neurosci Biobehav Rev.* 1993;17(4):459–467.
19. Rohrschneider K, Burk RO, Volcker HE. [Follow-up examinations of papillary morphology with laser scanning tomography]. *Ophthalmologe.* 1994; 91(6):811–819.
20. Tomita G, Honbe K, Kitazawa Y. Reproducibility of measurements by laser scanning tomography in eyes before and after pilocarpine treatment. *Graefes Arch Clin Exp Ophthalmol.* 1994;232(7):406–408.
21. Weinreb RN. Laser scanning tomography to diagnose and monitor glaucoma. *Curr Opin Ophthalmol.* 1993;4(2):3–6.
22. Rohrschneider K, Burk RO, Volcker HE. [Papilledema. Follow-up using laser scanning tomography]. *Fortschr Ophthalmol.* 1990;87(5):471–474.
23. Rohrschneider K, Burk RO, Volcker HE. Reproducibility of topometric data acquisition in normal and glaucomatous optic nerve heads with the laser tomographic scanner. *Graefes Arch Clin Exp Ophthalmol.* 1993;231(8):457–464.
24. Burk RO, Rohrschneider K, Noack H, et al. [Volumetric analysis of the optic papilla using laser scanning tomography. Parameter definition and comparison of glaucoma and control papilla]. *Klin Monatsbl Augenheilkd.* 1991;198(6):522–529.
25. Burk RO, Rohrschneider K, Noack H, et al. Are large optic nerve heads susceptible to glaucomatous damage at normal intraocular pressure? A three-dimensional study by laser scanning tomography. *Graefes Arch Clin Exp Ophthalmol.* 1992;230(6): 552–560.
26. Burk RO. [3-dimensional topographic analysis of the papilla as a component of glaucoma diagnosis]. *Ophthalmologe.* 1992;89(3):190–203.
27. Burk RO, Rohrschneider K, Völcker HE, et al. Laser scanning tomography and stereophotogrammetry in three-dimensional optic disc analysis. *Graefes Arch Clin Exp Ophthalmol.* 1993;231(4):193–198.
28. Burk RO, König J, Rohrschneider K, et al. [3-dimensional topography of the optic papilla with laser scanning tomography: clinical correlation of cluster analysis]. *Klin Monatsbl Augenheilkd.* 1994;204(6):504–512.
29. Rohrschneider K, Burk RO, Bornfield N, et al. [Capillary hemangioma of the retina. Laser scanning tomography follow-up after radiotherapy]. *Fortschr Ophthalmol.* 1991;88(6):623–628.
30. Rohrschneider K, Burk RO, Volcker HE. Depth position of spontaneous venous pulsations in ocular hypertensives and control-group discs. *Ger J Ophthalmol.* 1992;1(3–4):188–192.
31. Thomson S. Retinal topography with the Heidelberg Retina Tomograph. *J Audiov Media Med.* 1994;17(4):156–160.
32. Weinberger D, Stiebel H, Gaton D, et al. Three-dimensional measurements of central serous chorioretinopathy using a scanning laser tomograph. *Am J Ophthalmol.* 1996;122(6):864–869.
33. Weinberger D, Stiebel H, Gaton D, et al. Three-dimensional measurements of idiopathic macular holes using a scanning laser tomograph. *Ophthalmology.* 1995;102(10): 1,445–1,449.
34. Yoshikawa K, Ujikawa M, Iijima T, et al. [Reproducibility of the topographic parameters of the optic disk with the scanning laser tomograph]. *Nippon Ganka Gakkai Zasshi.* 1995;99(4):469–474.
35. Rohrschneider K, Burk RO, Kruse FE, et al. Reproducibility of the optic nerve head topography with a new laser tomographic scanning device. *Ophthalmology.* 1994; 101(6):1,044–1,049.
36. Mikelberg FS, Wijsman K, Schulzer M. Reproducibility of topographic parameters obtained with the Heidelberg Retina Tomograph. *J Glaucoma.* 1993;2:101–103.
37. Hatch WV, Flanagan JG, Williams-Lyn DE, et al. Interobserver agreement of Heidelberg retina tomograph parameters. *J Glaucoma.* 1999;8(4):232–237.
38. Bartz-Schmidt KU, Jonescu-Cuypers CP, Thumann G, et al. [Effect of the contour line on cup surface using the Heidelberg Retina Tomograph]. *Klin Monatsbl Augenheilkd.* 1996;209(5): 292–297.
39. Orgul S, Cioffi GA, Bacon DR, et al. Sources of variability of topometric data with a scanning laser ophthalmoscope. *Arch Ophthalmol.* 1996;114(2): 161–164.
40. Orgul S, Croffi GA, Van Buskirk EM. Variability of contour line alignment on sequential images with the Heidelberg Retina Tomograph. *Graefes Arch Clin Exp Ophthalmol.* 1997;235(2):82–86.
41. Chauhan BC, Blanchard JW, Hamilton DC, et al. Technique for detecting serial topographic changes in the optic disc and peripapillary retina using scanning laser tomography. *Invest Ophthalmol Vis Sci.* 2000;41(3):775–782.
42. Mikelberg FS, Parfitt CM, Swindale NV, et al. Ability of the Heidelberg Retina Tomograph to detect early glaucomatous visual field loss. *J Glaucoma.* 1995;4:242 247.
43. Iester M, Mikelberg FS, Drance SM. The effect of optic disc size on diagnostic precision with the Heidelberg retina tomograph. *Ophthalmology.* 1997;104(3):545–548.
44. Bathija R, Zangwill L, Berry CC, et al. Detection of early glaucomatous structural damage with confocal scanning laser tomography. *J Glaucoma.* 1998;7(2):121–127.
45. Wollstein G, Garway-Heath DF, Hitchings RA. Identification of early glaucoma cases with the scanning laser ophthalmoscope. *Ophthalmology.* 1998;105(8):1,557–1,563.
46. Uchida H, Brigatti L, Caprioli J. Detection of structural damage from glaucoma with confocal laser image analysis. *Invest Ophthalmol Vis Sci.* 1996; 37(12):2,393–2,401.
47. Brigatti L, Caprioli J. Correlation of visual field with scanning confocal laser optic disc measurements in glaucoma. *Arch Ophthalmol.* 1995;113(9): 1191–1194.
48. Teesalu P, Vihanninjoki K, Airaksinen PJ, et al. Correlation of blue-on-yellow visual fields with scanning confocal laser optic disc measurements. *Invest Ophthalmol Vis Sci.* 1997;38(12):2,452–2,459.
49. Iester M, Swindale NV, Mikelberg FS. Sector-based analysis of optic nerve head shape parameters and visual field indices in healthy and glaucomatous eyes. *J Glaucoma.* 1997;6(6):370–376.
50. Iester M, Mikelberg MS, Courtright P, et al. Correlation between the visual field indices and Heidelberg retina tomograph parameters. *J Glaucoma.* 1997;6(2):78–82.
51. Tsai CS, Zangwill L, Sample PA, et al. Correlation of peripapillary retinal height and visual field in glaucoma and normal subjects. *J Glaucoma.* 1997;6(4):221–230.
52. Eid TM, Spaeth GL, Katz LJ, et al. Quantitative estimation of retinal nerve fiber layer height in glaucoma and the relationship with optic nerve head topography and visual field. *J Glaucoma.* 1997;6(4):221–230.

53. Lee KH, Park KH, Kim DM, et al. Relationship between optic nerve head parameters of Heidelberg Retina Tomograph and visual field defects in primary open-angle glaucoma. *Korean J Ophthalmol.* 1996;10(1):24–28.

54. Lusky M, Bosem ME, Weinreb RN. Reproducibility of optic nerve head topography measurements in eyes with undilated pupils. *J Glaucoma.* 1993;2:104–109.

55. Caprioli J, Park HJ, Ugurlu S, et al. Slope of the peripapillary nerve fiber layer surface in glaucoma. *Invest Ophthalmol Vis Sci.* 1998;39(12):2,321–2,328.

56. Zangwill L, Irak I, Berry CC, et al. Effect of cataract and pupil size on image quality with confocal scanning laser ophthalmoscopy. *Arch Ophthalmol.* 1997;115(8): 983–990.

57. Chauhan BC, McCormick TA. Effect of the cardiac cycle on topographic measurements using confocal scanning laser tomography. *Graefes Arch Clin Exp Ophthalmol.* 1995;233(9):568–572.

58. Bartsch DU, Freeman WR. Axial intensity distribution analysis of the human retina with a confocal scanning laser tomograph. *Exp Eye Res.* 1994;58(2):161–173.

59. Hudson C, Flanagan JG, Turner GS, et al. Scanning laser tomography Z profile signal width as an objective index of macular retinal thickening. *Br J Ophthalmol.* 1998;82(2): 121–130.

60. Hee MR, Izatt JA, Swanson EA, et al. Optical coherence tomography of the human retina. *Arch Ophthalmol.* 1995;113(3):325–332.

61. Michelson G, Schmauss B, Langhans MJ, et al. Principle, validity, and reliability of scanning laser Doppler flowmetry. *J Glaucoma.* 1996;5(2): 99–105.

62. Michelson G, Welzenbach J, Pal I, et al. Automatic full field analysis of perfusion images gained by scanning laser Doppler flowmetry. *Br J Ophthalmol.* 1998;82(11):1,294–1,300.

63. Michelson G, Welzenbach J, Pal I, et al. Functional imaging of the retinal microvasculature by scanning laser Doppler flowmetry. *Int Ophthalmol.* 2001;23(4–6):327–335.

64. Chauhan BC, Smith FM. Confocal scanning laser Doppler flowmetry: experiments in a model flow system. *J Glaucoma.* 1997;6(4):237–245.

65. Nicolela MT, Hnik P, Drance SM. Scanning laser Doppler flowmeter study of retinal and optic disk blood flow in glaucomatous patients. *Am J Ophthalmol.* 1996;122(6):775–783.

66. Nicolela MT, Hnik P, Schulzer M, et al. Reproducibility of retinal and optic nerve head blood flow measurements with scanning laser Doppler flowmetry. *J Glaucoma.* 1997;6(3):157–164.

67. Lietz A, Hendrickson P, Flammer J, et al. Effect of carbogen, oxygen and intraocular pressure on Heidelberg retina flowmeter parameter 'flow' measured at the papilla. *Ophthalmologica.* 1998;212(3):149–152.

68. Griesser SM, Lietz A, Orgul S, et al. Heidelberg retina flowmeter parameters at the papilla in healthy subjects. *Eur J Ophthalmol.* 1999;9(1):32–36.

69. Avila CP, Bartsch DU, Bitner DG, et al. Retinal blood flow measurements in branch retinal vein occlusion using scanning laser Doppler flowmetry. *Am J Ophthalmol.* 1998;126(5):683–690.

70. Mullner-Eidenbock A, Rainer G, Strenn K, et al. High-altitude retinopathy and retinal vascular dysregulation. *Eye.* 2000;14 Pt 5:724–729.

71. Paris G, Sponsel WE, Sandoval SS, et al. Sildenafil increases ocular perfusion. *Int Ophthalmol.* 2001;23(4–6):355–358.

72. Shinoda K, Kimura I, Eshita T, et al. Microcirculation in the macular area of eyes with an idiopathic epiretinal membrane. *Graefes Arch Clin Exp Ophthalmol.* 2001;239(12):941–945.

73. Bohdanecka Z, Orgul S, Prunte C, et al. Influence of acquisition parameters on hemodynamic measurements with the Heidelberg Retina Flowmeter at the optic disc. *J Glaucoma.* 1998;7(3):151–157.

74. Kagemann L, Harris A, Chung HS, et al. Heidelberg retinal flowmetry: factors affecting blood flow measurement. *Br J Ophthalmol.* 1998;82(2):131–136.

75. Jonescu-Cuypers CP, Chung HS, Kagemann L, et al. New neuroretinal rim blood flow evaluation method combining Heidelberg retina flowmetry and tomography. *Br J Ophthalmol.* 2001;85(3):304–309.

76. Kagemann L, Harris A, Chung HS, et al. Photodetector sensitivity level and heidelberg retina flowmeter measurements in humans. *Invest Ophthalmol Vis Sci.* 2001;42(2):354–357.

77. Hayashi N, Tomita G, Kitazawa Y. Optic disc blood flow measured by scanning laser-Doppler flowmetry using a new analysis program. *Jpn J Ophthalmol.* 2000;44(5):573–574.

78. Sampaolesi J, Tosi J, Darchuk V, et al. Antiglaucomatous drugs effects on optic nerve head flow: design, baseline and preliminary report. *Int Ophthalmol.* 2001;23(4–6):359–367.

79. Rawji MH, Flanagan JG. Intraocular and interocular symmetry in normal retinal capillary perfusion. *J Glaucoma.* 2001;10(1):4–12.

80. Michelson G, Patzelt A, Harazny J. Flickering light increases retinal blood flow. *Retina.* 2002;22(3):336–343.

81. Scheider A, Schroedel C. High resolution Indocyanine green angiography with a scanning laser ophthalmoscope. *Am J Ophthalmol.* 1989;108:458–459.

82. Scheider A, Plesch A. Indozyaningrün-Angiographie der Aderhaut mittels Infrarot- Scanning-Laser-Ophthalmoskopie. *Augenaerztl Fortb.* 1991;1(11):11–13.

83. Scheider A, Voeth A, Kaboth A, et al. Fluorescence characteristics of indocyanine green in the normal choroid and in subretinal neovascular membranes. *Ger J Ophthalmol.* 1992;1(1):7–11.

84. Scheider A. [Indocyanine green angiography with an infrared scanning laser ophthalmoscope. Initial clinical experiences]. *Ophthalmologe.* 1992;89(1):27–33.

85. Scheider A, Nasemann JE, Lund OE. Fluorescein and indocyanine green angiographies of central serous choroidopathy by scanning laser ophthalmoscopy. *Am J Ophthalmol.* 1993;115(1):50–56.

86. Bischoff PM, Niederberger HJ, Torok B, et al. Simultaneous indocyanine green and fluorescein angiography. *Retina.* 1995;15(2):91–99.

87. Holz FG, Bellmann C, Dithmar S, et al. [Simultaneous fluorescein and indocyanine green angiography with a confocal laser ophthalmoscope]. *Ophthalmologe.* 1997;94(5):348–353.

88. Rivero ME, Bartsch DU, Otto T, et al. Automated scanning laser ophthalmoscope image montages of retinal diseases. *Ophthalmology.* 1999;106(12):2,296–2,300.

89. Flower RW, Csaky KG, Murphy RP. Disparity between fundus camera and scanning laser ophthalmoscope indocyanine green imaging of retinal pigment epithelium detachments. *Retina.* 1998;18(3):260–268.

90. Garcia CR, Rivero ME, Bartsch DU, et al. Oral fluorescein angiography with the confocal laser scanning ophthalmoscope. *Ophthalmology.* 1999;106(6):1,114–1,118.

91. Bartsch DU, Elmusharaf A, El-Bradey M, et al. Oral fluorescein angiography in patients with choroidal neovascularization and macular degeneration. *Ophthalmic Surg Lasers Imaging.* 2003;34(1):17–24.

92. Kwiterovich KA, Maguire MG, Murphy RP, et al. Frequency of adverse systemic reactions after fluorescein angiography. Results of a prospective study. *Ophthalmology.* 1991;98(7):1,139–1,142.

93. Yannuzzi LA, Rohrer KT, Tindel LJ, et al. Fluorescein angiography complication survey. *Ophthalmology.* 1986;93(5):611–617.

94. Watson AP, Rosen ES. Oral fluorescein angiography: reassessment of its relative safety and evaluation of optimum conditions with use of capsules. *Br J Ophthalmol.* 1990;74(8):458–461.

95. Balogh VJ. The use of oral fluorescein angiography in idiopathic central serous choroidopathy. *J Am Opt Asso.* 1986;57(12):909–913.

96. Azad R, Nayak BK, Tewari HK, et al. Oral fluorescein angiography. *Ind J Ophthalmol.* 1984;32(5):415–417.

97. Sullivan TJ. Drug allergy. In: Middleton E Jr, et al., eds. *Allergy: Principles and Practice.* St. Louis: Mosby; 1993:V.II chap. 69.

98. Jensen O. Malignant melanomas of the human uvea. 25-year-follow-up of cases in Denmark. 1943–1952. *Acta Ophthalmol.* 1982;60:161–182.

99. Singh A, Topham A. Incidence of uveal melanoma in the United States: 1973–1997. *Ophthalmology.* 2002;109:AAO abstract.

100. Mueller AJ, Bartsch DU, Folberg R, et al. Imaging the microvasculature of choroidal melanomas with confocal indocyanine green scanning laser ophthalmoscopy. *Arch Ophthalmol.* 1998;116(1):31–39.

101. Mueller AJ, Bartsch DU, Schaller U, et al. Imaging the microcirculation of untreated and treated human choroidal melanomas. *Int Ophthalmol.* 2001;23(4–6):385–393.

102. Mueller AJ, Folberg R, Freeman WR, et al. Evaluation of the human choroidal melanoma rabbit model for studying microcirculation patterns with confocal ICG and histology. *Exp Eye Res.* 1999;68(6):671–678.

103. Mueller AJ, Freeman WR, Folberg R, et al. Evaluation of microvascularization pattern visibility in human choroidal melanomas: comparison of confocal fluorescein with indocyanine green angiography. *Graefes Arch Clin Exp Ophthalmol.* 1999;237(6):448–456.

104. Mehaffey MG, Folberg R, Meyer M, et al. Relative importance of quantifying area and vascular patterns in uveal melanomas. *Am J Ophthalmol.* 1997;123(6):798–809.

105. Rummelt V, Folberg R, Woolson RF, et al. Relation between the microcirculation architecture and the aggressive behavior of ciliary body melanomas. *Ophthalmology.* 1995;102:844–851.

106. Folberg R, Pe'er J, Gruman LM, et al. The morphologic characteristics of tumor blood vessels as a marker of tumor progression in primary human uveal melanoma: a matched case-control study. *Hum Pathol.* 1992;23(11):1,298–1,305.

107. Folberg R, Rummelt V, Parys-Van Ginderdeuren R, et al. The prognostic value of tumor blood vessel morphology in primary uveal melanoma. *Ophthalmology.* 1993;100(9): 1,389–1,398.

108. Folberg R. Tumor progression in ocular melanomas. *J Invest Dermatol.* 1993;100(3):326S–331S.

109. Mueller A, Maniotis AJ, Freeman WR, et al. An orthotopic model for human uveal melanoma in SCID mice. *Microvasc Res.* 2002;64(2):207.

110. Mueller AJ, Freeman WR, Folberg R, et al. [The Munich/San Diego/Iowa City Collaboration (MuSIC). MuSIC report I: design characteristics of the collective and preliminary results]. *Ophthalmologe.* 2002;99(3):193–199.

111. Mueller AJ, Freeman WR, Schaller UC, et al. Complex microcirculation patterns detected by confocal indocyanine green angiography predict time to growth of small choroidal melanocytic tumors: MuSIC Report II. *Ophthalmology.* 2002;109(12): 2,207–2,214.

112. Schaller UC, Mueller AJ, Bartsch DU, et al. [Correlation between ICG angiography verified networks in uveal melanomas and rate of tumor regression after brachytherapy]. *Ophthalmologe.* 2002;99(7):545–548.

113. Stave J, Zinser G, Grummer G, et al. [Modified Heidelberg Retinal Tomograph HRT. Initial results of in vivo presentation of corneal structures]. *Ophthalmologe.* 2002;99(4):276–280.

114. Van de Velde FJ, Timberlake GT, Jalkh AE, et al. [Static microperimetry with the laser scanning ophthalmoscope]. *Ophthalmologie.* 1990;4(3):291–294.

115. Schneider U, Kuck H, Kreissig I. Fixation and central visual field after perifoveal krypton laser treatment of subfoveal neovascularizations. *Eur J Ophthalmol.* 1993;3(4):193–200.

116. Sjaarda RN, Frank DA, Glaser BM, et al. Assessment of vision in idiopathic macular holes with macular microperimetry using the scanning laser ophthalmoscope. *Ophthalmology.* 1993;100(10):1,513–1,518.

117. Sjaarda RN, Frank DA, Glaser BM, et al. Resolution of an absolute scotoma and improvement of relative scotomata after successful macular hole surgery. *Am J Ophthalmol.* 1993;116(2):129–139.

118. Varano M, Scassa C. Scanning laser ophthalmoscope microperimetry. *Semin Ophthalmol.* 1998;13(4):203–209.

119. Ishiko S, Ogasawara H, Yoshida A, et al. The use of scanning laser ophthalmoscope microperimetry to detect visual impairment caused by macular photocoagulation. *Ophthalmic Surg Lasers.* 1998;29(2):95–98.

120. Fujikado T, Ohji M, Hayashi A, et al. Anatomic and functional recovery of the fovea after foveal translocation surgery without large retinotomy and simultaneous excision of a neovascular membrane. *Am J Ophthalmol.* 1998;126(6):839–842.

121. Rohrschneider K, Bultmann S, Gluck R, et al. Scanning laser ophthalmoscope fundus perimetry before and after laser photocoagulation for clinically significant diabetic macular edema. *Am J Ophthalmol.* 2000;129(1):27–32.

122. Rohrschneider K, Becker M, Schumacher N, et al. Normal values for fundus perimetry with the scanning laser ophthalmoscope. *Am J Ophthalmol.* 1998;126(1):52–58.

123. Rohrschneider K, Bultmann S, Kiel R, et al. [Diagnosis of retinal diseases. Comparison between multifocal ERG and fundus perimetry—a case study]. *Ophthalmologe.* 2002;99(9):695–702.

124. Rohrschneider K, Fendrich T, Becker M, et al. Static fundus perimetry using the scanning laser ophthalmoscope with an automated threshold strategy. *Graefes Arch Clin Exp Ophthalmol.* 1995;233(12):743–749.

125. Rohrschneider K, Gluck R, Becker M, et al. Scanning laser fundus perimetry before laser photocoagulation of well defined choroidal neovascularisation. *Br J Ophthalmol.* 1997;81(7):568–573.

126. Sutter EE, Tran D. The field topography of ERG components in man—I. The photopic luminance response. *Vision Res.* 1992;32(3):433–446.

127. Bultmann S, Martin M, Rohrschneider K. [Follow-up on MEWDS by fundus perimetry and multifocal ERG with the SLO]. *Ophthalmologe.* 2002;99(9):719–723.

128. Seeliger MW, Narfstrom K. Functional assessment of the regional distribution of disease in a cat model of hereditary retinal degeneration. *Invest Ophthalmol Vis Sci.* 2000;41(7):1,998–2,005.

129. Seeliger MW, Narfstrom K, Reinhard J, et al. Continuous monitoring of the stimulated area in multifocal ERG. *Doc Ophthalmol.* 2000;100(2–3):167–184.

130. Holz FG, Bellman C, Staudt S, et al. Fundus autofluorescence and development of geographic atrophy in age-related macular degeneration. *Invest Ophthalmol Vis Sci.* 2001;42(5):1,051–1,056.

131. Rudolph G, Bechmann M, Berninger T, et al. [Topographic mapping of retinal function with a scanning laser ophthalmoscope and multifocal electroretinography using short M-sequences]. *Vestn Oftalmol.* 2001;117(2):32–35.

132. Rudolph G, Kalpadakis P, Bechmann M, et al. Scanning laser ophthalmoscope-evoked multifocal-ERG (SLO-m-ERG) by using short m-sequences. *Eur J Ophthalmol.* 2002;12(2):109–116.

133. Bultmann S, Rohrschneider K. Reproducibility of multifocal ERG using the scanning laser ophthalmoscope. *Graefes Arch Clin Exp Ophthalmol.* 2002;240(10):841–845.

134. Poloschek CM, Rupp V, Krastel H, et al. Multifocal ERG recording with simultaneous fundus monitoring using a confocal scanning laser ophthalmoscope. *Eye.* 2003;17(2):159–166.

135. Kalpadakis P, Rudolph G. Multifocal ERG with the scanning laser ophthalmoscope: query on the ideal configuration for attaining high resolution and result stability. *Graefes Arch Clin Exp Ophthalmol.* 2003;241(6):522; author reply 523.

136. Babcock HW. The possibility of compensating astronomical seeing. *Pub Astronom Soc Pac.* 1953;65:229–236.

137. Dreher AW, Bille JF, Weinreb RN. Active optical depth resolution improvement of the laser tomographic scanner. *Applied Optics.* 1989;28(4):804–808.

138. Miller DT, Williams DR, Morris GM, et al. Images of cone photoreceptors in the living human eye. *Vision Res.* 1996;36(8):1,067–1,079.

139. Liang J, Williams DR, Miller DT. Supernormal vision and high-resolution retinal imaging through adaptive optics. *J Opt Soc Am A.* 1997;14(11):2,884–2,892.

140. Roorda A, Romero-Borja F, Donnelly III WJ, et al. Adaptive optics scanning laser ophthalmoscopy. *Optics Express.* 2002;10(9):405–412.

141. Hammer DX, Ferguson RD, Magill JC, et al. Compact scanning laser ophthalmoscope with high-speed retinal tracker. *Appl Opt.* 2003;42(22):4,621–4,632.

142. Podoleanu AG, Dobre GM, Cucu RG, et al. Combined multiplanar optical coherence tomography and confocal scanning ophthalmoscopy. *J Biomed Opt.* 2004;9(1):86–93.

143. Podoleanu AG, Dobre GM, Cucu RG, et al. Sequential optical coherence tomography and confocal imaging. *Opt Lett.* 2004;29(4):364–366.

144. Podoleanu A, Charalambous I, Plesea L, et al. Correction of distortions in optical coherence tomography imaging of the eye. *Phys Med Biol.* 2004;49(7):1,277–1,294.

145. Schmidt-Erfurth U, Teschner S, Noack J, et al. Three-dimensional topographic angiography in chorioretinal vascular disease. *Invest Ophthalmol Vis Sci.* 2001;42(10):2,386–2,394.

146. Schmidt-Erfurth U, Noack J, Teschner S, et al. [Confocal indocyanine green angiography with 3-dimensional topography. Results in choroid neovascularization (CNV)]. *Ophthalmologe.* 1999;96(12):797–804.

147. Schmidt-Erfurth U, Michels S, Barbazetto I, et al. Photodynamic effects on choroidal neovascularization and physiological choroid. *Invest Ophthalmol Vis Sci.* 2002;43(3):830–841.

148. Schmidt-Erfurth UM, Michels S. Changes in confocal indocyanine green angiography through two years after photodynamic therapy with verteporfin. *Ophthalmology.* 2003;110(7):1,306–1,314.

149. Teschner S, Noack J, Birngruber R, et al. Characterization of leakage activity in exudative chorioretinal disease with three-dimensional confocal angiography. *Ophthalmology.* 2003;110(4):687–697.

Antioxidants, Free Radicals, and the Retina

14

Siobhan E. Moriarty-Craige   *Paul Sternberg, Jr.*

INTRODUCTION

Oxidative stress has been implicated in age-related macular degeneration (AMD), as well as in many other chronic degenerative disease states, such as cardiovascular and neurodegenerative diseases, cataracts, and diabetes. The eye is especially susceptible to oxidative processes because of its function and location. The eye has a variety of chromophores or photosensitizers, such as melanin, rhodopsin, and lipofuscin. It is subject to high light incidence and, in conjunction with these photosensitizers, has the ability to produce a multitude of harmful reactive oxygen intermediates (ROI) (Fig. 14.1).

Much evidence suggests that oxidative stress may be associated with AMD. Since there is currently no clinical treatment for most cases of AMD, many scientists have focused on a nutritional approach; specifically, antioxidants for retarding progression of disease. There are considerable data indicating that the morphologic changes occurring in the eye with aging and disease are due to oxidative stress. In addition, observational studies have noted an inverse relationship between the intake of fruits and vegetables (especially those high in antioxidants) and AMD. This suggests that antioxidants may be able to mitigate the effect of ROI on the eye, thus slowing the progression of disease. Although oxidative stress is suspected to be involved in other eye diseases, such as cataract, this chapter will focus on the current data implicating oxidative stress in AMD, and the potential role of antioxidants in prevention of the disease.

OXIDATIVE STRESS

Reactive Oxygen Intermediates (ROI)

Oxygen is necessary for aerobic life, but is potentially toxic and can form harmful molecules known as ROI. This term describes free radicals, singlet oxygen, and hydrogen peroxide (H_2O_2) (Table 14.1). Free radicals contain one or more unpaired electrons in the outer orbital, which makes them unstable and capable of attracting electrons from other molecules in order to achieve a stable state. H_2O_2 is more stable than free radicals, but forms the highly reactive hydroxyl radical (OH) when it obtains another electron (Fig. 14.2). If one of the electrons of the two outer orbitals of molecular oxygen is inverted, the highly reactive singlet oxygen is formed. Singlet oxygen can form as the result of light acting on oxygen in the presence of a photosensitizer such as rhodopsin (Fig. 14.1). This reactive molecule is able to rapidly oxidize other molecules, including membrane polyunsaturated fatty acids (PUFAs) (Table 14.2).

Oxidative Stress

Although oxidants are constantly generated for essential biologic functions, excess generation of oxidants or an imbalance between oxidants and antioxidants can produce a common pathophysiologic condition termed oxidative stress. Oxidative stress contributes significantly to age-related diseases such as atherosclerosis, chronic lung disease, Alzheimer's disease, and AMD (1–4). Oxidative stress is associated with low antioxidant levels, lipid peroxidation, protein modification, and DNA damage (5–8). In addition to exogenous sources, such as pollution and smoking, ROI are formed through normal cellular reduction–oxidation (redox) reactions (Table 14.1) (9).

Many cellular components, such as lipids, proteins, and nucleic acids, can be damaged by ROI. Lipid peroxidation can be initiated by hydroxyl radical, hydroperoxyl radical, or singlet oxygen (Table 14.2); it often occurs as a propagating chain of events that culminates in destruction of organelles and plasma membrane. Toxic compounds that result from lipid peroxidation, such as malondialdehyde

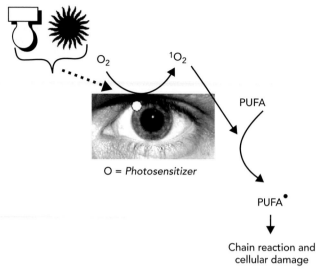

O = *Photosensitizer*

Figure 14.1 The eye contains many photosensitizers, such as rhodopsin, melanin, cytochrome c oxidase, protoporphyrin IX (hemoglobin precursor supplied to the eye via the choroid), and lipofuscin. These photosensitizers are able to react with light to form singlet oxygen or other ROI that can then attack PUFAs or cause other cellular damage.

(MDA), can cause inflammation at the site of formation or at other sites by diffusion. In proteins, the oxidation of sulfhydryl-containing enzymes by ROI often causes inactivation of enzymes or changes in protein function. ROI can cause DNA damage or inhibition of transcription and translation through base hydroxylation and cross-linking of DNA strands (10).

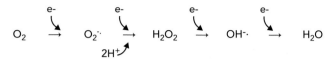

Figure 14.2 The sequential one-electron transfer of oxygen to water. In biological systems, superoxide usually forms hydrogen peroxide only in the presence of the enzyme super oxide dismutase. In addition, hydrogen peroxide forms the hydroxyl radical in the presence of a metal catalyst such as Fe^{2+}. e^-, electron.

Aging

Aging is associated with a higher incidence of degenerative diseases of the eye, such as AMD, cataract, glaucoma, and diabetic retinopathy (11). In fact, age is the primary risk factor for AMD. In a recent study in which Medicare beneficiaries over the age of 65 were followed for a 9-year period, the incidence of AMD climbed from 5% to 27% (12).

The commonality of aging implies that its cause is similar in all species. The free radical theory of aging identifies ROI as causing cumulative damage to DNA and other macromolecules, leading to senescence, cell death, disease, and ultimate organism death (13). Several studies show that plasma thiol/disulfide redox state becomes oxidized with aging (14,15). Among the changes that are well-documented are decreased glutathione (GSH), increased cystine (CySS), and increased total homocysteine (Hcys). In a study that examined the redox of individual thiol/disulfide couples in human plasma, there was a clear oxidation in association with age (Fig. 14.3). In addition, a linear oxidation of about 0.2 mV/year was found for cysteine/cystine (Cys/CySS), whereas the glutathione/glutathione disulfide

TABLE 14.1

MANY ROI CAN BE FORMED ENDOGENOUSLY THROUGH NORMAL METABOLISM. DEPICTED HERE ARE THE MOST COMMON ROI AND EXAMPLES OF THEIR POSSIBLE PRODUCTION SITES.

Potentially Harmful ROI	Name	Sources
$O_2^{\cdot-}$	Superoxide anion radical	Auto-oxidations, oxidases, electron transport chain, respiratory burst, light + lipofuscin
H_2O_2	Hydrogen peroxide	Electron transport chain, light + lipofuscin
$OH^{\cdot}$	Hydroxyl radical	Fenton reaction, Haber-Weiss reaction
$ROO^{\cdot}$	Peroxide radical	Hydroxyl attack of rod and cone PUFAs after RPE phagocytosis
$^1O_2$	Singlet oxygen	Light acting on molecular oxygen in the presence of photosensitizers (i.e., lipofuscin)

TABLE 14.2

LIPID PEROXIDATION CAN BE DIVIDED INTO THREE PHASES: INITIATION, PROPAGATION, AND TERMINATION.

Possible Schematic of Events in PUFA Oxidation

RH R⋅	Initiation
R⋅ + O_2 ROO⋅	
ROO⋅ + RH ROOH + R⋅	Propagation
R⋅ (or ROO⋅) + vitamin E	Termination
(or other antioxidant)	
RH + vitamin E⋅	

During the propagation phase, lipid radicals rapidly react with oxygen to form the peroxyl radical, which then reacts with another lipid to form the more stable hydroperoxide. This chain of events can continue until the PUFAs are completely consumed or the chain is broken, as shown in the termination phase by an antioxidant such as vitamin E, which is one of the most effective chain-breaking antioxidants.

(GSH/GSSG) redox was maintained until 45 years of age, after which it rapidly declined by 0.7 mV/year (14,15). Similar oxidation of plasma thiols is seen with chemotherapy, HIV, diabetes, and AMD (16–18).

OXIDATIVE STRESS AND AMD

The relationship between the development and progression of AMD and oxidative stress is supported by many layers of evidence. These include risk factors for the disease,

the pathoanatomic changes associated with the disease, as well as the primary involvement of the retinal pigment epithelium (RPE) in disease development.

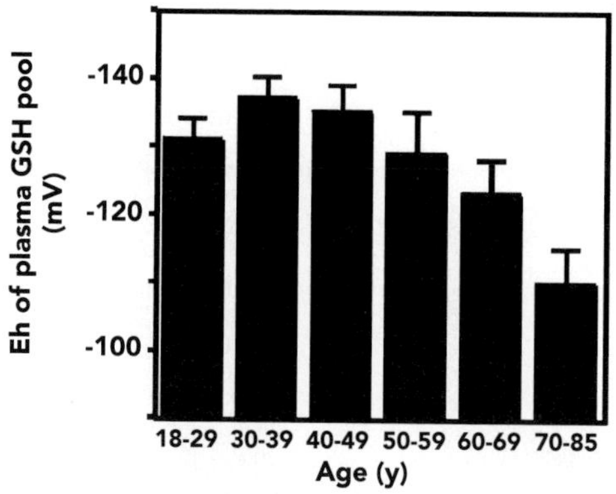

AMD Risk Factors

A number of studies have investigated risk factors for AMD, several of which reflect oxidative stress as playing a causal role. Currently the primary risk factor is aging, but other risk factors such as smoking, light exposure, iris color, and macula pigment density have also been associated.

Cigarette smoke contains an extremely high concentration of free radicals (19) causing an increased state of oxidative stress in the body. A meta-analysis of three large population-based studies on three different continents found an odds ratio for all types of AMD of 3.12 for current smokers compared to nonsmokers (20). This study concluded that smoking is the main preventable risk factor associated with AMD. Another review of the literature examined the effect of smoking on cataract and AMD and also reported a causal relationship between smoking and both age-related diseases (21). The Australian Blue Mountains eye study showed that smokers have an increased 5-year incidence of late-AMD lesions and retinal pigmentary abnormalities; smokers also developed late AMD earlier than nonsmokers (22). A recent study determined that the plasma concentrations of GSH and Cys are lower and the GSH/GSSG and Cys/CySS redox status is oxidized in smokers compared to nonsmokers (23), possibly because cigarette smoke contains compounds (e.g., acrolein) that react with GSH (24), as well as ROI that oxidize GSH to GSSG.

Figure 14.3 There is an age-related oxidation of the plasma redox state that may effect susceptibility to disease states such as AMD. Eh, ; GSH,. (Reprinted with permission from Jones DP, Mody VC Jr, Carlson JL, et al., Redox analysis of human plasma allows separation of pro-oxidant events of aging from decline in antioxidant defenses. *Free Radic Biol Med.* 2002;33:1290–1300.)

In addition to smoking, there are studies suggesting other risk factors associated with AMD could be linked to oxidative stress. The primary one is light exposure, which includes ionizing radiation, UV light, and visible light. Such exposure can initiate free radical formation that can then lead to lipid peroxidation of the photoreceptor outer segment (POS) membranes (25,26), suggesting an association between oxidative stress and AMD. Sunlight exposure could increase the amount of cumulative incident and focused light on the macula and increase the likelihood of oxidative injury. Indeed, it has been implicated as a risk factor (27), but its association with AMD has not consistently been found to be significant.

There are a variety of animal models utilizing light-induced retinal and RPE damage to simulate AMD. However, most of these studies employed short-duration exposures of high-intensity light. Hence, the effects demonstrated in these studies may not be an accurate modeling of the clinical setting, with long-term exposure to lower-intensity light.

Cross-sectional studies examining AMD and iris color have observed a higher prevalence of AMD in subjects with light-colored irises than those with dark-colored irises, suggesting that light iris pigmentation is associated with more severe AMD (28,29). In the Beaver Dam Eye Study, iris color was associated with an increased 10-year incidence of pigmentary abnormalities in the RPE, but the findings relating to disease outcome were inconsistent (30). A similar longitudinal study, the Blue Mountains Eye Study, came to the conclusion that there was no significant association between iris color and AMD.

The data on macula pigment density is inconclusive, and is difficult to interpret because other AMD risk factors, such as smoking and iris color, also affect macula pigment density (31,32). One study demonstrated that, with aging, the macula pigment density decreased; healthy eyes predisposed to AMD had a lower macula pigment density than those who were not at risk (33). However, other studies have not demonstrated conclusive evidence in this area.

Pathoanatomic Changes with AMD

In AMD the macula region of the retina deteriorates, ultimately leading to death of photoreceptors, which impacts central vision. The neurosensory retina and the RPE contain an abundance of photosensitizers. Because the retina is subject to high levels of light irradiation and the consumption of O_2 in the retina is greater than any other tissue, this tissue is prone to oxidative stress and damage (34–37). AMD changes include geographic atrophy, detachment of the RPE, and choroidal neovascularization, all of which are associated with photoreceptor damage and loss. The pathologic changes in the macula with AMD suggest that the primary cause of the disease is due to RPE damage, followed by photoreceptor damage and retina deterioration. Therefore, much research has focused on the oxidative changes seen in the RPE with aging and disease onset.

Retinal Pigment Epithelium

The etiology of AMD is poorly understood. However, it is likely that the RPE plays a critical role in the pathogenesis of the disease. Clinically, in patients with early stages of AMD, RPE atrophy, which leads to alteration of photoreceptor function, is associated with a difficulty in form recognition (38). It is thought that AMD could be due to oxidative insult to the RPE, thus contributing to cell loss.

The RPE functions both to deliver nutrients to the photoreceptors from the choroid, as well as to take waste material from the photoreceptors and deliver it to the choroid (Fig. 14.4). By phagocytosing shed POS, the RPE plays a crucial role in photoreceptor maintenance. As a result of its location and various functions, the RPE is subjected to considerable oxidative stress. The combination of a high incidence of focused light, high oxygen tension, and phagocytosed POS rich in PUFAs, creates an excellent environment for lipid peroxidation (39). There is a significantly higher concentration of lipid peroxidation products in AMD subjects versus controls (40), indicating oxidative stress and, specifically, a buildup of oxidized PUFAs from the POS. These can lead to the accrual of basal laminar material and drusen beneath the RPE, which likely results in inefficient nutrient and waste transfer to and from the choroid (Fig. 14.5) (41). This may lead to further RPE dysfunction, additional oxidative stress, and further accumulation of drusen. This cycle may ultimately lead to AMD.

In the aging human, the RPE is a nondividing monolayer of cells. Most in vitro modeling for AMD has involved primary or immortalized RPE cells that are capable of proliferation. However, a recent in vitro model of long-term, nondividing human RPE cells (Fig. 14.6) similar to the in vivo setting, demonstrated that these cells are more sensitive to oxidant-induced injury than proliferating human RPE cells (42). This suggests that the postmitotic RPE in vivo could be more susceptible with age to oxidative stress and oxidant-related injury. Additionally, the oxidants tBH

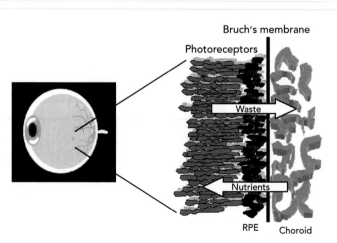

Figure 14.4 The RPE is located between Bruch's membrane and the photoreceptors. The RPE is involved in transporting nutrients to the photoreceptors from the choroid, and wastes from the photoreceptors to the choroid.

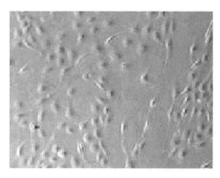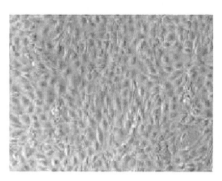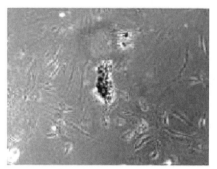

Figure 14.5 The normal RPE is a monolayer of cells. With age, waste builds up under the RPE. This drusen formation can enlarge and eventually cause RPE loss and dysfunction.

and H_2O_2 can induce apoptosis in RPE. The mechanism of RPE damage and subsequent cell death by oxidants is likely related to mitochondrial dysfunction and activation of cell surface death receptors. (39,43–45).

Lipofuscin

Age is the strongest risk factor for AMD and correlates with RPE lipofuscin content. For example, at the age of 90, approximately 19% of the RPE cells are occupied by lipofuscin, compared with only 1% in the first 10 years of life (46,47). Lipofuscin is a brownish, autofluorescent pigment that accumulates from the breakdown of POS in the lysosomes of the RPE. Lipofuscin is present in many other cell types, including brain, heart muscle, and liver. It is also referred to as the "aging" pigment. Lipofuscin accumulation in the RPE is a hallmark of AMD, and much greater

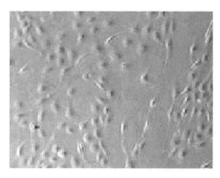

Normal RPE

↓

Drusen formation

↓

RPE loss and dysfunction

Figure 14.6 An in vitro model of physiologic conditions. **A.** Actively proliferating RPE. **B.** Confluent RPE. **C.** RPE after remaining in culture for one month.

amounts of lipofuscin are seen in atrophic AMD than in normal eyes (48).

Photoreceptor loss was found to directly correlate with adjacent RPE lipofuscin accumulation (49). This finding suggests that the increased phagocytic and metabolic load on the RPE causes an accumulation of lipofuscin in the RPE, resulting in photoreceptor death. The photoreceptors likely undergo some oxidation due to the high proportion of the easily oxidized PUFAs (Table 14.2) and therefore yield changed products that are not easily digested by the RPE cells (50). Higgins et al. recently showed that expression of chemotactic and angiogenic factors was stimulated by the phagocytosis of oxidized POS in bovine RPE (51). This suggests that oxidized POS products may buildup over time and add to the susceptibility of the RPE to oxidative damage, the accumulation of waste underneath the retina (drusen), and onset of AMD.

Aging RPE accumulates lipofuscin, which includes N-retinylidene-N-retinylethanolamine (A2E) as a major autofluorescent component. RPE cells that contain an abundance of lipofuscin high in the proportion of the fluorophore A2E exhibit cell membrane blebbing and cytoplasmic extrusion into Bruch's membrane (52) (Fig. 14.5). Furthermore, cells with a high quantity of A2E are more susceptible to blue–light-induced damage and subsequent apoptosis through the mitochondrial pathway, which can be regulated by Bcl-2 (53). The accumulation of A2E also interferes with inhibition of lysosomal degradative capacity, loss of membrane integrity, and phototoxicity to the RPE (54,55). A2E seems to be formed from oxidized POS, and this has been demonstrated in vitro (56,57). Hence, the accumulation of lipofuscin and A2E may increase the susceptibility of the RPE to oxidative stress.

Mitochondria

Since the RPE cells are very metabolically active, a decrease in mitochondrial function may contribute to the compromised cell function and ultimate cell death seen in AMD.

Mitochondrial dysfunction could be caused by mitochondrial DNA (mtDNA) damage by harmful ROI. The mtDNA encodes 13 proteins that are all part of oxidative phosphorylation. Mitochondria create ATP through oxidative phosphorylation, which is essential for all normal cell processes. Through this process they also produce harmful ROI; over time, electron transport becomes less efficient with a greater leakage of ROI, which may cycle back, causing mitochondrial or other cellular damage, leading to a further decrease in efficiency (58). Mitochondrial efficiency declines with age in many postmitotic tissues, and has been theorized to play a role in the free radical theory of aging (58,59).

The mtDNA is more susceptible to oxidant-induced injury than is nuclear DNA for a variety of reasons. The mtDNA is attached to the mitochondrial inner membrane where ROI are created through the activity of the electron transport chain. Also, the mtDNA lacks protection by histones or from other DNA-binding proteins, and the mitochondrion has a limited ability to repair its DNA. In vitro, the addition of H_2O_2 and POS to cultured RPE cells induces mtDNA damage, indicating mtDNA mutations may indeed play a role in the pathogenesis of AMD (60,61). Furthermore, a common 4977-bp deletion in mtDNA ($\Delta mtDNA^{4977}$) is found in many degenerative diseases and aging postmitotic tissues (62,63). This common deletion also accumulates in hRPE cells with age (64). The aging process is also associated with point mutations in the D-loop, which accumulate over time and suggest functional impairment in the mitochondrial genetic machinery (65).

As previously mentioned, the fluorophore A2E can act as a proapoptotic molecule via a mitochondria-related mechanism. This is possibly through the targeting of A2E (a cation) to cytochrome oxidase (COX). Inhibition of mitochondrial function may cause a loss of RPE cell viability, or at least a metabolic disruption in the RPE, which may lead to RPE atrophy and subsequent cell loss in the central retina (66). These studies augment existing data implicating mtDNA damage as having a significant role in aging. Yet, there remains much that is not known about this increase in mtDNA mutations and its importance in aging and age-related diseases and, specifically, in AMD.

ANTIOXIDANTS

Oxidative stress has been postulated to be a mechanism of AMD. There have been a number of studies looking at the potential role for antioxidants in protecting against development of the disease or limiting its progression. For example, one study has shown that intake of fruits and vegetables, which are high in antioxidants can be inversely correlated with AMD (67,68). The Age-Related Eye Disease Study (AREDS) showed that supplemental antioxidants (vitamin C, vitamin E, and beta-carotene) and zinc can significantly retard the progression of AMD (69,70). This was a 7-year study that examined 5,000 men and women ages 55 to 80 years. Patients were assigned to placebo, zinc alone, antioxidants alone, and zinc plus antioxidants. The study demonstrated that antioxidant and zinc supplementation reduce the risk of progression from intermediate AMD to advanced AMD by 25%. This result provides strong support for a link between AMD and oxidative injury.

The Baltimore Longitudinal Study of Aging (BLSA) also found that there was a protective effect for antioxidants. In this study, the investigators generated an antioxidant index, which was composed of plasma ascorbic acid (vitamin C), alpha-tocopherol (vitamin E), and beta-carotene levels (71). Individuals with a higher antioxidant index had a lower incidence of AMD. There have been a large number of other human clinical and epidemiological studies; although results vary, these studies, in conjunction with tissue culture and animal studies, provide considerable support for the importance of antioxidant status and antioxidant supplementation for AMD. For example, studies have deprived animals (including primates) of antioxidants and found that they are much more prone to retinal degeneration than controls, while animals supplemented with antioxidants have demonstrated increased resistance to retinal degeneration (26,72–75).

Vitamin C (Ascorbate)

Vitamin C is a potent, water-soluble reducing agent that has antioxidant activity, acting as an electron donor. It is thought to play a major role in many degenerative disorders associated with oxidative stress. This antioxidant is found in high concentrations in the eye (76).

Organisciak et al. found that rats given vitamin C prior to light exposure were protected against light-induced retinal damage (72). Furthermore, cyclic–light-reared rats lost 50% to 55% of their visual cells; this loss was decreased to 30% to 35% by supplementation with vitamin C before intense light exposure (77). Vitamin C treatment also protected against hypoxia-induced apoptosis (less DNA fragmentation) in RPE cells (78).

A study of the distribution of vitamin C in the retina demonstrated that vitamin C seems to move from the vitreous cavity into the subretinal space (79). This study also demonstrated that the retina was permeable to vitamin C. As observed in cat, bovine, and bullfrog RPE, this is probably through a sodium-dependent carrier system (80–82). Interestingly, only the oxidized form, dehydroascorbate, was observed in the RPE, suggesting the presence of oxidative reactions in that cell layer, in which vitamin C is necessary (79).

The normal RPE contains large numbers of phagosomes formed by invagination of the plasma membrane from RPE phagocytosis of shed POS. The frequency of phagosome production is thought to serve as an index for light damage and oxidative stress. Phagosome frequency is decreased with vitamin C supplementation (83).

Epidemiologic data on AMD and vitamin C have been variable. The National Health and Nutrition Examination

Survey I (NHANES I) reported that a diet high in vitamins A and C was negatively associated with AMD. However, this association disappeared after adjusting for demographic and medical factors (68). The Eye Disease Case-Control Study (EDCCS) found that blood concentration of vitamin C was not indicative of the prevalence of AMD (84).

Vitamin E (Alpha-Tocopherol)

Vitamin E is a lipid-soluble antioxidant that passes through membranes and is often incorporated into membranes. It functions to convert superoxide anion, hydroxyl radical, and lipid peroxyl radical to less-reactive forms by donating a hydrogen ion. Typically, vitamin E acts as a chain-breaking antioxidant by rapidly reacting with peroxyl radicals (more quickly than PUFAs), which prevents the propagation of free radical damage to lipids in biologic membranes (Table 14.2) (85). The retina contains high quantities of vitamin E in the POS. Because POS are high in PUFAs, the main role of vitamin E is most likely to maintain the integrity of these lipids and scavenge ROI.

Organisciak et al. found that vitamin E concentration in the retina increases with age, and postulated that this might be due to increased oxidative stress in the retina over time (86). In vitro studies have demonstrated that vitamin E significantly reduces the amount of damage to the POS when challenged with an oxidative insult (87,88). Studies in monkeys have demonstrated that vitamin E deficiency leads to retinal degeneration (26). Yet, human studies have reported inconsistent results. The BLSA (n = 976) demonstrated a protective effect for high plasma vitamin E concentrations (71). However, in a recent study of 1193 health volunteers between the ages of 55 and 80, vitamin E supplementation was not seen to prevent the development or progression of early or later stages of AMD (89).

Carotenoids

The macula region is yellow in color (thus its name, macula lutea, or yellow spot), but it was only in the mid-1980s that the reason for this coloration was completely understood. Bone et al. and Handelman et al. discovered that the macula is composed of two very similar carotenoids, lutein and zeaxanthin (90–93). Humans absorb very high amounts of carotenoids from the diet. It is estimated that people who eat diets high in fruits and vegetables may consume more than several milligrams of carotenoids every day. Therefore, it seems that these carotenoids must have some other function than the coloration of the macula alone, and most likely they play multiple physiologic roles.

A protective effect for beta-carotene was seen in BLSA, but this was not statistically significant (71). In the EDCCS (n: neovascular AMD = 421, control = 615) a protective association was seen between carotenoid concentration and the severe form of AMD. This study found that with a medium carotenoid level, there was $\frac{1}{2}$ the risk of AMD. With a high carotenoid level, there was $\frac{1}{3}$ the risk of AMD

(94). This same study demonstrated an inverse association between carotenoid intake and neovascular AMD (84).

Speculation as to the exact function of these carotenoids abounds, but it is hypothesized that they play a critical role in scavenging ROI (84). People who report the consumption of diets rich in lutein and zeaxanthin have a lower incidence of macular degeneration (84). There is some evidence that oral intake of lutein and zeaxanthin can increase the concentration of these pigments in the macula of patients, and many pharmaceutical companies have advocated that AMD patients take such. However, to date there are no clinical trials demonstrating that these carotenoids are protective.

Other Antioxidants

GSH is an essential endogenous antioxidant system that functions both directly and indirectly to eliminate toxicants. One direct mechanism to remove harmful reactive oxygen species occurs via a family of GSH peroxidases. GSH also reacts with superoxide and reactive aldehydes generated during lipid peroxidation. Indirect functions include reduction of dehydroascorbate to vitamin C. Free radical termination reactions of vitamin C generate semidehydroascorbate, which in turn undergoes spontaneous dismutation to form vitamin C and dehydroascorbate. Reduction of dehydroascorbate is key to maintaining the vitamin C pool. Vitamin C, in turn, maintains vitamin E pools by reducing the free radical form of vitamin E (generated during radical chain termination) (95). GSH may function similar to vitamin C and vitamin E in the protection and maintenance of the eye.

Rats subjected to intense light exposure demonstrate a significant increase in retinal GSH (77). Studies have demonstrated that GSH and its amino acid precursors are able to protect against oxidative injury to cultured human RPE. Under hypoxic conditions, N-acetyl-cysteine (NAC) (a GSH precursor) treatment protected against apoptosis (78). In addition, compounds that induce the synthesis of GSH, such as dimethylfumarate (DMF), sulforaphane, and the antischistosomal agent, oltipraz, are also able to protect the RPE from oxidative injury and death (96–98).

SUMMARY, CONCLUSIONS, AND FUTURE DIRECTIONS

There is considerable evidence to support the hypothesis that oxidative stress plays an important role in the pathogenesis of AMD. The macula is subject to high levels of focused light, has an oxygen-rich environment, and undergoes constant turnover of POS that are rich in PUFAs. As a result, the aging macular RPE may become less metabolically active, leading to buildup of basal laminar material and drusen. This can lead to a cycle of further damage and increased susceptibility to oxidative insult.

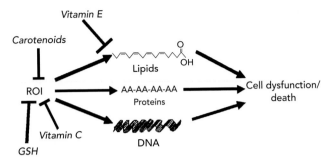

Figure 14.7 An overview of the effects of harmful ROI on macromolecules and the ability of antioxidants to prevent these occurrences.

The body contains a number of antioxidants designed to protect cells such as the RPE from oxidative injury. These include vitamin C, vitamin E, carotenoids, and GSH (Fig. 14.7). A number of epidemiological studies have suggested that antioxidant supplementation could be beneficial for AMD. Recently, AREDS demonstrated the benefit of beta-carotene, vitamin C, vitamin E, and zinc in reducing the risk of AMD progression. Further studies are planned to explore the possible benefit of the carotenoids, lutein and zeaxanthin, as well as other agents that may protect by augmenting GSH levels. It is hoped that interventions such as these can have a significant impact on the prevalence and progression of this blinding disease.

ACKNOWLEDGMENTS

We would like to thank Michael Orr for aiding in the figures.

REFERENCES

1. Traber MG, van der Vliet A, Reznick AZ, et al. Tobacco-related diseases. Is there a role for antioxidant micronutrient supplementation? *Clin Chest Med.* 2000;21:173–187, x.
2. Rao AV, Balachandran B. Role of oxidative stress and antioxidants in neurodegenerative diseases. *Nutr Neurosci.* 2002;5:291–309.
3. Husain D, Ambati B, Adamis AP. et al. Mechanisms of age-related macular degeneration. *Ophthalmol Clin North Am.* 2002;15:87–91.
4. Maxwell S, Greig L. Anti-oxidants—a protective role in cardiovascular disease? *Expert Opin Pharmacother.* 2001;2:1,737–1,750.
5. Bridges AB, Scott NA, Parry GJ, et al. Age, sex, cigarette smoking and indices of free radical activity in healthy humans. *Eur J Med.* 1993;2:205–208.
6. Godschalk R, Nair J, van Schooten FJ, et al. Comparison of multiple DNA adduct types in tumor adjacent human lung tissue: effect of cigarette smoking. *Carcinogenesis.* 2002;23:2,081–2,086.
7. Mayne ST. Antioxidant nutrients and chronic disease: use of biomarkers of exposure and oxidative stress status in epidemiologic research. *J Nutr.* 2003;133:Suppl 3:933s–940s.
8. Nishio E, Watanabe Y. Cigarette smoke extract inhibits plasma paraoxonase activity by modification of the enzyme's free thiols. *Biochem Biophys Res Commun.* 1997;236:289–293.
9. Barja G. Endogenous oxidative stress: relationship to aging, longevity and caloric restriction. *Ageing Res Rev.* 2002;1:397–411.
10. Barja G. Rate of generation of oxidative stress-related damage and animal longevity. *Free Radic Biol Med.* 2002;33:1,167–1,172.
11. Jackson GR, Owsley C. Visual dysfunction, neurodegenerative diseases, and aging. *Neurol Clin.* 2003;21:709–728.
12. Lee PP, Feldman ZW, Ostermann J, et al. Longitudinal prevalence of major eye diseases. *Arch Ophthalmol.* 2003;121:1,303–1,310.
13. Harman D. Aging: a theory based on free radical and radiation chemistry. *J Gerontol.* 1956;11:298–300.
14. Jones DP, Mody VC, Jr., Carlson JL, et al. Redox analysis of human plasma allows separation of pro-oxidant events of aging from decline in antioxidant defenses. *Free Radic Biol Med.* 2002;33:1,290–1,300.
15. Cudkowicz ME, Sexton PM, Ellis T, et al. The pharmacokinetics and pharmaco-dynamics of Procysteine in amyotrophic lateral sclerosis. *Neurology.* 1999;52:1,492–1,494.
16. Buhl R, Jaffe HA, Holroyd KJ, et al. Systemic glutathione deficiency in symptom-free HIV-seropositive individuals. *Lancet.* 1989;2:1,294–1,298.
17. Costagliola C, Iuliano G, Menzione M, et al. Systemic human diseases as oxidative risk factors in cataractogenesis. I. Diabetes. *Ophthalmic Res.* 1988;20:308–316.
18. Samiec PS, Drews-Botsch C, Flagg EW, et al. Glutathione in human plasma: decline in association with aging, age-related macular degeneration, and diabetes. *Free Radic Biol Med.* 1998;24:699–704.
19. Pryor WA, Prier DG, Church DF. Electron-spin resonance study of mainstream and sidestream cigarette smoke: nature of the free radicals in gas-phase smoke and in cigarette tar. *Environ Health Perspect.* 1983;47:345–355.
20. Smith W, Assink J, Klein R, et al. Risk factors for age-related macular degeneration: pooled findings from three continents. *Ophthalmology.* 2001;108:697–704.
21. DeBlack SS. Cigarette smoking as a risk factor for cataract and age-related macular degeneration: a review of the literature. *Optometry.*2003;74:99–110.
22. Mitchell P, Wang JJ, Smith W, et al. Smoking and the 5-year incidence of age-related maculopathy: the Blue Mountains Eye Study. *Arch Ophthalmol.* 2002;120:1,357–1,363.
23. Moriarty SE, Shah JH, Lynn M, et al. Oxidation of glutathione and cysteine in human plasma associated with smoking. *Free Radic Biol Med.* 2003;35:1,582–1,588.
24. Reddy S, Finkelstein EI, Wong PS, et al. Identification of glutathione modifications by cigarette smoke. *Free Radic Biol Med.* 2002;33:1,490–1,498.
25. Feeney L, Berman ER. Oxygen toxicity: membrane damage by free radicals. *Invest Ophthalmol.* 1976;15:789–792.
26. Hayes KC. Retinal degeneration in monkeys induced by deficiencies of vitamin E or A. *Invest Ophthalmol.* 1974;13:499–510.
27. Young RW. Solar radiation and age-related macular degeneration. *Surv Ophthalmol.* 1988;32:252–269.
28. Frank RN, Puklin JE, Stock C, et al. Race, iris color, and age-related macular degeneration. *Trans Am Ophthalmol Soc.* 2000;98:109–115; discussion 115–107.
29. Sandberg MA, Gaudio AR, Miller S, et al. Iris pigmentation and extent of disease in patients with neovascular age-related macular degeneration. *Invest Ophthalmol Vis Sci.* 1994;35:2,734–2,740.
30. Tomany SC, Klein R, Klein BE. The relationship between iris color, hair color, and skin sun sensitivity and the 10-year incidence of age-related maculopathy: the Beaver Dam Eye Study. *Ophthalmology.* 2003;110:1,526–1,533.
31. Hammond BR, Jr., Fuld K, Snodderly DM. Iris color and macular pigment optical density. *Exp Eye Res.* 1996;62:293–297.
32. Hammond BR Jr., Wooten BR, Snodderly DM. Cigarette smoking and retinal carotenoids: implications for age-related macular degeneration. *Vision Res.* 1996;36:3,003–3,009.
33. Beatty S, Murray IJ, Henson DB, et al. Macular pigment and risk for age-related macular degeneration in subjects from a northern European population. *Invest Ophthalmol Vis Sci.* 2001;42:439–446.
34. Alm A, Bill A. Ocular and optic nerve blood flow at normal and increased intraocular pressures in monkeys (*Macaca irus*]): a study with radioactively labelled microspheres including flow determinations in brain and some other tissues. *Exp Eye Res.* 1973;15:15–29.
35. Delmelle M. Retinal sensitized photodynamic damage to liposomes. *Photochem Photobiol.* 1978;28:357–360.
36. Gaillard ER, Atherton SJ, Eldred G, et al. Photophysical studies on human retinal lipofuscin. *Photochem Photobiol.* 1995;61:448–453.
37. Rozanowska M, Jarvis-Evans J, Korytowski W, et al. Blue light-induced reactivity of retinal age pigment. In vitro generation of oxygen-reactive species. *J Biol Chem.* 1995;270:18,825–18,830.
38. Tolentino MJ, Miller S, Gaudio AR, et al. Visual field deficits in early age-related macular degeneration. *Vision Res.* 1994;34:409–413.
39. Cai J, Nelson KC, Wu M, et al. Oxidative damage and protection of the RPE. *Prog Retin Eye Res.* 2000;19:205–221.
40. Nowak M, Swietochowska E, Wielkoszynski T, et al. Changes in blood antioxidants and several lipid peroxidation products in women with age-related macular degeneration. *Eur J Ophthalmol.* 2003;13:281–286.
41. Beatty S, Koh H, Phil M, et al. The role of oxidative stress in the pathogenesis of age-related macular degeneration. *Surv Ophthalmol.* 2000;45:115–134.
42. Jiang S, Moriarty SE, Grossniklaus H, et al. Increased oxidant-induced apoptosis in cultured nondividing human retinal pigment epithelial cells. *Invest Ophthalmol Vis Sci.* 2002;43:2,546–2,553.
43. Jin GF, Hurst JS, Godley BF. Hydrogen peroxide stimulates apoptosis in cultured human retinal pigment epithelial cells. *Curr Eye Res.* 2001;22:165–173.
44. Richter C. Insight into age-related macular degeneration: new vision in sight. *Cell Death Differ.* 2001;8:207–209.
45. Jiang S, Wu MW, Sternberg P, et al. Fas mediates apoptosis and oxidant-induced cell death in cultured hRPE cells. *Invest Ophthalmol Vis Sci.* 2000;41:645–655.
46. Feeney-Burns L, Hilderbrand ES, Eldridge S. Aging human RPE: morphometric analysis of macular, equatorial, and peripheral cells. *Invest Ophthalmol Vis Sci.* 1984;25:195–200.
47. Feeney-Burns L, Eldred GE. The fate of the phagosome: conversion to 'age pigment' and impact in human retinal pigment epithelium. *Trans Ophthalmol Soc UK.* 1983;103 (Pt 4):416–421.
48. Sarks JP, Sarks SH, Killingsworth MC. Evolution of geographic atrophy of the retinal pigment epithelium. *Eye.* 1988;2 (Pt 5):552–577.

49. Dorey CK, Wu G, Ebenstein D, et al. Cell loss in the aging retina. Relationship to lipofuscin accumulation and macular degeneration. *Invest Ophthalmol Vis Sci.* 1989;30:1,691–1,699.

50. Akeo K, Hiramitsu T, Kanda T, et al. Comparative effects of linoleic acid and linoleic acid hydroperoxide on growth and morphology of bovine retinal pigment epithelial cells in vitro. *Curr Eye Res.* 1996;15:467–476.

51. Higgins GT, Wang JH, Dockery P, et al. Induction of angiogenic cytokine expression in cultured RPE by ingestion of oxidized photoreceptor outer segments. *Invest Ophthalmol Vis Sci.* 2003;44:1,775–1,782.

52. Eldred GE, Lasky MR. Retinal age pigments generated by self-assembling lysosomotropic detergents. *Nature.* 1993;361:724–726.

53. Sparrow JR, Cai B. Blue light-induced apoptosis of A2E-containing RPE: involvement of caspase-3 and protection by Bcl-2. *Invest Ophthalmol Vis Sci.* 2001;42:1,356–1,362.

54. Schutt F, Davies S, Kopitz J, et al. Photodamage to human RPE cells by A2-E, a retinoid component of lipofuscin. *Invest Ophthalmol Vis Sci.* 2000;41: 2,303–2,308.

55. Holz FG, Schutt F, Kopitz J, et al. Inhibition of lysosomal degradative functions in RPE cells by a retinoid component of lipofuscin. *Invest Ophthalmol Vis Sci.* 1999;40:737–743.

56. Liu J, Itagaki Y, Ben-Shabat S, et al. The biosynthesis of A2E, a fluorophore of aging retina, involves the formation of the precursor, A2-PE, in the photoreceptor outer segment membrane. *J Biol Chem.* 2000;275:29,354–29,360.

57. Mata NL, Weng J, Travis GH. Biosynthesis of a major lipofuscin fluorophore in mice and humans with ABCR-mediated retinal and macular degeneration. *Proc Natl Acad Sci USA.* 2000;97:7,154–7,159.

58. Lenaz G, D'Aurelio M, Merlo Pich M, et al. Mitochondrial bioenergetics in aging. *Biochim Biophys Acta.* 2000;1459:397–404.

59. Hagen TM, Moreau R, Suh JH, et al. Mitochondrial decay in the aging rat heart: evidence for improvement by dietary supplementation with acetyl-L-carnitine and/or lipoic acid. *Ann NY Acad Sci.* 2002;959:491–507.

60. Jin GF, Hurst JS, Godley BF. Rod outer segments mediate mitochondrial DNA damage and apoptosis in human retinal pigment epithelium. *Curr Eye Res.* 2001;23:11–19.

61. Ballinger SW, Van Houten B, Jin GF, et al. Hydrogen peroxide causes significant mitochondrial DNA damage in human RPE cells. *Exp Eye Res.* 1999;68:765–772.

62. Soong NW, Hinton DR, Cortopassi G, et al. Mosaicism for a specific somatic mitochondrial DNA mutation in adult human brain. *Nat Genet.* 1992;2:318–323.

63. Wallace DC. Mitochondrial DNA sequence variation in human evolution and disease. *Proc Natl Acad Sci USA.* 1994;91:8,739–8,746.

64. Barreau E, Brossas JY, Courtois Y, et al. Accumulation of mitochondrial DNA deletions in human retina during aging. *Invest Ophthalmol Vis Sci.* 1996;37:384–391.

65. Khaidakov M, Heflich RH, Manjanatha MG, et al. Accumulation of point mutations in mitochondrial DNA of aging mice. *Mutat Res.* 2003;526:1–7.

66. Suter M, Reme C, Grimm C, et al. Age-related macular degeneration. The lipofuscin component N-retinyl-N-retinylidene ethanolamine detaches proapoptotic proteins from mitochondria and induces apoptosis in mammalian retinal pigment epithelial cells. *J Biol Chem.* 2000;275:39,625–39,630.

67. Hammond BR Jr., Wooten BR, Snodderly DM. Preservation of visual sensitivity of older subjects: association with macular pigment density. *Invest Ophthalmol Vis Sci.* 1998;39:397–406.

68. Goldberg J, Flowerdew G, Smith E, et al. Factors associated with age-related macular degeneration. An analysis of data from the first National Health and Nutrition Examination Survey. *Am J Epidemiol.* 1988;128:700–710.

69. The age-related eye disease study: a clinical trial of zinc and antioxidants-age-related eye disease study report no. 2. *J Nutr.* 2000;130:1,516S–1,519S.

70. A randomized, placebo-controlled, clinical trial of high-dose supplementation with vitamins C and E, beta carotene, and zinc for age-related macular degeneration and vision loss: AREDS report no. 8. *Arch Ophthalmol.* 2001; 119:1,417–1,436.

71. West S, Vitale S, Hallfrisch J, et al. Are antioxidants or supplements protective for age-related macular degeneration? *Arch Ophthalmol.* 1994;112: 222–227.

72. Organisciak DT, Wang HM, Li ZY, et al. The protective effect of ascorbate in retinal light damage of rats. *Invest Ophthalmol Vis Sci.* 1985;26: 1,580–1,588.

73. Ham WT Jr., Mueller HA, Ruffolo JJ Jr., et al. Basic mechanisms underlying the production of photochemical lesions in the mammalian retina. *Curr Eye Res.* 1984;3:165–174.

74. Tso MO, Woodford BJ, Lam KW. Distribution of ascorbate in normal primate retina and after photic injury: a biochemical, morphological correlated study. *Curr Eye Res.* 1984;3:181–191.

75. Katz ML, Parker KR, Handelman GJ, et al. Effects of antioxidant nutrient deficiency on the retina and retinal pigment epithelium of albino rats: a light and electron microscopic study. *Exp Eye Res.* 1982;34:339–369.

76. Varma SD, Chand D, Sharma YR, et al. Oxidative stress on lens and cataract formation: role of light and oxygen. *Curr Eye Res.* 1984;3:35–57.

77. Organisciak DT, Wang HM, Kou AL. Ascorbate and glutathione levels in the developing normal and dystrophic rat retina: effect of intense light exposure. *Curr Eye Res.* 1984;3:257–267.

78. Castillo M, Bellot JL, Garcia-Cabanes C, et al. Effects of hypoxia on retinal pigmented epithelium cells: protection by antioxidants. *Ophthalmic Res.* 2002;34:338–342.

79. Lai YL, Fong D, Lam KW, et al. Distribution of ascorbate in the retina, subretinal fluid and pigment epithelium. *Curr Eye Res.* 1986;5:933–938.

80. Khatami M, Stramm LE, Rockey JH. Ascorbate transport in cultured cat retinal pigment epithelial cells. *Exp Eye Res.* 1986;43:607–615.

81. DiMattio J, Streitman J. Active transport of ascorbic acid across the retinal pigment epithelium of the bullfrog. *Curr Eye Res.* 1991;10:959–965.

82. Khatami M. Na+-linked active transport of ascorbate into cultured bovine retinal pigment epithelial cells: heterologous inhibition by glucose. *Membr Biochem.* 1987;7:115–130.

83. Blanks JC, Pickford MS, Organisciak DT, Ascorbate treatment prevents accumulation of phagosomes in RPE in light damage. *Invest Ophthalmol Vis Sci.* 1992;33:2,814–2,821.

84. Seddon JM, Ajani UA, Sperduto RD, et al. Dietary carotenoids, vitamins A, C, and E, and advanced age-related macular degeneration. *Eye Disease Case-Control Study Group. Jama.* 1994;272:1,413–1,420.

85. Evstigneeva RP, Volkov IM, Chudinova VV. Vitamin E as a universal antioxidant and stabilizer of biological membranes. *Membr Cell Biol.*1998;12:151–172.

86. Organisciak DT, Berman ER, Wang HM, et al. Vitamin E in human neural retina and retinal pigment epithelium: effect of age. *Curr Eye Res.* 1987;6: 1,051–1,055.

87. Farnsworth CC, Dratz EA. Oxidative damage of retinal rod outer segment membranes and the role of vitamin E. *Biochim Biophys Acta.* 1976;443: 556–570.

88. Ueda T, Armstrong D. Preventive effect of natural and synthetic antioxidants on lipid peroxidation in the mammalian eye. *Ophthalmic Res.* 1996;28: 184–192.

89. Taylor HR, Tikellis G, Robman LD, et al. Vitamin E supplementation and macular degeneration: randomised controlled trial. *Bmj.* 2002;325:11.

90. Bone RA, Landrum JT, Tarsis SL. Preliminary identification of the human macular pigment. *Vision Res.* 1985;25:1,531–1,535.

91. Bone RA, Landrum JT, Fernandez L, et al. Analysis of the macular pigment by HPLC: retinal distribution and age study. *Invest Ophthalmol Vis Sci.* 1988;29:843–849.

92. Handelman GJ, Dratz EA, Reay CC, et al. Carotenoids in the human macula and whole retina. *Invest Ophthalmol Vis Sci.* 1988;29:850–855.

93. Handelman GJ, Snodderly DM, Adler AJ, et al. Measurement of carotenoids in human and monkey retinas. *Methods Enzymol.* 1992;213:220–230.

94. Antioxidant status and neovascular age-related macular degeneration. Eye Disease Case-Control Study Group. *Arch Ophthalmol.* 1993;111:104–109.

95. Buettner GR. The pecking order of free radicals and antioxidants: lipid peroxidation, alpha-tocopherol, and ascorbate. *Arch Biochem Biophys.* 1993;300:535–543.

96. Nelson KC, Armstrong JS, Moriarty S, et al. Protection of retinal pigment epithelial cells from oxidative damage by oltipraz, a cancer chemopreventive agent. *Invest Ophthalmol Vis Sci.* 2002;43:3,550–3,554.

97. Nelson KC, Carlson JL, Newman ML, et al. Effect of dietary inducer dimethylfumarate on glutathione in cultured human retinal pigment epithelial cells. *Invest Ophthalmol Vis Sci.* 1999;40:1,927–1,935.

98. Gao X, Dinkova-Kostova AT, Talalay P. Powerful and prolonged protection of human retinal pigment epithelial cells, keratinocytes, and mouse leukemia cells against oxidative damage: the indirect antioxidant effects of sulforaphane. *Proc Natl Acad Sci USA.* 2001;98:15,221–15,226.

Laser Photocoagulation of Eyes with Soft Drusen

Marta S. Figueroa   *Thomas R. Friberg*

Age-related macular degeneration (AMD) is the leading cause of blindness in developed countries among patients older than 60 years of age (1–3). The wet, or exudative, form is typically secondary to the growth of new vessels from the choroidal and accounts for about 12% of the cases. However, this form is responsible for the vast majority of visual loss, with 80% of patients with wet AMD having visual acuities equal to or worse than 20/200 (3–6).

While therapeutic approaches to the advanced stages of AMD are becoming more numerous, none to date reliably improves visual acuity after it has decreased. Hence, an effective prophylactic treatment that alters the natural course of AMD would be invaluable as it could prevent blindness in tens of thousands of patients.

Histological studies have shown that the growth of new vessels from the choroid occurs mainly within areas of large, confluent drusen (7–9). Similarly, several clinical studies have shown that certain characteristics of soft drusen are associated with a higher risk of neovascularization. These factors include a drusen size greater than 100 μm, a confluence of drusen, location in the fovea, and an association with focal hyperpigmentation (Fig. 15.1) (10,11). The risk of progression to the exudative form of AMD also depends on the condition of the fellow eye. It is estimated that the risk of developing wet AMD within 3 years is between 13% and 18% for those with soft bilateral drusen (12,13). The presence of a choroidal neovascular membrane in one eye increases the risk of developing wet AMD by nearly 60% in the fellow eye within 5 years (10).

If soft drusen could be made to disappear, the risk of evolution towards the exudative form of AMD and the atrophic form of AMD might be reduced. In addition, drusen resorption could possibly prevent secondary atrophy of the overlying retinal pigment epithelium (RPE), thus averting the atrophy of the overlying photoreceptors and underlying choriocapillaries.

PHOTOCOAGULATION OF DRUSEN

In 1973, Gass reported the disappearance of drusen adjacent to laser spots when studying the efficacy of photocoagulation on RPE detachment in AMD (14). Since this finding was made, several authors have attempted to not only confirm this result, but also to identify the most suitable photocoagulation parameters and techniques to produce this effect. Several clinical trials were conducted using various laser types including the blue-green argon laser wavelength, green argon (15–28), krypton (27,28), and yellow dye laser (29). In addition, attempts to minimize tissue damage led to the use of threshold and subthreshold 810 nm diode laser lesions for the same purpose (30).

There have been two primary approaches to photocoagulation of eyes with drusen. The first is the application of the laser to the drusen themselves, which is known as the *direct* technique. Photocoagulation of the retina adjacent to the drusen, the *indirect* technique, has also been used. Proponents of the first technique suggest that the energy of the laser is partially absorbed by the drusen, thus reducing the collateral effects on adjacent structures. This attenuating effect would explain why laser-induced scars are practically invisible, their location and size only determinable by fluorescein

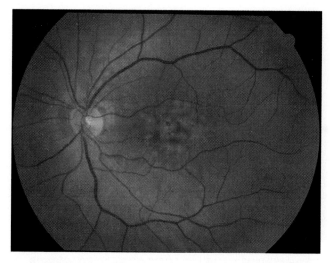

Figure 15.1   Soft confluent drusen with focal hyperpigmentation.

angiography (15–18,21–23,27,28,31). Advocates of indirect treatment favor photocoagulation in a grid pattern using either annular or horseshoe patterns (15,19,20,24,25, 29,30). Two findings have lent support to this technique: first, the discovery of new vessels in large soft drusen (7–9), which should be avoided by the laser; secondly, the fact that direct photocoagulation results in the disappearance over time not only of the treated drusen, but also those located far from laser scars (16). Moreover, treating the drusen-free retina allows for application of the laser far from the center of the foveal vascular zone, which is particularly useful when dealing with large drusen or drusenoid RPE detachments at less than 750 μm from the foveal center (Fig. 15.2). Keeping laser spots at a distance from the fovea prevents the visual loss that might result from late enlargement of laser scars through mechanisms such as apoptosis. Similarly, if choroidal neovascular membranes appear as a complication of the laser treatment itself, the vessels can be treated with less risk of secondary visual loss than if the fovea were involved.

The characteristics of the different spot sizes, application duration, and intensities of laser treatment have been quite similar in all studies. Laser spot sizes are typically between 100 and 200 μm for 0.05 to 0.2 seconds, with power settings low enough to create only a slight change of color in the retina immediately after application. Subthreshold treatment is even more mild, with no color change noted upon treatment (30). To prevent extension of laser scars affecting the fovea, a minimum distance of 500 μm from the center of the foveal vascular zone should be maintained during laser treatment (27). Some authors have suggested that this distance should be as much as 750 μm (24).

RESULTS OF PHOTOCOAGULATION TO EYES WITH DRUSEN

Laser photocoagulation leads not only to disappearance of treated drusen, but also of drusen located far from laser scars. This disappearance progresses outward from treated areas to untreated ones. When the laser is applied only in the temporal half of the retina, this progression becomes quite evident, as temporal drusen disappear first, then the subfoveal ones and finally those in the nasal quadrants of the macula (Figs. 15.3, 15.4) (16,17). In one study, the last drusen to disappear were those located in the superonasal part of the macula, though the cause of this finding is not clear (17).

One of the advantages of treating only the temporal half of the macular is the lower number of spots necessary, which reduces the risk of treatment-related complications. However, some authors have reported the reappearance of drusen in areas where laser treatment was not applied, despite initial disappearance. In our experience, the reappearance of drusen can occur either in treated areas or in areas located far from the laser application. The pattern of drusen reappearance was annular in many such cases and it occurred several years after photocoagulation (Fig. 15.5).

While different types of laser treatment lead to disappearance of drusen, green argon laser produces this effect in the shortest time. Disappearance of treated drusen has been reported after 3 months, while disappearance of those located far from laser scars after 10 months (16–18,32). In contrast, the 810 nm diode laser has been embraced by some authors because its penetration of the sensory retina to the retinal pigment epithelium and choroid allows for easier titration and placement of mild lesions. Application of diode laser also shows differences when comparing visible and sub-threshold modes. Time of disappearance of 50% of drusen area is prolonged when treatment is performed in a non-visible or sub-threshold mode, compared to the threshold mode (18 versus 12 months) (30).

Many hypotheses have been advanced to explain the disappearance of drusen following photocoagulation. Several different processes could play a role, including a

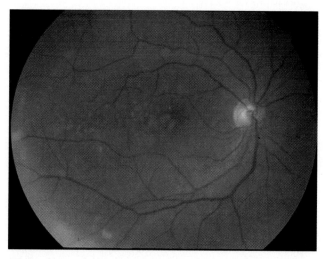

Figure 15.2   Laser spots applied far from the drusen in the center of the foveal vascular zone.

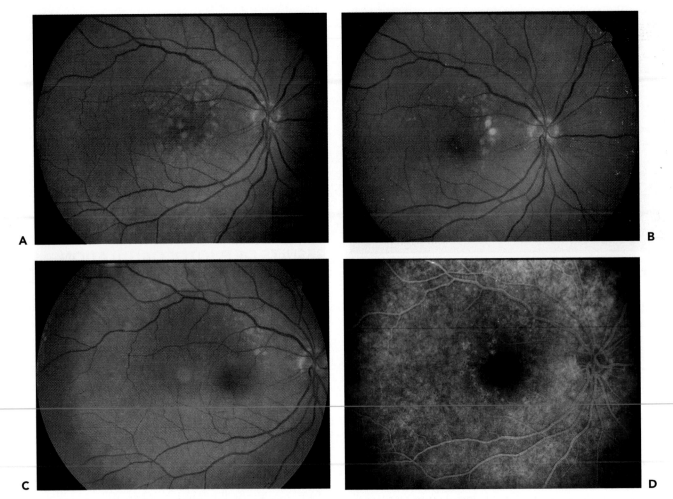

Figure 15.3 **A.** Preoperative appearance. **B.** Seven months after treatment: both treated and subfoveal drusen have disappeared. **C.** Fundus 1 year after photocoagulation. **D.** Fluorescein angiography showing laser spots that are not visible in the color photograph.

reduction in the inflow of debris that eventually develops into drusen and an increase in the outflow of debris from the drusen themselves.

Decreased deposition of debris could occur by the destruction of aged RPE cells and their replacement by newer healthier cells. Aged RPE cells may be responsible for the recycling of receptor waste products, which then accumulate under the basal membrane of the RPE in the form of drusen. New, healthy cells presumably have a normal enzymatic function, which may decrease debris deposition in the region.

There are several possible arguments for the greater outflow of debris from the drusen after photocoagulation. The following are some of the most important ones:

1. Following photocoagulation, new and healthier RPE cells with increased phagocytic capacity grow from the margins of scars.
2. The arrival of cells with phagocytic capacity follows photocoagulation. Histological studies in monkeys have shown that photocoagulation can lead to the disappearance of drusen owing to the action of cells with

phagocytic capacity that were identified as choriocapillary pericytes (33). Other studies have also reported the phagocytic capacity of the endothelial cells from the choriocapillaries (19).

3. An increase in the transport capacity through Bruch's membrane. Sigelman (23) postulated that laser scars might aid the drainage of debris by reducing resistance to outflow through an abnormally thick Bruch's membrane. This effect may be secondary to a laser-induced modification in the characteristics of lipids in Bruch's membrane. Little (21), in contrast, attributed this lowered resistance to the opening of small pores caused by the contraction of elastic and collagen fibers in the membrane.

If the disappearance of drusen re-establishes a more normal macular architecture, we can speculate on how this could lead to a reduced risk of progression to the exudative form of AMD. One possible explanation for the reduction of this risk would be that drusen disappearance leads to reattachment of the RPE basal membrane to the rest of Bruch's membrane, thereby causing the disappearance of

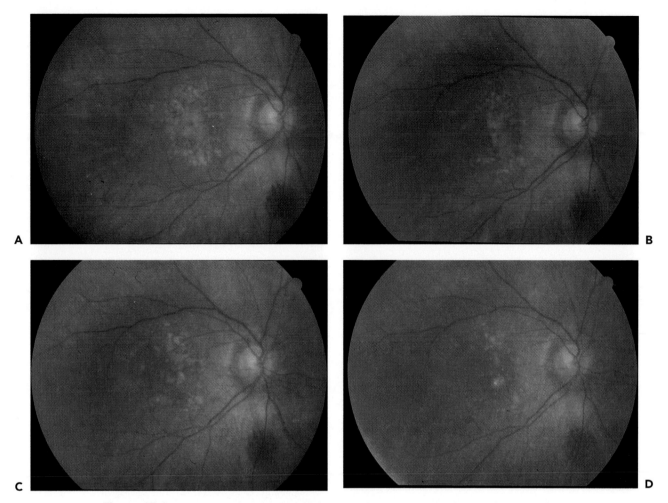

Figure 15.4 **A.** Preoperative. **B.** Treated drusen in the temporal macula have disappeared. **C.** Disappearance of subfoveal drusen. **D.** One year after treatment, nasal drusen persist.

the cleavage plane produced by the drusen. This may help prevent the extension of a pre-existing membrane or even the involution of small new vessels that underlie drusen (9). Also, the reduction of this metabolic debris between the external retina and the choroid may lower the angiogenic stimulus.

Whatever the mechanisms are, no large randomized controlled studies to date have shown that the disappearance of drusen is clearly associated with a lower incidence of choroidal neovascular membranes. Figueroa and colleagues, as well as many others, were unable to find a statistically significant difference between treated and untreated eyes, even though the average follow-up was 7 years (15,17,21,24, 28,29,33). Indeed, only one randomized prospective study has shown a beneficial effect, but it was small in scope, as it compared the results in 17 treated patients to 19 untreated controls (31). None of the treated patients developed new vessels following an average follow-up of 2.5 years, compared to 5 of the controls ($P = 0.03$). The laser parameters used were not substantially different than those used in other studies: 200 µm, 0.05 seconds at low intensity; application of the laser both on and between drusen; and an average of 100 spots per eye.

In contrast, to date three studies have reported a negative impact of laser treatment when comparing treated and untreated eyes (25,26,34). In these multicenter group studies, two groups of patients were followed over time: one with bilateral soft drusen in which one eye was treated and the other used as a control; and a second group with high-risk drusen in one eye and a choroidal neovascular membrane in the fellow eye (which was randomized to treatment or observation). The highest incidence of membranes among treated eyes was found in the group of patients with membranes in the fellow eye, that is, in the high-risk group. At 12 months, the incidence was approximately five-times higher in treated eyes than in observed eyes (23% vs. 5%). However, by month 30 the cumulative incidence was nearly the same in treated and observed eyes (33% vs. 32%). The parameters used were generally similar to those of other studies, with the number of laser spots per eye ranging from 20 to 24. Differences included the use of higher energy settings and retreatment guidelines.

In a study presented at the 2003 American Academy of Ophthalmology meeting, patients who had multiple drusen in one eye and a disciform process in the other were randomized to treatment using the 810 nm diode laser.

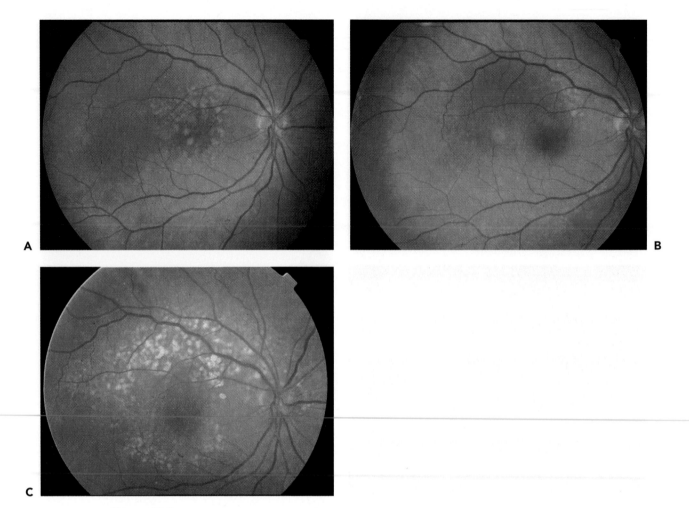

Figure 15.5 **A.** Preoperative. **B.** Fundus following drusen disappearance. **C.** Drusen reappeared in an annular pattern 10 years after photocoagulation.

Treatment consisted of a one-time grid placement of 48 spots, 125 μm in diameter, avoiding the fovea. The intensity of the laser lesions was so mild that the lesions could not be seen directly after placement. The rate of choroidal neovascularization in treated eyes consistently exceeded the rate in observed eyes, and at 18 months were 18% in treated eyes versus 10% in observed eyes (p < 0.05).

The available data do not support laser treatment of soft drusen for preventing exudative AMD. On the contrary, the larger studies argue strongly against laser application in the fellow eyes of patients who already have choroidal neovascularization in the fellow eye. Results for bilaterally eligible patients in these two trials have not been released.

Can evolution toward the atrophic form of AMD be prevented? It may be assumed that if laser-induced drusen disappearance occurs before the atrophy of the overlying RPE, we might possibly prevent progression to the atrophic form of the disease. Unfortunately, no studies have yet shown that prophylactic treatment is beneficial for the atrophic form of the disease.

Visual results following laser-induced disappearance of drusen are somewhat more encouraging than prevention of choroidal neovascularization. Improvements in vision

of 30% to 40% have been reported in treated eyes (16–18, 20–24). Though improvements are generally small—no more than two lines in visual acuity—several studies have found statistically significant differences in visual acuity between treated eyes and the control group (21,24,29,35). Visual improvements usually occur in eyes with large drusen located in the center of the fovea. These drusen can form drusenoid-like detachments of the RPE, which may flatten out after photocoagulation. Another possibility is that the disappearance of drusen is accompanied by an improvement in hydraulic conductivity through Bruch's membrane, facilitating the exchange of nutrients between the RPE and the choriocapillaries, thereby improving retinal function.

However, the Drusen Laser Study has recently reported a higher incidence of visual acuity loss in the treatment group than in the control group (33).

TREATMENT-RELATED COMPLICATIONS

The most common complication when applying laser treatment in the macular area is the radial expansion of

RPE atrophy from the laser lesions. Unlike the photocoagulation advocated for pathologies such as diabetes, the technique used for drusen treatment produces minimal lesions that are practically undetectable without fluorescein angiography. These thinning spots on the RPE can be seen in fluorescein angiography as hyperfluorescent areas in the early stages of the angiogram, with no late leakage.

Other complications that have been described following photocoagulation are subretinal fibrosis (36,37), choroidal neovascular membranes (38), accidental burns to the fovea, choroidal and retinal bleeding, venous retinal occlusion, and preretinal macular membranes. Visual deterioration has also been reported secondary to the deposit of an orange-colored hyperfluorescent material in the subfoveal area following photocoagulation of drusen. The nature and origin of this pigment remains unknown (39).

In addition to these complications, photocoagulation of soft drusen involves laser treatment of eyes already at high risk for the development of exudative AMD. Indeed, the pigmentary changes often observed in association with this type of drusen suggest macrophage movement below Bruch's membrane, and this is associated with an activation of the underlying choroidal capillaries. Owing to the inflammatory reaction it provokes, photocoagulation may speed up this cellular response and induce the release of angiogenic factors. In this way, the laser may strengthen the angiogenic stimulus already present in these high-risk eyes.

In most studies, the application of laser to or around the drusen is usually performed after fluorescein angiography has confirmed the absence of choroidal neovascularization. Nevertheless, some studies with indocyanine green angiography have shown that among patients with membranes, up to 10% of fellow eyes with soft drusen and a normal fluorescein angiography show exudative changes (40). Far from stabilizing the disease, using photocoagulation on these eyes might exacerbate the AMD. Thus, some advocate initial angiography with indocyanine green to avoid treating eyes containing an exudative component (41).

Considering the lack of clear efficacy, laser photocoagulation of soft drusen should be considered a treatment under investigation as of this writing. Despite disappearance of drusen, laser photocoagulation has so far yielded no distinct benefits in terms of AMD progression. Longer follow-up times may show that early treatment is capable of reducing the incidence of the atrophic form.

At present, two fully enrolled, major multicenter studies are following patients with drusen in both eyes, of which one eye has been treated. The Complication of AMD Prevention Trial (CAPT) is following randomized patients with soft bilateral drusen that were treated with green argon laser. In contrast, in the bilateral arm of the Prophylactic Treatment of Age-Related Macular Degeneration study, a subthreshold 810 nm diode laser was used as a one-time prophylactic treatment for non-exudative AMD. These studies may add new data to what has been described and analyzed in this brief overview.

Therefore, the only treatment yet proven to ameliorate the development of choroidal neovascularization and visual loss in patients with dry AMD is the use of specific nutritional supplements (42).

REFERENCES

1. Banks CN, Hutton WK. Blindness in New South Wales: an estimate of the prevalence and some of the contributing causes. *Aust J Ophthalmol.* 1982;9:285.
2. Khan HA, Moorhead HB. Statistics on blindness in the model reporting areas, 1969–1970. Department of Health, Education and Welfare publication #73-427. Washington DC: *United States Government Printing Office*; 1973.
3. Leibowwitz H, Krueger DE, Maunder LR, et al. The Framingham Eye Study Monograph; an ophthalmological and epidemiological study of cataract, glaucoma, diabetic retinopathy, macular degeneration and visual acuity in a general population of 2631 adults. *Surv Ophthalmol.* 1980; 24:335–610.
4. Ferris FL III, Fine SL, Hyman LA. Age-related macular degeneration and blindness due to neovascular maculopathy. *Arch Ophthalmol.* 1984;102:1,640–1,642.
5. Hyman LG, Lilienfeld AM, Ferris FL III, Fine SL. Senile macular degeneration: a case control study. *Am J Epidemiol.* 1983;118:213–227.
6. Klein BE, Klein R. Cataracts and macular degeneration in older Americans. *Arch Ophthalmol.* 1982;100:571–576.
7. Green WR, Key SN. Senile macular degeneration: a histopathologic study. *Trans Am Ophthalmol Soc.* 1977;75:180–254.
8. Green WR, McDonnell PH, Yeo JH. Pathologic features of senile macular degeneration. *Ophthalmology.* 1985;92:615–627.
9. Sarks SH. Drusen and their relationship to senile macular degeneration. *Aust J Ophthalmol.* 1980;8:117–130.
10. Bressler SB, Maguire MG, Bressler NM, et al. Relationship of drusen and abnormalities of the retinal pigment epithelium to the prognosis of neovascular macular degeneration: the Macular Photocoagulation Study Group. *Arch Ophthalmol.* 1990;108:1,442–1,447.
11. Bressler NM, Bressler SB, Seddon JM, et al. Drusen characteristics in patients with exudative versus non-exudative age-related macular degeneration. *Retina.* 1998;8:109–114.
12. Holz FG, Wolfensberger TJ, Piguer B, et al. Bilateral macular drusen in age-related macular degeneration: prognosis and risk factors. *Ophthalmology.* 1994;101:1,522–1,528.
13. Smiddy WE, Fine SL. Prognosis of patients with bilateral macular drusen. *Ophthalmology.* 1984;92:271–276.
14. Gass JDM. Drusen and disciform macular detachment and degeneration. *Arch Ophthalmol.* 1973:206–217.
15. Cleasby GW, Nakanishi AS, Norris JL. Prophylactic photocoagulation of the fellow eye in exudative senile maculopathy: a preliminary report. *Mod Probl Ophthalmol.* 1979:141–147.
16. Figueroa MS, Regueras A, Bertrand J. Laser photocoagulation to treat macular soft drusen in age-related macular degeneration. *Retina.* 1994:391–396.
17. Figueroa MS, Regueras A, Bertrand J, et al. Laser photocoagulation for macular soft drusen: up-dated results. *Retina.* 1997;17:378–384.
18. Frennesson JC, Nilsson Seg. Laser photocoagulation of soft drusen in early age-related maculopathy (ARM). The one year results of the prospective randomized trial. *Eu J Ophthalmol.* 1996.
19. Guymer RH, Gross-Jendroska M, Owens SL, et al. Laser treatment in subjects with high-risk clinical features of age-related macular degeneration. *Ach Ophthalmol.* 1997;115:595–603.
20. Haut J, Renard Y, Kraiem S. Traitement prophylactique per laser de la DMLA de l'oeil adelphe après DMLA du premier oeil. *J Fr Ophthalmol.* 1991;14:473–476.
21. Little H, Showman JM, Brown BW. A pilot randomized controlled study on the effect of laser photocoagulation of confluent soft macular drusen. *Ophthalmology.* 1997;104:623–631.
22. Ruiz JM, Alió JL. Tratamiento de la maculopatía por drusas blandas con fotocoagulación directa perifoveal. *Arch Soc Esp Oftalmol.* 1995;68:73–78.
23. Sigelman J. Foveal drusen resorption one year after perifoveal laser photocoagulation. *Ophthalmology.* 1991;98:1,379–1,383.
24. Sarks SH, Arnold JJ, Sarks JP, et al. Prophylactic perifoveal laser treatment of soft drusen. *Aust N Zealand J Ophthalmol.* 1996;24(1):15–26.
25. The Choroidal Neovascularization Prevention Trial Research Group. Laser treatment in eyes with large drusen. *Ophthalmology.* 1998;105:11–23.
26. The Choroidal Neovascularization Prevention Trial Research Group. Choroidal neovascularization in the Choroidal Neovascularization Prevention Trial. *Ophthalmology.* 1998;105:1,364–1,372.
27. Wetzig PC. Treatment of drusen-related aging macular degeneration by photocoagulation. *Trans Am Ophthalmol Soc.* 1988:299–306.
28. Wetzig PC. Photocoagulation of drusen-related macular degeneration: a long-term outcome. *Trans Am Ophthalmol Soc.* 1994:299–306.
29. Bressler SB, Vitale J, Hawtons BS. Laser to drusen trial an assessment of short term safety within a randomized prospective, controlled clinical trial. *Invest Ophthalmol Vis Sci.* 1995;36:1,028.
30. Olk Jr, Friberg TR, Stickney KL, et al. Therapeutic benefits of infrared (810 nm) diode laser macular grid photocoagulation in prophylactic treatment of

nonexudative age-related macular degeneration. *Ophthalmology.* 1999;106: 2,082–2,090.

31. Frennesson C, Nilsson Seg. Significant decrease in exudative complications after prophylactic laser treatment of soft drusen maculopathy in a randomized study. *Invest Ophthalmol Vis Sci.* 1997;38:18.

32. Duvall J, Tso MOM. Cellular mechanisms of resolution of drusen after laser photocoagulation: an experimental study. *Arch Ophthalmol.* 1985;103: 694–703.

33. Owens SL, Bunce C, Branon AJ, et al. Drusen Laser Study Group. Prophylactic laser treatment appears to promote choroidal neovascularization in high-risk ARM: results of an interim analysis. *Eye.* 2003;17:623–627.

34. The Choroidal Neovascularization Prevention Trial Research Group. Laser treatment in fellow eyes with large drusen: updated findings from a pilot randomized clinical trial. *Ophthalmology.* 2003;110:971–978.

35. Ho A, Maguire M, Yoken J, et al. Laser-induced drusen reduction improves visual function at 1 year. *Ophthalmology.* 1999;106:1,367–1,373.

36. Guyer Dr, D'Amico DJ, Smith CW. Subretinal fibrosis after laser photocoagulation for diabetic macular edema. *Am J Ophthalmol.* 1992;113:652–656.

37. Han DP, Meiler WF, Burton TC. Submacular fibrosis after photocoagulation for diabetic macular edema. *Am J Ophthalmol.* 1992;113:513–521.

38. Lewis H, Schachat AP, Haimann MH, et al. Choroidal neovascularization after laser photocoagulation for diabetic macular edema. *Ophthalmology.* 1990;97:503–511.

39. Hyver SW, Schatz H, McDonald HR, et al. A case of visual acuity loss following laser photocoagulation for macular drusen. *Arch Ophthalmol.* 1997; 115:554.

40. Guyer Dr, Hanutsaha P, Yannuzzi La, et al. Indocyanine green video angiography of drusen as a possible predictive indicator of exudative maculopathy. *Invest Ophthalmol Vis Sci.* 1996;37:413.

41. Brancato R, Trabucchi G, Introini U. Hyperfluorescent plaque lesions in the late phases of indocyanine green angiography: a possible contraindication to the laser treatment of drusen. *Am J Ophthalmol.* 1997;124:554–557.

42. Age-Related Eye Disease Study Research Group. A randomized, placebo-controlled, clinical trial of high-dose supplementation with vitamins C and E and beta carotene for age-related cataract and vision loss: AREDS report no. 9. *Arch Ophthalmol.* 2001;119:1,439–1,452.

Choroidal Neovascularization and the Macular Photocoagulation Study

16

James M. Weisz   Stephen R. O'Connell

INTRODUCTION

The term choroidal neovascularization (CNV) refers to the ingrowth of fibrovascular tissue from the choroidal circulation into or underneath the retina. Choroidal neovascular lesions may occur whenever there is disruption of Bruch's membrane. Age-related macular degeneration (AMD) is the most common predisposing condition to the development of CNV; however, CNV lesions are also associated with other conditions, such as the ocular histoplasmosis syndrome, multifocal choroiditis, pathologic myopia, and choroidal rupture from trauma. Choroidal neovascular lesions typically progress to fibrovascular disciform scars, which, when located in the fovea, cause devastating and irreversible vision loss. Unfortunately, CNV lesions tend to either present subfoveally or grow posteriorly toward the fovea. In fact, while CNV occurs in only 8% of patients with AMD, it is responsible for 85% of the severe visual loss caused by AMD (1). The results of the Age Related Eye Disease Study (AREDS) have shown that high-dose supplements of β–carotene, vitamin C, vitamin E, and zinc can reduce the risk of advanced AMD complications, including CNV, in medium- and high-risk AMD by 25% (2). However, at this time, there is no known treatment that can reliably prevent the development of CNV. The investigations of the Macular Photocoagulation Study (MPS) Group, however, have demonstrated that laser photocoagulation can, in certain cases, favorably alter the natural history of CNV lesions. More recently, photodynamic therapy with verteporfin has been shown to reduce the risk of vision loss in selected subfoveal cases. This chapter will attempt to distill the published findings of the MPS and provide guidelines for thermal laser treatment of CNV lesions in light of recent findings on photodynamic therapy (PDT).

PATIENT EVALUATION

Choroidal neovascularization should be suspected in anyone complaining of metamorphopsia or scotoma, especially if they are over the age of 65 and are known to have non-neovascular AMD (3). When a patient presents with a CNV lesion, biomicroscopy may reveal retinal elevation from fluid, blood or lipid, retinal pigment epithelial (RPE) elevation from sub-RPE fluid, blood or fibrovascular tissue, intraretinal blood or lipid, or cystic edema of the neurosensory retina. Other causes of subretinal hemorrhage, such as macroaneurysms, choroidal rupture from trauma, lacquer cracks from pathologic myopia, or choroidal tumors, should be considered and ruled out. The fundus, however, may appear to be normal in spite of the presence of CNV, especially if the only sign present is subretinal fluid. A contact lens examination demonstrating an increased distance between the inner and outer aspect of a focused slit beam may be the only means to detect subretinal fluid or subtle retinal edema. When CNV is suspected, a fluorescein angiogram is needed to evaluate its presence, and it will determine if the patient fits treatment guidelines.

Evaluation with Intravenous Fluorescein Angiography

Choroidal neovascularization may have a variety of appearances on fluorescein angiography. The basic patterns currently recognized are termed classic and occult. Distinguishing between these two patterns is important because MPS and PDT treatment guidelines and prognosis depend upon their properly differentiating the two (4–7). Classic CNV is characterized by bright, well-demarcated areas of hyperfluorescence in the early (transit) phase, with significant leakage apparent in the later frames as the dye pools in the subretinal space and obscures the boundary of the hyperfluorescence (Fig. 16.1). The lacy vessels occasionally visualized in the early phase are the best known feature of classic CNV, but are not required for a

lesion to be considered classic. In fact, this appearance is more typically present in classic CNV lesions associated with OHS rather than AMD, and may also be seen in lesions judged by fluorescein pattern to be occult CNV.

Occult CNV refers to two types of hyperfluorescent patterns seen in eyes with CNV. The first pattern, termed a fibrovascular pigment epithelial detachment (FVPED), is characterized by irregular elevation of the RPE associated with stippled hyperfluorescent dots. It is best appreciated stereoscopically at approximately 1 to 2 minutes after dye injection (Fig. 16.2). Staining or leakage is evident in the late phase as fluorescein collects within the fibrous tissue or pools in the subretinal space overlying the FVPED. The exact boundary of an FVPED is often not well demarcated because the elevation slopes gradually down to normal RPE. Thus, the FVPED boundary determination is dependent upon the fluorescent outline of the elevated RPE, the quality of the stereo photograph, and the thickness of the fibrovascular tissue.

The second pattern of occult CNV, late leakage of an undetermined source (LLUS), refers to late choroidal leakage

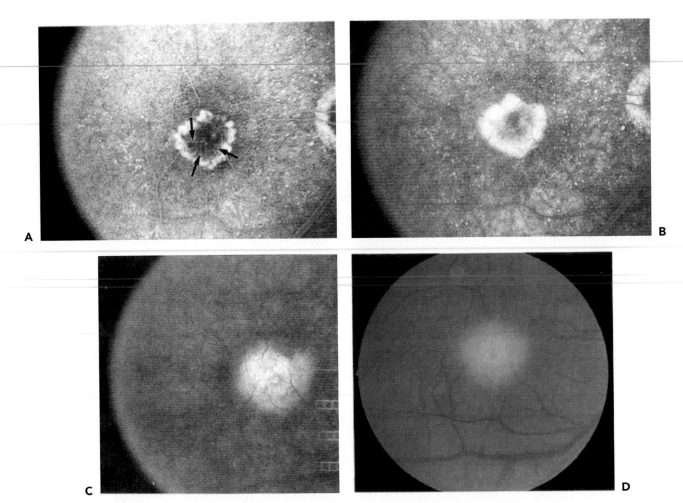

Figure 16.1 Classic choroidal neovascularization (CNV). **A.** Early phase of fluorescein angiogram shows early filling of CNV with central feeder vessels (*arrows*). **B.** Middle phase, 1 minute after fluorescein injection shows fluorescein leakage from CNV. **C.** Late phase of angiogram shows pooling of dye in subsensory retinal space, obscuring the boundaries demarcated in the early phase. **D.** Uniform whitening of retina 12 to 48 hours after laser photocoagulation of this classic CNV lesion. (Reprinted with permission of the American Medical Association from *Arch Ophthalmol*. 1991;109:1,242–1,257.)

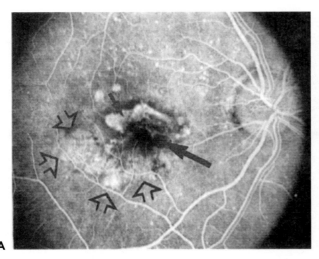
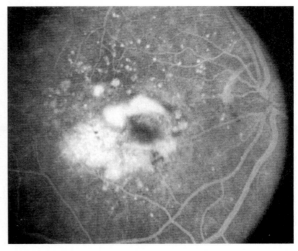

Figure 16.2 Classic choroidal neovascularization (CNV), laser scar, and occult CNV occurring as a fibrovascular pigment epithelial detachment (FVPED). **A.** Early phase of fluorescein angiogram shows an area of classic CNV (*small arrow*), scar from previous laser treatment (*large arrow*), and irregular elevation of the RPE with stippled hyperfluorescence (*open arrows*) representing a FVPED inferior and temporal to the scar. **B.** One minute after fluorescein injection, there is already leakage from the classic CNV component and increased intensity of the stippled hyperfluorescence from the FVPED component. (Reprinted with permission of the American Medical Association from *Arch Ophthalmol.* 1991;109:1,242–1,257.)

in which there is no clearly identifiable classic CNV or FVPED in the early or middle phase of the angiogram to account for an area of leakage in the late phase (Fig. 16.3). Often, this pattern of occult CNV can appear as speckled hyperfluorescence with pooling of dye in the subretinal space overlying the speckles. By definition, the boundaries of LLUS are not well demarcated, and a lesion with this component should not be considered for thermal laser treatment.

SUMMARIZED MPS RESULTS BY LESION LOCATION

Extrafoveal and Juxtafoveal CNV

The MPS studied the efficacy of laser treatment for CNV lesions found to be in an extrafoveal (defined as CNV with the posterior boundary >200 μm from the foveal center) or a juxtafoveal (defined as CNV with the posterior border 1 to 199 μm from the foveal center, or extrafoveal CNV with blood or blocked fluorescence within 200 μm of the foveal center) location.

The long-term (5-year) results of a randomized prospective trial designed to evaluate the effectiveness of laser for extrafoveal choroidal neovascularization was published in 1991 (5). It reported a statistically significant relative risk (RR = 1.5) of losing six or more lines of baseline level visual acuity among untreated eyes compared with laser treated eyes from 6 months through 5 years after entry (*P* = .001). Untreated eyes lost a mean of 7.1 lines of visual acuity, while laser treated eyes lost 5.2 lines. Unfortunately, persistent or recurrent CNV was observed in 54% of treated eyes, usually on the foveal (posterior) side of the treated lesion. Eyes with persistence or recurrence were associated with significant visual loss.

The 5-year results for juxtafoveal lesions in AMD were published in 1994 (6). They also demonstrated the benefit of laser photocoagulation over observation. The RR of losing six or more lines of visual acuity from baseline to any follow-up examination from 6 months through 5 years after enrollment was 1.2 (*P* = 0.04). The baseline level of visual acuity was maintained in 25% of the treated eyes, compared to 15% of the untreated eyes over the study period. In addition, more than twice as many treated patients as untreated patients retained visual acuity of 20/40 or better. Unfortunately, by the 5-year follow-up examination, 78% of those treated had either persistent or recurrent CNV involving the foveal center. Since retreatment may be beneficial with laser photocoagulation or PDT (see below), close follow-up is recommended to detect potentially treatable recurrences before significant growth has occurred. This will allow experts to provide retreatment that can be applied to as small an area as possible. Each visit within 1 to 2 years after treatment should include both contact lens biomicroscopy and fluorescein angiography to detect these recurrences at the earliest possible time. Biomicroscopy alone is probably inadequate to detect all recurrent CNV. In a prospective study comparing slit lamp examination alone to examination with fluorescein angiography, questionable or definite recurrence was seen in 12% of those cases considered inactive by biomicroscopy (7). Most of these cases had recurrences for which additional treatment was recommended and applied.

New Subfoveal CNV

The MPS reports have been important milestones in the therapy of CNV, especially with respect to subfoveal CNV, which is the most common presentation (8–12). Subfoveal

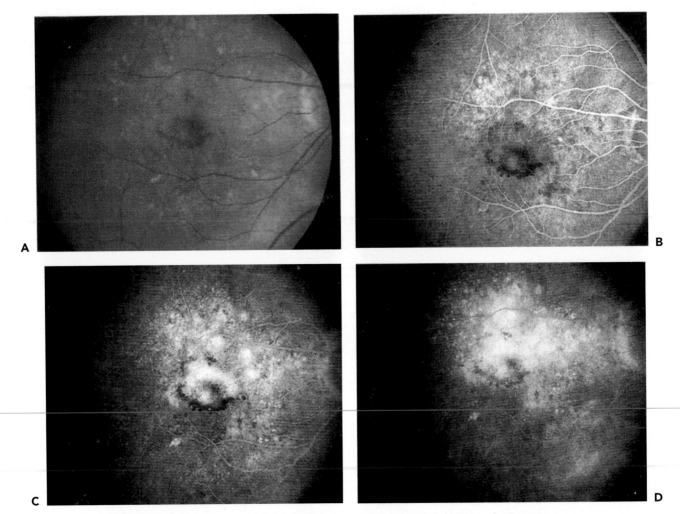

Figure 16.3 Occult choroidal neovascularization (CNV) causing late leakage of unknown source (LLUS). **A.** Subretinal hemorrhage, fluid, and drusen. **B.** Early phase of angiogram. **C.** Middle phase of angiogram shows pinpoint areas of speckled hyperfluorescence and larger areas of hyperfluorescence, with accumulation of fluorescein leakage in overlying sensory retinal space. **D.** In the late phase of the angiogram, there are additional areas of leakage whose source cannot be discerned from either the early (3a) or middle phase (3b). (Reprinted with permission of the American Medical Association from *Arch Ophthalmol.* 1991;109:1,242–1,257.)

lesions, even when small, make many ophthalmologists hesitant to use the destructive modality of laser photocoagulation because of the immediate reduction in visual acuity—although an untreated lesion may eventually cause even greater loss of vision. The MPS reports establish the benefits of treatment over observation for eligible lesions, and have provided a proven therapy for this debilitating disease.

The randomized prospective clinical trial for "new" subfoveal CNV (i.e. no prior laser photocoagulation) was initiated in 1986 (8). Eligible lesions were assigned randomly to photocoagulation or observation. The essential criteria to determine eligibility for the trial were as follows:

1. Classic CNV present as one component of the lesion, although occult CNV could be present as well.
2. Well-demarcated lesion boundaries, including the boundaries of any occult CNV, if present.

3. The size of the total lesion ≤3.5 MPS disc areas (Fig. 16.4).

The impact of treating these lesions with photocoagulation is given below; however, PDT with verteporfin may be considered for many of these lesions.

In the initial MPS report on treatment of new subfoveal lesions, laser-treated eyes on average retained better levels of visual acuity, reading speed, and contrast sensitivity compared to untreated eyes after 2 years of follow-up (8). An immediate decrease in vision, however, usually occurred in laser-treated patients, and on average photocoagulated eyes had worse visual acuity than untreated eyes during the first 3 to 6 months after treatment. The benefits of treatment were realized 1 to 2 years after treatment as vision continued to decline in the eyes randomized to observation. This did not occur in eyes randomized to laser treatment. Additional follow-up at 4 years continued to

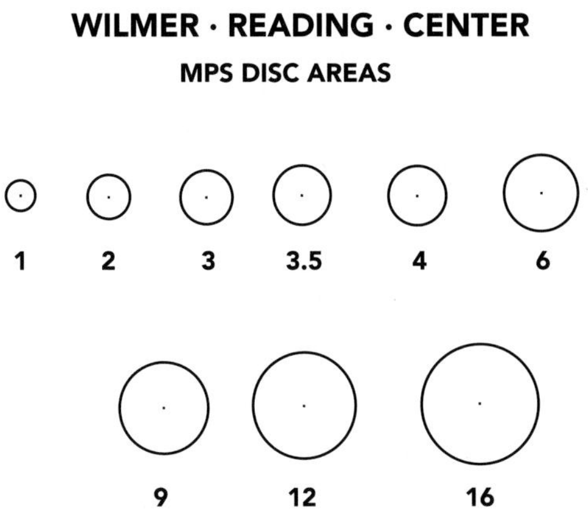

WILMER · READING · CENTER

MPS DISC AREAS

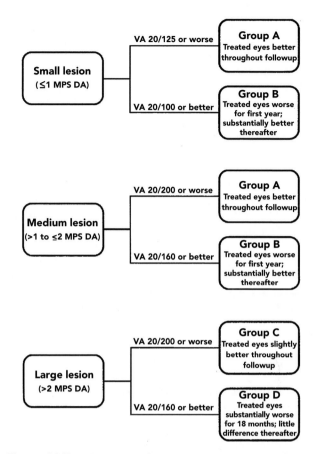

Figure 16.4 A drawing of a current MPS disc areas template (actual size not depicted here). One MPS disc area (D = 4.5 mm), 2 MPS disc areas (D = 6.4 mm), 3.5 MPS disc areas (D = 8.4 mm), 4 MPS disc areas (D = 9.0 mm), 6 MPS disc areas (D = 11.0 mm), 16 MPS disc areas (D = 18.0 mm), as measured in the case of this template on a 35-degree fundus photograph from a camera with a magnification factor of 2.5×. An average disc diameter of 1.5 mm is used to calculate the diameters of the various circles.

Figure 16.5 Schematic aid for determining the pattern of visual loss in eyes with new subfoveal choroidal neovascularization treated according to MPS criteria. DA, disc area; VA, visual acuity. (Reprinted with permission of the American Medical Association from *Arch Ophthalmol.* 1994;112:480–488.)

show this same trend, despite both treated and untreated eyes losing additional lines of visual acuity (11). At 4 years, the majority of treated eyes maintained visual acuity better than 20/400, compared to the untreated eyes with the majority having visual acuity of 20/400 or worse. Looking at the data from another perspective, 47% of 83 untreated eyes had lost six or more lines of visual acuity from baseline compared to 22% of 77 laser treated eyes ($P = 0.002$). Both reading speed and contrast sensitivity were found to be better in the treated group at 4 years.

Influence on Outcome of Initial Lesion Size and Visual Acuity

After the first reports, a subsequent analysis of all patients enrolled in the new subfoveal CNV study was performed with respect to subgroups divided by initial lesion size and visual acuity to identify characteristics that might influence the outcome (12). Overall, treatment benefit diminished with increasing size of the lesion and the average visual acuity loss was greatest for those eyes treated with relatively good visual acuity at baseline. Subgroups were analyzed according to three lesion sizes and three levels of initial visual acuity; four outcome patterns were recognized among the various groups (Fig. 16.5).

In the first pattern, (A), treated eyes fared better at every visit starting from 3 months and continuing throughout follow-up. These eyes, which have smaller lesions (less than one MPS disc area) and poorer acuities (20/200 or worse), appear to be excellent candidates for treatment and should be strongly considered accordingly at their initial presentation.

The second pattern, (B), includes treated eyes with lesions one to two disc areas in size and visual acuity of 20/160 or better, and lesions less than one MPS disc area in size and visual acuity of 20/100 or better. Pattern B eyes

fared worse than untreated eyes for the first year, then did substantially better thereafter and are thus good candidates for treatment as well. The immediate loss of visual acuity with treatment, however, may be unacceptable to the treating ophthalmologist or the patient in this group. If treatment for these lesions is not performed, it may be appropriate to recommend careful follow-up at short intervals (10 to 14 days). Should visual acuity fall or lesion size increase, treatment may be reconsidered.

The third pattern, (C), includes eyes with large lesions (>2.0 but <3.5 MPS disc areas) and visual acuity of 20/200 or worse. Pattern C treated eyes were only slightly better than untreated eyes throughout follow up. These eyes are still good candidates for treatment when one considers that from the 3-month visit to the end of the 4-year follow-up, the risk of further severe vision loss was lower with treatment.

The fourth pattern, (D), includes eyes with large lesions and visual acuity of 20/160 or better. Pattern D eyes were substantially worse with treatment for 18 months, demonstrating little difference thereafter. Throughout the 4-year follow-up, there was no appreciable treatment benefit. Thus, these eyes are poor treatment candidates. Nevertheless, they still should be followed closely for a few months because if visual acuity were to decline, they might be reclassified into a pattern C—for which treatment could be considered beneficial.

Though observation may be a viable option for all groups, the patient and the ophthalmologist should be aware that lesion size could change appreciably between follow-up examinations before the patient suffers visual acuity loss that's so significant that laser treatment is no longer a viable option and the opportunity to improve on the natural course is irretrievably lost. Should treatment be considered, the patient should understand that laser treatment would not restore vision. If the foveal center is involved with treatment, there likely will be an immediate reduction in vision—but that reduction would be less severe than it would if the disease were allowed to progress on its natural course. Patients should also know that further neovascular complications could and do occur frequently in spite of treatment. Some patients, even if they might have a pattern A lesion, may be poor candidates for laser photocoagulation if they cannot accept or understand these facts.

Recurrent Subfoveal Choroidal Neovascularization

In more than half of laser-treated patients with extrafoveal and juxtafoveal CNV, persistence or recurrence of neovascularization occurs within 2 years following initial treatment (13–15). Areas of persistent and recurrent CNV usually involve the foveal center and are associated with severe vision loss when compared to eyes that do not have persistence or recurrence.

Persistent CNV is defined in the MPS as active fluorescein leakage at the border of treatment within 6 weeks of initial treatment. The development of persistent leakage *within* the border of a laser-treated area (leakage that does not extend beyond the confines of the laser-treated area even in the later phase frames) has been called central leakage. It is not associated with subsequent extension of the CNV beyond the treated area. Compared to eyes that do not have evidence of central leakage within 6 weeks of treatment, eyes with this change are no more likely to go on to develop subsequent vision loss.

Recurrent CNV is defined as new fluorescein leakage after 6 week in an eye that was previously documented to have inactive treatment borders by 6 weeks after treatment. Because recurrence and persistence after initial treatment of extrafoveal and juxtafoveal CNV lesions has dire consequences, a companion trial to the *new* subfoveal lesion study, the *recurrent* subfoveal lesion study, was also begun in 1986 (9). The principal eligibility criteria were similar to the new trial with the following additional considerations:

1. No prior laser treatment to the center of the foveal avascular zone.
2. Involvement of the geometric center of the fovea by the recurrent CNV.

3. Total size of the recurrent neovascular lesion and prior treatment area not to exceed 6 disc areas—with some area of uninvolved retina within 1 disc diameter of the foveal center—if treatment were to be applied per protocol to the entire lesion.

The mean visual acuity of the laser-treated eyes in the recurrent study at 3 years after enrollment was 20/250, one line better than the mean of 20/200 in the untreated eyes (9). More than twice as many treated eyes, however, had a visual acuity better than 20/200 at the 3-year examination, and less than half as many treated eyes as untreated eyes had visual acuity of 20/400 or worse. Thus, treatment is recommended for lesions that meet the above criteria. Subgroup analysis of the recurrent trial showed that treatment was beneficial regardless of the initial visual acuity, in contrast to similar subgroup analysis for the "new" subfoveal trial.

Recurrent CNV also is seen frequently in eyes that have previously undergone subfoveal photocoagulation. Close to half of the eyes treated for subfoveal CNV have persistent or recurrent CNV within 3 years (14). In addition, a new independent area of CNV develops in 3% of treated eyes within 3 years. Subgroup analysis shows that the development of persistent, recurrent, or independent CNV in these patients has little additional deleterious effect on visual function. At 3 years, the visual acuity for subfoveally treated eyes without persistence or recurrence is 20/320. For treated eyes with persistence it is 20/400, and for treated eyes with recurrence it is 20/250. About half of the eyes in the "new" subfoveal study were eligible for retreatment using the above criteria (except that laser photocoagulation had already been applied to the foveal center). However, the number of eyes with recurrence following subfoveal laser that did or did not receive re-treatment, for which the recurrence did or did not include classic CNV with well-demarcated boundaries and size less than or equal to 6 MPS disc areas, is too small to draw conclusions regarding recommendations for retreatment. Nonetheless, if a recurrence following subfoveal laser treatment has classic CNV, well-demarcated boundaries, and a total size less than or equal to six MPS disc areas, retreatment should be considered.

TREATMENT GUIDELINES

By MPS criteria, all fluorescein angiograms used to guide treatment should be less than 96 hours old because CNV can grow rapidly over a period of days (4). The major component (>50%) of the lesion should be CNV (classic or occult) excluding any area of prior laser treatment scar. Consequently, a lesion that is >50% serous PED would not have met criteria for the MPS trials and the treatment benefits identified in these trials might not apply to such lesions. The entire boundary of the lesion to be treated should be well demarcated, and the lesion should contain at least some classic CNV. Photocoagulation is applied with a spot size of 200 to 500 μm for a duration of 0.2 to 0.5 seconds and with a power of between 200 to 500 mW. The border of the lesion starting on the foveal side is treated first with 200 μm burns, followed by overlapping 200 to 500 μm burns to the interior. The treatment endpoint should be a uniform white photocoagulation burn over the entire extent of the CNV lesion, including all classic and occult CNV and any features that obscure the boundary of the CNV lesion (Fig. 16.1D). These features may include abnormal hypofluorescence, blood, or serous pigment epithelial detachments, and are included in the area of treatment because they may harbor hidden parts of the CNV lesion. In addition, in an attempt to insure complete ablation of the CNV, the treatment area is generally extended beyond these boundaries, with different guidelines depending upon the location of the CNV lesion. This extension is 100 μm for extrafoveal CNV lesions and for the non-foveal side of juxtafoveal lesions. On the foveal side of juxtafoveal lesions, the treatment is extended 100 μm beyond any blood if the posterior edge of the CNV lesion is greater than 100 μm from the fovea; otherwise the treatment is just to the edge of hyperfluorescence. For subfoveal lesions, the treatment is extended 100 μm beyond all lesion features except blood. In addition, if it is a recurrent subfoveal lesion, the treatment extends 300 μm into the area of prior treatment at its interface with the recurrent lesion, and feeder vessels, if present, are treated 300 μm beyond their border radially, and 100 μm beyond their border laterally. A feeder vessel is a choroidal vessel apparent during the transit phase of the angiogram, and is connected unequivocally to the leaking recurrent choroidal neovascular complex. Feeder vessels typically extend across the perimeter of the laser-treated area to the area of recurrent CNV (3). Retrobulbar anesthesia should be administered when deemed necessary, to ensure globe stability. It is also recommended that during treatment, the angiogram be projected onto an appropriate device to allow for repeated verification of vascular landmarks with respect to the location of the CNV. Following treatment, a photograph of the fundus, taken with the same camera, should be compared to the pretreatment angiogram to ensure complete coverage of the lesion by laser of the proper intensity. Data from several MPS trials have shown that eyes in which laser treatment did not completely cover the CNV on the foveal side, or did not meet the required level of intensity, had approximately three times the risk of developing persistent CNV compared to eyes in which the CNV was properly covered and completely covered by intense confluent white burns. This may be especially important for juxtafoveal lesions where even the most experienced ophthalmologist might be hesitant to adequately treat the foveal side. If the extent of the lesion on a pretreatment angiogram shows any areas of inadequate coverage compared to the extent of laser treatment on a posttreatment photograph, then additional treatment to incompletely treated areas should be performed as necessary.

Additional Information Important to the Management of CNV

Occult Choroidal Neovascularization

When the original studies demonstrating the benefit of laser photocoagulation for extrafoveal and juxtafoveal CNV were initiated, a distinction was not made in the pattern of CNV between occult and classic. Subsequent reanalysis of all fluorescein angiograms from the juxtafoveal MPS trial have strengthened the conclusion that laser treatment of lesions composed entirely of classic CNV with no occult CNV is beneficial compared to observation when treatment covers the entire lesion (15). Furthermore, the reanalysis found that treatment of only the classic CNV portion of classic and occult CNV legions provides no benefit over observation. Reanalysis of the handful of eyes entered into the study with only occult CNV found too few such eyes, and with too much lesion coverage variability, to draw conclusions about the benefit of treatment in this subgroup. Nevertheless, 41% of the eyes with occult CNV only that were not treated lost significant vision by 1 year after study entry, usually following the development of classic CNV.

When an eye with only occult CNV that does not extend into the foveal center is well demarcated in a symptomatic patient, it is probably reasonable to consider photocoagulation. Laser treatment may reduce the likelihood that the CNV will eventually extend into the center of the fovea; however, because the natural history of lesions with occult CNV is not known precisely at this time, it is not wrong to observe without treatment in this circumstance.

A close follow-up to monitor for the development of classic CNV, which might benefit from photocoagulation, may be appropriate for subfoveal lesions with occult CNV—but only if the entire lesion is less than 3.5 MPS disc areas, or is a recurrent lesion ≤6 MPS disc areas. Follow-up, then, for subfoveal occult CNV lesions should be perhaps every few months until either classic CNV develops or until the lesion becomes too large to consider for laser treatment.

Subfoveal occult CNV-only lesions do not always have a bad outcome, however; approximately 25% of the eyes with such lesions maintaining baseline visual acuity after 3 years. Therefore, if an eye with occult CNV only does extend into the foveal center, treatment is not recommended because laser photocoagulation is likely to cause significantly more vision loss than the disease itself.

Peripapillary Choroidal Neovascularization

Peripapillary CNV involving the papillomacular bundle is most typically seen in patients with the ocular histoplasmosis syndrome, but idiopathic causes, as well as AMD, may also present with such lesions. Some ophthalmologists are hesitant to treat peripapillary CNV because they fear that the photocoagulation may lead to damage of the nerve fiber layer in the papillomacular bundle, and result in a central scotoma outside the area of the treatment. Other ophthalmologists are hesitant because they believe that the natural course of such lesions might be more benign than the treatment. The MPS group has reported a subgroup analysis on photocoagulation of peripapillary CNV (17). In this study, it was seen that untreated peripapillary CNV can cause substantial vision loss. Almost one fourth of the untreated eyes had a visual acuity of 20/500 or worse by 3 years after study entry, with 26% of the untreated eyes during the 3-year follow-up losing six or more lines of vision compared to 14% of treated eyes. More specifically, a substantial benefit was seen in those eyes that had large peripapillary CNV lesions nasal to the fovea and underlying the papillomacular bundle, with 44% of treated eyes compared to 29% of untreated eyes having a visual acuity of 20/40 or better at 3 years follow-up. In addition, only 9% of treated eyes compared to 54% of untreated eyes lost six or more lines of visual acuity in this group. No treated eye in this group lost significant central vision unless recurrent CNV extended into the foveal center, implying that no central scotoma developed from nerve fiber layer photocoagulation damage to fibers serving the fovea. Thus, laser photocoagulation should be considered in lesions of this type, yet it is still prudent to caution the patient that this has in the past resulted in instances of central vision loss. However, the risk of vision loss caused by thermal damage to the papillomacular bundle appears to be far outweighed by the risk of visual loss from untreated CNV.

Pigment Epithelial Detachments

Various lesions in AMD will result in elevation of the pigment epithelial layer of the retina. A FVPED is a type of occult choroidal neovascularization described above. Treatment of such lesions is considered, as described above, if a well-demarcated FVPED lesion does not involve the foveal center or, if it does involve the foveal center, it is well demarcated, has a classic CNV component, and is relatively small.

A serous detachment of the RPE is distinguishable angiographically from a FVPED by the appearance of early phase, well-circumscribed, bright uniform hyperfluorescence, with persistence of bright fluorescence in the later phases and with little, if any, leakage into the subretinal space. Although the clinical course is variable, most of these patients will develop evidence of CNV within 1 to 2 years (18). Some of these lesions have a notched edge, which is believed to be a sign of occult CNV in the notch. Rarely, a patient may present with extrafoveal classic CNV, which is associated with a subfoveal serous PED. Treatment of the extrafoveal lesion only has resulted in the resolution of the serous PED and in improved vision in selected cases (19). Nevertheless, recurrence of CNV in the vicinity of the serous PED is frequent, and a patient being considered for such treatment must be informed of the high likelihood of recurrence.

A hemorrhagic PED decreases the ability to detect CNV beneath the blood. The appearance of a hemorrhagic PED sometimes may mimic a choroidal melanoma, but the lack of low internal reflectivity on an ultrasound examination will assist in this distinction. A subset of patients with a hemorrhagic PED fit the profile of the "posterior uveal bleeding syndrome" (20). That syndrome is also known as "multiple serosanguineous pigment epithelial detachments" or "idiopathic polypoidal choroidal vasculopathy" (21,22). Kleiner first described it in 1984 (20). Afflicted individuals are usually middle-aged, female, hypertensive, have darkly pigmented skin, and exhibit multiple sanguineous or serosanguineous pigment epithelial detachments (23). The etiology and prognosis of this syndrome is still being investigated, and may be different from AMD. The only clinicopathologic correlation to date has demonstrated extensive subretinal fibrovascular tissue formation, with no abnormalities of the choroidal vessels. When choroidal neovascularization develops outside the foveal center in this syndrome, treatment with laser photocoagulation might be considered to reduce the risk of severe vision loss from potential growth of the fibrovascular tissue under the fovea.

A drusenoid PED is an extensive area of large, soft, and confluent drusen. In contrast to a serous PED, a drusenoid PED fluoresces faintly during the transit phase and does not progress to bright hyperfluorescence until the later phases. In addition, the boundaries of a drusenoid PED are less distinct and are somewhat more irregular than a serous PED. In contrast to a FVPED, a drusenoid PED shows no stippled hyperfluorescence. Biomicroscopically, reticulated pigment clumping is frequently seen overlying a drusenoid PED. These PEDs, however, are not to be included in the confluent treatment of CNV.

Wavelength Considerations

Use of a green versus red laser wavelength was investigated in MPS trials (24). Patients randomized to receive treatment for subfoveal CNV were randomized also to treatment with either an argon green or krypton red laser. Overall, there were no clinically significant differences in any of the visual outcome measures between the two groups. Rates of persistent or recurrent CNV were similar, and therefore, a treating ophthalmologist should select whatever wavelength will permit penetration of the ocular media best, and provide the required uniformly intense white burn. When the patient has significant nuclear sclerosis, for example, a yellow wavelength may facilitate penetration of the lens and allow the use of a lower power to achieve the recommended intensity.

Photodynamic Therapy with Verteporfin

PDT is discussed in detail in other chapters. However, it is important to summarize here the reported 1- and 2-year results from several treatment study groups because of the potential implications these results have upon one's decision to treat CNV. Those study groups are the treatment of age-related macular degeneration with PDT (TAP) study group (TAP report no. 1 and no. 2) and the Verteporfin in Photodynamic Therapy (VIP) Study Group (VIP report no. 2) (25–27). Verteporfin (Visudyne,

Novartis Ophthalmics/ QLT) is one of a group of photo-sensitive dyes that are being investigated for their potential use in the selective treatment of choroidal neovascular tissue. The TAP study is a double-blind, randomized, and placebo-controlled trial of verteporfin therapy for patients with subfoveal classic CNV. The VIP study is similar to the TAP study, but it included MPS-excluded occult lesions without classic CNV if they contained hemorrhage or demonstrated recent progression. The TAP reports no. 1 and no. 2 report a statistically significant reduction in the risk of moderate vision loss at 12 and 24 months for verteporfin-treated eyes versus placebo. The VIP report no. 2 reports a smaller but still statistically significant reduction in the risk of moderate vision loss at 24 months for verteporfin-treated eyes versus placebo. Moderate vision loss for these studies was defined as a loss of 15 letters on the Early Treatment of Diabetic Retinopathy (ETDRS) standardized chart and is roughly equivalent to three lines of Snellen acuity. These reports also showed that in order to achieve this visual acuity benefit, periodic (every 3 months) re-treatments may be needed. Subgroup analysis from TAP report no. 1 demonstrated that the visual acuity benefit of verteporfin therapy is for eyes with predominantly classic CNV lesions. Predominantly classic is a new definition of CNV, and it refers to those lesions demonstrated by fluorescein angiography to be composed of classic CNV for more than 50% of the total area of all lesion components. This definition does not involve the use of indocyanine green (ICG) angiography, and ICG is not needed for the consideration of verteporfin treatment. Lesions that were not predominantly classic (<50% classic CNV) did not show a significant visual acuity benefit from verteporfin treatment. Subgroup analysis from VIP report no. 2 suggest that smaller lesions (4 disc areas or less) or lesions with worse visual acuity (Snellen equivalent of 20/50[-1] or less) have a greater benefit. Further analysis reported in the TAP and VIP report no. 1 indicates that lesion size alone (4 disc areas or less) is a better predictor of the magnitude of the benefit of verteporfin treatment than either lesion composition or initial acuity (28).

The results from TAP reports no. 1 and no. 2 demonstrate that PDT with verteporfin should be considered for predominantly classic subfoveal lesions that previously would have undergone subfoveal laser ablation because they also fit the subfoveal MPS criteria. Other MPS-eligible lesions, which are predominantly classic, may also be considered for PDT.

Risk of Fellow Eye Involvement

Development of CNV in the fellow eye is often devastating because it is likely that there has been substantial vision

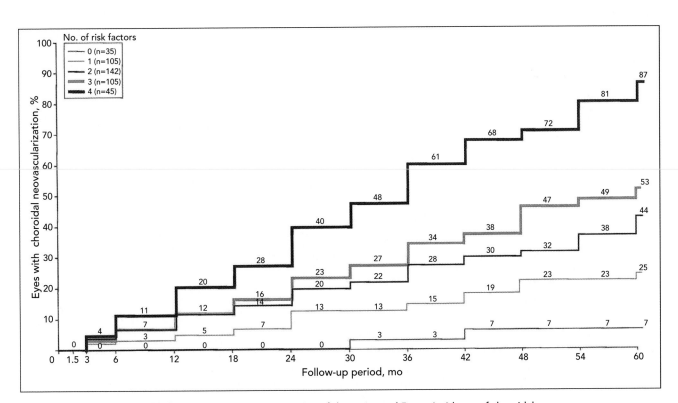

Figure 16.6 Kaplan-Meier representation of the estimated 5-year incidence of choroidal neovascularization (CNV) in the second eye of patients with juxtafoveal or subfoveal CNV secondary to AMD, based upon the number of risk factors present in the second eye. Risk factors include five or more drusen, one or more large (>63 μm) drusen, focal hyperpigmentation within 1,500 μm of the foveal center, and definite systemic hypertension (defined as systolic blood pressure Δ160 mm Hg, diastolic blood pressure Δ95 mm Hg, or use of antihypertensive medications). (Reprinted with permission of the American Medical Association from *Arch Ophthalmol.* 1997;115:741–747.)

loss in the first eye, and patients who are functioning quite well with good vision in their remaining eye are abruptly confronted for the first time with severe lifestyle impairment. It is therefore important to discover and treat second eye CNV as soon as possible in order to maximize the possibility of extrafoveal involvement only. Since symptoms may not appear until the fovea has become involved, it would be useful to stratify risk based on fundus appearance, and perhaps employ more aggressive monitoring strategies in those deemed to be at high risk. Therefore, the MPS group reviewed the eyes of 670 patients enrolled in the trials of laser therapy for juxtafoveal and subfoveal CNV to identify fundus characteristics that might be predictive of CNV development in the uninvolved fellow eyes (29). Follow up ranged from 3 to 5 years and revealed an overall incidence of 35%, which is consistent with previously reported figures (30). Application of life table estimation methods to these data yielded cumulative incidence rates of 10%, 28%, and 42% at 1, 3, and 5 years follow-up, respectively. Three characteristics of the central macula, defined as an area around the foveal center subtended by a circle of 1500 μm in radius, and one systemic factor were associated independently with an increased risk of developing CNV in the fellow eye: the presence of five or more drusen of any size, one or more large (>63 μm) drusen, focal hyperpigmentation, and systemic hypertension. A substantial difference in prognosis was noted depending on the number of risk factors present. The estimated 5-year incidence rates ranged from 7% for the subgroup with no risk factors to 87% for the subgroup with all four risk factors (Fig. 16.6). The presence of classic versus occult CNV in the first eye appeared to have no effect on the rate of CNV development in the fellow eye. These figures, do not apply to those with only non-neovascular changes in both eyes, but are very important in counseling the AMD patient who has just experienced the initial development of CNV in one eye.

CONCLUSIONS

The several MPS reports and the recent TAP and VIP reports outline a rational approach, based upon systematic experimental observations, to the management of the devastating consequences of CNV from AMD. Unfortunately, although substantial progress has been made in understanding the manifestations and treatment of CNV, the only interventions proven beneficial thus far, laser photocoagulation and PDT with verteporfin, are palliative. Often, a good post-treatment result is acuity of 20/160 to 20/200, and many patients are not candidates for either treatment. Current investigations (reviewed in other chapters) may provide an ophthalmologist with tools that can selectively destroy neovascular tissue without harming adjacent structures, or prevent it from forming in the first place. Until these new interventions are available and are proven effective, the management of CNV is limited to

patient education and examining eyes at risk for CNV in order to identify cases which may benefit from laser photocoagulation or photodynamic therapy over observation. In addition, one can determine when AMD (neovascular or non-neovascular)—rather than other ocular causes (such as cataracts)—might be contributing to decreased vision. When any patient, especially over the age of 65, experiences symptoms of metamorphopsia or visual change, a prompt examination by an ophthalmologist skilled in the recognition of neovascular complications is paramount. Early detection in such patients may limit the severe vision loss that AMD might otherwise cause.

REFERENCES

1. Klein R, Klein BE, Linton KL. Prevalence of age-related maculopathy: The Beaver Dam Eye Study. *Ophthalmology*. 1992;99:933–943.
2. Age-Related Eye Disease Study Research Group. A randomized, placebo-controlled, clinical trial of high-dose supplementation with vitamins C and E, beta carotene, and zinc for age-related macular degeneration and vision loss. AREDS report no. 8 *Arch Ophthalmol*. 2001;119:1,417–1,436.
3. Bressler NM, Bressler SB, Fine SL. Age-related macular degeneration. *Surv Ophthalmol*. 1988;32:375–413.
4. Macular Photocoagulation Study Group. Subfoveal neovascular lesions in age-related macular degeneration. Guidelines for evaluation and treatment in the macular photocoagulation study. *Arch Ophthalmol*. 1991;109:1,242–1,257.
5. Macular Photocoagulation Study Group. Argon laser photocoagulation for neovascular maculopathy: five year results from randomized clinical trials. *Arch Ophthalmol*. 1991;109:1,109–1,114.
6. Macular Photocoagulation Study Group. Laser photocoagulation for juxtafoveal choroidal neovascularization. Five-year results from randomized clinical trials. *Arch Ophthalmol*. 1994 Apr;112:500–509.
7. Sykes SO, Bressler NM, Maguire MG, et al. Detecting recurrent choroidal neovascularization. Comparison of clinical examination with and without fluorescein angiography. *Arch Ophthalmol*. 1994;112:1,561–1,566.
8. Macular Photocoagulation Study Group. Laser photocoagulation of subfoveal neovascular lesions in age-related macular degeneration. Results of a randomized clinical trial. *Arch Ophthalmol*. 1991;109:1,220–1,231.
9. Macular Photocoagulation Study Group. Laser photocoagulation of subfoveal recurrent neovascular lesions in age-related macular degeneration. Results of a randomized clinical trial. *Arch Ophthalmol*. 1991;109:1,232–1,241.
10. Macular Photocoagulation Study Group. Subfoveal neovascular lesions in age-related macular degeneration. Guidelines for evaluation and treatment in the macular photocoagulation study. *Arch Ophthalmol*. 1991;109:1,242–1,257.
11. Macular Photocoagulation Study Group. Laser photocoagulation of subfoveal neovascular lesions of age-related macular degeneration. Updated findings from two clinical trials. *Arch Ophthalmol*. 1993;111:1,200–1,209.
12. Macular Photocoagulation Study Group. Visual outcome after laser photocoagulation for subfoveal choroidal neovascularization secondary to age-related macular degeneration. The influence of lesion size and initial visual acuity. *Arch Ophthalmol*. 1994;112:480–488.
13. Macular Photocoagulation Study Group. Persistent and recurrent neovascularization after krypton laser photocoagulation for neovascular lesions of age-related macular degeneration. *Arch Ophthalmol*. 1990;108:825–831.
14. Macular Photocoagulation Study Group. Persistent and recurrent neovascularization after laser photocoagulation for subfoveal choroidal neovascularization in age-related macular degeneration. *Arch Ophthalmol*. 1994;112:489–499.
15. Macular Photocoagulation Study Group. Pretreatment fundus characteristics as predictors of recurrent choroidal neovascularization. *Arch Ophthalmol*. 1991;109:1,193–1,194.
16. Macular Photocoagulation Study Group. Occult Choroidal Neovascularization. Influence on visual outcome in patients with age-related macular degeneration. *Arch Ophthalmol*. 1996;114:400–412.
17. Macular Photocoagulation Study Group. Laser photocoagulation for neovascular lesions nasal to the fovea associated with ocular histoplasmosis or idiopathic causes. *Arch Ophthalmol*. 1995;113:56–61.
18. Gass JDM. Serous retinal pigment epithelial detachment with a notch. A sign of occult choroidal neovascularization. *Retina*. 1984;4:205–220.
19. Maguire JI, Benson WE, Brown GC. Treatment of foveal pigment epithelial detachments with contiguous extrafoveal choroidal neovascular membranes. *Am J Ophthalmol*. 1990;109:523–529.
20. Kleiner RC, Brucker AJ, Johnston RL. The posterior uveal bleeding syndrome. *Retina*. 1990;10:9–17.
21. Stern RM, Zakov AN, Zegarra H, et al. Multiple recurrent serosanguineous retinal pigment epithelial detachments in black women. *Am J Ophthalmol*. 1985;10:560–569.

22. Yannuzzi LA, Sorenson J, Spaide RF, et al. Idiopathic polypoidal choroidal vasculopathy (IPCV). *Retina.* 1990;10:1–8.

23. Perkovich BT, Zakov N, Berlin LA, et al. An update on multiple recurrent serosanguineous retinal pigment epithelial detachments in Black women. *Retina.* 1995;5:100–110.

24. Macular Photocoagulation Study (MPS) Group. Evaluation of argon green vs. krypton red laser for photocoagulation of subfoveal choroidal neovascularization in the macular photocoagulation study. *Arch Ophthalmol.* 1994:112:1,176–1,184.

25. Treatment of Age-Related Macular Degeneration with Photodynamic Therapy (TAP) Study Group. Photodynamic therapy of subfoveal choroidal neovascularization in age-related macular degeneration with verteporfin. One-year results of 2 randomized clinical trials-TAP report 1. *Arch Ophthalmol.* 1999;117:1,329–1,345.

26. Treatment of Age-Related Macular Degeneration with Photodynamic Therapy (TAP) Study Group. Photodynamic therapy of subfoveal choroidal neovascularization in age-related macular degeneration with verteporfin: two-year results of 2 randomized clinical trials—TAP report 2. *Arch Ophthalmol* 2001;119:198–207.

27. Verteporfin in Photodynamic Therapy Study Group. Verteporfin therapy of subfoveal choroidal neovascularization in age-related macular degeneration: two-year results of a randomized clinical trial including lesions with occult with no classic choroidal neovascularization—Verteporfin in Photodynamic Therapy report 2. *Am J Ophthalmol.* 2001;131:541–560.

28. Treatment of Age-Related Macular Degeneration With Photodynamic Therapy (TAP) Study Group, Verteporfin in Photodynamic Therapy (VIP) Study Group. Effect of baseline lesion size, visual acuity, and lesion composition on visual acuity change from baseline with and without verteporfin therapy in choroidal neovascularization secondary to age-related macular degeneration—TAP and VIP report No. 1. *Am J Ophthalmol.* 2003 Sep;136(3):407–418.

29. Macular Photocoagulation Study Group. Risk factors for choroidal neovascularization in the second eye of patients with juxtafoveal or subfoveal choroidal neovascularization secondary to age-related macular degeneration. *Arch Ophthalmol.* 1997;115:741–747.

30. Bressler SB, Maguire MG, Bressler NM, et al. Macular Photocoagulation Study Group. Relationship of drusen and abnormalities of the retinal pigment epithelium to the prognosis of neovascular macular degeneration. *Arch Ophthalmol.* 1990;108:1,442–1,447.

Photodynamic Therapy for Choroidal Neovascularization and Age-Related Macular Degeneration

Lluis Arias Barquet   *Jordi M. Monés*   *Alejandro J. Lavaque*
Joan Miller   *Evangelos S. Gragoudas*

INTRODUCTION

Age-related macular degeneration (AMD) is the leading cause of severe vision loss in people aged 65 or older in developed countries. The strategies for the management of this disease can be divided into those that seek to prevent the development of AMD or retard its progression and those that seek to improve our therapy of the neovascular form. This first category includes genetic linkage and therapy studies, epidemiologic studies, and preventive treatments including nutritional therapy, laser for drusen, and modification of scleral rigidity. The second category incorporates variations of thermal laser photocoagulation, submacular surgery, radiation, photodynamic therapy (PDT), and pharmacologic therapy.

PDT is an innovative therapy for the treatment of Choroidal Neovascular Membranes (CNV) secondary to AMD and other less frequent etiologies. The main indications for PDT were legitimized by carefully designed and developed clinical trials.

Currently, PDT is a treatment that is constantly changing. While this book was written and edited, several studies were under development, paving the way for techniques and treatments in the near future.

PDT is a two-phase treatment. First, it is necessary to inject a photosensitizing agent (chromophore) intra-venously that later, in the second phase, is activated with a laser that has the same band of light absorption as the drug. The photosensitizer is activated after it absorbs the energy from the light source (laser) and is activated, which then triggers a cascade of events that originates a selective damage of the tissue that contains the dye (choroidal neovasculatures).

The first experience with the use of PDT in ophthalmology was in 1994 (1). The performance of the technique in the treatment of intraocular tumors and subretinal neovessels was reported (2). The propitious results obtained in the treatment of choroidal melanomas initiated the study of PDT in animal models of CNV (3–5). In 1998, the results of 61 patients with subfoveal CNV secondary to AMD treated with PDT were published (3). A temporary closing of the CNV was observed, and a stabilization of the visual acuity was achieved. Based on this experiment, phase III clinical trials were designed and developed during the past few years.

MECHANISM OF ACTION

Lasers in ophthalmology can produce a thermal burn (photocoagulation) or a mechanical tear (photodisruption), or can induce chemical changes (photodynamic therapy). Cellular and tissue changes produced by PDT can occur in a natural environment during exposure to a light source under particular circumstances (4). The light by itself has the capability to interact with the cells and produce oxidative reactions leading to the alteration in the basic structures of the cells (organelles) and the target tissue. PDT is based on the intravenous (usually an antecubital vein) administration of a photosensitizer drug that reaches the target tissue via the bloodstream. Subsequently, the photosensitizer is activated locally by light irradiation at an absorption maximum of the dye. The absorption spectrum of the photosensitizer dictates the wavelengths of the radiation that may be suitable for PDT. Generally, the wavelength selected coincides with the absorption maximum of the photosensitizer. The light-dye interaction elevates the photosensitizer from its electronic ground state to a higher-level (excited) triplet state. The excited photosensitizer quickly returns to the ground state and, in the process, transfers energy to other molecules. If this energy is transferred to molecular oxygen, singlet oxygen is formed, which then reacts with proteins, nucleic acids, and lipid membranes. On the other hand, if the excited photosensitizer transfers energy to other compounds, superoxide, hydroxyl, and other free radicals may be formed. The effects of PDT can vary depending on the nature of the agent used, but all have some characteristics in common. The effective penetration depth of the PDT treatment is dependent upon the wavelength of the light and the optical properties of the tissue. Typically, the effective penetration depth is 2 to 3 mm at 630 nm, and increases to 5 mm to 7 mm at 700 nm to 800 nm. Cellular injury mediated by singlet oxygen is the predominant pathway of tissue injury secondary to PDT, and requires adequate levels of oxygen in the target tissues (5). It is important to stress that photodynamic reactions are oxygen-dependent, so the penetration of the membrane is requisite in order to incite the treatment. Both types of reactions, singlet oxygen and the formation of free radicals, can occur in an instantaneous or separate fashion, depending upon the photosensitizer's chemical structure and photodynamic characteristics used during the treatment. Although difficult to demonstrate, the singlet oxygen is highly unstable and has a very short half-life (in order of nanoseconds), which is why this chemical phenomenon has not been possible to register (6).

The physical and chemical reactions that follow the formation of the intravascular free radicals are not completely known. It is established that at least three mechanisms of action exist that are interrelated and produce the therapeutic effect. These phenomena would occur at different levels, and involve cellular, vascular, and immunologic reactions (7).

At the cellular level, the free radicals generated would develop a cytotoxic effect mainly by interacting with the mitochondria, lysosomes, and other intracellular organelles (8). The cellular destruction occurs by an apoptotic process (a progression of cellular death characterized by the activation of a series of enzymes that leads to the fragmentation of the nuclear DNA and the disintegration of the cell into small particles that are digested by the neighboring cells) (9).

Photodynamic tissue effects are not dependent upon increasing the temperature of the target tissue, and thus they differ from conventional thermal photocoagulation of dye-enhanced thermal photocoagulation.

It is believed that the main mechanism of action in PDT is the vascular lesions that the treatment produces. The generated free radicals produce breaks in the intraluminal membranes of the vascular endothelial cells. This reaction alters the internal configuration of the neovasculature, which consequently leads to the destruction of the vascular endothelium. With the alteration of the endothelial cells, the basal membrane of the capillary vessel is exposed. The basal membrane interacts with the blood in the luminal space, triggering a platelet aggregation (10). The activated platelets liberate diverse mediators of inflammation (thromboxane, histamine, and others). These substances produce thrombosis of the vascular lumen and a temporary closing of the CNV (11). Experimental studies indicate that the vascular closing would be limited to the CNV with slight effects on the surrounding microcirculation, which is key to explaining the selectivity of PDT (12).

Through the utilization of certain photosensitizers, an immunomodulator effect is observed. For instance, the application of low dose PDT to the cutaneous tissue increases the survival rate of the skin implants significantly (13).

The effectiveness and selectivity of PDT depend upon disparate factors. The most important are: the photodynamic characteristics of the chromophore used, the administered dose, infusion parameters, the type and wavelength of laser used, the total dose of light irradiation, and the time lapsed between the beginning of the infusion and the drug activation. Although different types of light sources could be used to activate the dye during PDT, the laser systems present many advantages over other forms of light emission. Generally, modern lasers are easy to handle, produce a monochrome light in the spectrum required, allow the diameter of the spot to be easily modified, and have a very precise fiberoptic system of light delivery. In PDT, it is critical to obtain a uniform emission of laser over the treatment area. Currently, there are many types of lasers available in the field of ophthalmology—but the diode lasers are the most preferred. The ideal wavelength for the treatment must coincide with the peak of light absorption of the photosensitizer used (14). The penetration of light in the target tissue is contingent upon the amount of dispersion (scattering) of light and the absorption by the lens. Below the 600 nm range, the light dispersion is high and the probability of light absorption by endogenous chromophores, such as melanin and hemoglobin, increases. Conversely, in a range exceeding 900 nm, the depth penetration of the light decreases because the ocular fluids absorb the light. Unfortunately, very long wavelengths are energetically weak and limit the formation of the necessary amount of free radicals for a satisfactory treatment. Other important factors that affect the penetration of the light are the light absorption by the photosensitizer (self-shielding) and the inactivation of the dye during the exposure to the light (photobleaching) (8).

PHOTOSENSITIZERS

Several major classes of photosensitizers have been used in vitro and in vivo in animal models for investigations of photodynamic therapy. Among these agents, the tetrapyrroles, phthalocyanines, benzophenoxazines, and xanthenes have been used for ocular applications (Table 17.1). Porphyrin derivates, such as hematoporphyrin derivates (HPD) and porfimer sodium, are the most widely studied photodynamic agents.

The physical and chemical properties of the photosensitizer help greatly in determining the effectiveness of PDT. In particular, the properties, which aid greatly in the determination of the efficacy of PDT, are the pharmacokinetic profile and the wavelength of maximum light absorption (15).

The chemical composition of the dye and the affinity for different tissues play an important role in the treatment strategy. Hydrophilic molecules diffuse easily into the interstitial space, while lipophilic compounds are confined longer in the intravascular space. Furthermore, the bolus administration of the photosensitizer increases its selectivity and concentration in the choroidal neovascular tissue (16).

The photosensitizing dye diffuses into the bloodstream and adheres to the plasmatic low-density lipoproteins (LDL). These lipoproteins have abundant receptors in the cytoplasmic membranes of tumoral cells, as well as in the vascular endothelium. The photosensitizer-LDL complex is incorporated into the cell by endocytosis. Once in the cytoplasmic space, the dye becomes vulnerable to being activated by a laser with the appropriate wavelength (17).

To minimize the adverse effects, it is important to bear in mind the pharmacokinetic profile of the dye. A short half-life is desirable because it diminishes the risk of systemic and skin photosensitivity after the treatment (18).

Thomas et al. was the first group that used a photosensitizing dye, dihematoporphyrin, with the idea of enhancing the therapeutic effects after the application of a low-intensity argon laser (19). The results were not favorable due to the increased temperature reached by the laser, which was high enough to produce intense burns in the retina. In later research, several drugs were tested with various results. With the introduction of the new generation of photosensitizing dyes, the effectiveness and security increased (20,21). PDT has become the treatment of choice in the management of CNV secondary to AMD and myopia (22). The discovery of verteporfin (benzoporphyrin derivate) created a revolution in the field of the PDT. Presently, several photosensitizers are being investigated for use in PDT protocols in the future. The principal characteristic of this group could be summarized as follows:

Verteporfin

Verteporfin (Visudyne) is a tetrapyrrole derived from the benzoporphyrin (BPD-MA: benzoporphyrin derivative monoacid TO) (23,24). Currently, verteporfin is a unique

TABLE 17.1
THERAPEUTIC PHOTOSENSITIZERS USED FOR PHOTODYNAMIC THERAPY IN OPHTHALMOLOGY
Xanthene derivates: Rose Bengal

Tetrapyrrole derivates:
    Hematoporphyrin derivate (HPD)
    Photofrin (porfimer sodium/dihematoporphyrin ether)
    Benzoporphyrin derivate
    Tin etiopurpurin
    Lutetium texaphyrin

Chlorins and bacteriochlorins:
    Chlorin e6
    Bacteriochlorin a

Phthalocyanines:
    Chloroaluminum sulfonated phthalocyanine
    Zinc phthalocyanine

(Modified from Miller JW, Gragoudas ES. Photodynamic therapy for choroidal neovascularization and age-related macular degeneration. In: Quiroz-Mercado H, Alfaro VD, Liggett PE, Tano Y, de Juan Jr eds. *Macular Surgery.* Lippincott Williams & Wilkins; 2000.)

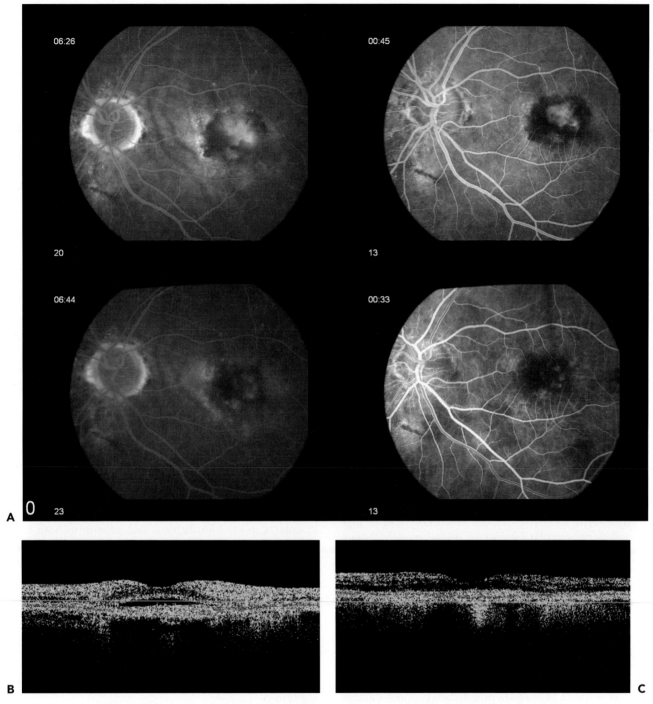

Figure 17.1 A. *Top right*: Early phase of the FA shows an early hyperfluorescence compatible with a subfoveal CNV. *Top left*: FA, late phase. Leakage from an active CNV. Visual acuity: 20/200. *Bottom right*: Early phase of the FA 4 weeks after one treatment with PDT. *Bottom left*: Late phase of the FA. There is no leakage and the hyperfluorescence area is less evident. Visual acuity: 20/80. **B.** OCT line before the treatment with PDT shows the presence of subfoveal fluid. Macular thickness: 298u. **C.** OCT line 4 weeks after one treatment with PDT. The fluid was reabsorbed and the fovea remains flat. Macular thickness: 226u.

photosensitizer for PDT approved by the US Food and Drug Administration (FDA) for the treatment of CNV secondary to AMD and pathologic myopia (Fig. 17.1).

Verteporfin possesses some characteristics that make it a suitable drug for PDT protocols:

1. It is a potent photosensitizer that has the capability to reach significant concentrations in the target tissue with relatively low doses (25).
2. It courses through the bloodstream attached to LDL (26). This characteristic permits a high level of accumulation

in the endothelial cells of the neovascular membrane (27). This effect can be enhanced if verteporfin is delivered with liposomes (28). For clinical use, the dye is administered intravenously as a liposomic formula.

3. It presents two peaks of luminous absorption. One peak is near the ultraviolet spectrum (around 400 nm) and the second is near the long wavelengths (680 to 695 nm) (29). For the activation of verteporfin during PDT, it is advisable to use longer wavelengths since they can effectively penetrate blood and other fluids (30). Moreover, by using this spectrum of light irradiation, the dye could be activated using a laser with low thermal effects.

4. Its half-life is approximately 4 to 6 hours and its effectiveness wears off in 24 to 48 hours. The metabolism is mainly hepatic and it is eliminated by the digestive system. Less than 0.01% of the dose is recovered in the urine. After the infusion of verteporfin, the patient must avoid skin exposure to direct solar or artificial light for 48 hours (31).

5. Verteporfin selectively debilitates the capillaries of the CNV (32). The treatment carried out under the recommended standards produces minimal damage in the choroids and retina. The integral point for verteporfin activation was established 15 minutes after the commencement of the dye infusion. At this particular moment, the drug reaches the maximum concentration level in the neovascular net. Due to the high lipid concentration and the presence of receptors for LDL, verteporfin accumulates immediately after its administration in the retinal pigment epithelial (RPE) cells, photoreceptors, and choroids. For this reason, the activation of the drug should be avoided during an earlier time period (33).

6. Verteporfin has demonstrated its effectiveness by producing neovascular closings in animal models. Angiographic studies have shown an early hypofluorescence in the treated area that begins 24 hours after the treatment and lasts approximately 4 weeks. This hypofluorescence is interpreted as a closure of the neovessels. This phenomenon was corroborated using optic and electronic microscopy. After PDT, the RPE could suffer transitory and/or permanent changes. This collateral damage could be related with the dose used, exposure time, and the moment of light irradiance. Repetitive treatments of PDT apparently do not produce damage in the normal retina (32).

7. The vascular closure does not occur immediately after treatment. During the first 24 hours, the permeability in the CNV increases. This initial exudative phase is followed by the occlusion of the vascular channels during the first week. Both phases have been demonstrated clearly by the optical coherent tomography (OCT), fluorescein, and indocyanine green (ICG) angiograms.

8. The effectiveness of verteporfin for the treatment of subfoveal CNV in patients with AMD has been investigated in rigorous clinical trials. A retreatment scheme has also been evaluated (31,32).

9. The laser should be delivered 15 minutes after the intravenous infusion of verteporfin (6 mg/m^2 during 10 minutes). The dye is activated with a non-thermal diode laser (689 nm), using the following parameters: a duration of 83 seconds, a dose of 50 J/cm^2, and an intensity of 600 mW/cm^2.

Other Photosensitizing Dyes

With the onset of PDT, many first-generation photosensitizer dyes were used. For instance, Photofrin, a purified derivate from hematoporphyrin, was approved in different countries for the treatment of cancer. Due to its slow, 3- to 6-week elimination and its limited penetration, its use was abandoned in ophthalmology. Phthalocyanine, a second-generation photosensitizer, could not be used in ophthalmology due its significant secondary systemic effects (34).

Other photosensitizers have shown variable performance:

1. Tin ethyl etiopurpurin (SnET2, Purlytin) is a lipophilic dye administered as an emulsion. Its maximum peak of light absorption is around 664 nm. In experimental studies, Purlytin was effective in sealing CNV. The initial results were promising. Stabilization or improvement of visual acuity was observed in 64% of the patients enrolled in the study. After the enrollment of 900 patients in a phase III clinical trial, it was determined that the drug did not achieve the desired results in the treatment of CNV secondary to AMD (35–39).

2. Lutetium texaphyrin (Lu-Tex) is soluble in water and has peaks of light absorption at 475 and 732 nm. It circulates in the bloodstream and adheres to both HDL and LDL. Experimental studies demonstrated its effectiveness in the treatment of neovascular nets secondary to AMD. An intriguing point to note is the synergistic effect produced when administered in conjunction with antiangiogenic drugs (40–42).

3. Mono-L-aspartyl chlorin e6 (NPe6) and ATX-S10(Na) are soluble in water and absorb light energy at 664 nm and 670 nm, respectively (43,44).

Experimental studies in animals have shown encouraging results.

CLINICAL TRIALS WITH VERTEPORFIN

In order to evaluate the effectiveness of verteporfin for the treatment of CNV secondary to AMD and pathologic myopia, phase III clinical trials were developed (45–50).

The Treatment of AMD with Photodynamic Therapy (TAP) Study and the Verteporfin in Photodynamic Therapy (VIP) Study are randomized, multicenter, and double-blind clinical trials developed to study the performance of verteporfin in the management of subretinal neovascular disease.

TAP

The inclusion criteria for this study were:

1. Subfoveal CNV secondary to AMD.
2. Area of CNV $\geq$50% of the lesion.
3. Evidences of classic component (with or without occult component) of the CNV.
4. Visual acuity of 20/40 to 20/200.
5. Lesion with a diameter $\leq$5,400 microns.

The TAP study was conformed by two arms (IIIa and IIIb) with identical design. The study was carried out in 22 centers in Europe and the United States. The participants were randomized in a proportion of two to one (verteporfin to placebo), so that of the 609 patients, 402 were in the former and 207 were in the latter group. All of them were recruited between December 1996 and October 1997.

The patients received a constant volume of 30 mL of either verteporfin or placebo intravenously for 10 minutes. The drug was activated 15 minutes after the initiation of the infusion by an infrared laser. Patients were followed for 2 years. Based upon the results of the fluorescein angiogram at each visit, which indicated CNV activity, re-treatments were scheduled.

The main objective of the TAP study was to determine if the treatment with verteporfin was able to diminish the risk of moderate visual loss (three or more lines of visual acuity) during the follow-up.

The results at 12 months were the following:

1. The average number of treatments needed was 3.4 per patient during the first year. The maximum was four treatments. The requirement of re-treatments diminished during the follow-up: 90% at 3 months, 80% at 6 months, 70% at 9 months, and 64% at 12 months.
2. Moderate visual loss was observed in 39% of the patients in the verteporfin group and 54% in the placebo group (P <0.001).
3. Sixty-one percent of patients treated with verteporfin maintained a stable vision (loss of less than three lines of visual acuity) compared to 46% in the placebo group.
4. Sixteen-percent of the patients treated with verteporfin improved vision (experienced an increase of one or more lines of visual acuity) compared to 7% in the placebo group.
5. Severe visual loss (more than six lines of visual acuity) was observed in 15% of the patients treated with verteporfin and 24% in the placebo group.
6. The loss of contrast sensitivity was more evident in the placebo group.
7. Verteporfin showed better results in predominately classic lesions (classic component $\geq$50%) than in minimally classic lesions (classic component smaller than 50%). A moderate loss of vision in the predominantly classic lesions was observed in 33% in those treated with verteporfin) compared to 61% in those treated with the placebo (P <0.001). In minimally classic

lesions, a moderate loss of vision was observed in 44% of the verteporfin group versus 45% in the placebo group (P = 0.92).

These data show that PDT with verteporfin reduces the risk of moderate and severe visual loss in patients with predominantly classic subfoveal CNV secondary to AMD (Fig. 17.1).

The results of the TAP study following a 24-month time period revealed:

1. The average number of treatments during the second year was 2.2; the maximum was four. The average during 24 months of follow-ups was 5.6 treatments, and the maximum was eight.
2. A moderate loss of vision (greater than three lines of visual acuity) occurred in 47% of the patients treated with verteporfin and in 62% of the patients in the placebo group (P <0.001).
3. At the end of the follow-up, patients with predominately classic lesions had better results than patients with minimally classic lesions. A moderate loss of vision in the predominantly classic lesions was observed in 41% of the verteporfin group versus 69% in the placebo group (P <0.001). The respective percentages in the minimally classic group were 53% and 56% (P = 0.58).
4. Fifty-nine percent of the patients treated with verteporfin had better vision, compared to 31% in those in the placebo group.

These data show that the visual benefits observed in subfoveal CNV secondary to AMD continued during the 24 months. An extension to 36 months of the TAP study demonstrated that the visual results in the group of patients with predominantly classic lesions treated with verteporfin remained stable. The average number of treatments during this extension was 1.1.

VIP

This clinical trial enrolled patients with CNV secondary to pathologic myopia and occult subfoveal CNV secondary to AMD.

The study began in 1998 and included 459 patients recruited in 28 centers in Europe and the United States. It was conformed by two phase-III arms: IIIa (120 patients with CNV secondary to myopia) and IIIb (339 patients with occult CNV secondary to AMD). The patients included in the VIP study were randomized and followed with the same diagram used in the TAP trial.

VIP in occult CNV secondary to AMD:

1. The main objective of the study was to determine if treatment with verteporfin diminished the risk of moderate visual loss (greater than three lines of visual acuity) during the follow-up.
2. At the end of the first year, verteporfin did not perform any better than letting the disease run its natural course. (51% verteporfin versus 55% placebo) (P = 0.52).

3. At the end of the second year, a smaller percentage of the group treated with verteporfin suffered from moderate vision loss (55% compared to 68%, $P = 0.023$).

4. At the end of the follow-up, the average number of treatments was five, and the maximum was eight.

5. Secondary to an unknown cause, 4% of the patients treated with verteporfin suffered a severe decrease of visual acuity (loss ≥ 20 letters) during the first 7 days after the treatment.

6. Analyzing the group with occult active CNV secondary to AMD (membranes associated with recent loss of vision and increased size or bleeding) the results showed a benefit when the patient received the treatment with verteporfin in the following circumstances:
   a. Small lesion (less than four MPS disc diameters) with independence of the visual acuity.
   b. Visual acuity >20/50, with independence of the size of the lesion.

The group of patients that had occult lesions with diameters greater than four MPS disc diameters, and with visual acuities >20/50 had a greater risk of moderate and severe visual loss after the treatment.

VIP in CNV Secondary to Pathologic Myopia:

The aim of the study was to evaluate the number of patients with CNV secondary to pathologic myopia who lost <1.5 lines of visual acuity after the treatment with verteporfin. The results were:

1. At 12 months, 72% of the patients treated with verteporfin lost <1.5 lines of vision compared with 44% of the patients in the placebo group ($P = 0.003$).

2. Although not statistically significant, at 24 months the patients in the verteporfin group maintained better visual acuities than those in the control group.

3. At the conclusion of the second year, 39% of the patients treated with verteporfin (13% in the placebo group) gained at least one line of visual acuity.

4. The average number of treatments in the verteporfin group was 5.1 (3.4 during the first year and 1.7 in the second).

New Clinical Trials

After the TAP and VIP studies were reported and with the intention of optimizing the treatment, different groups developed diverse protocols and assessed the therapy in other pathologies different than AMD and pathologic myopia. They included:

1. Verteporfin in Ocular Histoplasmosis (VOH) Study. The aim was to evaluate the effectiveness of the treatment with verteporfin in CNV secondary to ocular histoplasmosis. Twenty-six patients were recruited and followed up for 12 months. After the treatment, a mean of seven lines of improvement was observed (51,52).

2. Visudyne Early Retreatment (VER) Trial. The goal was to determine if earlier re-treatments reduced the risk of moderate visual loss in patients with subfoveal predominantly classic CNV secondary to AMD. The patients were retreated every 6 weeks during the first 6 months and later every 3 months until 2 years. After 12 months of follow-up examinations, no significant differences were observed when comparing the results with the control group.

3. Visudyne in Minimally Classic CNV (VIM) Trial. In a retrospective analysis, the group of patients with minimally classic CNV secondary to AMD (with lesions measuring less than four MPS Disc Diameters and visual acuities <20/50) lost less vision when they were treated with verteporfin compared to patients that didn't receive PDT (42% versus 63% in the placebo group). Previous studies suggested that diminishing light, fluence could maximize the photodynamic effects of verteporfin. For this reason, a phase II study was designed to compare the application of PDT with verteporfin using standard fluence (600 mW/cm^2) to reduced fluence (300 mW/cm^2). After 12 months, it was observed that the group treated with verteporfin had better visual acuities than the control group (PDT with reduced light fluence compared to placebo $P = 0.02$; PDT with standard light fluence compared to placebo $P = 0.08$; PDT with verteporfin group compared to placebo $P = 0.01$) (53).

4. Visudyne with Altered (delayed) Light in Occult CNV Trial (VALIO). In phase I and II clinical trials, a benefit was observed in occult CNV when the laser was delivered 30 minutes after the beginning of the infusion of verteporfin. In classic CNV, the most substantial benefit was obtained after 15 minutes. Bearing in mind the possibility to optimize the treatment in this particular subgroup, a phase II study was designed in order to determine if delayed laser application (30 minutes) had a positive impact in the visual and angiographic results. The results at 6 months did not indicate any differences (54).

5. Visudyne In Occult with Non-classic CNV Trial (VIO). The aim of this phase III study is to analyze whether or not the treatment with verteporfin reduces the risk of visual loss in patients with occult subfoveal CNV secondary to AMD.

6. Photodynamic Therapy in Occult-Only Lesions (POOL) Study. The main objective of this phase IV study is to evaluate the effect of the treatment with verteporfin in patients with occult lesions without the classic component of subfoveal CNV secondary to AMD. This study will be developed exclusively in Europe. Presently, the study is in its recruiting phase.

MAIN INDICATIONS FOR PHOTODYNAMIC THERAPY

Currently, the main candidates for treatment with verteporfin can be summarized as follows:

1. Classic subfoveal CNV secondary to AMD.

2. Active occult CNV secondary to AMD (new blood, increased size, or visual loss in the last 3 months) with the following characteristics:

a. Lesion less than or equal to four MPS disc diameter areas, without considering the visual acuity.

b. Visual acuity <20/50, without considering the size of the lesion.

3. Subfoveal CNV secondary to pathological myopia.

4. Subfoveal CNV secondary to ocular histoplasmosis (Pending approval by the FDA).

Some clinical evidence shows that PDT could be useful in the management of other conditions that involve the retina, including:

1. Choroidal Hemangioma. Various authors have demonstrated the beneficial effect of PDT in the management of the exudative retinal detachments related to the presence of choroidal hemangiomas (55,56). Schmidt-Erfurth et al. published a series of 15 patients who had complete remission of the lesions as well as the exudative manifestations after treatment with verteporfin. The number of treatments needed varied from one to four. The mean visual acuity before treatment was 20/125 and improved to 20/80 following treatment (57).

2. Inflammatory diseases and idiopathic CNV. A recent study reported 32 cases with CNV secondary to ocular histoplasmosis treated with PDT (58). An improvement was obtained in 69% of the cases. Another small series reported on the benefit of verteporfin in CNV secondary to multifocal choroiditis with panuveitis. In a series of 7 patients and after a mean of 2 treatments, an improvement in the visual acuities of 0.86 lines was obtained (59). Adverse effects related to the treatment were not reported. In another study of eight patients with the diagnosis of idiopathic CNV, after a mean follow-up of 13.5 months, 63% of the patients improved their visual acuity by an average of 3.6 lines on the Snellen chart (60). A second trial that grouped 19 cases of idiopathic and inflammatory CNV was presented. Resolution of the exudative manifestation was observed in the majority of the patients (61).

3. CNV secondary to angioid streaks. Preliminary reports indicated the possibility to treat the CNV associated with angioid streaks with PDT. In this particular group the results were highly variable (62). A great tendency for recurrence was observed (63).

4. Idiopathic juxtafoveal retinal telangiectasis. Verteporfin has shown to be effective in the treatment of this pathology. As in other pathologies, re-treatments are necessary (64,65).

5. Polypoidal CNV. Chorioretinal disease characterized by the presence of aneurysmal dilations of the choroidal vessels usually complicated with recurrent serous and hemorrhagic detachments of the retina and RPE cells. PDT with verteporfin usually seals the dilated vessel and permits the resolution of the exudative manifestations. Good visual results were reported (66–68).

6. Central serous chorioretinopathy (CSCR). Encouraging results have been reported after the treatment of this entity with PDT (69). Yanuzzi et al. obtained an improvement in 20 eyes of 12 patients by guiding the treatment with ICG angiographies (ICGA). Undesirable secondary effects have not been reported after the treatment (70).

7. Diabetic retinopathy. It is well known that patients with diabetic retinopathy are at risk for developing subretinal neovessels. These patients are susceptible to treatment with Verteporfin. However, it is important to take into consideration that diabetes mellitus could make the retinal vessels more sensitive to the treatment. CNV secondary to laser photocoagulation in diabetic patients has been treated successfully with PDT (71,72).

8. Retinal dystrophies. Isolated reports comment on the beneficial effects of verteporfin in the management of CNV associated with fundus flavimaculatus, Sorsby disease, pattern dystrophies, and *malattia leventinese* (73–77).

9. Others. Verteporfin has been used in the treatment of retinal angiomatous proliferation (RAP), retinal capillary hemangiomas, CNV secondary to choroidal osteoma and rubeolic retinopathy (78–81). Furthermore, PDT could be used with advantages in the treatment of iris and corneal neovascularizations (82,83).

CONTRAINDICATIONS AND CAUTIONS

Two absolute contraindications exist for the realization of PDT with verteporfin:

1. Presence of Porphyria or hypersensitivity to the porphyrin.

2. Severe hepatic insufficiency (84).

There are some drugs that could influence the results of the treatment. For example, calcium channel blockers and polymyxin B can increase the concentration of verteporfin in the vascular endothelium. Alternatively, some well-known photosensitizing drugs, such as tetracycline, sulfonylurea, and diuretics can increase the possibilities of an undesirable skin photoreaction. Antioxidant agents or drugs that neutralize the free radicals reactions as β-carotene, ethanol, and mannitol can reduce the intravascular activity of verteporfin. Drugs that inhibit platelet aggregation, such as the inhibitors of the thromboxane A2, can diminish the effectiveness of the treatment.

SECONDARY EFFECTS

During the development of the clinical trials, significant adverse reactions were not evidenced. The 12-month TAP report showed the following complications (45):

1. Transitory visual alterations (17.7% verteporfin versus 11.6% placebo).

2. Local reactions in the site of the injection (13.4% versus 3.4%).

3. Reversible transitory photosensitization (3% versus 0%).
4. Back pain related with verteporfin infusion (2.2% versus 0%).
5. Allergic reactions (1.2% versus 3.4%).

The adverse reactions in the TAP 24-month report were similar (46). Skin reactions were observed in 14 of 402 patients (3.5%) treated with verteporfin. Most of the reactions occurred during the first 24 hours after the treatment, and they were secondary to skin exposure to intense light. Diabetic patients have a larger risk of skin reactions (85).

The back pain that appeared in some patients during the drug infusion is of unknown etiology (86). It was transitory and customarily disappeared at the end of the infusion. Previous hydration did not prevent this complication. The administration of intravenous diphenhydramine minimized the pain (87). Serious systemic adverse reactions can occur sporadically (88,89).

Retinal complications related with the treatment were:

1. Tears of the RPE have been reported in myopic patients as well as in AMD. The mechanisms that trigger this complication are not well known. Fragility of the RPE cells associated with contractile changes in the CNV after the treatment is suspected (90,91).
2. Massive macular hemorrhages. The risk of this complication is <2%. It occurs during the first 48 hours after the treatment with PDT and is considered a direct consequence of the treatment (92).
3. Presence of hot spots in the ICGA. After the treatment with PDT, some patients exhibit the presence of hot spots in the choroidal circulation in the ICGA. Fibrin accumulation secondary to a localized vasculitis induced by the treatment is suspected (93).
4. Macular hole formation has been identified during the first month after the treatment and could be related with secondary changes in the retinovitreal interface (94).
5. Vitreous hemorrhages. In the TAP study, four cases of vitreous hemorrhage were reported in the verteporfin group (1%) and 1 case in the placebo group (0.5%) (46). The causes of this complication are unknown.
6. Visual hallucinations. Five percent of the patients treated with Visudyne presented structured transitory visual hallucinations (Charles Bonnet syndrome) (95).

RECOMMENDATION FOR TREATMENT

Inclusion criteria are:

1. Lesion composition. PDT is indicated in the treatment of CNV secondary to AMD in:
   a. Predominantly classic lesions
   b. Occult small active lesions with low vision. In minimally classic lesions, it is possible to consider the treatment in lesions less than or equal to four MPS disc diameters and vision <20/50. In patients with pathological myopia, the composition of the lesion should not influence the patient selection (45,46).
2. Size of the lesion. The TAP and VIP studies did not include lesions bigger than 5,400 microns (nine MPS disc diameters) partially due to the impossibility of obtaining treatment spots bigger than 6,400 microns in diameter. Nevertheless, the current lasers and contact lenses used for laser treatment help to obtain spots up to 8000 microns in diameter; thus bigger lesions can be treated. A distance of 200 microns between the spot and the optic disc is desirable (96).
3. Localization of the lesion. The treatment with verteporfin is suitable mainly in subfoveal lesions, although in certain circumstances, lesions in other localizations could benefit with the treatment. For instance, PDT should be indicated in the treatment of juxtafoveal lesions in myopic patients (97,98).
4. Visual acuity. At the moment, there is no clear limit of visual acuity in which the treatment is not recommended (99).
5. Age. Although there is less experience, treatment in children has shown good visual results, and undesirable secondary effects have not been reported (100,101).

RE-TREATMENTS

During the TAP and VIP studies, re-treatments were scheduled in 3-month intervals (102). Some new considerations were added after the inception of the studies:

1. A new session of PDT can be applied 12 weeks (±2) after the last treatment. In general, it is considered that if a well-documented vision loss occurs during the follow-up, or if the fluorescein angiogram (FA) detects a significant increase in the size of the CNV, the requirement of a new treatment before the third month should be considered. However, some authors have not been able to demonstrate beneficial effects when using shorter intervals (103).
2. The re-treatments should be indicated when the FA shows persistent leakage in the late frames of the test.
3. A lesion should not be retreated when the FA indicates:
   a. Minimum leakage (the leakage occupies <50% of the initial treated area)
   b. Absence of leakage (leakage is not appreciated in the CNV area and the hyperfluorescence observed in the FA corresponds with staining of the scar tissue).
4. Very big lesions should not be treated because the beneficial effect of the treatment would be minimal or not at all useful (104).
5. The patient should be examined every 3 months during the first 2 years. Each visit must include an FA. If the patient reaches the semester without indication for

retreatment, the intervals between visits could be longer.

PROGNOSTIC FACTORS

Prognostic factors can be summarized as follows:

1. Early detection. The main objective of PDT is to reduce the risk of visual loss associated with the presence of a CNV. For that reason, early diagnosis and treatment is desirable. PDT is more effective during the early stages of the disease when the neovascular component of the membrane is greater than the scar tissue. An early derivation of the patient to specialized centers of diagnosis and treatment is of capital importance (105).
2. Size of the lesion. It appears that lesions smaller than four MPS disc diameters respond better to the treatment (Fig. 17.2). It is possible that in the near future the greatest diameter of the CNV will be of more importance than the composition (107).
3. Visual acuity. Poor visual acuities at the beginning are related with poor visual outcomes after the treatment. The predominantly classic CNV usually has a satisfactory response to PDT; nevertheless these lesions frequently arise in conjunction with poor visual acuities. In these cases, a reduction of the size of the scotoma and an improvement of the contrast sensitivity are the main objectives (104).
4. Chorioretinal anastomosis. The presence of a communication between the choroidal and retinal circulations carries a poor prognosis. These patients usually do not respond to PDT treatment (108).
5. Etiology of the CNV. CNV secondary to pathological myopia usually responds better than CNV associated with AMD (109). The visual outcome seems to be related with the age of the patients. Patients under the age of 55 respond better to the therapy. On the other hand, CNV associated with angioid streaks do not respond favorably to the treatment with PDT (63).

SOCIOECONOMIC IMPACT OF PHOTODYNAMIC THERAPY

AMD is the leading cause of severe vision loss in people 65 years and older in Western countries (110–112). Margherio et al. demonstrated that 17% of the patients remitted with the diagnosis of CNV secondary to AMD have the subfoveal predominantly classic form of the disease, which could be treated with PDT (113). Other studies show that only 20% to 30% of the patients with CNV secondary to AMD could be treated with verteporfin (114).

Presently, the main indicator in deciding the treatment is the classification of CNV based upon results from the FA. A correct evaluation of the FA in each case is mandatory to indicate the potentiality of treatment. Nevertheless, the interpretation of the FA is not always obvious. Different patterns of presentation can be interpreted in different ways (115).

The first economic analysis of the use of PDT with verteporfin was published in the 2001 (116). This study analyzed the cost-effectiveness of treatment in AMD patients who had a disciform scar in one eye and a recent diagnosis of predominantly classic CNV in the fellow eye. The study showed that the initial visual acuity at the moment of the diagnosis in the second eye was the main indicator of the cost-effectiveness relationship.

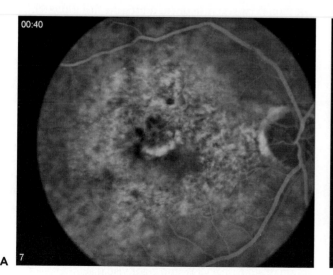
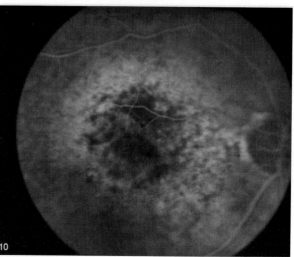

Figure 17.2 A. Early frame of the FA shows generalized atrophy and remodeling of the RPE in the macular area associated with an early hyperfluorescence compatible with a CNV. **B.** Two weeks after one treatment with PDT the FA shows a round area of hypofluorescence in the treated site. No exudative manifestations are visible.

NEW FUNCTIONAL AND HISTOPATHOLOGICAL DATA

Histopathological studies of neovascular membranes extracted surgically after the application of PDT confirm the damage of the endothelial cells in the neovascular net with thrombus formation and secondary vascular occlusion. Other authors have demonstrated a possible harmful effect of the treatment on the RPE cells (119).

A recent study analyzed eight patients with CNV that received submacular surgery after PDT. The histopathological results reveal that PDT does not completely close the capillaries of the CNV; instead the greater the diameter of the neovessel, the greater difficulty there is in closing it. This would be related with the clinical observation that smaller lesions have a better response to such treatment (121,122).

The real effectiveness of PDT and the benefit that the treatment brings to the quality of life of the patients have been evaluated (123). PDT is not able to prevent the loss of central fixation in the majority of the cases, but stabilizes visual acuity (124). PDT stabilizes the reading speed during a minimum period of 9 to 12 months. The results are greater in patients with pathological myopia than in patients with AMD (125). The size of the scotoma would be directly related to the reading speed. PDT preserves and improves the contrast sensitivity (126). The TAP study demonstrated that the patients treated with verteporfin maintained a better contrast sensitivity compared to the control group. Scientific evidence demonstrates that the contrast sensitivity and the visual field are crucial for the visual orientation and the mobility of these patients. It is possible that this phenomenon has a positive impact on the visual function of the patients who receive PDT treatment.

NEW PERSPECTIVES IN PHOTODYNAMIC THERAPY

Contribution of complementary tests:

1. FA. During the first days after PDT treatment, a hypofluorescence in the treated area was observed. This phenomenon was secondary to the occlusion of the choroidal and neovascular vessels associated with a blockage at the level of the RPE. At the end of the first week, absence of neovascular activity was observed in most of the patients (127,128).
2. ICGA. Specifically useful for the study of the choroidal circulation. Successive treatments produce a significant reduction in the size of the CNV and the area of leakage (129). The studies with ICGA suggest that the re-treatments with PDT should be sufficiently spaced in order to guarantee a full recovery of the choroidal perfusion. Moreover, early re-treatments could be:
   a. Ineffective, as the choroidal hypoperfusion may not contribute enough oxygen to trigger the cascade of events that follow the verteporfin activation.
   b. Counteractive, as early re-treatments could produce a choroidal ischemic effect that may favor the liberation of angiogenic factors (130).
3. Multifocal electroretinogram. This variant of electroretinogram provides the opportunity to analyze the electric activity of the macular area. Some studies have evaluated the macular electrical response after PDT in patients with AMD and myopia. The increment of electrical activity in the foveal and parafoveal areas is evident, particularly in myopic patients (131,132).
4. OCT. Rogers et al. analyzed the results of the OCT in 90 cases of predominantly classic subfoveal CNV secondary to AMD treated with PDT (133). They suggested a 5-stage classification:
   a. Stage I. Acute inflammatory response with increase of the subretinal fluid during the first days after the treatment.
   b. Stage II. Near-normal recovery of the foveal silhouette, with decrease of the subretinal fluid. This occurs in weeks 1 to 4.
   c. Stage III. Takes place among the 4- and 12-week periods following treatment. This stage can be divided into two subgroups:
      i. Stage IIIa. There is more subretinal fluid than fibrosis. This indicates active CNV.
      ii. Stage IIIb. There is more fibrosis than subretinal fluid.
   d. Stage IV. Presence of cystic macular edema.
   e. Stage V. Resolution of the subretinal exudation, with irreversible damage of the choroid and neurosensory retina.

A recent study using OCT displayed what occurs during the application of PDT with verteporfin. In the first 2 hours after treatment, an increase of the permeability of the CNV was observed. At the conclusion of the first week, there is a marked reduction of the subretinal fluid, with a recovery of the foveal contour. Relapses are frequent during the first trimester.

TREATMENT COMBINATION

The following treatments incorporating PDT have recently been proposed:

1. Macular translocation (MT) and PDT. MT could be done before or after PDT (135,136). MT is an intricate surgical technique with significant intrinsic surgical risks. Nonetheless, it was the only treatment that proved to be effective in enhancing the visual acuity in patients with CNV. In one study, 48% of the patients with subfoveal CNV secondary to AMD treated with MT gained more than two lines of vision (137). This combined therapy would be designated in unique eyes containing small subfoveal CNV and poor visual acuities.
2. Treatment of the feeder vessel and PDT. The application of PDT increases the percentage of detection of the feeder vessel in patients with CNV (84% of the cases).

The possibility to combine both therapies would reduce the number of re-treatments (138).

3. Antiangiogenic therapy and PDT. Currently, most of the antiangiogenic therapies are in the developmental phase. Nevertheless, the combination of PDT and the intravitreal injection of triamcinolone acetonide in patients with AMD has shown encouraging results (139).

Further studies in PDT for neovasculature may include studies of new photosensitizers developed specifically for neovasculature rather than tumors, targeting photosensitizers by binding them to targeting molecules, and combining PDT with other treatment modalities, including antiangiogenic therapy, radiation, and surgery.

REFERENCES

1. Schmidt-Erfurth U, Hasan T, Flotte T. Photodynamic therapy of experimental intraocular tumors with benzoporphyrin-lipoprotein. *Ophthalmology.* 1994;91:348–356.
2. Schmidt-Erfurth U, Hasan T, Gragoudas ES, et al. Vascular targeting in photodynamic occlusion of subretinal vessels. *Ophthalmology.* 1994;101: 1,953–1,961.
3. Schmidt-Erfurth U, Miller J, Sickenberg M, et al. Photodynamic therapy of subfoveal choroidal neovascularization:clinical and angiographic examples. *Graefes Arch Clin Exp Ophthalmol.* 1998;236:365–374.
4. Organisciak DT, Darrow RM, Barsalou L, et al. Light history and age-related changes in retinal light damage. *Invest Ophthalmol Vis Sci.* 1998;39:1107–1116.
5. Schmidt-Erfurth U, Hasan T. Mechanisms of action of photodynamic therapy with verteporfin for the treatment of age-related macular degeneration. *Surv Ophthalmol.* 2000;45:195–214.
6. Rodgers MA. On the problems involved in detecting luminescence from singlet oxygen in biological specimens. *J Photochem Photobiol B* 1988;1: 371–373.
7. Henderson BW, Dougherty TJ. How does photodynamic therapy work? *Photochem Photobiol.* 1992;55:145–157.
8. Jori G, Reddi E. The role of lipoproteins in the delivery of tumor-targeting photosensitizers. *Int J Biochem.* 1993;25:1,369–1,375.
9. Granville DJ, Jiang H, McManus BM, et al. Fas ligand and TRAIL augment the effect of photodynamic therapy on the induction of apoptosis in JURKAT cells. *Int Immunopharmacol.* 2001;1:1,831–1,840.
10. Schmidt-Erfurth U, Bauman W, Gragoudas ES, et al. Photodynamic therapy of experimental choroidal melanoma using lipoprotein-delivered benzoporphyrin. *Ophthalmology.* 1994;101:89–99.
11. Fingar VH. Vascular effects of photodynamic therapy. *J Clin Laser Med Surg.* 1996;14:323–328.
12. Fingar VH, Kik PK, Haydon PS, et al. Analysis of acute vascular damage after photodynamic therapy using benzoporphyrin derivative. *Br J Cancer.* 1999;79:1,702–1,708.
13. Obochi MO, Ratkay LG, Levy JG. Prolonged skin allograft survival after photodynamic therapy associated with modification of donor skin antigenicity. *Transplantation.* 1997;63:810–817.
14. Svaasand LO, Gomer CJ, Morinelli E. On the physical rationale of photodynamic therapy. Future directions and applications in pharmacodynamic therapy. *IS6 SPIE Institute Series.* 1990;233–248.
15. Aveline B, Hasan T, Redmond RW. Photophysical and photosensitizing properties of benzoporphyrin derivative monoacid ring A. *Photochem Photobiol.* 1994;59:328–335.
16. Jori G. Factors controlling the selectivity and efficiency of tumor damage in photodynamic therapy. *Lasers Med Sci.* 1990;5:115–120.
17. Kramer M, Kenney AG, Delori F, et al. Imaging of experimental choroidal neovascularization using liposomal benzoporphyrin derivative mono-acid angiography. *Invest Ophthalmol Vis Sci.* 1995;36:S236.
18. Schmidt-Erfurth U, Diddens H, Birngruber R, et al. Photodynamic targeting of human retinoblastoma cells using covalent low-density lipoprotein conjugates. *Br J Cancer.* 1997;75:54–61.
19. Thomas EL, Langhofer M. Closure of experimental subretinal neovascular vessels with dihematoporphyrin ether augmented argon green laser photocoagulation. *Photochem Photobiol.* 1987;46:881–886.
20. Miller H, Miller B. Photodynamic therapy of subretinal neovascularization in the monkey eye. *Arch Ophthalmol.* 1993;111:855–860.
21. Richter AM, Cerruti-Sola S, Sternberg ED, et al. Biodistribution of tritiated benzoporphyrin derivative (3H-BPD-MA), a new potent photosensitizer, in normal and tumor-bearing mice. *J Photochem Photobiol B.* 1990;5: 231–244.
22. Fogelman AM, Berliner JA, Van Lenten BJ, et al. Lipoprotein receptors and endothelial cells. *Semin Thromb Hemost.* 1988;14:206–209.
23. Richter AM, Waterfield E, Jain AK, et al. Liposomal delivery of a photosensitizer, benzoporphyrin derivative monoacid ring A (BPD), to tumor tissue in a mouse tumor model. *Photochem Photobiol.* 1993;57:1,000–1,006.
24. Richter AM, Kelly B, Chow J, et al. Preliminary studies on a more effective phototoxic agent than hematoporphyrin. *J Natl Cancer Inst.* 1987;79: 1,327–1,332.
25. Richter AM, Waterfield E, Jain AK, et al. Photosensitising potency of structural analogues of benzoporphyrin derivative (BPD) in a mouse tumor model. *Br J Cancer.* 1991;63:87–93.
26. Haimovici R, Kramer M, Miller JW, et al. Localization of lipoprotein-delivered benzoporphyrin derivative in the rabbit eye. *Curr Eye Res.* 1997;16:83–90.
27. Kramer M, Miller JW, Michaud N, et al. Liposomal benzoporphyrin derivative verteporfin photodynamic therapy. Selective treatment of choroidal neovascularization in monkeys. *Ophthalmology.* 1996;103:427–438.
28. Husain D, Miller JW, Michaud N, et al. Long-term effect of photodynamic therapy (PDT) using liposomal benzoporphyrin derivative (BPD) on experimental choroidal neovascularization (CNV) and normal retina and choroids. *Invest Ophthalmol Vis Sci.* 1996;37:S223.
29. Reinke MH, Canakis C, Husain D, et al. Verteporfin photodynamic therapy retreatment of normal retina and choroid in the cynomolgus monkey. *Ophthalmology.* 1999;106:1,915–1,923.
30. Michels S, Schmidt-Erfurth U. Sequence of early vascular events after photodynamic therapy. *Invest Ophthalmol Vis Sci.* 2003;44:2,147–2,154.
31. Miller JW, Schmidt-Erfurth U, Sickenberg M, et al. Photodynamic therapy with verteporfin for choroidal neovascularization by age-related macular degeneration:results of a single treatment in a phase I and II study. *Arch Ophthalmol.* 1999;117:1,161–1,173.
32. Schmidt-Erfurth U, Miller JW, Sickenberg M, et al. Photodynamic therapy with verteporfin for choroidal neovascularization caused by age-related macular degeneration: results of retreatment in a phase I and II study. *Arch Ophthalmol.* 1999;117:1,177–1,187.
33. Gomer CJ. Preclinical examination of first and second-generation photosensitizers used in photodynamic therapy. *Photochem Photobiol.* 1991;54: 1,093–1,107.
34. Kliman GH, Puliafito CA, Stern D, et al. Phthalocyanine photodynamic therapy: new strategy for closure of choroidal neovascularization. *Lasers Surg Med.* 1994;15:2–10.
35. Peyman GA, Moshfeghi DM, Moshfeghi A, et al. Photodynamic therapy for choriocapillaris using tin ethyl etiopurpurin (SnET2). *Ophthalmic Surg Lasers.* 1997;28:409–417.
36. Baumal C, Puliafito C, Pierrot L, et al. Photodynamic therapy (PDT) of experimental choroidal neovascularization with tin ethyl etiopurpurin. *Invest Ophthalmol Vis Sci.* 1996;37:S122.
37. Thomas EL, Rosen R, Murphy R, et al. Visual acuity stabilizes after a single treatment with SnET2-photodynamic therapy in patients with subfoveal choroidal neovascularization. *Invest Ophthalmol Vis Sci.* 1999;40:S401.
38. Hunt DW. Rostaporfin (Miravant Medical Technologies). *Drugs.* 2002;5: 180–186.
39. Woodburn KW, Fan Q, Kessel D, et al. Phototherapy of cancer and atheromatous plaque with texaphyrins. *Clin Laser Med Surg.* 1996;14:343–348.
40. Blumenkranz MS, Woodburn K, Quin F, et al. Lutetium texaphyrin (Lutex):a potential new agent for ocular fundus angiography and photodynamic therapy. *Am J Ophthalmol.* 2000;129:495–500.
41. Miller JW. Other photodynamic therapy drugs. Presented at the annual meeting of the American Academy of Ophthalmology, New Orleans, 2001.
42. Woodburn KW, Engelman CJ, Blumenkranz MS. Photodynamic therapy for choroidal neovascularization: a review. *Retina.* 2002;22:391–405.
43. Mori K, Yoneya S, Ohta M. Angiographic and histologic effects of fundus photodynamic therapy with a hydrophilic sensitizer (mono-L-aspartyl chlorin e6). *Ophthalmology.* 1999;106:663–668.
44. Obana A, Gohto Y, Kanai M, et al. Selective photodynamic effects of the new photosensitizer ATX-S10(Na) on choroidal neovascularization in monkeys. *Arch Ophthalmol.* 2000;118:650–658.
45. Treatment of AMD with PDT Study Group. Photodynamic therapy of subfoveal choroidal neovascularization in AMD with verteporfin: one-year results of 2 randomized clinical trials—TAP report 1. *Arch Ophthalmol.* 1999;117:1,329–1,345.
46. Treatment of Age-Related Macular Degeneration with Photodynamic Therapy (TAP) Study Group. Photodynamic therapy of subfoveal choroidal neovascularization in age-related macular degeneration with verteporfin. Two-year results of 2 randomized clinical trials—TAP report 2. *Arch Ophthalmol.* 2001;119:198–207.
47. Treatment of Age-Related Macular Degeneration with Photodynamic Therapy (TAP) Study Group. Verteporfin therapy for subfoveal choroidal neovascularization in age-related macular degeneration. Three-year results of an open label extension of 2 randomized clinical trials—TAP report no. 5. *Arch Ophthalmol.* 2002;120:1,307–1,314.
48. Verteporfin in Photodynamic Therapy (VIP) Study Group. Verteporfin therapy of subfoveal choroidal neovascularization in age-related macular degeneration:2-year results of a randomized clinical trial including lesions with occult with no classic choroidal neovascularization—VIP report 2. *Am J Ophthalmol.* 2001;131:541–560.
49. Verteporfin in Photodynamic Therapy (VIP) Study Group. Photodynamic therapy of subfoveal choroidal neovascularization in pathologic myopia with verteporfin: 1-year results of a randomized clinical trial—VIP report 1. *Ophthalmology.* 2001;108:841–853.

50. Verteporfin in Photodynamic Therapy (VIP) Study Group. Verteporfin therapy of subfoveal choroidal neovascularization in pathologic myopia: two-year results of a randomized clinical trial—VIP report 3. *Ophthalmology.* 2003;110:667–673.

51. Saperstein DA, Rosenfeld PJ, Bressler NM, et al. Verteporfin in Ocular Histoplasmosis (VOH) Study Group. Photodynamic therapy of subfoveal choroidal neovascularization with verteporfin in the ocular histoplasmosis syndrome: one-year results of an uncontrolled, prospective case series. *Ophthalmology.* 2002;109:1,499–1,505.

52. Bressler NM. New photodynamic therapy investigations. Presented at the annual meeting of the American Academy of Ophthalmology, New Orleans, 2001.

53. Rosenfeld PJ for TAP Study Group. Visual outcomes in patients with minimally classic choroidal neovascularization (CNV): rationale for the Visudyne in Minimally Classic CNV (VIM) Trial. *Invest Ophthalmol Vis Sci.* 2001;42:S512.

54. Kaiser PK. Photodynamic therapy update: update on verteporfin ocular photodynamic therapy clinical trials. Presented at the annual meeting of the American Academy of Ophthalmology, Anaheim, 2003.

55. Barbazetto I, Schmidt-Erfurth U. Photodynamic therapy of choroidal hemangioma: two case reports. *Graefes Arch Clin Exp Ophthalmol.* 2000;238:214–221.

56. Landau IM, Steen B, Seregard S. Photodynamic therapy for circumscribed choroidal hemangioma. *Acta Ophthalmol Scand.* 2002;80:531–536.

57. Schmidt-Erfurth U, Michels S, Kusserow C, et al. Photodynamic therapy for symptomatic choroidal hemangioma: visual and anatomic results. *Ophthalmology.* 2002;109:2,284–2,294.

58. Busquets MA, Shah GK, Wickens J, et al. Ocular photodynamic therapy with verteporfin for choroidal neovascularization secondary to ocular histoplasmosis syndrome. *Retina.* 2003;23:299–306.

59. Spaide RF, Freund KB, Slakter J, et al. Treatment of subfoveal choroidal neovascularization associated with multifocal choroiditis and panuveitis with photodynamic therapy. *Retina.* 2002;22:545–549.

60. Spaide RF, Martín ML, Slakter J, et al. Treatment of idiopathic subfoveal choroidal neovascular lesions using photodynamic therapy with verteporfin. *Am J Ophthalmol.* 2002;134:62–68.

61. Rogers AH, Duker JS, Nichols N, et al. J. Photodynamic therapy of idiopathic and inflammatory choroidal neovascularization in young adults. *Ophthalmology.* 2003;110:1,315–1,320.

62. Sickenberg M, Schmidt-Erfurth U, Miller JW, et al. A preliminary study of photodynamic therapy using verteporfin for choroidal neovascularization in pathologic myopia, ocular histoplasmosis syndrome, angioid streaks, and idiopathic causes. *Arch Ophthalmol.* 2000;118:327–336.

63. Shaikh S, Ruby AJ, Williams GA. Photodynamic therapy using verteporfin for choroidal neovascularization in angioid streaks. *Am J Ophthalmol.* 2003;135:1–6.

64. Potter MJ, Szabo SM, Chan EY, et al. Photodynamic therapy of a subretinal neovascular membrane type 2A idiopathic juxtafoveolar retinal telangiectasis. *Am J Ophthalmol.* 2002;133:149–151.

65. Hershberger VS, Hutchins RK, Laber PW. Photodynamic therapy with verteporfin for subretinal neovascularization secondary to bilateral idiopathic acquired juxtafoveolar telangiectasis. *Ophthalmic Surg Lasers Imaging.* 2003;34:318–320.

66. Rogers AH, Greenberg PB, Martidis A, et al. Photodynamic therapy of polypoidal choroidal vasculopathy. *Ophthalmic Surg Lasers Imaging.* 2003;34:60–63.

67. Quaranta M, Mauget-Faysse M, Coscas G. Exudative idiopathic polypoidal choroidal vasculopathy and photodynamic therapy with verteporfin. *Am J Ophthalmol.* 2002;134:277–280.

68. Spaide RF, Donsoff I, Lam DL, et al. Treatment of polypoidal choroidal vasculopathy with photodynamic therapy. *Retina.* 2002;22:529–535.

69. Bataglia Parodi M, Da Pozzo S, Ravalico G. Photodynamic therapy in chronic central serous chorioretinopathy. *Retina.* 2003;23:235–237.

70. Yannuzzi LA, Slakter J, Gross NE, et al. Indocyanine green angiography-guided photodynamic therapy for treatment of chronic central serous chorioretinopathy: a pilot study. *Retina.* 2003;23:288–298.

71. Ladd BS, Solomon SD, Bressler NM, et al. Photodynamic therapy with verteporfin for choroidal neovascularization in patients with diabetic retinopathy. *Am J Ophthalmol.* 2001;132:659–667.

72. Shah GK. Photodynamic therapy for choroidal neovascularization after thermal laser photocoagulation for diabetic macular edema. *Am J Ophthalmol.* 2003;135:114–116.

73. Valmaggia C, Niederberger H, Helbig H. Photodynamic therapy for choroidal neovascularization in fundus flavimaculatus. *Retina.* 2002;22:111–113.

74. Wong SC, Fong KC, Lee N, et al. Successful photodynamic therapy for subretinal neovascularization due to Sorsby's fundus dystrophy: 1-year follow-up. *Br J Ophthalmol.* 2003;87:796–797.

75. Menchini U, Giacomelli G, Cappelli S, et al. Photodynamic therapy in adult-onset vitelliform macular dystrophy misdiagnosed as choroidal neovascularization. *Arch Ophthalmol.* 2002;120:1761–1763. *Arch Ophthalmol.* 2003;121:417.

76. Battaglia Parodi M, Da Pozzo S, Ravalico G. Photodynamic therapy for choroidal neovascularization associated with pattern dystrophy. *Retina.* 2003;23:171–176.

77. Dantas MA, Slakter JS, Negrao S, et al. Photodynamic therapy with verteporfin in malattia leventinese. *Ophthalmology.* 2002;109:296–301.

78. Rodríguez-Coleman H, Spaide RF, Yannuzzi LA. Treatment of angiomatous lesions of the retina with photodynamic therapy. *Retina.* 2002;22:228–232.

79. Schmidt-Erfurth U, Kusserow C, Barbazetto IA, et al. Benefits and complications of photodynamic therapy of papillary capillary hemangiomas. *Ophthalmology.* 2002;109:1,256–1,266.

80. Battaglia Parodi M, Da Pozzo S, Toto L, et al. Photodynamic therapy for choroidal neovascularization associated with choroidal osteoma. *Retina.* 2001;21:660–661.

81. Wang LK, Kansal S, Pulido JS. Photodynamic therapy for the treatment of choroidal neovascularization secondary to rubella retinopathy. *Am J Ophthalmol.* 2002;134:790–792.

82. Muller VA, Ruokonen P, Schellenbeck M, et al. Treatment of rubeosis iridis with photodynamic therapy with verteporfin. A new therapeutic and prophylactic option for patients with the risk of neovascular glaucoma? *Ophthalmic Res.* 2003;35:60–64.

83. Fossarello M, Peiretti E, Zucca I, et al. Photodynamic therapy of corneal neovascularization with verteporfin. *Cornea.* 2003;22:485–488.

84. Fine SL, Berger JW, Maguire MG. Age-related macular degeneration. *N Engl J Med.* 2000;342:483–492.

85. Asensio Sanchez VM, Corral Azor A, Garcia Pascual A. Verteporfin and photosensitivity in diabetics. *Arch Soc Esp Oftalmol.* 2003;78:277–279.

86. Borodoker N, Spaide RF, Maranan L, et al. Verteporfin infusion-associated pain. *Am J Ophthalmol.* 2002;133:211–214.

87. Tornambe PE. Using intravenous diphenhydramine to minimize back pain associated with photodynamic therapy with verteporfin. *Arch Ophthalmol.* 2002;120:872.

88. Noffke AS, Jampol LM, Weinberg DV, et al. A potentially life-threatening adverse reaction to verteporfin. *Arch Ophthalmol.* 2001;119:143.

89. Kang SW, Kang SJ, Kim HO, et al. Photodynamic therapy using verteporfin-induced minimal change nephrotic syndrome. *Am J Ophthalmol.* 2002;134:907–908.

90. Gelisken F, Inhoffen W, Partsch M, et al. Retinal pigment epithelial tear after photodynamic therapy for choroidal neovascularization. *Am J Ophthalmol.* 2001;131:518–520.

91. Srivastava SK, Sternberg P Jr. Retinal pigment epithelial tear weeks following photodynamic therapy with verteporfin for choroidal neovascularization secondary to pathologic myopia. *Retina.* 2002;22:669–671.

92. Theodossiadis GP, Panagiotidis D, Georgalas IG, et al. Retinal hemorrhage after photodynamic therapy in patients with subfoveal choroidal neovascularization caused by age-related macular degeneration. *Graefes Arch Clin Exp Ophthalmol.* 2003;241:13–18.

93. Battaglia Parodi M, Da Pozzo S. Hot spots after photodynamic therapy for choroidal neovascularization in age-related macular degeneration. *Retina.* 2002;22:671–673.

94. Mansour AM, Husseini ZM, Schakal AR. Macular hole following photodynamic therapy. *Ophthalmic Surg Lasers.* 2002;33:511–513.

95. Cohen SY, Bulik A, Tadayoni R, et al. Visual hallucinations and Charles Bonnet syndrome after photodynamic therapy for age-related macular degeneration. *Br J Ophthalmol.* 2003;87:977–979.

96. Treatment of Age-Related Macular Degeneration with Photodynamic Therapy (TAP) Study Group. Verteporfin therapy of subfoveal choroidal neovascularization in patients with age-related macular degeneration. Additional information regarding baseline lesion composition's impact on vision outcomes—TAP report no. 3. *Arch Ophthalmol.* 2002;120:1,443–1,454.

97. Jampol LM, Scott L. Treatment of juxtafoveal and extrafoveal choroidal neovascularization in era of photodynamic therapy with verteporfin. *Am J Ophthalmol.* 2002;134:99–101.

98. Cohen SY, Bulik A, Dubois L, et al. Photodynamic therapy for juxtafoveal choroidal neovascularization in myopic eyes. *Am J Ophthalmol.* 2003;136:371–374.

99. Packo KH, Dwarakanathan S, Orth DH, et al. Comparison of standardized MPS protocol visual acuity and non-standardized Snellen acuity in age-related macular degeneration. *Invest Ophthalmol Vis Sci.* 2001;42:S449.

100. Farah ME, Costa RA, Muccioli C, et al. Photodynamic therapy with verteporfin for subfoveal choroidal neovascularization in Vogt-Koyanagi-Harada syndrome. *Am J Ophthalmol.* 2002;134:137–139.

101. Mimouni KF, Bressler SB, Bressler NM. Photodynamic therapy with verteporfin for subfoveal choroidal neovascularization in children. *Am J Ophthalmol.* 2003;135:900–902.

102. Verteporfin roundtable 2000 and 2001 participants. Treatment of Age-Related Macular Degeneration with Photodynamic Therapy (TAP) Study Group principal investigators, Verteporfin in Photodynamic Therapy (VIP) Study Group principal investigators. Guidelines for using verteporfin in photodynamic therapy to treat choroidal neovascularization due to age-related macular degeneration and other causes. *Retina.* 2002;22:6–18.

103. Eter N, Vogel A, Inhetvin-Hutter C, et al. Interval reduction of photodynamic therapy in age-related macular degeneration is not advantageous. A pilot project. *Ophthalmologe.* 2003;100:314–317.

104. Gelisken F, Bartz-Schmidt KU. Visual prognosis and patient selection. *Ophthalmologe.* 2002;99:144–149.

105. Bressler NM. Early detection and treatment of neovascular age-related macular degeneration. *J Am Board Fam Pract*. 2002;15:142–152.

106. Haddad WM, Coscas G, Soubrane G. Eligibility for treatment and angiographic features at the early stage of exudative age-related macular degeneration. *Br J Ophthalmol*. 2002;86:663–669.

107. Rubin GS, Bressler NM, The Treatment of Age-Related Macular Degeneration with Photodynamic Therapy (TAP) Study Group. Effects of verteporfin therapy on contrast sensitivity. Results from the Treatment of Age-Related Macular Degeneration with Photodynamic Therapy (TAP) investigation—TAP report no. 4. *Retina*. 2002;22:536–544.

108. Kusserow C, Michels S, Schmidt-Erfurth U. Chorioretinal anastomosis as unfavourable prognostic factor during photodynamic therapy. *Ophthalmologe*. 2003;100:197–202.

109. Montero JA, Ruiz-Moreno JM. Verteporfin photodynamic therapy in highly myopic subfoveal choroidal neovascularization. *Br J Ophthalmol*. 2003;87:173–176.

110. La Cour M, Kiilgaard JF, Nissen MH. Age-related macular degeneration: epidemiology and optimal treatment. *Drugs Aging*. 2002;19:101–133.

111. Landy J, Brown GC. Update on photodynamic therapy. *Curr Opin Ophthalmol*. 2003;14:163–168.

112. Mandal N, Chisholm IH. Identifying the proportion of age-related macular degeneration patients who would benefit from photodynamic therapy with verteporfin. *Br J Ophthalmol*. 2002;86:118–121.

113. Margherio RR, Margherio AR, De Santis ME. Laser treatments with verteporfin therapy and its potential impact on retinal practices. *Retina*. 2000;20:325–330.

114. Rechtman E, Ciulla TA, Criswell MH, et al. An update on photodynamic therapy in age-related macular degeneration. *Expert Opin Pharmacother*. 2002;3:931–938.

115. Kaiser RS, Berger JW, Williams GA, et al. Variability in fluorescein angiography interpretation for photodynamic therapy in age-related macular degeneration. *Retina*. 2002;22:683–690.

116. Sharma S, Brown GC, Brown MM, et al. The cost-effectiveness of photodynamic therapy for fellow eyes with subfoveal choroidal neovascularization secondary to age-related macular degeneration. *Ophthalmology*. 2001;108:2,051–2,059.

117. Meads C, Salas C, Roberts T, et al. Clinical effectiveness and cost-utility of photodynamic therapy for wet age-related macular degeneration: a systematic review and economic evaluation. *Health Technol Assess*. 2003;7:1–108.

118. Soubrane G, Bressler NM. Treatment of subfoveal choroidal neovascularization in age-related macular degeneration: a focus on clinical application of verteporfin photodynamic therapy. *Br J Ophthalmol*. 2001;85:483–495.

119. Ghazi NG, Jabbour NM, De La Cruz ZC, et al. Clinicopathologic studies of age-related macular degeneration with classic subfoveal choroidal neovascularization treated with photodynamic therapy. *Retina*. 2001;21:478–486.

120. Schnurrbusch UE, Welt K, Horn LC, et al. Histological findings of surgically excised choroidal neovascular membranes after photodynamic therapy. *Br J Ophthalmol*. 2001;85:1,086–1,091.

121. Moshfeghi DM, Kaiser PK, Grossniklaus HE, et al. Clinicopathologic study after submacular removal of choroidal neovascular membranes treated with verteporfin ocular photodynamic therapy. *Am J Ophthalmol*. 2003;135:343–350.

122. Arroyo JG, Michaud N, Jakobiec FA. Choroidal neovascular membranes treated with photodynamic therapy. *Arch Ophthalmol*. 2003;121:898–903.

123. Anand R, Bressler NM, Bressler SB, et al. "Improvement after verteporfin therapy" writing committee for TAP Study Group. Improvement after verteporfin therapy. *Arch Ophthalmol*. 2003;121:415–416.

124. Elsner H, Schmidt-Erfurth U. Photodynamic therapy of subfoveal choroidal neovascularization. Analysis of fixation behavior. *Ophthalmologe*. 2002;99:620–624.

125. Tholen AM, Bernasconi PP, Fierz AB, et al. Reading ability after photodynamic therapy for age-related macular degeneration and for high myopia. *Ophthalmologe*. 2003;100:28–32.

126. Ergun E, Maar N, Radner W, et al. Scotoma size and reading speed in patients with subfoveal occult choroidal neovascularization in age-related macular degeneration. *Ophthalmology*. 2003;110:65–69.

127. Parodi MB, Da Pozzo S, Ravalico G. Angiographic features after photodynamic therapy for choroidal neovascularization in age-related macular degeneration and pathological myopia. *Br J Ophthalmol*. 2003;87:177–183.

128. Tan W, Beaumont PE, Chang AA. Case series outcomes at 1 week following verteporfin photodynamic therapy. *Retina*. 2003;23:166–170.

129. Michels S, Barbazetto I, Schmidt-Erfurth U. Changes in neovascular membranes and normal choroid blood vessels after multiple photodynamic therapy treatments. *Ophthalmologe*. 2002;99:96–100.

130. Schmidt-Erfurth U, Michels S, Barbazetto I, et al. Photodynamic effects on choroidal neovascularization and physiological choroid. *Invest Ophthalmol Vis Sci*. 2002;43:830–841.

131. Ruther K, Breidenbach K, Schwartz R, et al. Testing central retinal function with multifocal electroretinography before and after photodynamic therapy. *Ophthalmology*. 2003;100:459–464.

132. Moschos MN, Panayotidis D, Moschos MM, et al. A preliminary assessment of macular function by MF-ERG in myopic eyes with CNV with complete response to photodynamic therapy. *Eur J Ophthalmol*. 2003;13:461–467.

133. Rogers AH, Martidis A, Greenberg PB, et al. Optic coherence tomography findings following photodynamic therapy of choroidal neovascularization. *Am J Ophthalmol*. 2002;134:566–576.

134. Costa RA, Farah ME, Cardillo JA, et al. Immediate indocyanine green angiography and optical coherence tomography evaluation after photodynamic therapy for subfoveal choroidal neovascularization. *Retina*. 2003;23:159–165.

135. Grossniklaus HE, Brooks HL Jr, Sippy BD, et al. Retinal translocation and photodynamic therapy for age-related macular degeneration with classic choroidal neovascularization: a clinicopathologic case report. *Retina*. 2002;22:818–824.

136. Fujii GY, de Juan E Jr, Humayun MS, et al. Limited macular translocation for the management of subfoveal choroidal neovascularization after photodynamic therapy. *Am J Ophthalmol*. 2003;135:109–112.

137. Pieramici DJ, de Juan E, Fujii GY et al. Limited inferior macular translocation for the treatment of subfoveal choroidal neovascularization secondary to age-related macular degeneration. *Am J Ophthalmol*. 2000;130:419–428.

138. Piermarocchi S, Lo Giudice G, Sartore M, et al. Photodynamic therapy increases the eligibility for feeder vessel treatment of choroidal neovascularization caused by age-related macular degeneration. *Am J Ophthalmol*. 2002;133:572–555.

139. Spaide RF, Sorenson J, Maranan L. Combined photodynamic therapy with verteporfin and intravitreal triamcinolone acetonide for choroidal neovascularization. *Ophthalmology*. 2003;110:1,517–1,525.

Transpupillary Thermotherapy for the Treatment of Choroidal Neovascularization Associated with Age-Related Macular Degeneration

18

Peter E. Liggett   *Alejandro J. Lavaque*   *Eric P. Jablon*   *Elias Reichel*
Hugo Quiroz-Mercado

INTRODUCTION

Age-related macular degeneration (AMD) is the leading cause of central vision loss in patients older than 65 years of age in the developed world, and the third leading cause in developing countries. Although most patients with AMD have the geographic, or dry form, approximately 25% will develop choroidal neovascularization (CNV) (1,2). Choroidal neovascular membranes invade the subretinal pigmented epithelium (sub-RPE) and subretinal spaces through cracks in Bruch's membrane, and cause mechanical and cellular damage to the outer retina. If left untreated, CNV can lead to progressive and irreversible loss of sight. In particular, subfoveal CNV may cause profound central vision disruption.

Until recently, the only options available to patients with AMD and subfoveal CNV were observation or thermal laser treatment of the neovascular membrane. Argon laser photocoagulation treatment for classic CNV reduces the incidence of severe vision loss in patients with extrafoveal and juxtafoveal neovascular membranes. However, few patients meet the strict guidelines established by the Macular Photocoagulation Study Group for treatment of subfoveal CNV, and those treated often had an immediate decline in visual acuity (5). With limited exceptions, the natural course of CNV leads to irreversible disciform scarring in the macula and a dense central scotoma. Because of these devastating consequences of CNV, numerous medical and surgical therapeutic alternatives have been proposed (6–20).

Photodynamic therapy (PDT) involves the intravenous administration of a photosensitizing drug followed by the application of nonthermal laser light to the affected tissue, which incites a local photochemical reaction and thrombosis within the abnormal choroidal vascular membranes. PDT does not affect normal retinal vasculature, and thus offers a potential treatment for subfoveal CNV without the immediate loss of central vision induced by the thermal laser. Unfortunately, PDT has been found to be beneficial only for patients with a predominantly classic CNV or a purely occult CNV. Moreover, patients who receive PDT for purely occult CNV do not seem to fare any better than untreated patients (7). In patients treated with PDT for occult CNV, only 34% had stable or improved visual acuity at 12 months, while in the control group, 23% had stable or improved visual acuity. Another problem is the lack of insurance coverage for PDT in patients with other forms of CNV who require treatment.

For patients with minimally classic lesions, recent trials indicate that transpupillary thermotherapy (TTT) is effective in stabilizing CNV as well visual acuity (10,11). TTT is a treatment modality that uses a large spot size, low irradiance (810 nm), and long exposure times with infrared light, which increases the fundus temperature and creates a selective, irreversible cytotoxic effect. TTT creates a subthreshold photocoagulation in retinal and choroidal tissue with no visible endpoint and no ophthalmoscopically apparent damage to the posterior pole. Heating the retina and choroid results in CNV closure and the resorption of intraretinal and subretinal fluid in a significant number of cases (Fig. 18.1) (10,19,20,24,25).

BASICS

Effects of Laser Energy on the Retina and Choroid

Near-infrared irradiation is well suited for treating macular disease because it has high tissue penetration and minimal ocular media absorption. In addition, it is poorly absorbed by hemoglobin and xanthophylls, allowing transmission through preretinal and subretinal hemorrhage, and reducing nerve fiber layer damage (6). In general, retinal absorption of radiation can produce (a) photomechanical disruption, (b) thermal injury, and (c) phototoxicity. Photomechanical retinal damage may occur when intense laser irradiance produces plasma, vapor, or acoustic waves, which can cause rapid chorioretinal distortion. An Nd:YAG laser exerts its therapeutic effect by producing mechanical light damage. Thermal injury occurs when radiation from lasers and other intense light sources causes denaturation of chorioretinal proteins and damage to other thermosensitive molecular components of the retina. Conventional short-pulse argon laser photocoagulation is a suprathreshold procedure that elevates retinal temperatures 40°C to 60°C above the normal body temperature of 37°C. Suprathreshold photocoagulation produces instantaneous tissue damage and results in retinal scar formation. Retinal phototoxicity may occur after prolonged exposure to intense blue light or ultraviolet radiation, which leads to photochemical reactions that damage the retina (26).

Unlike conventional short-pulse retinal photocoagulation, TTT uses lengthy exposure times and large retinal spot sizes to produce subthreshold retinal irradiances, as shown in Table 18.1 (26). Characteristics of long-pulse irradiance include: (a) deeper chorioretinal tissue penetration than visible light, (b) decreased photoreceptor pigment bleaching, (c) less energy transmission to bipolar cell axons within the macula, and (d) negligible risk of retinal phototoxicity. Melanin in the RPE and choroid converts laser radiation into heat energy, which increases the temperature of the treated tissue (Fig. 18.2). The photothermal effect produced by a laser beam is a function of laser power, spot size, power density (irradiance in W/cm²), the wavelength dependent coefficient of absorption for the specific tissue, and the duration of the irradiation. Power density, or irradiance, is the concentration of laser beam power in terms of power per unit area and is expressed as W/cm².

$$(P \times 100)/\pi r^2 = W/cm^2$$

P: represents the laser power in Watts.

r: is the radius of the laser spot in mm.

This formula indicates that the laser spot radius and power density (or irradiation) have an inverse relationship. As the radius spot increases, power density decreases. Therefore, larger optical spots require greater power to maintain proper irradiance.

While irradiance is laser power per unit area, radiant exposure is energy per unit area. Radiant exposure represents the density of laser beam energy and is defined as the energy per unit area incident upon a surface and is expressed in units of J/cm².

$$[Q(J) \times 100]/\pi r^2 = J/cm^2$$

Moreover, energy is the capacity to perform work over a period of time. Energy is measured by determining the delivery of power over intervals of time and is expressed as:

$$Energy = Power \times Time$$

Laser light energy is measured in J, with one J equal to one W/sec. If the power decreases and the time interval remains the same, energy will decrease. Energy may remain constant with corresponding changes in both power and time. For example, 1 J of energy can be delivered with 2 W of power in 0.5 second or by 0.5 W of power in 2 seconds.

$$Irradiance = power/area = W/cm^2$$
$$Radiant\ exposure = [power \times time]/area = J/cm^2$$

Retinal temperature rise in laser therapy is proportional to retinal irradiance for a particular spot size, exposure duration, and wavelength. TTT is a low irradiance, large spot size, long-pulse (continuous wave mode), infrared laser photocoagulation protocol.

Effects of Transpupillary Thermotherapy on the Retina and Choroid

Transpupillary thermotherapy may produce different and synergetic mechanisms against choroidal neovascularization (19).

Thermal Obliteration

TTT may result in thermal obliteration of the choroidal vasculature. Near infrared wavelengths are not significantly

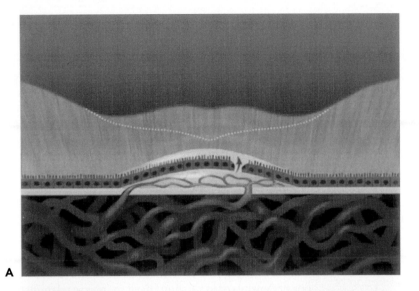

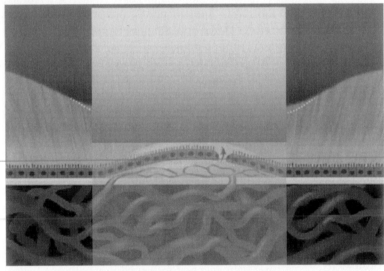

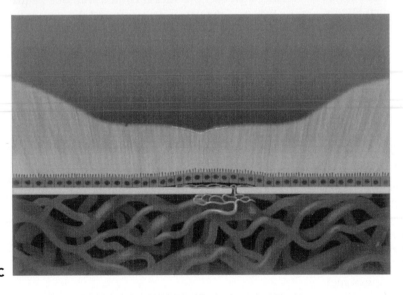

Figure 18.1 **A**. Eyes with vision loss due to subfoveal occult CNV (fibrovascular RPE detachments and late leakage of undetermined source). **B**. Hyperthermia induced by laser absorption by natural pigments located primarily in RPE. **C**. Reduction in leakage and resorption of exudation. The fovea flattens and vision may stabilize or improve. (Images courtesy of IRIDEX Corporation, Mountain View, CA.)

absorbed by hemoglobin. Therefore, vascular damage most likely occurs by heat conversion from the pigmented targets of the radiation, including RPE cells and choroidal melanocytes. In other words, the light absorption centers lie outside the vessel lumen, and vascular endothelium is damaged by heat radiating from melanin granules toward the vessel wall. Blood flow in the microcirculation during TTT is bimodal, with blood flow increasing at temperatures between 40°C to 43°C and decreasing above 43°C (27). During a therapeutic treatment of CNV, TTT increases the retinal temperature approximately 10°C over the normal body temperature of

	PDT (Photodynamic Therapy)	TTT (Transpupillary Thermotherapy)	Conventional Short-pulse Photocoagulation
Wavelength	Diode red laser (689 nm)	Diode infrared laser (819 nm)	Green, yellow, red and infrared lasers (514–810 nm)
Pulse duration	83 sec	60 sec	Microseconds to a few seconds
Laser-tissue irradiance	Photochemical (drug activation)	Photothermal (photocoagulation)	Photothermal (photocoagulation)
Maximal retinal temperature rise	2°C (65 mW, 83 sec, 3 mm spot diameter)	10°C (800 mW, 60 sec, 3 mm spot diameter)	42°C (514–810 nm, ±150 mW, ±0.1 sec, ±200 u spot diameter)

TABLE 18.1

THERAPEUTIC LASERS: TRANSPUPILLARY THERMOTHERAPY, PHOTODYNAMIC THERAPY, AND CONVENTIONAL SHORT-PULSE RETINAL PHOTOCOAGULATION

(Modified from Mainster MA, Reichel E. Transpupillary thermotherapy for age-related macular degeneration: long-pulse photocoagulation, apoptosis, and heat shock proteins. *Ophthalmic Surg Lasers.* 2000;31:359–373.)

37°C. A threshold laser burn is a retinal lesion that is just barely visible ophthalmoscopically during treatment. Considering that the threshold temperature is approximately 46°C to 47°C in the normal retina (28), TTT may either be a threshold or subthreshold photocoagulation procedure. In those cases where CNV exists, the threshold could rise for two reasons: (a) the neovascular net may hinder transmission of the laser light to the RPE cells and the choroid (highest source of energy absorption), and (b) the presence of subretinal fluid can attenuate the transmission of heat to the retina. In these instances, a higher power setting may be necessary to achieve the desired therapeutic result.

RPE Activities

RPE may undergo transformation, proliferation, migration, and secretion in response to TTT. TTT may stimulate RPE proliferation from viable cells at the edges of breaks in Bruch's membrane. Proliferated RPE cells tightly envelope newly formed vessels, and probably assist in reabsorbing any accumulated subretinal fluid (29). Moreover, in vitro cultures of human retinal pigment epithelial cells released

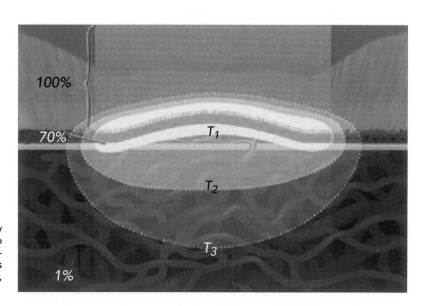

Figure 18.2 Downward heat sink effect by choroidal circulation, (<10°C rise, $T_1 > T_2 > T_3$). No ophthalmoscopic or FA evidence of retinal damage. Secondary effect on CNV membrane. (Images courtesy of IRIDEX Corporation, Mountain View, CA.)

higher levels of an inhibitor of neovascularization (30). The combination of these two special activities could close or limit the growth of certain CNV.

Intravascular Thrombosis

TTT probably results in tissue hyperthermia, which stimulates the production of free radicals that cause endothelial cell damage. In turn, endothelial damage leads to thrombogenesis and clot formation inside the vessel lumen. There is evidence that pH may decrease during hyperthermia, causing increased rigidity of red blood cell membranes, which directly impacts the viscosity of blood. Lower pH also renders the endothelial cells more sensitive to heat. Endothelial cell swelling reduces the effective diameter of the blood vessels and reduces flow. Other associated inflammatory effects of TTT include leukocyte adhesion and increased vascular permeability (28). Leukocyte adhesion to vessel walls also decreases their functional diameter (27).

Gradient Pressure

Choroidal neovascularization probably requires a threshold pressure gradient to remain open. TTT could close feeder arteriolar vessels and veins from the choroid that supply and drain the neovascular complex. As a result, choriocapillaris blood flow underlying the CNV is also reduced, thus increasing the resistance in the interior of the neovascular complex, inducing closure (31). On the other hand, flow resistance in the choriocapillaris and the CNV might also be increased by interstitial pressure and edema caused by extravasated fluid after hyperthermia. Ciulla and Harris demonstrated the changes that TTT produced in choroidal perfusion as well as in posterior ciliary arteries with the consequent redistribution of blood flow in the posterior eye circulation (32). Treatment repetition, with coherent intervals, could induce the progressive closure of the neovascular net through transient changes in perfusion dynamics.

Neovascular Apoptosis

Recent studies have speculated that low-subthreshold hyperthermia may destroy target cells by apoptosis rather than accidental cell death. Accidental cell death is a passive process in which there is cytoplasmic swelling, rupture of cell membranes, and local inflammation caused by leakage of cellular debris into the extracellular space. On the other hand, apoptosis is a programmed, active, energy-dependent process associated with cytoplasmic shrinkage. Packaged cellular debris produced in apoptosis is removed with a comparatively mild inflammatory reaction by adjacent cells that are typically not primary phagocytes. Accidental cell death and apoptosis both lead to necrosis. Apoptosis plays an important role in the involution of choroidal neovascularization (26).

Heat Shock Proteins

Heat shock proteins (HSPs), also called "stress proteins," are a group of proteins that are present in all cells in all life forms. They are induced when a cell undergoes various types of environmental stressors, such as heat, cold, or oxygen deprivation (33). HSPs are also present in cells under perfectly normal conditions. Hyperthermia induces cellular stress and the consequent production of HSPs in surviving cells (34). HSPs provide transient protection for surviving cells against a new, higher dose of heat (thermotolerance). The photoreceptor layer (26) and choroidal vessels (34) are the primary sites of HSP production after hyperthermic stress. Thus, hyperthermia transiently protects the surviving retina against subsequent photodamage. This protection is greatest 18 hours after hyperthermia, coinciding with the time of maximal HSP production. This phenomenon opens the door for new therapeutic strategies. For example, the application of a standard TTT treatment (810 nm wavelength, 3 mm spot diameter, 60-second exposure duration) may produce an increase in photoreceptor thermotolerance. Subsequently, if a therapeutic 800 mW TTT treatment for CNV were performed 18 to 24 hours later, previously induced thermotolerance might help protect the outer retina from thermal injury (26). Increased HSP production after TTT probably decreases the amount of necrosis and inflammation within the choroidal tissue, leading to a decrease in the stimulus for neovascularization. The continuous improvement in exudation that is observed for months after a TTT procedure in some patients would be consistent with the hypothesis that the treatment may interrupt a vicious cycle (34). Nevertheless, it is important to keep in mind that, in some patients, the window of efficiency of the temperature elevation is slightly below the photocoagulation threshold. The term *heat dose* is often used to emphasize that both the magnitude of the hyperthermia and the duration of exposure determine the final cellular effect. According to this notion, with low temperatures, the duration of exposure has to be increased in order to reach the same degree of HSP hyperexpression and thermotolerance (35). Some authors have proposed that decreased levels of heat shock proteins in the retina during aging may contribute to the apparent increased susceptibility of photoreceptors to age-acquired retinal disease (36).

Inhibition of Angiogenesis

Laser-irradiated RPE may produce antiangiogenic factors that could possibly play a role in the inhibition of new vessel formation (37). Moreover, HSP hyperexpression could be one of the first steps toward production of cytokines (36).

Fluorescein and Indocyanine Green Angiography After Transpupillary Thermotherapy

TTT induces a dynamic sequence of vascular changes demonstrable on fluorescein angiography (FA) and indocyanine green angiography ICGA (27). Within 1 hour after treatment, FA and ICGA demonstrate hyperfluorescence

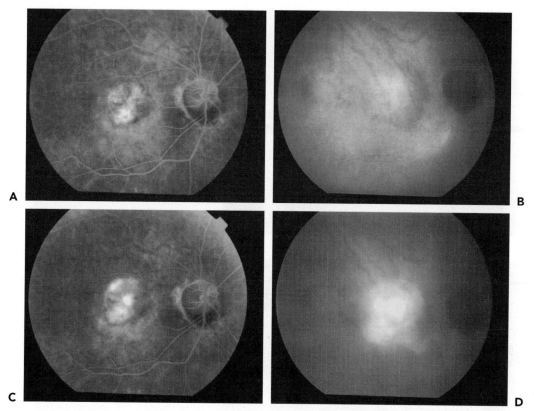

Figure 18.3   FA and ICGA before (**A** and **B**) and 1 hour after (**C** and **D**) TTT of occult CNV due to AMD. Both FA and ICGA show increased leakage activity. The margins of the treated area corresponding to the laser spot are well delineated by ICGA after treatment. (From Lanzetta P, Michieletto P, Pirracchio A, et al. Fluorescein and indocyanine green angiography after transpupillary thermotherapy of choroidal neovascularization. Early vascular changes. *Semin Ophthalmol.* 2001;16:97–100.)

caused by increased leakage of new vessels and choroidal vasculature (Figs. 18.3 and 18.4). After 1 week, FA and ICGA showed hypofluorescence covering the entire irradiated area, and the leakage from CNV membranes subsided (Figs. 18.5 and 18.6). Follow-up at 1 and 3 weeks demonstrated that the vascular closing continued. At 4 weeks after TTT, FA showed mottled hyperfluorescence of the treated area and the absence of angiographic leakage.

Vascular changes associated with TTT include local and general variations in the choroidal and posterior ciliary arterial blood flow. Dose changes include a transiently decreased volumetric blood flow in the retinal circulation 24 hours after treatment. In the posterior ciliary arteries, there are no changes observed at 24 hours. However, at 1 month, there is a decrease in the mean end diastolic velocity (EDV) and an increase in the resistive index (RI) in both the nasal and temporal sides of the choroids (32).

Importance of Melanin Concentration in the Ocular Fundus

The presence of melanin in the normal human eye is perhaps more important than the presence of melanin in the skin. Since the pigmented cells in the eye are mostly nondividing and practically no melanin renewal is known to occur, the ocular pigmentation once constituted must last for a person's entire life. Thus, the biological consequences of any structural modification that may occur in eye melanin as a result of environmental insults, or simply of aging, are potentially much more severe than those of skin melanin modification (38).

While some authors conclude that eyes with a high concentration of melanin have less risk of developing AMD (39–41), others have not been able to demonstrate this protective effect (42,43). Notwithstanding, it is clear that the two most important risk factors for AMD are age and advanced disease in the fellow eye (43).

The human RPE contains two classes of pigment— melanin and lipofuscin—that are quite different in terms of development and function. In contrast to melanin, RPE lipofuscin develops after birth and continues to increase with age. Lipofuscin is thought to represent the endproducts of oxidative damage to lipids, possibly derived from the phagocytosis, and the digestion of photoreceptors. An inverse relationship exists between melanin and lipofuscin in the RPE. While the amounts of both choroidal and RPE melanin tend to decrease with aging, the amount of RPE lipofuscin tends to increase (44).

Lipofuscin content in the RPE increases from the equator to the posterior pole, with a consistent dip in the macular

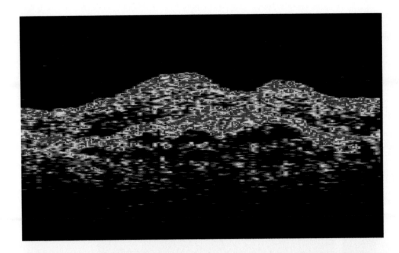

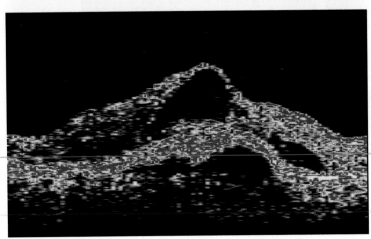

Figure 18.4 OCT before (*top*) and 1 hour after (*bottom*) TTT in the same patient shown in Fig. 18.1. Before treatment, CNV can be appreciated beneath the fovea. A discrete amount of subretinal and intraretinal fluid is also present. Immediately after treatment, OCT shows an acute inflammatory response with increased thickening of the treated area due to the accumulation of subretinal and intraretinal fluid. (From Lanzetta P, Michieletto P, Pirracchio A, et al. Fluorescein and indocyanine green angiography after transpupillary thermotherapy of choroidal neovascularization. Early vascular changes. *Semin Ophthalmol.* 2001;16:97–100.)

area. In contrast, RPE melanin decreases from the equator to the posterior pole, with a consistent peak at the macula. Choroidal melanin, like RPE, increases gradually from the equator to the posterior pole, with the highest levels located in the submacular choroid (40). In addition, melanin and lipofuscin are distributed differently within the RPE cells. Melanin has a higher concentration in the apical aspect of the cell, whereas lipofuscin is concentrated more basally. This polarity of both pigments is more pronounced in younger eyes than adult ones. While the RPE melanin concentration tends to decrease with age in Whites and Blacks, lipofuscin increases as an effect of aging. In other words, there is an inverse relationship between RPE melanin and lipofuscin concentration in the elderly patient (39,43).

Black individuals have a significantly greater total choroidal melanin concentration than Whites. Choroidal melanin concentrations are approximately 2.5 times higher in the outer choroid (half near the sclera) than in the inner choroid (half adjacent to the RPE). Although the melanin of the RPE and choroid are superimposed upon each other, it is useful to know their optical density in relation to each other when exposed to light in vivo (44). Altogether, the concentration of ocular pigment and its topographic distribution under the macular area has profound implications in the absorption of laser light and the generation of heat during TTT.

Histopathology after Transpupillary Thermotherapy

TTT is a subthreshold photocoagulation treatment with no visible endpoint and no ophthalmoscopically apparent choroidal or retinal damage. However, histologic changes have been demonstrated after subthreshold retinal hyperthermia. Under experimental conditions, TTT produces the following changes (45–47):

1. Nerve fiber layer edema and ganglion cell damage.
2. Pyknotic and vacuolization changes in the inner and outer nuclear layers.
3. Damage in the outer photoreceptor segments with separation from the RPE.
4. Focal disruption of cellular membranes.
5. Accumulation of subretinal fluid.
6. Disruption of the RPE layer with areas of separation from Bruch's membrane.
7. Dispersion of pigment granules among the outer segments of photoreceptors cells.

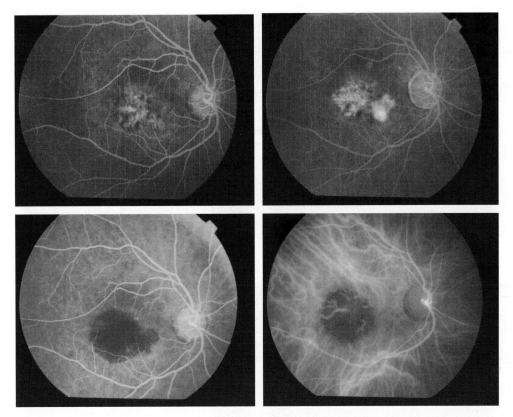

Figure 18.5 TTT of occult CNV due to AMD. *Top left* and *right*: Early and late phases of FA before TTT. *Bottom left* and *right*: FA and ICGA 1 week after TTT. Both FA and ICGA show the exact contour of the treated area that appears homogeneously hypofluorescent with FA. Large choroidal vessels within the dark spot can be seen with ICGA. (From Lanzetta P, Michieletto P, Pirracchio A, et al. Fluorescein and indocyanine green angiography after transpupillary thermotherapy of choroidal neovascularization. Early vascular changes. *Semin Ophthalmol.* 2001;16:97–100).

8. Choriocapillaris congestion and vessel closure.
9. Large choroidal vessels appear normal.

Extrapolating this experimental data to eyes with exudative AMD has limitations. Eyes with CNV have subretinal fluid and other exudative materials such as lipid and blood in the subretinal or sub-RPE space. On the other hand, there is abnormal fibrovascular tissue at the level of the RPE. It is highly likely that these pathologic features would influence the effects of the local temperature increase induced by TTT. Subretinal fluid, for example, probably helps to minimize any excessive heat damage by TTT to the neurosensory retina (46).

STRATEGIES, PARAMETERS, TECHNIQUE, AND THERMODYNAMICS

Although TTT offers advantages over conventional thermal lasers for the treatment of subfoveal CNV, one problem with TTT is that it is difficult to titrate. The 810 nm wavelength (diode laser) selectively affects pigmented structures. Melanosomes are the initial target of hyperthermia. The observation that structures containing melanin are affected by higher temperatures, while nonmelanized tissues are spared, demonstrates that diode laser irradiation is absorbed by melanin (48). In other words, a challenge of TTT is selecting laser power levels that are neither too low nor too excessive, but that are sufficient to alter the natural history of the lesions and trigger the desired pathophysiologic and therapeutic responses (27). For this reason, it is important to determine the melanin concentration in a patient's fundus before initiating treatment.

Determining the Pigmentation of the Ocular Fundus

At the moment, our methods for evaluating fundus pigmentation are still rudimentary, and all of the potential parameters at our disposal, including skin pigmentation, hair color, and fundoscopy, should be used to determine laser power settings until more quantitative methods are routinely available. In general, laser power settings must be progressively diminished with increasing patient pigmentation because the amount of energy absorbed by tissue is proportional to pigmentation levels. The dividing line between heating and burning depends on the concentration of RPE and choroidal pigment. The laser parameters

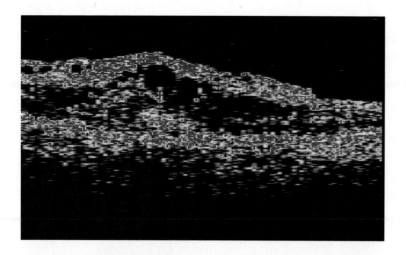

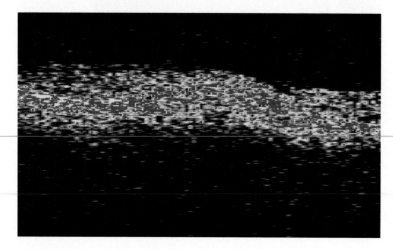

Figure 18.6 OCT before (*top*) and 1 week after (*bottom*) TTT of CNV. Before treatment, the exam shows retinal fluid associated with the CNV. One week after treatment, fluid has completely reabsorbed and a more normal contour is noted. Note also that the retina has increased its reflectivity homogeneously. This pattern might represent the sequelae of the inflammatory response to treatment. (From Lanzetta P, Michieletto P, Pirracchio A, et al. Fluorescein and indocyanine green angiography after transpupillary thermotherapy of choroidal neovascularization. Early vascular changes. *Semin Ophthalmol.* 2001;16:97–100)

recommended for the treatment of CNV in AMD have been established based on a Caucasian, lightly pigmented population, and should probably be readjusted for individual patients according to the amount of fundus pigmentation.

Fundus pigmentation closely corresponds to iris pigmentation (39) and could be categorized as:

1. Darkly pigmented fundus.
2. Medium-light pigmented fundus.
3. Lightly pigmented fundus (42).

On the other hand, the skin phototype and chromotype are important variables. The skin phototype could be assessed according to the Fitzpatrick Classification (49), with individual patients recalling burning tendency and tanning ability following 2 hours of unprotected sun exposure around noon on a sunny day in early summer. Based on this assessment, six skin types could be defined:

1. Always burn, never tan.
2. Usually burn, tan less than the average.
3. Sometimes burn mildly, tan about average.
4. Rarely burn, tan more than average.
5. Brown-skinned.
6. Black-skinned.

The Fitzpatrick Classification has some weak points, but skin typing has found widespread use in clinical and epidemiological studies because it is quick and easy, and can be performed without any equipment (50).

In white-haired people, the original pigmentary status should be part of the patient history. Information on juvenile (25 years of age) hair color could be recorded as:

1. Red or blond
2. Brown
3. Black

Eye color, defined as the dominant color of the iris, could be assessed during the interview using a clinical, three-point scale:

1. Blue
2. Green or gray
3. Brown or dark

With these data, we can develop a practical strategy for parameters and laser settings (Table 18.2). If the patient has dark hair and/or eyes, it would be wise to diminish the diode laser power by 100 mW for each variable. For example, a patient with skin phototype 3 would require 700 to

TABLE 18.2

PRACTICAL APPROACH FOR PATIENT PARAMETERS AND LASER SETTINGS

Skin Phototype	Constitutive or Unexposed Skin Color	Sunburn and Tanning History	Melanin Pigmentation		Laser Power in mW[a] (Diode 810 nm)
			Immediate Pigment Darkening (IPD)	Delayed Tanning (DT)	
I	Ivory white (pale white)	Burns easily, never tans	None	None	850–1,000
II	White	Burns easily, tans minimally	Weak, IPD ±	Minimal to weak, DT ± or +	750–900
III	White	Burns and tans moderately and uniformly	Definite, low IPD + (light tan)	Low, DT + or ++ (light brown)	700–850
IV	Beige or lightly tanned	Burns minimally, tans easily and moderately	Moderate, IPD ++ (light brown)	Moderate, DT ++ (brown)	650–750
V	Moderate brown or tanned	Rarely burns, tans profusely (dark brown)	Intense, IPD +++ (brown)	Strong, intense DT +++ (dark brown)	550–700
VI	Dark brown or black	Never burns, tans profusely (deep brown or black	Intense, IPD +++ (dark brown)	Strong, intense DT +++ (dark brown)	450–650

[a] If the patient has dark hair and/or dark eyes, the laser power should be diminished 100 mW for each variable.
+++, strong reaction; ++, moderate reaction; +, weak reaction; ±, minimal reaction.

850 mW of laser power over 60 seconds. However, if the patient also had dark hair and iris pigmentation, 200 mW would be subtracted from the initial power. Thus, the first treatment would be carried out with a power of 500 to 650 mW. Of course, this is a conservative algorithm on which diverse adjustments may be conducted, depending on the patient and the experience of the surgeon.

Other Strategies for TTT

For proper realization of this technique, several other parameters should be kept in mind:

1. *Strategies for a correct treatment.* Before beginning the technique, the patient must be properly prepared. TTT should not be performed if the pupil is not sufficiently dilated or if the lesion is too anterior to be reached with a wide-field contact lens. Clarity of the media is also important to maintain effective treatment, because the presence of opacities affects the amount of energy that reaches the retina.
2. *Ocular settings.* Proper ocular settings must be used to ensure that the retinal spot size selected is actually obtained. These settings are easily determined by fogging each eye independently with plus power until the surface of the focusing spot is seen sharply (26).
3. *Power and spot size.* The power needed to produce a particular retinal temperature rise is proportional to the

diameter rather than the area of the laser spot on the retina. Thus, to achieve a particular target temperature rise, laser power must be doubled or halved if spot size is doubled or halved.
4. *Beam circularity.* It is important to maintain a circular laser spot during TTT because any deviation from this could cause increased and irregular tissue target irradiance. An exaggerated contact lens tilt might cause an astigmatic laser spot of the retina, with higher irradiance and overtreatment on one side of the laser spot, and lower irradiance and undertreatment on the other side. It is also important to avoid excessive pressure on contact ophthalmoscopic lenses, which could alter choroidal perfusion and hence heat convection (26)—although the latter seems to be of less importance (45).
5. *Absorption of laser energy.* Melanin is the most effective chorioretinal light absorber. Chorioretinal heat generation is proportional to light absorption, so laser-induced temperature increases are higher for a particular retinal irradiance in more darkly pigmented fundi than in lightly pigmented ones (26). The color of the normal human fundus varies with individual genetic constitution, and could be heterogeneous in the same patients. Thus, light absorption in pigment clumps from prior focal photocoagulation can cause local hot spots in large TTT treatment fields. Moreover, the presence of areas of atrophic choriocapillaris adjacent to the treatment zone may diminish the important *heat*

sink role of the choroidal vessels, allowing the retinal temperature to rise into the range necessary to produce a coagulation necrosis (51). The presence of a subretinal hemorrhage can also cause variations in temperature during treatment. A thin layer of hemoglobin might not impair the treatment, but a hemorrhage of sufficient thickness will hinder the absorption of energy at the choriocapillaris, thus diminishing the effectiveness of TTT and increasing the possibilities of retinal thermal damage.

6. *Localization and etiology of the CNV.* If the lesion is predominantly classic or classic (type II) CNV, preliminary clinical experience has shown that classic CNV secondary to AMD typically requires only 66% of the power needed for occult CNV. Furthermore, CNV membranes due to pathologic myopia are usually smaller and more pigmented, and typically require only 50% of the power used for occult CNV.

7. *Size of the CNV.* Two different strategies can be used to treat lesions fully when their greatest linear dimension is greater than 3 mm. First, a lower magnification may be used with a contact ophthalmoscopic lens with a wider field. There are several laser lenses that provide spot sizes ranging from 3 to 6 mm. Second, overlapping 3 mm diameter exposures may be used, but the doctor must be careful to minimize overlapping regions. Treatment in the central macula should never be repeated in an overlapping exposure.

8. *Media opacity.* Treatment may be limited by fundus visibility and by the ability to observe subtle fundus changes. Laser parameters may require adjustment depending on the density of any cataract present. Retinal irradiance decreases with increasing ocular media opacification because of the increased scattering and light absorption during the beam's intraocular transit. In general, to achieve similar clinical endpoints in different eyes, TTT power should be adjusted with respect to the patient's media clarity, fundus pigmentation, RPE atrophy, and even choroidal circulation (26).

9. *Pseudophakic eyes.* Careful monitoring is particularly important in pseudophakic eyes, which may have higher transmission and lower scattering of laser radiation than eyes with an aged crystalline lens.

10. *Interrupted treatment.* When the treatment is interrupted momentarily (e.g., for patient movement) the treatment should be completed so that a patient's total laser exposure is 60 seconds in duration.

Technique

Transpupillary thermotherapy is administered through a slit lamp-mounted delivery system attached to a modified infrared diode laser at 810 nm with an adjustable beam width of 1.2, 2.0, or 3.0 mm, depending on the diameter of the CNV. A topical anesthetic such as 0.5% proparacaine is applied before placement of a three-mirror Goldmann lens, or an equivalent fundus lens, for use with the diode laser. The beam width may be further enlarged through contact lens magnification. For example, an area centralis lens magnifies the laser spot 0.94×, and a quadraspheric lens magnifies the laser spot 1.97×, resulting in a laser spot size of 5.91 mm in the latter. Continuous observation through the slit lamp ensures fixation. Treatment is initiated with one spot for 60 seconds duration at a power setting ranging from 360 to 1,000 mW, such that no visible change—or a barely detectable light-gray appearance to the lesion—is present at the end of the treatment. Power settings should be proportional to the spot size, with larger spots requiring higher energy levels. In general, for a 3.0 mm spot, the initial power level is 650 to 1000 mW. If any retinal whitening is observed, or if retinal whitening continues to be observed, the power setting is again decreased by 100 mW. Care must be taken to ensure that the entire lesion border is covered with the treatment beam. A security area of 500 to 1,000 μm from the border of the lesion is desirable (10). Other adjustments may be necessary depending on (a) the degree of neurosensory retinal detachment (amount of subretinal fluid), (b) the amount of subretinal hemorrhage, and (c) the location of the CNV.

Evaluation

Follow up is arranged at 2, 4, and 6 weeks, and at 3, 6, 9, 12, and 18 months. At each visit, visual acuity and retinal examinations must be performed with fundus photography and fluorescein angiography. Retreatment can be considered when no change in subretinal elevation is seen on slit lamp biomicroscopy and when persistent leakage is observed on late-phase fluorescein angiograms. Retreatment should never be performed earlier than 6 or 8 weeks after the initial treatment. If indicated, retreatment is often performed 8 to 12 weeks after initial therapy for occult CNV or 6 weeks after treatment of classic CNV. Four weeks is the artificial limit to consider CNV as persistent or recurrent. Approximately 20% of treated eyes require additional therapy.

RESULTS

In the literature, TTT has been used in patients of both genders, in patients older than 45 years of age, and in patients with the occult (10,52–57) and subfoveal (10,52,53,55–57) forms of AMD (type II). Also, there are reports of it being used in cases that are classic (type I), (54,57,58) predominantly classic (59), and minimally classic (53,59). The average of numbers of treatments in the different series varies from 1.2 to 1.9 times (1–3,10,53,55,59). The minimum time of follow up is 6 months with an average of 6.1 to 13.8 (10,54,56,57,59).

At the moment, the main indication for TTT is the treatment of occult neovascular membranes (10,52–57). In occult cases, PDT was shown to be less effective than for

TABLE 18.3

VISUAL ACUITY AFTER TTT IN OCCULT CNV SECONDARY TO AMD

Author	Initial Visual Acuity	Percentage Stabilization	Percentage Improving	Percentage Losing	Number of Treatment	Follow Up (month)
Reichel et al. (10)	≥20/400	56%	19%	25%	1–3 (mean 1.25)	6–25 (mean 13)
Salinas et al. (53)	20/200 to 20/50	50%	30%	20%	1–2 (mean 1.2)	≥6
Karel et al. (54)	Mean 20/100	57.9%	5.3%	36.8%	1–2	6–18 (mean 9.5)
Thach et al. (55)	Mean 20/177	81% (3 month) 71% (12 month)		29%	1–3 (mean 1.9)	≥6
Auer et al. (56)	Mean 20/80	72% (12 month)		28%	1–3	Mean 14.28

classical CNV (10,7,60). Transpupillary thermotherapy stabilizes the visual acuity in a significant number of patients, and the clinical results seem to be both clearly superior to the natural evolution of AMD (3,4) and comparable with PDT (Tables 18.3 and 18.4).

High closure rates have been obtained in the other forms of neovascularization (classic, predominantly classic, and minimally classic) after TTT due to regression of the neovascular membranes. The closure of the CNV is associated with a stabilization or improvement in vision in a high percentage of patients (53,54,58,59).

Cardillo Piccolino et al. evaluated the effectiveness of a single low-power (350 mW) transpupillary thermotherapy application in treating juxtafoveal recurrent choroidal neovascularization after conventional laser photocoagulation in patients with AMD. A high rate of closure was noted after the first treatment, but recurrences occurred in all eyes between 1 and 7 months (60). Hass et al. assessed the effectiveness of a single treatment of TTT in patients with exudative AMD, using 800 mW for 60 seconds, and found no beneficial effect on the spontaneous course of the CNV after one treatment in patients with AMD (57). In summary, TTT is particularly indicated in patients with occult CNV. However it could be considered in the other forms of CNV. In general, patient tolerance is good, but retreatment may be necessary.

TABLE 18.4

COMPARISON OF VISUAL ACUITY RESULTS TO OTHER TREATMENT TRIALS

Study	Patients with Stable or Improved Visual Acuity	Patients with a Loss of Two or More Lines of Visual Acuity
Natural history (9–12 mo) (4)	38%	62%
Photodynamic therapy (PDT)		
Predominantly classic (12 mo) (7)	38%	62%
Predominantly classic control (12 mo) (7)	24%	76%
Occult (12 mo) (6)	34%	66%
Occult control (12 mo) (6)	23%	77%
Transpupillary thermotherapy (TTT)		
Classic (58)	87.5%	12.5%
Predominantly classic (59)	66%	34%
Minimally classic (53,59)	70–72%	30–28%
Occult (10,52–57)	70–75%	25–30%

INDOCYANINE GREEN-ENHANCED DIODE LASER TRANSPUPILLARY THERMOTHERAPY

Background

Puliafito et al. first described indocyanine green-enhanced diode laser photocoagulation TTT (i-TTT) for the treatment of CNV (61,62). This technique involves the intravenous injection of a photosensitizing agent that accumulates in neovascular tissue. This photosensitized tissue is then irradiated by light at the absorption peak of the dye, which leads to vascular toxicity. This suggests that indocyanine green (ICG), as well as other chromophores, such as SnET2 (Miravant Study), could be used as photosensitizers in the treatment of CNV.

ICG is an anionic tricarbocyanine dye with a large protein-bound component that provides a selective intravascular retention advantage with a peak absorption of 805 nm, which is close to the peak emission (810 nm) of the conventional diode laser. Other important characteristics of ICG are: (63)

1. Low skin phototoxicity.
2. High tissue targetability.
3. Rapid biodistribution and clearance.
4. Easy administration and monitoring.

Therefore, i-TTT may permit the selective ablation of ICG-retaining choroidal neovascular membranes with relative sparing of the neighboring neurosensory retina (64).

Intravenous ICG pretreatment can be used to lower the TTT threshold fluence and irradiance required to create angiographically visible lesions in the choroid. A dose-dependent relationship exists between TTT fluence thresholds and ICG concentrations, such that the higher the ICG concentration, the lower the TTT fluence threshold (65).

This method has three advantages:

1. Infrared diode laser energy transmits readily through turbid retina as well as through retina and subretinal hemorrhages.
2. This method includes occlusion of relatively deep choroidal vessels, including CNV.
3. In exudative AMD, there is less melanin pigment in the proliferative pigment epithelium that covers the CNV, and this less-pigmented RPE absorbs little laser light. However, the therapy is still effective because ICG becomes a new chromophore and absorbs the infrared light (66).

At a histological level, the changes are summarized as follows: (67,68)

1. Occlusion of the choriocapillaris.
2. Destruction and loss of endothelial cells of large choroidal vessels.
3. Stroma edema.
4. Disappearance of large choroidal vessels.

5. Large choroidal vessel damage could be less intense in pigmented patients.
6. The effect is more marked in the large choroidal vessels (with a great concentration of ICG) than in the retinal vessels.

Technique

ICG is infused as a bolus injection of 15 mL of a 5 mg/mL ICG solution. Diode laser irradiation (810 nm) is initiated 5 minutes after the bolus infusion with an exposure time of 60 to 90 seconds, a starting power of 550 to 1,000 mW, and a spot size of 1.0 to 3.0 mm. The laser beam must irradiate the entire CNV. No change should be observed in the deep retina during the treatment (subthreshold therapy). Immediately following treatment, ICGA can be conducted without further ICG administration, and the treatment effect can be confirmed when hypofluorescence of the treated area is observed. Roizenblatt et al. described a trimodal (photocoagulation, transpupillary thermotherapy, and photodynamic therapy) application laser device coupled to a single light source. Its main benefits are wider treatment spot dimensions, longer treatment alternatives, and a Joule meter. It also features microprocessor connectivity (69).

Results

Initial visual acuity, functional outcome, number of treatments, and follow up are summarized in Table 18.5. Prognostic indicators for visual acuity of 20/200 or better after i-TTT are:

1. A relatively short distance between the edge of the laser burns and the center of the foveal avascular zone.
2. Good preoperative visual acuity (66).

TTT and i-TTT seem to be effective in stabilizing visual acuity in patients with CNV related to AMD. Results with both techniques are quite similar, and possible explanations for this might include differences between adjustments in ICG concentration during i-TTT, laser power, and/or the timing of laser application following ICG infusion.

Other Techniques

Costa et al. described two variants of the enhancing technique applicable for CNV: photodynamic therapy with ICG (i-PDT) (63,70) and neovascular ingrowth site photothrombosis (71). Photodynamic therapy with ICG begins with a highly concentrated bolus injection of 2.5 mL of ICG (1.5 mg/kg) in the cubital vein, followed immediately by a 5.0 mL saline flush. Two minutes after the injection, the dye is activated by the application of a 3,000 mW/cm^2 diode laser light (810 nm) for 95 seconds. The spot must be sufficient to cover the entire neovascular net under the retina.

TABLE 18.5

VISUAL ACUITY AFTER I-T T T IN CNV SECONDARY TO AMD

Author	Initial Visual Acuity	Percentage Stabilization	Percentage Improving	Percentage Losing	Number of Treatment	Follow Up (months)
Liggett et al. (ARVO 2003)	20/25–20/200	66.7%	16.7%	25%	1–6 (mean 2.0)	3–85 (mean 24)
Obana et al. (66)	≥20/250	42.1%	26.3%	31.6%	1–4 (mean 1.5)	6–51 (mean 26.5)
Shah et al. (ARVO 2003)	20/50–20/125	56%	–	–	1–3 (mean 1.7)	>6

The neovascular ingrowth site photothrombosis has different steps. After the identification of the feeder vessel in the choroidal neovascular net, ICG at a dose of 2 mg/kg body weight is dissolved in 4 mL of distilled water and administered in the cubital vein as follows: a loading dose of 2.0 mL of the ICG solution is infused as a bolus, followed immediately by a 5.0 mL saline flush; 20 minutes after the first dose, a single 0.8 mm diode laser spot is positioned in the center of the neovascular ingrowth site, and a second injection of the remaining ICG solution (2.0 mL) is administered, followed by a 5.0 mL saline flush. The diode laser emitting light at 810 nm and with an irradiance of 30 mW/cm² is started 10 seconds after the end of the second saline flush infusion. Laser light is applied over an interval of 80 seconds. Ten minutes after first light delivery, a second (and last) laser application using identical parameters is performed (71).

TRANSPUPILLARY THERMOTHERAPY AND ANTIANGIOGENIC DRUGS

Angiogenesis has been implicated as the main problem in wet AMD. Indeed, excised human CNV tissue after experimental submacular surgery has shown elevated levels of vascular endothelial growth factor (VEGF). Recent studies have suggested that pharmacologic intervention with antiangiogenic therapy may be useful to treat various forms of ocular neovascularization. Anti-VEGF therapy may be useful in two ways: (a) inhibiting the formation, and (b) diminishing the permeability of the new blood vessels.

Anti-VEGF therapy may, therefore, represent a two-pronged attack on CNV by means of its antiangiogenic and antipermeability properties (72). These benefits could be combined with other therapies, such as PDT or TTT.

Recently, a pilot study was conducted to examine combined modality treatment, including i-TTT and 4 mg of intravitreal triamcinolone acetonide for CNV secondary to AMD (Table 18.5). Patients in the study were not candidates for PDT with Visudyne. Of the 16 eyes treated with

this combination, 11 (69%) maintained or had improved visual acuity at the third month of the treatment, with the trend continuing in longer-term follow-up (Liggett et al., unpublished data).

SUBMACULAR HEMORRHAGE AND TRANSPUPILLARY THERMOTHERAPY

In order to improve the prognosis of submacular hemorrhage (SMH) in AMD with subretinal CNV, it is necessary to treat both the consequence—SMH—and the cause: CNV. Using a limited posterior vitrectomy with removal of the posterior hyaloid in order to improve the flexibility of the retina, allows maximal capability of blood displacement, and an intravitreal injection of SF6 (100%) is performed followed by a prone position for 8 hours (pneumatic displacement). After 8 hours, the patient is instructed to alternate between the prone and upright positions with short walks, allowing active and quick blood displacement. Several days later, when the CNV can be identified, TTT is performed (2003).

COMPLICATIONS

Reports of complications during or after TTT are low. The most important complications include:

1. *Intratreatment and posttreatment hemorrhage* (73). Bleeding can occur at the moment of treatment or soon after. A vitreous hemorrhage may be present. In cases where bleeding occurs, the thermal affect of the laser may damage a main choroidal vessel, causing a hemorrhage of variable dimensions before the clotting cascade can close the vascular lumen.

2. *Retinal pigmented epithelium tears* (74,55). The thermal effect from the infrared laser may cause the choroidal neovascular membrane to shrink during, or shortly, after treatment, leading to an RPE tear. This complication is especially feared in the presence of a serous pigment

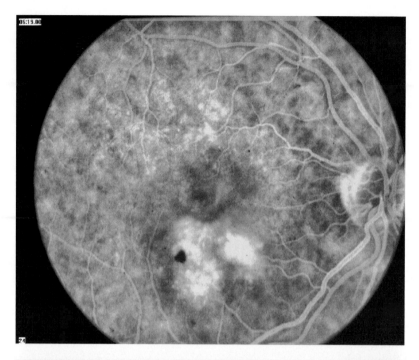

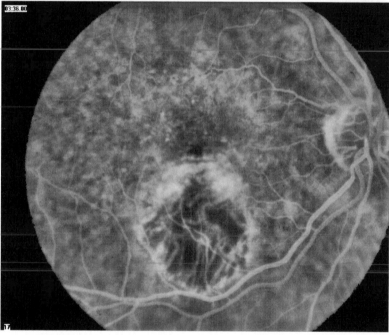

Figure 18.7 *Top*: Fluorescein angiography demonstrates occult choroidal neovascularization associated with age-related macular degeneration before transpupillary thermotherapy. The visual acuity was 20/200. *Bottom*: Fluorescein angiography clearly showing chorioretinal atrophy 2 months later. Because the superior border of the atrophy is under the fixation point, the visual acuity is 20/100.

epithelial detachment (PED) associated with the CNV. In these cases, TTT must be performed under a conservative protocol, or other therapeutic alternatives must be considered. For example, the feeder vessel or neovascular ingrowth site may be treated with photothrombosis.

3. *Progression of occult to classic membranes* (75,56). This transformation usually appears 1 or 2 months after TTT. In such cases, the hyperthermia may lead to an occlusion of the choroidal vessels. The resultant hypoxia could stimulate the production of cytokines, such as vascular endothelial growth factor, which could result

in the development of the neovascularization. This complication can be managed by observation alone (75), or PDT could be used as an alternative treatment in particular cases (56).

4. *Macular infarction* (51). Macular infarction manifests clinically with a marked whitening of the macula area and closure of the perifoveal capillaries on FA. Mild whitening is evident immediately after treatment, but if more severe yellow-white discoloration (coagulation necrosis) develops several hours after treatment, macular infarction must be considered. The presence of geographic retinal pigment epithelium atrophy or a

previous laser treatment scar in the macular region may predispose patients to this complication.

5. *Overtreatment* (56,76). Highly pigmented patients are prone to suffer this complication. Clinically, overtreatment manifests as a central scotoma of variable intensity that shows a tendency to recover with time (56) (Fig. 18.7). Serous PEDs larger than 25% of the lesion could predispose a patient to this complication (76).

6. *Detachment of subfoveal neovascularization* (77). This probably occurs secondary to scarring and contraction of the central portion of the CNV. Large membranes localized between the retina and the RPE (type II) may be predisposed to this evolution.

7. *Retinal angiomatous proliferation (RAP) and TTT* (78). RAP, a distinct form of neovascular AMD originating from the sensory retina, may occur after a conventional TTT treatment. Afflicted eyes respond with excessive scaring, retinal folds, and RPE tears.

8. *Acute vision loss* (51,76). Although acute vision loss is rare after TTT, it remains a possibility, about which patients should be informed.

9. *Others*. Other complications, such as vascular occlusion, secondary tractions, and retinal neovascularization have been described after the use of TTT for the treatment of intraocular tumors (79), and these complications should be kept in mind during TTT for exudative AMD.

FINAL WORDS

TTT may be useful, not only as independent therapy, but also as an adjunct to PDT, antiangiogenic drugs, and ionizing radiation therapy in the management of neovascular AMD. For example, the thermal susceptibility of CNV might be increased by local hypoxia from PDT; one of the reasons that hyperthermia and PDT are synergistic if PDT is administered before, but not after, hyperthermia (26). Synergism with other therapeutic modalities could achieve efficacy at lower fluences without significant damage to the neural retina (64,80).

Recent studies show that TTT is a safe procedure when is applied to juxtapapillary CNV located near the disc in patients with a healthy optic nerve (Chu et al., ARVO 2003), but other evidence suggests that TTT could be a jeopardizing procedure in patients with glaucomatous neuropathy (Reichel et al., ARVO 2003).

REFERENCES

1. Klein R, Klein BE, Linton KL. Prevalence of age-related maculopathy: the Beaver Dam Eye Study. *Ophthalmology.* 1992;99:933–934.
2. Leibowitz HM, Krueger DE, Maunder LR, et al. The Framingham Eye Study Monograph: VI. macular degeneration. *Surv Ophthalmol.* 1980;24(suppl): 428–457.
3. Bressler NM, Frost LA, Bressler SB, et al. Natural course of poorly defined choroidal neovascularization associated with macular degeneration. *Arch Ophthalmol.* 1988;106:1,537–1,542.
4. Stevens TS, Bressler NM, Maguire MG, et al. Occult choroidal neovascularization in age-related macular degeneration. A natural history study. *Arch Ophthalmol.* 1997;115:345–350.
5. Macular Photocoagulation Study Group. Laser photocoagulation of subfoveal neovascular lesions of age-related macular degeneration: results of a randomized clinical trial. *Arch Ophthalmol.* 1991;109:1,220–1,231.
6. Macular Photocoagulation Study Group. Laser photocoagulation of subfoveal neovascular lesions of age-related macular degeneration. Update findings from two clinical trials. *Arch Ophthalmol.* 1993;111:1,200–1,209.
7. Verteporfin in Photodynamic Therapy Study Group. Verteporfin therapy of subfoveal choroidal neovascularization in age-related macular degeneration: two years results of a randomized clinical trial including lesions with occult no classic choroidal neovascularization. Verteporfin in Photodynamic Therapy report 2. *Am J Ophthalmol.* 2001;131:541–560.
8. Treatment of Age-Related Macular Degeneration with Photodynamic Therapy (TAP) Study Group. Photodynamic therapy of subfoveal choroidal neovascularization in age-related macular degeneration with verteporfin: one year results of 2 randomized clinical trials. TAP report 1. *Arch Ophthalmol.* 1999;117:1,329–1,345.
9. Pharmacological Therapy for Macular Degeneration Study Group. Interferon alfa-2a is ineffective for patients with choroidal neovascularization secondary to age-related macular degeneration. Results of a prospective randomized placebo-controlled clinical trial. *Arch Ophthalmol.* 1997;115:865–872.
10. Reichel E, Berrocal AM, Ip M, et al. Transpupillary thermotherapy of occult subfoveal choroidal neovascularization in patients with age-related macular degeneration. *Ophthalmology.* 1999;106:1,908–1,914.
11. Ip M, Kroll A, Reichel E. Transpupillary thermotherapy. *Semin Ophthalmol.* 1999;14:11–18.
12. Fung WE. Interferon alfa-2a for treatment of age-related macular degeneration. *Am J Ophthalmol.* 1991;112:349–350.
13. Lewis ML, Davis J, Chuang E. Interferon alfa-2a in the treatment of exudative age-related macular degeneration. *Graefes Arch Clin Exp Ophthalmol.* 1993;231:615–618.
14. Danis RP, Ciulla TA, Pratt LM, et al. Intravitreal triamcinolone acetonide in exudative age-related macular degeneration. *Retina.* 2000;20: 244–250.
15. Lambert HM, Capone A Jr, Aeberg TM, et al. Surgical excision of subfoveal neovascular membrane in age-related macular degeneration. *Am J Ophthalmol.* 1992;113:257–262.
16. Ormerod LD, Puklin JE, Frank RN. Long-term outcomes after the surgical removal of advanced subfoveal neovascular membranes in age-related macular degeneration. *Ophthalmology.* 1994;101:1,201–1,210.
17. Machemer R, Steinhorst UH. Retinal separation, retinotomy, and macular relocation: II a surgical approach for age-related macular degeneration? *Graefes Arch Clin Exp Ophthalmol.* 1993;231:635–641.
18. Lewis H, Kaiser PK, Lewis S, Estafanous M. Macular translocation for subfoveal choroidal neovascularization in age-related macular degeneration: a prospective study. *Am J Ophthalmol.* 1999;128:135–146.
19. Hooper CY, Guymer RH. New treatments in age-related macular degeneration. *Clin Experiment Ophthalmol.* 2003;3:376–391.
20. Algvere PV, Seregard S. Age-related maculopathy: pathogenetic features and new treatment modalities. *Acta Ophthalmol Scand.* 2002;80:136–143.
21. Journee-de Kover JG, Oosterhuis JA, Kakebeeke-Kemme HM, et al. Transpupillary thermotherapy (TTT) by infrared irradiation of choroidal melanoma. *Doc Ophthalmol.* 1992;82:185–191.
22. Shields JA, Shields CL. Management of posterior uveal melanoma. *Surv Ophthalmol.* 1991;36:161–195.
23. De Potter P, Shields CL, Shields JA. New treatment modalities for uveal melanoma. *Curr Opin Ophthalmol.* 1996;7:27–32.
24. Algvere PV, Libert C, Lindgarde G, et al. Transpupillary thermotherapy of predominantly occult choroidal neovascularization in age-related macular degeneration with 12 months follow-up. *Acta Ophthalmol Scand.* 2003;81:110–117.
25. Subramanian ML, Reichel E. Current indications of transpupillary thermotherapy for the treatment of posterior segment diseases. *Curr Opin Ophthalmol.* 2003;14:155–158.
26. Mainster MA, Reichel E. Transpupillary thermotherapy for age-related macular degeneration: long-pulse photocoagulation, apoptosis, and heat shock proteins. *Ophthalmic Surg Lasers.* 2000;31:359–373.
27. Lanzetta P, Michieletto P, Pirracchio A, et al. Early vascular changes induced by transpupillary thermotherapy of choroidal neovascularization. *Ophthalmology.* 2002;109:1,098–1,104.
28. Miura S, Nishiwaki H, Ieki Y, et al. Noninvasive technique for monitoring chorioretinal temperature during transpupillary thermotherapy, with a thermosensitive liposome. *Invest Ophthalmol Vis Sci.* 2003;44: 2,716–2,721.
29. Miller H, Miller B, Ryan SJ. The role of the retinal pigment epithelium in the involution of subretinal neovascularization. *Invest Ophthalmol Vis Sci.* 1986;27:1,644–1,652.
30. Glaser BM, Campochiaro PA, Davis JL Jr, et al. Retinal pigment epithelial cells release inhibitors of neovascularization. *Ophthalmology.* 1987;94: 780–784.
31. Flower RW, Von Kerczek C, Zhu L, et al. Theoretical investigation of the role of choriocapillaris blood flow in treatment of subfoveal choroidal neovascularization associated with age-related macular degeneration. *Am J Ophthalmol.* 2001;132:85–93.
32. Ciulla TA, Harris A, Kagemann L. Transpupillary thermotherapy for subfoveal occult choroidal neovascularization: effect on ocular perfusion. *Invest Ophthalmol Vis Sci.* 2001;42:3,337–3,340.

33. Krebs RA, Feder ME. Tissue-specific variations in Hsp70 expression and thermal damage in *Drosophila melanogaster* larvae. *J Exp Biol.* 1997;14: 2,007–2,015.

34. Desmettre T, Maurage CA, Mordon S. Heat shock protein hyperexpression on chorioretinal layers after transpupillary thermotherapy. *Invest Ophthalmol Vis Sci.* 2001;42:2,976–2,980.

35. Desmettre T, Maurage CA, Mordon S. Transpupillary thermotherapy (TTT) with short duration laser exposures induce heat shock protein (HSP) hyperexpression on choroidoretinal layers. *Lasers Surg Med.* 2003;33:102–107.

36. Bernstein SL, Liu AM, Hansen BC, et al. Heat shock cognate-70 expression decline during normal aging of the primate retina. *Invest Ophthalmol Vis Sci.* 2000;41:2,857–2,862.

37. Ogata N, Ando A, Uyama M, et al. Expression of cytokines and transcription factors in photocoagulated human retinal pigment epithelial cells. *Graefes Arch Clin Exp Ophthalmol.* 2001;239:87–95.

38. Tadeusz S. Properties and function of the ocular melanin. A photobiophysical view. New trends in photobiology. *J Photochem Photobiol Biol.* 1992;12: 215–258.

39. Weiter JJ, Delori FC, Wing GL, et al. Relationship of senile macular degeneration to ocular pigmentation. *Am J Ophthalmol.* 1985;99:185–187.

40. Wing GL, Blanchard GC, Weiter JJ. The topography and age relationship of lipofuscin concentration in the retinal pigment epithelium. *Invest Ophthalmol Vis Sci.* 1978;17:600–605.

41. Gregor Z, Joffe L. Senile macular changes in the Black African. *Br J Ophthalmol.* 1978;62:547–551.

42. Vinding T. Pigmentation of the eye and hair in relation to age-macular degeneration. An epidemiological study of 1000 aged individuals. *Acta Ophthalmol.* 1990;68:53–58.

43. Beatty S, Murray IJ, Henson DB, et al. Macular pigment and risk for age-related macular degeneration in subjects from a Northern European population. *Invest Ophthalmol Vis Sci.* 2001;42:439–446.

44. Weiter JJ, Delori FC, Wing GL, et al. Retinal pigment epithelial lipofuscin and melanin and choroidal melanin in human eyes. *Invest Ophthalmol Vis Sci.* 1986;27:145–152.

45. Peyman GA, Genaidy M, Moshfeghi DM, et al. Transpupillary thermotherapy threshold parameters: funduscopic, angiographic, and histologic findings in pigmented and nonpigmented rabbits. *Retina.* 2003;23:371–377.

46. Connolly BP, Regillo CD, Eagle RC Jr, et al. The histopathologic effects of transpupillary thermotherapy in human eyes. *Ophthalmology.* 2003;110: 415–420.

47. Robertson DM, Salomao DR. The effect of transpupillary thermotherapy on the human macula. *Arch Ophthalmol.* 2002;120:652–656.

48. Procaccini EM, Riccio M, Belloci M, et al. The effects of a diode laser (810 nm) on pigmented guinea pig skin. *Laser Med Sci.* 2001;16:171–175.

49. Fitzpatrick TB. The validity and practicality of sun-reactive skin type I through VI. *Arch Dermatol.* 1988;124:869–871.

50. Lock-Andersen J, Wulf HC, Knudstorp ND. Interdependence of eye and hair colour, skin type and skin pigmentation in a Caucasian population. *Acta Derm Venérelo* (Stockh). 1998;78:214–219.

51. Benner JD, Ahuja RM, Butler JW. Macular infarction after transpupillary thermotherapy for subfoveal choroidal neovascularization in age-related macular degeneration. *Am J Ophthalmol.* 2002;134:765–768.

52. Rogers AH, Reichel E. Transpupillary thermotherapy of subfoveal occult choroidal neovascularization. *Curr Opin Ophthalmol.* 2001;12:212–215.

53. Salinas-Alaman A, Garcia Layana A, Juberias Sanchez JR, et al. Transpupillary thermotherapy in occult subretinal neovascularization in age-related macular degeneration. Preliminary results. *Arch Soc Esp Oftalmol.* 2002;77:617–622.

54. Karel I, Zahlava J, Boguszakova J, et al. Transpupillary thermotherapy in age-related macular degeneration. Preliminary results. *Cesk Slov Oftalmol.* 2002;58:215–223.

55. Thach AB, Sipperley JO, Dugel PU, et al. Large-spot size transpupillary thermotherapy for the treatment of occult choroidal neovascularization associated with age-related macular degeneration. *Arch Ophthalmol.* 2003;121: 817–820.

56. Auer C, Tao Tran V, Herbort CP. Transpupillary thermotherapy for occult subfoveal neovessels in age-related macular degeneration: importance of patient pigmentation for the determination of laser settings. *Klin Monatsbl Augenheilkd.* 2002;219:250–253.

57. Haas A, Feigl B, Weger M. Transpupillary thermotherapy in exudative, age-related macular degeneration. *Ophthalmologe.* 2003;100:111–114.

58. Pasechnikova NV, Teslenko AS. Transpupillary thermotherapy of classic choroidal neovascular membranes. *Vestn Oftalmol.* 2002;118:30–32.

59. Newsom RS, McAlister JC, Saeed M, et al. Transpupillary thermotherapy (TTT) for the treatment of choroidal neovascularisation. *Br J Ophthalmol.* 2001;85:173–178. Erratum In: *Br J Ophthalmol.* 2001;85:505.

60. Cardillo Piccolino F, Eandi CM, Ventre L, et al. Transpupillary thermotherapy of juxtafoveal recurrent choroidal neovascularization. *Eur J Ophthalmol.* 2003;13:453–460.

61. Puliafito CA, Destro M, To K, et al. Dye-enhanced photocoagulation of choroidal neovascularization. *Invest Ophthalmol Vis Sci.* 1988;29(Suppl): 414.

62. Puliafito CA, Guyer DR, Mones JM, et al. Indocyanine green digital angiography and dye-enhanced diode laser photocoagulation of choroidal neovascularization. *Invest Ophthalmol Vis Sci.* 1991;32(Suppl):712.

63. Costa RA, Farah ME, Freymuller E, et al. Choriocapillaris photodynamic therapy using indocyanine green. *Am J Ophthalmol.* 2001;132:557–565.

64. Reichel E, Puliafito CA, Duker JS, et al. Indocyanine green dye-enhanced diode laser photocoagulation of poorly defined subfoveal choroidal neovascularization. *Ophthalmic Surg.* 1994;25:195–201.

65. Peyman GA, Genaidy M, Yoneya S, et al. Transpupillary thermotherapy threshold parameters: effect of indocyanine green pretreatment. *Retina.* 2003;23:378–386.

66. Obana A, Gohto Y, Nishiguchi K, et al. A retrospective pilot study of indocyanine green enhanced diode laser photocoagulation for subfoveal choroidal neovascularization associated with age-related macular degeneration. *Jpn J Ophthamol.* 2000;44:668–676.

67. Matsumoto M, Miki T, Obana A, et al. Indocyanine green enhanced photocoagulation in the pigmented rabbit. *Nippon Ganka Gakkai Zasshi.* 1992;96:742–748.

68. Suh JH, Miki T, Obana A, et al. Effects of indocyanine green dye enhanced diode laser photocoagulation in non-pigmented rabbit eyes. *Osaka City Med J.* 1991;37:89–106.

69. Roizenblatt R, Farah ME, Castro J, et al. Diode laser modifications for treatment of choroidal neovascularisation. *Lasers Med Sci.* 2003;18:43–44.

70. Costa RA, Farah ME, Cardillo JA, et al. Photodynamic therapy with indocyanine green for occult subfoveal neovascularization caused by age-related macular degeneration. *Curr Eye Res.* 2001;23:271–275.

71. Costa RA, Rocha KM, Calucci D. Neovascular ingrowth site photothrombosis in choroidal neovascularization associated with retinal pigment epithelial detachment. *Graefe's Arch Clin Exp Ophthalmol.* 2003;241:245–250.

72. The Eyetech Study Group. Anti-vascular endothelial growth factor therapy for subfoveal choroidal neovascularization secondary to age-related macular degeneration. *Ophthalmology.* 2003;110:979–986.

73. Greuloch K, Lai WW, Pulido JS. Hemorrhage in patients who have received transpupillary thermotherapy for subfoveal choroidal neovascularization. *Can J Ophthalmol.* 2003;38:308–311.

74. Thompson JT. Retinal pigment epithelial tear after transpupillary thermotherapy for choroidal neovascularization. *Am J Ophthalmol.* 2001;131: 662–664.

75. Kaga T, Fonseca RA, Dantas MA, et al. Transient appearance of classic choroidal neovascularization after transpupillary thermotherapy for occult choroidal neovascularization. *Retina.* 2001;21:172–173.

76. Salinas-Alaman A, Garcia-Layana A, Moreno-Montanes J. Overtreatment of transpupillary thermotherapy for choroidal neovascularization. *Acta Ophthalmol Scand.* 2003;81:197–198.

77. Rumelt S, Kaiserman I, Rehany U, et al. Detachment of subfoveal choroidal neovascularization in age-related macular degeneration. *Am J Ophthalmol.* 2002;13:822–827.

78. Kuroiwa S, Arai J, Gaun S, et al. Rapidly progressive scar formation after transpupillary thermotherapy in retinal angiomatous proliferation. *Retina.* 2003;23:417–420.

79. Kiratli H, Bilgic S. Choriovitreal neovascularization following transpupillary thermotherapy for choroidal melanoma. *Eye.* 2003;17:436–437.

80. Navajas EV, Costa RA, Farah ME, et al. Indocyanine green-mediated photothrombosis combined with intravitreal triamcinolone for the treatment of choroidal neovascularization in serpiginous choroiditis. *Eye.* 2003;17: 563–566.

Choroidal Feeder Vessel Photocoagulation Therapy

19

Bert Glaser *T. Mark Johnson*

INTRODUCTION

Feeder vessel therapy (FVT) is an effective and safe treatment to reduce the effects of choroidal neovascularization (CNV) occurring in numerous disorders including age-related macular degeneration (AMD).

The rationale for FVT is that a single vessel often controls the majority of blood flow to an area of neovascularization within the choroid. This rationale is the basis for the use of embolization treatment for solid tumors. Altering blood flow to the new blood vessels within a solid tumor slows growth and in some cases causes the tumor to shrink or involute (1,2).

High-speed dynamic video indocyanine green angiography (HSICGA) is essential for demonstrating feeder vessels in CNV. Laser-induced attenuation of feeder vessels results in the regression of the associated CNV and marked reduction in exudation (3).

Feeder vessels are long (often longer than a millimeter) afferent vessels traveling through the intermediate, Sattler's layer of the choroid, and are distinguished from the short blood vessels described in histopathologic studies, which penetrate through Bruch's membrane for only a few tenths of a millimeter (4,5).

Several studies have demonstrated that FVT can substantially improve vision in a significant portion of treated patients (3,6–9). We have observed that attenuation of the feeder vessel induces remodeling and maturation of the CNV complex resulting in resolution of exudative manifestations such as subretinal fluid, subretinal hemorrhage, and retinal edema (6,10). The remodeling and maturation occurs in much the same manner as is seen in the case of retinal neovascularization associated with proliferative diabetic retinopathy following panretinal photocoagulation.

FVT is distinguished from PDT and Macular Photocoagulation Study (MPS) laser treatment by the area treated. In the latter two treatment modalities, the entire lesion undergoes treatment, resulting in large areas of subretinal fibrosis and disruption of the normal retinochoroidal architecture. In the case of FVT, only a 75 to 200 μm area is typically treated, thereby substantially reducing the amount of subsequent fibrosis and disruption. This fact may play a role in limiting the amount of fibrosis that occurs following FVT.

FVT is not a new technique in ophthalmology, and has been around for more than 30 years (11). In fact it was recommended in the guidelines for MPS treatment published in 1991 (12). However, in the past its use has been limited by difficulties in identifying the actual feeder vessel. The development of HSICGA allows identification of these feeder vessels as the afferent or arteriolar arm of the CNV complex in the majority of eyes with CNV. HSICGA also allows the identification of the efferent or venous side of the CNV complex in many cases. When comparing these findings to the findings on simultaneous fluorescein angiograms (FA), the arteriolar arm or feeder vessel fills and empties within the first 10 or 20 seconds of the HSICGA, and is therefore missed on the FA. What is instead seen on the FA, when not obscured by blood or pigment, is the efferent or draining vessel of the CNV complex. It has been shown that treating the efferent vessel does not result in sustained regression of the CNV complex (13).

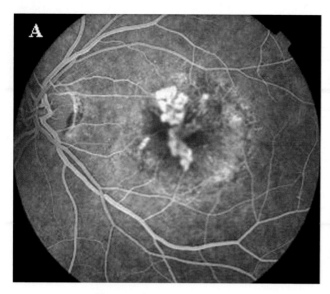
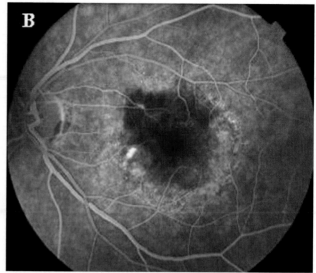

Figure 19.1   Classic and occult choroidal neovascular membrane (CNVM). **A.** Pretreatment fluorescein angiogram (FA) of CNVM. Visual acuity 20/200. **B.** One day post-treatment. FA shows almost total resolution of leakage. Visual acuity 20/40 and has remained stable for 2 years post treatment.

FVT works in eyes with a variety of types of CNV, including predominantly classic CNV and minimally classic CNV (Fig. 19.1).

IMAGING FOR FEEDER VESSEL THERAPY

Central to the choroidal FVT technique is the identification of the feeder vessel itself. To that end, imaging of the choroidal circulation is a vital step. In this situation both FA and indocyanine green (ICG) angiography serve a complimentary function (14). Although FA has been proven to be useful in establishing the extent of leakage of neovascular lesions in AMD, it has its limitations, particularly in the identification of the details of the vascular structures. In situations where choroidal neovascular membranes (CNVMs) are obscured by overlying hemorrhage, edema, or retinal pigment epithelial (RPE) hyperplasia, FA provides very little useful information with regards to choroidal vascular supply (15).

ICG has proven to be useful in the diagnosis and management of choroidal disorders such as AMD (16–18). Since the reports of human ICG angiograms were first published in 1970, there has been a continuous refinement of the technique, leading to increased spatial and temporal resolution of the images (19,20). With the advent of the ICG video angiogram in 1976, FVT of CNVM became more of a possibility (21–24). ICG angiography, and particularly HSICGA, can provide useful information with regard to the underlying vascular source to the neovascular complex (5,25).

The more recently developed scanning laser ophthalmoscope (SLO) allows real-time image capture at very low illumination levels (26–29). The typical exciter light source in such systems uses a small spot size (approximately 10 μm)

diode laser. This dynamic scanning system measures the reflectance of the retina as it is scanned by the laser beam (Fig. 19.2).

Confocal SLO systems are also capable of performing both FA and ICG angiography (30). Selection of light reflected from different focal planes in the retina is performed by moving the pinhole (31). The imaging capabilities of the SLO system in many instances provide added information to classifications such as classic, occult, or mixed types of the CNVM (32). HSICGA also allows for a more precise determination of reduced vascular perfusion postoperatively than is achievable with either FA or conventional ICG angiography.

Currently, the most commonly employed imaging system for FVT is the HSICGA. This SLO-based imaging technique allows for a capture rate of ICG angiography images to the level where directional flow through choroidal vessels can be identified (27,33–35). This approach to delineating the feeder vessels is superior to older techniques of dye accumulation, where later phases of the ICG angiography are examined for hyperfluorescence (36).

Methods for further refinement of the spatial resolution of ICG images involve the use of digital subtraction techniques and contrast enhancement (37–39). Similar in principal to those strategies employed in angiography of other vascular structures (e.g., cervical carotid circulation), these techniques allow for a greater resolution of CNV. This technique is still undergoing refinement. At present, most clinicians performing FVT depend on a technique based on the phi-motion phenomenon to temporally resolve the feeder vessel (40). This phenomenon describes the ability of the brain to analyze motion by observing rapidly flashing sequences of images. Typically, this is employed in video angiography to determine both the afferent and efferent supplies of the CNVM. This rapid-

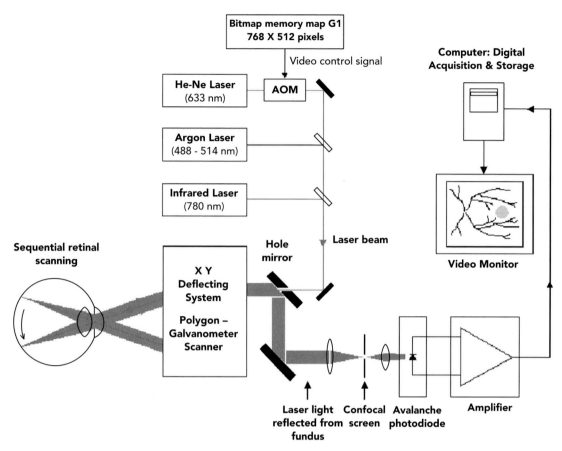

Figure 19.2   Schematic of scanning laser ophthalmoscope. (Adapted from Reinhard, J. 2003).

sequence viewing of high-resolution angiographic frames with control over the sequencing rates has provided a significant improvement in the analysis of the feeder vessels.

Static ICG angiography was divided into three phases (41). These phases focused attention on accumulation and leakage of ICG much in the same way as FA has been used. In sharp contrast, the period of most interest in FVT is the first 30 seconds of the dynamic HSICGA.

Interpretation of the HSICGA requires a moderate amount of experience (42). Understanding of the normal choroidal architecture is essential for successful identification of the feeder vessel (43). It is often best to begin by examining the FA to first determine the general area where a feeder vessel may be located. A careful examination of the HSICGA to identify the neovascular complex is then required. Once the extent of that complex has been determined, the next step is to identify the afferent and efferent feeder vessels. Detection of feeder vessels in exudative AMD has been reported to be from 22% to 86%, depending on the case series (3,9,10). Early studies of eyes with classic CNVMs showed that feeder vessels can be identified in at least 29% of cases using HSICGA (44). The advent of newer imaging devices and software has allowed the identification of feeder vessels in more than 90% of eyes with CNV regardless of the type of leakage.

There are several configurations of subretinal neovascular complexes in AMD that have been identified in

HSICGA. Delineation of a particular complex type can often be of assistance in locating the point of entry of the FV. For example a "sea fan" or "kidney bean" configuration, which is often seen in classic CNVMs, will more commonly have the feeder vessel located at the hilus of the complex. Similarly, a neovascular complex with a "medusa head" or "cartwheel" configuration will often have the feeder vessel entering centrally at the "hub."

INDICATIONS FOR FEEDER VESSEL THERAPY

The classification of CNVM in AMD as either classic or occult is based primarily upon FA features. This is particularly notable in those situations where an occult CNVM has been identified (45,46). Historically occult CNVMs have had a different visual acuity prognosis than classic (47). With FVT techniques, and particularly with imaging of the underlying subretinal and sub-RPE choroidal vasculopathy, the concern as to whether a CNVM is either classic or occult may become less important. What is critical is the identification and delineation of the feeder vessel themselves. Several studies have shown the presence of feeder vessels in occult CNVMs (3,48–50). FVT has been successfully applied to both classic and occult CNVMs in AMD (6–8,51,52). Indeed, success in the se of FVT has been reported (8,53).

Also, in several situations where a subfoveal CNVM exists, FVT has had a particular advantage since the feeder vessel itself is usually extrafoveal in location (3,9).

Pigment Epithelial Detachment

FVT has been applied to hemorrhagic and serosanguineous RPE detachments (54,55). These types of RPE detachments typically are associated with underlying CNV. More recently, pigment epithelial detachment (PED) in association with polypoidal choroidal vasculopathy (PCV) and retinal-choroidal anastomosis (RCA) in AMD patients have been described (56–58). Studies have demonstrated that ICG angiography can increase the identification of underlying CNVMs in PEDs (59–61). With the advent of ICG angiography, localization of the source of the hemorrhage or leak in PEDs was obtained at a much higher rate than with FA. Reports of ICG angiography-guided focal treatment of CNVMs in PED have yielded mixed results with regards to obliteration of the neovascular complex (52,55,59,62–64). The location of the CNVM in relation to the PED itself appears to significantly affect the outcome of laser treatment (62). In some recent, small studies that were able to identify feeder vessels in CNVMs associated with PEDs, the use of photothrombosis with ICG resulted in complete and sustained closure of the neovascular complex and resultant improvement in vision (54,65).

Recurrent Choroidal Neovascularization

The nearly 50% recurrence rate of conventional laser-treated CNVMs in AMD has made retreatment of these lesions a common event (66). FVT has been utilized in recurrent CNV following both conventional MPS-type laser photocoagulation and photodynamic therapy (PDT) (67). Not only has FVT been demonstrated to be successful at closure of recurrent CNVMs, but stabilization and improvement in visual acuity has also been demonstrated (67). The ability to delineate the feeder vessels through pigmented lesions give a particular advantage to both ICG angiography and FVT in those situations where there is recurrent neovascularization (50,68,69). Since the feeder vessel is almost always within the area of previous MPS or PDT treatment, laser directed at the feeder vessel cause no additional damage to untreated retina and choroid. It is important to note that treating ICG angiography-delineated hotspots in the immediate postlaser period is not warranted, as these are often transient and spontaneously disappear (70).

Retinal-Choroidal Anastomosis

Occasionally, abnormal communication between the choroidal and retinal circulation develops in AMD, either spontaneously or as a complication of focal laser therapy. This anastomotic complex, known as RCA can result in significant retinal edema with hard exudate formation. RCAs can be difficult to treat by FVT as well as by conventional laser photocoagulation (57,71,72). Recently described yellow-wavelength (568 nm) laser techniques have increased closure rates of RCA in AMD (73).

Polypoidal Choroidal Vasculopathy

PCV has been recently identified as a cause of recurrent macular subretinal and sub-RPE hemorrhages (74). Although this condition has been differentiated from CNV in AMD as a separate entity, clinically the two often coexist in the same patient (56,58,75–78). This condition, as mentioned earlier, can often be best visualized using ICG angiography (18,75,79). In those situations where there is CNV of the PCV lesions, the visual prognosis is poor (80–82). While successful closure of PCV lesions has been reported with conventional laser and PDT, good results have also been obtained with FVT (40,83–85). FVT might be most beneficial in those PCV lesions complicated by hemorrhagic PEDs, as their prognosis is poorer than other types of PCV (56,86,87).

Retinal Angiomatous Proliferation

Exudative AMD that is complicated by retinal angiomatous proliferation (RAP) lesions is also amenable to FVT. However, if the lesion is imaged with HSICGA, confluent yellow-laser treatment has been shown to be effective in ablating the entire lesion (88). Stage 2 or Stage 3 RAP lesions, where CNV exists within a vascularized PED and a RCA is present, are potential candidates for FVT (89). Some success has also been reported recently with surgical lysis of these lesions (90).

TECHNIQUES FOR FEEDER VESSEL THERAPY

Achieving regression of a CNVM with FVT requires several steps, including identification of the feeder vessel, selection of an appropriate laser to produce vascular attenuation, and employing an appropriate follow-up schedule to ensure that re-treatments are applied in a timely fashion. The goal of therapy is regression of the CNVM to achieve reduction of leakage and reabsorption of subretinal fluid with minimal subretinal fibrosis.

The concept of selective attenuation of feeder vessels to achieve regression of a choroidal neovascular complex has existed for many years. Direct treatment of feeder vessels was included in the MPS protocol for management of recurrent CNVM (12). Case reports of successful control of CNV following FVT have been reported in the literature (91,92). However, successful FVTs were uncommon prior to the advent of HSICGA.

Some confusion has existed as to the nature of feeder vessels. Pathological studies of exudative macular degeneration

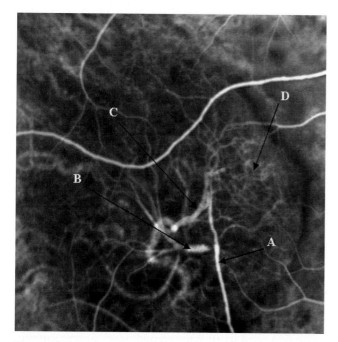

Figure 19.3 Choroidal neovascular membrane (CNVM) with afferent and efferent feeder vessels. **A.** Feeder vessel of the active lesion. **B.** Feeder vessel of an earlier regressed lesion. Note the presence of a penetrating vessel (**C**). **D.** Secondary and tertiary branches of the CNVM.

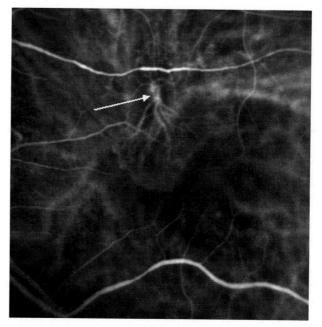

Figure 19.4 High-speed indocyanine green angiogram of a classic choroidal neovascularization with cartwheel pattern.

have frequently demonstrated vessels that penetrate Bruch's membrane as a component of the neovascular complex (93). These studies have reported that most CNVMs have three to five vessels penetrating Bruch's membrane (93). These penetrating vessels have often been erroneously considered feeder vessels. Feeder vessels represent vessels in the midlayers of the choroid that become preferential vascular supplies to areas of CNV. Because feeder vessels longitudinally traverse the choroid, they can be visualized on HSICGA while penetrating vessels, oriented perpendicular to Bruch's membrane, are not seen (Fig. 19.3).

Feeder vessels have certain characteristics that allow differentiation from normal choroidal vessels. They are smaller-diameter choroidal vessels that generally fill earlier than the surrounding choroidal vessels. Typically, a separate arterial and venous component can be detected, and in most cases these vessels may lie in close proximity.

Classic CNVMs are well-defined areas of early hyperfluorescence with exuberant late leakage from the lacy brush border on FA. Feeder vessels in classic CNVMs most commonly arise nasal to the CNVM in a "racquet like" pattern (3). Feeder vessels may also lie within the center of the neovascular complex and radiate outwards in a "cartwheel" or "umbrella" pattern to fill the brush border vessels. These central feeder vessels may be more difficult to discern, given that they lie beneath the neovascular complex (3). The draining vein is typically in close proximity to the arterial (Fig. 19.4). Recurrent CNVMs developing adjacent to a previous chorioretinal scar or previous MPS-type focal laser treatment are frequently classic in nature.

Feeder vessels run through the chorioretinal scar and extend into the recurrent neovascularization in a pattern reminiscent of a tennis racket (Fig. 19.5). Feeder vessels supplying occult CNVMs are typically long and linear, in comparison to the more tortuous course of normal choroidal vessels (33).

Atypical forms of CNV are also well demonstrated on HSICGA. RAP lesions are poorly demonstrated on FA,

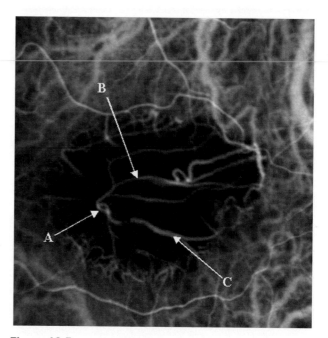

Figure 19.5 High-speed indocyanine green angiogram of recurrent choroidal neovascularization with racket pattern of feeder vessels.

appearing as ill-defined occult CNVMs. HSICGA clearly demonstrates the extent of the intraretinal neovascularization and clearly demonstrates the retinal-to-retinal anastomoses that are present in some of these cases (Fig. 19.6) (88). In one case series of 25 eyes with suspected RAP lesions, 88% had identifiable intraretinal neovascularization on HSICGA (94). Polypoidal neovascularization can also appear as occult leakage on FA. Static ICG imaging may demonstrate hot spots (78). HSICGA often clearly demonstrates an afferent arterial that supplies a cluster of dilated vascular lesions.

A variety of treatment protocols have been described to obtain closure or attenuation of feeder vessels. The goal of treatment is to cause resolution of subretinal fluid with minimal development of subretinal fibrosis. The neovascular complexes cease growing and the border of the neovascular tissue becomes more mature with fewer leaking vascular loops (Fig. 19.7).

All treatment techniques are designed to produce vascular modulation with minimal surrounding tissue trauma to minimize secondary scotomas. Pulsed applications of laser energy are applied to maximize the energy absorption in the target tissue (95). Laser spot sizes have varied from 75 to 200 μm, and application durations have varied from 100 to 200 msec. Initial laser energy is low, ranging from 50 to 100 mW. Protocols using 532 nm green, 810 nm red and 562 nm yellow laser have been described. No studies indicate that one wavelength produces preferable results (3,9,96,97). Some features of the feeder vessel may influence laser preference. Feeder vessels that are visible within previous chorioretinal scars have little surrounding pigmentation, and therefore use

of a wavelength that is optimally absorbed by oxyhemoglobin (yellow or green) is preferable. Feeder vessels that are not clinically visible and run under intact RPE are best treated using infrared wavelengths. Preferentially, treatment is applied to the arterial component of the feeder vessel, however, the anatomy of feeder vessels occasionally leads to treatment of both the artery and the vein (96).

The laser energy is gradually increased until a minimal reaction is observed in the underlying RPE. White burns of the retina should be avoided. In cases where the feeder vessel is visible, treatment should cause complete closure of flow. In some cases, the treatment endpoint is blanching of the entire complex; in other cases a posttreatment FA and HSICGA may be performed to confirm closure of the feeder vessel and the CNVM.

Some authors have utilized ICG as a photosensitizing dye to enhance feeder vessel closure. ICG is administered as a 50 mg loading dose followed by a second 50 mg dose 20 minutes later. Each infusion is followed by a flush of saline. Ten seconds after the second dose, an 800 μm 810 nm diode laser spot is applied to the feeder vessel ingrowth site for 80 seconds, delivering 30 W/cm². A second application is applied 10 seconds after the initial application (96). This technique has been used to obtain closure of CNV associated with angioid streaks and occult neovascularization in AMD (96,97).

FVT has been utilized in the treatment of recurrent leakage following PDT. In one trial of 20 patients with recurrent leakage following PDT, FVT was used to successfully obliterate the feeder vessel in 70% of cases, with 50% of cases remaining closed for 3 or more months (98). The

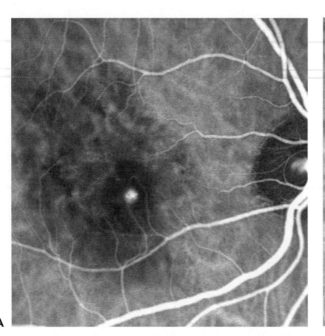
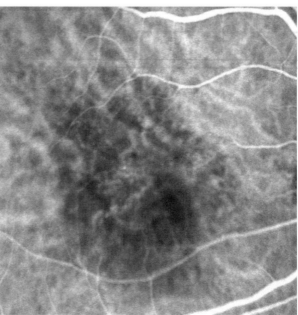

A   B

Figure 19.6 **A.** High-speed indocyanine green angiogram (HSICGA) of a RAP lesion. **B.** HSICGA of RAP lesion post feeder vessel therapy.

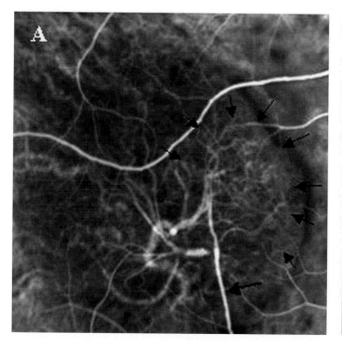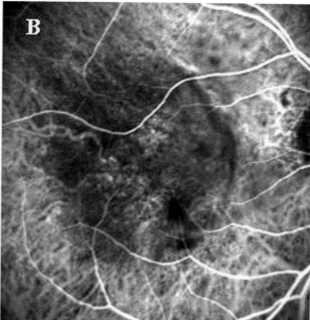

Figure 19.7   Pretreatment (**A**) and posttreatment (**B**) angiogram.

results suggested an improved functional outcome compared to an untreated control group (98).

Follow-up schedules for patients undergoing FVT are dictated by the biology of the neovascularization. Classic CNVMs tend to leak more profusely and grow more rapidly and therefore repeat examinations, and re-treatments when necessary, should be performed within 14 days of initial therapy. Occult lesions tend to be more indolent, and repeat examinations and treatment when necessary are more typically performed in 4 to 6 weeks.

FVT has an excellent safety profile given the low intensity of the treatment and the maintenance of treatment in an extra foveal location. In one early study of 37 patients, two subretinal hemorrhages were observed; however, both were considered negligible and reabsorbed spontaneously (9).

OUTCOMES OF FEEDER VESSEL THERAPY

Classic Choroidal Neovascularization

FVT is an effective treatment for AMD with classic CNV. The efficacy of FVT for classic CNV was first reported in 1998 (3,9). Two patterns of feeder vessels were described: umbrella or cartwheel, and racket. In these early reports, laser treatment was applied along the length of the feeder vessel for several hundred microns. After 1 year of follow up, Shiraga et al. observed visual improvement of more than two lines in 14 out of 37 (38%) eyes, and Staurenghi found similar improvement in eight out of 16 (50%) eyes (3,9). Shiraga reported recurrent CNV in seven out of 37 (19%) treated eyes, and Staurenghi noted recurrences in only two of 16 (13%) eyes after 1 year of follow up (3,9).

We reported a consecutive series of patients with FA evidence of classic CNV (6). Visual acuities were Snellen and/or ETDRS and were converted to ETDRS equivalents. Feeder vessels were identified and monitored using HSICGA guided by FA. Feeder vessel closure was accomplished using an 810 nm laser, set at a 75 to 200 μm spot size, pulse duration of 100 milliseconds, 50% duty cycle (millipulse mode), for an average total duration of 90 seconds. Laser energy was gradually increased to create graying of the RPE without visible retinal reaction. The endpoint of treatment was closure of the feeder vessel(s) on HSICGA.

Thirty-three eyes of 33 patients were followed for an average of 6 months after treatment. Only six out of 33 (18%) eyes lost the equivalent of more than three lines of vision, and just three out of 33 (9%) lost more than six lines. Vision improved by more than three lines in 11 out of 33 (33%) eyes (6).

Patients receiving FVT for AMD with classic CNV faired better than the natural history. In a recent report, 36% of patients with classic CNV lost more than three lines after 6 months (99). In contrast, only 18% of eyes receiving FVT in our current series lost more than three lines of vision (6). Even more striking is the finding that vision improved greater than three lines in 33% of eyes following FVT, compared to only 2.4% of eyes that might be expected to improve without treatment. FVT is a viable alternative for the management of classic CNV that can result in improved vision in a significant percentage of patients.

Occult Choroidal Neovascularization

Most patients with newly diagnosed exudative AMD present with a poorly defined lesion or occult CNV and do not meet the eligibility criteria for treatment with PDT (12,99). Recent evidence from the Verteporfin in Photodynamic Therapy (VIP) study group has shown that PDT only modestly reduces the risk of moderate and severe vision loss in this subgroup (100).

In a recent series we evaluated 37 eyes of 31 patients with newly diagnosed exudative AMD, with angiographic evidence of occult CNV. Eighty-one percent of the patients were female and 19% male (8). All patients were Caucasian with ages ranging from 62 to 92, with an average age of 77. All patients had a minimum of 1-year follow-up. Laser photocoagulation using an 810 nm diode laser was applied using the millipulse technique to a segment of each feeder vessel outside the fovea. Diode laser settings were 75 μm spot size, 0.10 second duration, 100 msec repeat mode, with incremental increases in power to create deep burns. After 1 year, ETDRS visual acuity was stable or improved in 24 out of 37 (64.8%) eyes. Nine eyes (24.3%) achieved greater than three lines of improvement in visual acuity. Eight eyes (21.6%) had worse visual acuity by one to three lines, and five eyes (13.5%) had loss of three to six lines of vision. The average number of treatments was 3.6. Overall, 75% of treatments were performed within the first 3 months (8). Determination of treatment adequacy was based on angiographic evidence of feeder vessel closure or attenuation.

The VIP Study Group reported 34% of their PDT-treated patients with occult with no classic CNV, having stable or improved vision, with only 3% having greater than three lines of visual improvement at 1 year (101). In our study, 64.8% of treated eyes had stable or improved vision, with 24.3% achieving greater than three lines of visual improvement (8). In this small series, FVT has been shown to yield resolution of exudative manifestations and stabilize or improve vision in a majority of the patients treated, and should be considered as a treatment option for occult with no classic CNV associated with AMD.

Recurrent Choroidal Neovascularization

The MPS has demonstrated the benefits of treatment of well-demarcated lesions for reduction of severe vision loss compared with no treatment (66,102). However, patients with subfoveal CNV experience immediate loss of vision after treatment, and up to 66% of patients have persistent or recurrent CNV within 3 years (66,102). Recurrent CNV has a poor prognosis and is usually associated with further vision loss, especially when the CNV recurs in the subfoveal area. The area of recurrence is typically adjacent to and extends from the existing scar. The relatively bare anatomy of an atrophic scar facilitates the identification and treatment of feeder vessels. Feeder vessels can often be identified within the margins of the scar by HSICGA, and treated by direct visualization. Treatment within an existing scar is advantageous because the ensuing laser damage is located in an area of nonfunctional retina, and so does not produce additional visual damage. Early treatment

results for recurrent CNV utilizing the ablation of the feeder vessel within the existing scar have been promising: visual acuities improved and remained stable over an 18 month period (67).

Retinal Angiomatous Proliferations

RAPs are a form of primary intraretinal neovascularization that may occur in 10% to 15% of patients with exudative macular degeneration. Patients present with cystoid retinal edema, intraretinal hemorrhages, and a focal hot spot on static ICG imaging (89). FA typically demonstrates occult neovascularization. HSICGA can be useful in clearly identifying the boundaries of the intraretinal neovascularization.

A prospective case series has been conducted of 12 eyes of 11 consecutive patients with macular degeneration and associated RAP lesions identified and treated using HSICGA (88). Confluent yellow laser (568 nm) was applied to completely ablate the intraretinal neovascularization and any associated intraretinal vascular anastomoses. HSICGA was required in all patients to clearly define the intraretinal neovascularization. HSICGA was essential for localization of early, small RAP lesions. A mean of 2.1 laser treatments per eye was required. With an average follow up of 4.8 months, 92% had a reduction or resolution of subretinal fluid and retinal edema; 84% had stable or improved visual acuity, with 42% gaining one or more lines (88).

HSICGA is an important method for the identification of RAP. HSICGA is able to localize early RAP lesions that are not well defined with traditional imaging techniques. Many RAP lesions present with excellent visual acuity; HSICGA allows for earlier identification and therapy, which may offer improved visual outcomes.

Retinal-Choroidal Anastomoses

RCAs are a common finding in advanced cases of AMD. These high-flow lesions are associated with extensive subretinal exudation. Improvement of visual acuity can be obtained with successful closure of the RCA and associated resolution of subretinal fluid, though some limitations in visual function exist due to associated subretinal fibrosis (71).

HSICGA clearly demonstrates that arterial and venous components of flow within the RCA. High-frequency, high-intensity yellow-wavelength laser can be utilized to obtain closure of the arterial component of the RCA. By utilizing high-frequency pulses of laser energy, absorption is maximized in the target area with minimal heat dissemination to the surrounding tissues. Associated reduction in flow can lead to successful reduction in subretinal fluid.

In one series of 19 eyes with RCA associated with macular degeneration, HSICGA was used to identify and treat the arterial component of the RCA (73). At mean follow up of 11.7 (2–23) months, patients had undergone an average of 3.52 (1–12) sessions of laser treatment. Final visual acuity remained within one line of baseline in all patients. Fifty-three percent had complete resolution of subretinal fluid. Forty-three percent had complete closure of RCAs while the remainder had attenuation of flow. No significant complications were encountered (73).

Polypoidal Choroidal Vasculopathy

Idiopathic PCV is an atypical form of CNV characterized by orange subretinal lesions associated with recurrent serosanguineous PED (78). FA may demonstrate pooling within polypoidal lesions or associated classic or occult CNV (78). Static ICG imaging shows focal hot spots corresponding to the polypoidal lesions (78). Initially these lesions were described to arise in a peripapillary region; however, some patients appear to have a macular variant that arises in a more central location (74,78). A variety of treatment approaches have been utilized in the management of exudative lesions, including direct photocoagulation and PDT.

HSICGA can be useful in the identification of polypoidal lesions. Typically the polypoidal cluster is fed by an arteriole that arises in a peripapillary location. In one series of 10 patients with polypoidal lesions identified on HSICGA, seven had definite feeder vessels (40). Regression of subretinal fluid, hemorrhage, and lipid, with attenuation or resolution of the polypoid dilatations 6 months after feeder vessel treatment, occurred in six of the seven treated PCV eyes. A mean number of 4.6 treatments were required. Visual acuity at the last follow-up of 1.5 to 22 (mean = 13.5 months) months following initial treatment remained within two lines of pretreatment vision in all eyes (40).

SUMMARY

The challenge in treating CNV is to reduce the areas of active leakage and hemorrhage, while minimizing collateral damage to the surrounding tissue. The MPS attempted this by treating only well-defined lesions (12). Surgical approaches to extract CNVs have been met with limited success. More recently, PDT proved useful in slowing visual deterioration in select patients with small, well-defined subfoveal CNVs (99). The rate of vision loss was slower in the study group compared to placebo; however, the mean visual acuity continued to deteriorate at subsequent visits. The concept of treating feeder vessels is based upon the concept that by treating only the afferent vessel, rather than the entire lesion, trauma to surrounding tissue is minimized.

REFERENCES

1. Gee M, Soulen MC. Chemoembolization for hepatic metastases. *Tech Vasc Interv Radiol.* 2002;5(3):132–140.
2. Takeuchi S, Tanaka R, Fujii Y, et al. Surgical treatment of hemangioblastomas with presurgical endovascular embolization. *Neurol Med Chir (Tokyo).* 2001;41(5):246–251; discussion 251–252.
3. Staurenghi G, Orzalesi N, La Capria A, et al. Laser treatment of feeder vessels in subfoveal choroidal neovascular membranes: a revisitation using dynamic indocyanine green angiography. *Ophthalmology.* 1998;105(12):2,297–2,305.
4. Flower RW. Experimental studies of indocyanine green dye-enhanced photocoagulation of choroidal neovascularization feeder vessels. *Am J Ophthalmol.* 2000;129(4):501–512.
5. Flower RW, von Kerczek C, Zhu L, et al. Theoretical investigation of the role of choriocapillaris blood flow in treatment of subfoveal choroidal neovascularization associated with age-related macular degeneration. *Am J Ophthalmol.* 2001;132(1):85–93.
6. Glaser BM, Baudo TA, Velez G, et al. Feeder vessel treatment for age-related macular degeneration with classic choroidal neovascular membranes. *Invest Ophthalmol Vis Sci.* 2001.
7. Murphy RP, Lin, Glaser BM. FV treatment for ARMD with subfoveal fibrovascular CNV. *Invest Ophthalmol Vis Sci.* 2001.
8. Roh ML, Glaser BM. Feeder vessel treatment of occult with no classic choroidal neovascularization in age-related macular degeneration. *ARVO Meeting Abstracts.* 2003;44(5):1,776.
9. Shiraga F, Ojima Y, Matsuo T, et al. Feeder vessel photocoagulation of subfoveal choroidal neovascularization secondary to age-related macular degeneration. *Ophthalmology.* 1998;105(4):662–669.
10. Glaser B, Murphy R, Lakhanpal R, et al. Identification and treatment of modulating choroidal vessels associated with occult choroidal neovascularization. *ARVO Meeting Abstracts.* 2000;41:S320.
11. Little HL, Zweng HC, Jack RL, et al. Techniques of argon laser photocoagulation of diabetic disk new vessels. *Am J Ophthalmol.* 1976;82(5):675–683.
12. Macular Photocoagulation Study Group. Subfoveal neovascular lesions in age-related macular degeneration. Guidelines for evaluation and treatment in the macular photocoagulation study. *Arch Ophthalmol.* 1991;109(9):1,242–1,257.
13. Staurenghi G, Flower RW. Clinical observations supporting a theoretical model of choriocapillaris blood flow in treatment of choroidal neovascularization associated with age-related macular degeneration. *Am J Ophthalmol.* 2002;133(6):801–808.
14. Srivastava S, Csaky KG. Fluorescein angiographic findings in choroidal neovascularization (CNV) immediately following feeder vessel closure. *ARVO Meeting Abstracts.* 2003;44(5):4,940–4,943.
15. Kramer M, Mimouni K, Priel E, et al. Comparison of fluorescein angiography and indocyanine green angiography for imaging of choroidal neovascularization in hemorrhagic age-related macular degeneration. *Am J Ophthalmol.* 2000;129(4):495–500.
16. Destro M, Puliafito CA. Indocyanine green videoangiography of choroidal neovascularization. *Ophthalmology.* 1989;96(6):846–853.
17. Obana A, Gohto Y, Matsumoto M, et al. Indocyanine green angiographic features prognostic of visual outcome in the natural course of patients with age related macular degeneration. *Br J Ophthalmol.* 1999;83(4):429–437.
18. Stanga PE, Lim JI, Hamilton P. Indocyanine green angiography in chorioretinal diseases: indications and interpretation: an evidence-based update. *Ophthalmology.* 2003;110(1):15–21; quiz 22–23.
19. Kogure K, David NJ, Yamanouchi U, et al. Infrared absorption angiography of the fundus circulation. *Arch Ophthalmol.* 1970;83(2):209–214.
20. Kulvin S, Stauffer L, Kogure K, et al. Fundus angiography in man by intracarotid administration of dye. *South Med J.* 1970;63(9):998–1,000.
21. Orth DH, Patz A, Flower RW. Potential clinical applications of indocyanine green choroidal angiography—preliminary report. *Eye Ear Nose Throat Mon.* 1976;55(1):15–28, 58.
22. Flower RW, Fryczkowski AW, McLeod DS. Variability in choriocapillaris blood flow distribution. *Invest Ophthalmol Vis Sci.* 1995;36(7):1,247–1,258.
23. Klein GJ, Baumgartner RH, Flower RW. An image processing approach to characterizing choroidal blood flow. *Invest Ophthalmol Vis Sci.* 1990;31(4):629–637.
24. Prunte C, Niesel P. Quantification of choroidal blood-flow parameters using indocyanine green video-fluorescence angiography and statistical picture analysis. *Graefes Arch Clin Exp Ophthalmol.* 1988;226(1):55–58.
25. Gelisken F, Inhoffen W, Schneider U, et al. Indocyanine green videoangiography of occult choroidal neovascularization: a comparison of scanning laser ophthalmoscope with high-resolution digital fundus camera. *Retina.* 1998;18(1):37–43.
26. Mainster MA, Timberlake GT, Webb RH, et al. Scanning laser ophthalmoscopy. Clinical applications. *Ophthalmology.* 1982;89(7):852–857.
27. Scheider A, Schroedel C. High resolution indocyanine green angiography with a scanning laser ophthalmoscope. *Am J Ophthalmol.* 1989;108(4):458–459.
28. Schneider U, Kuck H, Inhoffen W, et al. Indocyanine green angiographically well-defined choroidal neovascularization: angiographic patterns obtained using the scanning laser ophthalmoscope. *Ger J Ophthalmol.* 1995;4(2):67–74.
29. Wolf S, Wald KJ, Elsner AE, et al. Indocyanine green choroidal videoangiography: a comparison of imaging analysis with the scanning laser ophthalmoscope and the fundus camera. *Retina.* 1993;13(3):266–269.
30. Holz FG, Bellmann C, Dithmar S, et al. [Simultaneous fluorescein and indocyanine green angiography with a confocal laser ophthalmoscope]. *Ophthalmologe.* 1997;94(5):348–353.

31. Webb RH, Hughes GW, Delori FC. Confocal scanning laser ophthalmoscope. *Applied Optics.* 1987;26(8):1,492–1,499.
32. Rosenthal J. A perspective and editorial on ICG imaging and treatment of macular neovascularization. *Physician Center.* 2003:2001.
33. Staurenghi G, Musicco I, Salvetti P, et al. Anatomic and flow characteristics of feeder vessels in choroidal neovascular membranes. *ARVO Meeting Abstracts.* 2002;43(12):2,512.
34. Yamamoto Y. Measurement of blood flow velocity in feeder vessels of choroidal neovascularization by a scanning laser ophthalmoscope and image analysis system. *Jpn J Ophthalmol.* 2003;47(1):53–58.
35. Yamamoto Y. [Measurement of flow velocity in feeder vessels of choroidal neovascularization with a scanning laser ophthalmoscope and image analysis system.] *Nippon Ganka Gakkai Zasshi.* 2002;106(5):287–292.
36. Ashman RA, Reinholz F, Eikelboom RH. Differential imaging in scanning laser ophthalmoscopy. *Int Ophthalmol.* 2001;23(4–6):405–408.
37. Kohno T, De Laey JJ, Miki T. Detection of choroidal neovascularization in age-related macular degeneration using subtraction methods in indocyanine green angiography. *Bull Soc Belge Ophtalmol.* 1995;259:81–88.
38. Maberley DA, Cruess AF. Indocyanine green angiography: an evaluation of image enhancement for the identification of occult choroidal neovascular membranes. *Retina.* 1999;19(1):37–44.
39. Torok B, Hirschi R, Szekely G, et al. [Automatic measurement of dye filling of simultaneous digital ICG and fluorescein angiography sequences.] *Klin Monatsbl Augenheilkd.* 2000;216(5):268–271.
40. Somaiya M, Glaser B. High-speed phi-motion ICG characteristics and feeder vessel treatment of polypoidal choroidal vasculopathy in age-related macular degeneration. *ARVO Meeting Abstracts.* 2002;43(12):2,509.
41. Slakter J, Flower RW, Yannuzzi LA. *Indocyanine Green Angiography: Imaging of the Retina.* Mosby; 1997:359.
42. Salvetti P, Massacesi A, Viola F, et al. Feeder vessel identification: the learning curve. *ARVO Meeting Abstracts.* 2001;42:1,242.
43. Ito YN, Mori K, Young-Duvall J, et al. Aging changes of the choroidal dye filling pattern in indocyanine green angiography of normal subjects. *Retina.* 2001;21(3):237–242.
44. Gelisken F, Inhoffen W, Schneider U, et al. Indocyanine green angiography in classic choroidal neovascularization. *Jpn J Ophthalmol.* 1998;42(4):300–303.
45. Guyer DR, Yannuzzi LA, Slakter JS, et al. Digital indocyanine-green videoangiography of occult choroidal neovascularization. *Ophthalmology.* 1994;101(10):1,727–1,735; discussion 1,735–1,737.
46. Haddad WM, Coscas G, Soubrane G. Eligibility for treatment and angiographic features at the early stage of exudative age related macular degeneration. *Br J Ophthalmol.* 2002;86(6):663–669.
47. Stevens TS, Bressler NM, Maguire MG, et al. Occult choroidal neovascularization in age-related macular degeneration. A natural history study. *Arch Ophthalmol.* 1997;115(3):345–350.
48. Donati G, Kapetanios AD, Pournaras CJ. ICG-guided laser photocoagulation of juxtafoveal and extrafoveal occult choroidal neovascularization. *Graefes Arch Clin Exp Ophthalmol.* 1999;237(11):881–886.
49. Pece A, Introini U, Bolognesi G, et al. Indocyanine green angiography in age-related macular degeneration with occult neovascularization. *Ophthalmologica.* 1998;212(5):295–300.
50. Regillo CD, Blade KA, Custis PH, et al. Evaluating persistent and recurrent choroidal neovascularization. The role of indocyanine green angiography. *Ophthalmology.* 1998;105(10):1,821–1,826.
51. Mori R, Yuzawa M. [Utility of indocyanine green angiography guided laser photocoagulation of choroidal neovascularization in age-related macular degeneration.] *Nippon Ganka Gakkai Zasshi.* 2002;106(10):621–629.
52. Weinberger AW, Knabben H, Solbach U, et al. Indocyanine green guided laser photocoagulation in patients with occult choroidal neovascularisation. *Br J Ophthalmol.* 1999;83(2):168–172.
53. Sayag D, Coscas F, Coscas G, et al. Feeder vessel treatment with millipulse diode laser on occult subfoveal choroidal new vessels in age-related macular degeneration (AMD) using high speed ICG-angiography. *ARVO Meeting Abstracts.* 2003;44(5):1,762.
54. Costa KM, Rocha RA, Calucci D, et al. Neovascular ingrowth site photothrombosis in choroidal neovascularization associated with retinal pigment epithelial detachment. *Graefes Arch Clin Exp Ophthalmol.* 2003;241(3):245–250.
55. Stanescu D, Coscas G, Coscas F, et al. Feeder vessel treatment in age-related macular degeneration (AMD) with classic, occult choroidal neovascularization and vascularized retinal pigment epithelium detachment. *ARVO Meeting Abstracts.* 2002;43(12):1,226.
56. Muller C, Spital G, Radermacher M, et al. [Pigment epithelium detachments in AMD (age-associated macular degeneration) and *polypoid choroidal vasculopathy.* A fluorescein and indocyanine green angiography study.] *Ophthalmologe.* 2002;99(2):85–89.
57. Slakter JS, Yannuzzi LA, Schneider U, et al. Retinal choroidal anastomoses and occult choroidal neovascularization in age-related macular degeneration. *Ophthalmology.* 2000;107(4):742–753; discussion 753–754.
58. Tateiwa H, Kuroiwa S, Gaun S, et al. Polypoidal choroidal vasculopathy with large vascular network. *Graefes Arch Clin Exp Ophthalmol.* 2002; 240(5):354–361.
59. Baumal CR, Reichel E, Duker JS, et al. Indocyanine green hyperfluorescence associated with serous retinal pigment epithelial detachment in age-related macular degeneration. *Ophthalmology.* 1997;104(5):761–769.
60. Sallet G, Lafaut BA, De Laey JJ. Indocyanine green angiography and age-related serous pigment epithelial detachment. *Graefes Arch Clin Exp Ophthalmol.* 1996;234(1):25–33.
61. Yannuzzi LA, Hope-Ross M, Slakter JS, et al. Analysis of vascularized pigment epithelial detachments using indocyanine green videoangiography. *Retina.* 1994;14(2):99–113.
62. Brancato R, Introini U, Bolognesi G, et al. ICGA-guided laser photocoagulation of occult choroidal neovascularization in age-related macular degeneration. Indocyanine green angiography. *Retina.* 2000;20(2):134–142.
63. Da Pozzo S, Parodi MB, Ravalico G. A pilot study of ICG-guided laser photocoagulation for occult choroidal neovascularization presenting as a focal spot in age-related macular degeneration. *Int Ophthalmol.* 2001;24(4):187–189.
64. Gomez-Ulla F, Gonzalez F, Abelenda D, et al. Diode laser photocoagulation of choroidal neovascularization associated with retinal pigment epithelial detachment. *Acta Ophthalmol Scand.* 2001;79(1):39–44.
65. Rocha KM, Costa RA, Calucci D, et al. Neovascular ingrowth site photothrombosis in choroidal neovascularization associated with retinal pigment epithelial detachment. *ARVO Meeting Abstracts.* 2003;44(5):4,924.
66. Macular Photocoagulation Study Group. Laser photocoagulation of subfoveal neovascular lesions in age-related macular degeneration. Results of a randomized clinical trial. *Arch Ophthalmol.* 1991;109(9):1,220–1,231.
67. Luu J, Baudo T, Glaser B. Feeder vessel treatment of recurrent choroidal neovascularization (CNV). *ARVO Meeting Abstracts.* 2002;43(12):2,510.
68. Reichel E, Pollock DA, Duker JS, et al. Indocyanine green angiography for recurrent choroidal neovascularization in age-related macular degeneration. *Ophthalmic Surg Lasers.* 1995;26(6):513–518.
69. Sorenson JA, Yannuzzi LA, Slakter JS, et al. A pilot study of digital indocyanine green videoangiography for recurrent occult choroidal neovascularization in age-related macular degeneration. *Arch Ophthalmol.* 1994;112(4):473–479.
70. Chen CJ, Chen LJ, Miller KR. Clinical significance of postlaser indocyanine green angiographic hot spots in age-related macular degeneration. *Ophthalmology.* 1999;106(5):925–929; discussion 929–931.
71. Cialdini AP, Jalkh AE, Trempe CL, et al. Photocoagulation of chorioretinal anastomoses in far-advanced age-related macular degeneration. *Ophthalmic Surg.* 1989;20(5):316–320.
72. Mantel I, Zografos L. [Photocoagulation of the retinal feeder vessels of a chorioretinal anastomosis in age-related macular degeneration.] *J Fr Ophtalmol.* 2003;26(5):493–497.
73. Johnson T, Luu J, Glaser B. Micropulse laser modulation of retinal-choroidal anastomoses in exudative macular degeneration. *ARVO Meeting Abstracts.* 2002;43(12):2,506.
74. Moorthy RS, Lyon AT, Rabb MF, et al. Idiopathic polypoidal choroidal vasculopathy of the macula. *Ophthalmology.* 1998;105(8):1,380–1,385.
75. Escano MF, Fujii S, Ishibashi K, et al. Indocyanine green videoangiography in macular variant of idiopathic polypoidal choroidal vasculopathy. *Jpn J Ophthalmol.* 2000;44(3):313–316.
76. Lois N. Idiopathic polypoidal choroidal vasculopathy in a patient with atrophic age related macular degeneration. *Br J Ophthalmol.* 2001;85(8):1,011–1,012.
77. Scassellati-Sforzolini B, Mariotti C, Bryan R, et al. Polypoidal choroidal vasculopathy in Italy. *Retina.* 2001;21 (2):121–125.
78. Yannuzzi LA, Sorenson J, Spaide RF, et al. Idiopathic polypoidal choroidal vasculopathy (IPCV). *Retina.* 1990;10(1):1–8.
79. Ciardella AP, Donsoff IM, Yannuzzi LA. Polypoidal choroidal vasculopathy. *Ophthalmol Clin North Am.* 2002;15(4):537–554.
80. Iida T, Yannuzzi LA, Freund KB, et al. Retinal angiopathy and polypoidal choroidal vasculopathy. *Retina.* 2002;22(4):455–463.
81. Kimura T, Akita J, Nishijima K, et al. [Visual prognosis in polypoidal choroidal vasculopathy associated with subretinal hematoma.] *Nippon Ganka Gakkai Zasshi.* 2002;106(10):642–647.
82. Lafaut BA, Leys AM, Snyers B, et al. Polypoidal choroidal vasculopathy in Caucasians. *Graefes Arch Clin Exp Ophthalmol.* 2000;238(9):752–759.
83. Quaranta M, Mauget-Faysse M, Coscas G. Exudative idiopathic polypoidal choroidal vasculopathy and photodynamic therapy with verteporfin. *Am J Ophthalmol.* 2002;134(2):277–280.
84. Spaide RF, Donsoff I, Lam DL, et al. Treatment of polypoidal choroidal vasculopathy with photodynamic therapy. *Retina.* 2002;22(5):529–535.
85. Yuzawa M, Mori R, Haruyama M. A study of laser photocoagulation for polypoidal choroidal vasculopathy. *Jpn J Ophthalmol.* 2003;47(4):379–384.
86. Lakhanpal V, Glaser B, Murphy RP, et al. Observations and characteristics of polypoidal choroidal vasculopathy ("PCV") using HSICG: a pilot study. *Invest Ophthalmol Vis Sci.* 2000.
87. Uyama M, Wada M, Nagai Y, et al. Polypoidal choroidal vasculopathy: natural history. *Am J Ophthalmol.* 2002;133(5):639–648.
88. Johnson TM, Glaser BM. High speed ICG guided focal laser treatment of retinal angiomatous proliferations. *ARVO Meeting Abstracts.* 2003;44(5):5,034.
89. Yannuzzi LA, Negrao S, Iida T, et al. Retinal angiomatous proliferation in age-related macular degeneration. *Retina.* 2001;21(5):416–434.
90. Garg SJ, Sivalingam A, Martidis A. Six month follow-up of surgical ablation for Stage 2 retinal angiomatous proliferation. *ARVO Meeting Abstracts.* 2003;44(5):1791.

91. Deutman AF, Hendikse F, Hoyng C. [Treatment of choroidal neovascularization in degenerative myopia.] *Ophtalmologie.* 1989;3(4):299–301.

92. Melberg NS, Thomas MA. Successful feeder vessel laser treatment of recurrent neovascularization following subfoveal surgery. *Arch Ophthalmol.* 1996;114(2):224–226.

93. Green WR, Enger C. Age-related macular degeneration histopathologic studies. The 1992 Lorenz E. Zimmerman lecture. *Ophthalmology.* 1993;100 (10):1,519–1,535.

94. Bottoni F, Staurenghi G. Dynamic indocyanine green angiography (ICGA) for the detection of deep retinal vascular anomalous complexes (RVAC). *ARVO Meeting Abstracts.* 2001;42:3,780.

95. Garden JM, Tan OT, Kerschmann R, et al. Effect of dye laser pulse duration on selective cutaneous vascular injury. *J Invest Dermatol.* 1986;87(5): 653–657.

96. Costa RA, Calucci D, Cardillo JA, et al. Selective occlusion of subfoveal choroidal neovascularization in angioid streaks by using a new technique of ingrowth site treatment. *Ophthalmology.* 2003;110(6): 1,192–1,203.

97. Costa RA, Farah ME, Cardillo JA, et al. Photodynamic therapy with indocyanine green for occult subfoveal choroidal neovascularization caused by age-related macular degeneration. *Curr Eye Res.* 2001;23(4):271–275.

98. Staurenghi G, Sickenberg M, Massacesi A, et al. Combining photodynamic therapy and feeder vessel photocoagulation: a pilot study. *ARVO Meeting Abstracts.* 2001;42:1,241.

99. Group Toa-rmdwptTS. Photodynamic therapy of subfoveal choroidal neovascularization in age-related macular degeneration with verteporfin: one-year results of 2 randomized clinical trials—TAP report. Treatment of Age-Related Macular Degeneration with Photodynamic Therapy (TAP) Study Group. *Arch Ophthalmol.* 1999;117(10):1,329–1,345.

100. Bressler NM. Verteporfin therapy of subfoveal choroidal neovascularization in age-related macular degeneration: two-year results of a randomized clinical trial including lesions with occult with no classic choroidal neovascularization—verteporfin in photodynamic therapy report 2. *Am J Ophthalmol.* 2002;133(1):168–169.

101. Group ViPTVS. Verteporfin therapy of subfoveal choroidal neovascularization in age-related macular degeneration: two-year results of a randomized clinical trial including lesions with occult with no classic choroidal neovascularization—verteporfin in photodynamic therapy report 2. *Am J Ophthalmol.* 2001;131(5):541–560.

102. Macular Photocoagulation Study Group. Laser photocoagulation of subfoveal recurrent neovascular lesions in age-related macular degeneration. Results of a randomized clinical trial. *Arch Ophthalmol.* 1991;109(9): 1,232–1,241.

103. Piermarocchi S, Bertoja E, Lo Giudice G, et al. Photodynamic therapy ("PDT") increases the eligibility for FV treatment of CNV due to ARMD. *Invest Ophthalmol Vis Sci.* 2001.

104. Piermarocchi S, Lo Giudice G, Sartore M, et al. Photodynamic therapy increases the eligibility for feeder vessel treatment of choroidal neovascularization caused by age-related macular degeneration. *Am J Ophthalmol.* 2002;133(4):572–575.

105. Piermarocchi S, Pilotto E, Lo Giudice G, et al. Sequential combined photodynamic and feeder vessel treatment reduces the number of photodynamic re-treatments of choroidal neovascularization in age-related macular degeneration. *ARVO Meeting Abstracts.* 2002;43(12):3,981.

106. Staurenghi G, Massacesi A, Ilenia Musicco I, et al. Combining photodynamic therapy and feeder vessel photocoagulation: a pilot study. *Seminars in Ophthalmology.* 2001;16(4):233–236.

Pneumatic Displacement of Submacular Hemorrhage

Alejandro J. Lavaque   *Nauman Alam Chaudhry*   *Peter E. Liggett*

INTRODUCTION

Subretinal hemorrhage in the macular region can occur in association with a variety of systemic and ocular disorders, as well as from an idiopathic event. The commonly associated ocular conditions include the following: choroidal neovascularization (CNV) secondary to age-related macular degeneration (AMD), ocular histoplasmosis (OHS), myopia, ruptured macroaneurysms, sickle cell disease (1), trauma, Valsalva´s retinopathy, idiopathic central serous retinopathy, diabetic retinopathy, central retinal vein occlusion, choroidal rupture (2), and complications of subretinal fluid drainage during retinal detachment surgery. When the submacular hemorrhage (SMH) is large and involves the fovea, a potential threat to visual acuity occurs. Because of this poor outcome, interest has developed in alternatives that can improve the visual prognosis, all of them having the common goal of clearing the blood from the macula to minimize the degree of permanent damage in this area (1). In this chapter we focus on the characteristics and management of SMH secondary to wet AMD.

In AMD the cause of the SMH may be linked to (3):

1. Spontaneous bleeding from the CNV. New choroidal vessels are poorly formed and have weak intercellular junctions; therefore, bleeding may occur with an increase in intraluminal pressure (4). Moreover, a significant number of those patients use anticoagulant therapy, and this practice can be related to hemorrhagic events.

2. A tear in a vascularized retinal pigment epithelium (RPE) detachment. The RPE tear can be related to the retraction of the occult CNV. The sudden occurrence of RPE and choriocapillaris tears may result in extensive bleeding that hides the original rip (5).

3. Spontaneous hemorrhage in an area of RPE atrophy. The occurrence of subretinal hemorrhage within atrophic areas in patients with dry AMD, not related with neovessels, has been described. This type of hemorrhage can have a good prognosis after resolution (6).

Previously asymptomatic patients who lose vision abruptly because of thick SMH commonly conceal otherwise-inactive (nonleaking) fibrovascular pigment epithelium detachments. Hence, angiographic studies performed after blood displacement demonstrate that this is the most common neovascular lesion in these patients (7).

NATURAL HISTORY OF SUBMACULAR HEMORRHAGE

The natural history and visual prognosis in the eye with macular subretinal hemorrhage have been reviewed by a number of investigators (2,5,8,9).

These reports, although useful, do not provide us with accurate information on the natural history of SMH. They include a small number of patients, follow-up is limited, and all of them have retrospective designs.

From the limited information to date, it is likely that most patients with SMH associated with CNV, particularly in AMD, have a poor visual outcome. In addition, it seems that the amount of damage done to the retina by an intraretinal or subretinal hemorrhage is related to its size and the ability of the ocular tissue to clear the blood. Without intervention, thick macular hemorrhage associated with AMD usually leaves a large disciform scar in its wake, with a related severe loss of visual acuity (3).

Table 20.1 compares the results.

The visual acuity outcome of subretinal hemorrhage may vary depending on:

1. Extent and location of hemorrhage: The overall area of the subretinal hemorrhage may affect the visual prognosis. The total area affected helps to predict final visual acuity, with a larger hemorrhage leading to a worse visual outcome (5,9,10). The extent of the hemorrhage can be related in patients with systemic anticoagulation therapy, hypertension and cardiovascular diseases (2,11). Sometimes the bleed can occur concomitantly with a hypertensive attack (5).
2. Height of the clot: Hemorrhages thick enough to obscure underlying choroidal details are sufficiently important for assessing damage (3,9). Increased thickness of subretinal hemorrhage has been inversely correlated with visual acuity outcome; in other words, thicker hemorrhages have a poorer prognosis than thinner ones (5,12). The increased distance between neurosensorial retina and the RPE may act as a barrier that prevents nutrients from reaching the photoreceptors, thereby increasing the chance of permanent retinal damage.
3. Associated with CNV: Final visual acuity is worse in eyes with SMH from AMD-related CNV than in eyes with hemorrhage from other etiologies (2,12). Nevertheless, there are reports of relatively good visual recovery after resolution of SMH in eyes where neovascularization did not aggressively evolve. In previously asymptomatic patients who lose vision abruptly, thick SMHs commonly conceal otherwise inactive (nonleaking) fibrovascular pigment epithelium detachments. A portion of these lesions remains relatively quiescent for the long term, permitting significant visual recovery with

stability in some eyes (7). In other cases, the angiographic study shows CNV treatable with laser photocoagulation, photodynamic therapy (PDT), or transpupillary thermotherapy (TTT).
4. Idiopathic polypoidal choroidal vasculopathy: This condition may represent a variant of AMD-related CNV and seems to be more benign in its evolution.
5. State of the RPE and choriocapillaris before the hemorrhage: In advanced AMD the prognosis is poor because of the diseased RPE and choroids under the fovea (3). On the other hand, evidence exists that a healthy RPE and choroids have the capacity to reabsorb the hemorrhage and achieve visual recovery (13). The ability of the ocular tissue to clear the hemorrhage is directly related to the prognosis. A small amount of hemorrhage under the retina is capable of clearing with minimal damage (10).
6. Visual acuity after the hemorrhage: Bad visual acuities after the hemorrhage are associated with worse visual outcome (2).
7. Time of reabsorption: This period directly relates to the height of the clot and the capacity of reabsorption of the complex RPE/choriocapillaris. The trend is toward declining visual acuity with increasing reabsorption time. The time for clearing of the subretinal hemorrhage is highly variable, ranging from 2 months to 2 years, with a mean of 6 to 8 months (2,5). Recurrent episodes, which occur in 40% of cases, also portend a poor visual prognosis (5). In addition, the timing of the SMH treatment after onset of the hemorrhage is important for visual recovery. Earlier evacuation of subretinal hemorrhage has better results (14).
8. Compartmentalization of the blood—Sub-RPE, subretinal, and/or intravitreal hemorrhage. The sub-RPE component of the SMH is much more difficult to treat (3).

Without treatment, thick macular hemorrhages associated with AMD usually evolve into irreversible lesions of choroid, RPE, and retina. The natural long-term outcome of these lesions can be one of the following (5):

1. Fibrous tissue or disciform scars.
2. Widespread atrophy.

TABLE 20.1
STUDIES OF THE NATURAL HISTORY OF SUBMACULAR HEMORRHAGE

Author	Number of Eyes	Average Initial Visual Acuity	Percentage >20/100	Percentage Improving	Average Final Visual Acuity
Avery et al. (9)	41	20/125	26%	21%	—
Bennet et al. (12)	12	20/1,300	0%	25%	20/1,700
Berrocal et al. (2)	20	20/200	30%	40%	20/300
Scupola et al. (5)	60	20/400	<10%	—	20/1,250
Chen et al. (8)	86	—	—	10.5%	20/480

3. RPE rip.
4. Chorioretinal folds.
5. Diffuse RPE alterations.

MECHANISM OF RETINAL INJURY

1. Direct toxicity: Subretinal blood is toxic to the outer retina and has been documented to cause acute (within 24 hours), irreversible photoreceptor damage with edema and disintegration of the outer nuclear layer (15). Clearance of subretinal hemorrhage involves phagocytosis and fibrinolysis. Macrophages, RPE cells, and Muller cells phagocytose the hemorrhage and convert the intracellular hemosiderin into ferritin; once iron-binding proteins become saturated, residual free iron interferes with the function of intracellular enzymes.
2. Barrier effect: Subretinal blood clots form a direct mechanical barrier between the retina and the RPE. This inhibits metabolic exchange, which is essential for the health of the retinal tissue.
3. Tractional forceps in the subretinal space: Immediately after the hemorrhage and during clot formation, fibrin interacts with the neurosensorial epithelium forming fibrin-photoreceptor interdigitation. This produces tractional forceps, causing tearing of the photoreceptor's outer and inner segments (15). Later degeneration progresses to involve all retina layers overlying the densest areas of fibrin in the clot (14).
4. Subretinal fibrosis: During the process of blood clearing, a number of cells migrate under the subretinal space, producing inflammation and scar formation (10). The formation of fibrous tissue is directly proportional to the size of the hemorrhage. The blood stimulates connective tissue formation in the subretinal space by attracting macrophages and fibroblasts (5).

CLASSIFICATION

Depending on size (16):

1. Small hemorrhage: Less than 3 disc diameters in greatest linear dimension centered on the foveal avascular zone (FAZ) or, for larger ones, eccentric to the fovea. Small hemorrhages tend to be thin and patients have the possibility to develop a transitory alternative fixation point during recovery (5).
2. Medium Hemorrhage: Larger than 3 disc diameters but still mostly contained within the temporal vascular arcades.
3. Large Hemorrhage: Extending far beyond the arcades.

ANCILLARY TESTS

Current diagnostic methods allow the identification of the origin of the bleeding in only a few cases. But for these cases, identification can be of great help.

1. Fluorescein angiography (FA): Generally of limited use because of the blood. In the best scenarios only small areas of hyperfluorescence can be seen and the exact limit of the CNV remains obscured.
2. Indocyanine green angiography (ICGA): More useful than FA. ICGA allows the identification of the border of the CNV in half of cases (5).
3. Optical coherence tomography (OCT): OCT is analogous to ultrasound, except that the use of light rather than sound enables higher longitudinal resolution with a noncontact and noninvasive measurement. In positions where the blood allows, detachment of the neurosensory retina and RPE have distinct presentations on OCT and can be studied. Subretinal and intraretinal fluid cause changes in retinal thickness or elevation that can be quantified directly from the images. CNVs are evident in the tomograms as a thickening and fragmentation of a reflective layer, which corresponds to the RPE and choriocapillaris (17).
4. Ultrasound: Ocular echography can help to determine the height of the hemorrhage and identify RPE tears (5). Hemorrhagic disciform lesions are located in the subretinal pigment epithelial space and appear echographically as solid chorioretinal elevations characterized by a bumpy, lobulated surface with indistinct peripheral margins, irregular internal structure, and medium-to-high internal reflectivity. These lesions can be reliably differentiated from associated subretinal or suprachoroidal hemorrhage by ocular echography when the maximal height of the lesion is 1 mm or greater (18). Moreover, after the gas injection a number of patients can develop a vitreous hemorrhage, and in those cases the determination of displacement can be made echographically (19).

THE ROLE OF TISSUE PLASMINOGEN ACTIVATOR

The activation of plasminogen results in the formation of plasmin, a proteolytic enzyme that degrades fibrin, which is the principal structural component of a thrombus or a clot. Human tissue-type plasminogen activator (tPA) has become available through recombinant DNA technology in sufficient quantities to use this agent in patients. The characteristics that distinguish it from other thrombolytic agents is its specificity: tPA binds to fibrin (not fibrinogen) and in this bound form only converts plasminogen to plasmin (fibrin-selective plasminogen activation). Clot lysis is thereby initiated only at the site of the clot. tPA is also considered a native plasminogen activator because endothelial (and other) cells secrete it into the circulation (20).

Rapid removal or displacement of SMH caused by CNV is essential to restore visual function. Today, the use of tPA, both intravitreal with gas (19,21–30) or subretinal after a core vitrectomy (31–38), seems to be an effective treatment for the displacement or evacuation of subretinal hemorrhages. Hemorrhages into subretinal blebs containing tissue plasminogen activator do not form fibrin stands or cause photoreceptor tearing. These findings highlight the potential for improved retinal survival if organized subretinal clot can be eliminated soon after its formation (14).

The theoretical benefits of subretinal tPA are:

1. Liquefy previously formed subretinal thrombus.
2. Reduce thrombus thickness over time.
3. Hasten reabsorption of residual blood.
4. Dilute the concentration of toxins released by subretinal blood.
5. Decrease the barrier effect of solid hemorrhage on the overlying neurosensory retina.
6. Lyse interphotoreceptor fibrin.

However, controversy exists as to whether intravitreally injected tPA accesses the subretinal space in humans in sufficient quantities to achieve clot dissolution (38). Animal models show conflicting data (39). Early studies appear to show effective clot dissolution in experimental subretinal hemorrhage models, but a recent study using radiolabeled tPA in rabbits failed to demonstrate penetration of the drug through an intact internal limiting membrane (ILM) of the neurosensory retina (40). Furthermore, new experience in patients suggest that intravitreal gas alone may allow for sufficient subretinal blood displacement (41–43).

When it is injected in the vitreous cavity, the exact dose of tPA remains controversial. Toxic effects to the retina have been reported after intravitreal injection of tPA (50–100 µg/0.1 mL) in humans, causing RPE hyperpigmentation, reduction of scotopic b-wave amplitude, and exudative retinal detachment (21,44,45). These data have also been confirmed in animal experiments (46). This retinal toxicity seems to be dose dependent and cumulative; thus, tPA reinjections can be dangerous (44).

Some points must be kept in mind when an intravitreal tPA injection is performed:

1. Increased vitreous liquefaction in elderly patients facilitates tPA diffusion in the vitreous body, lowering toxic retinal effects close to the injection site (47). Nevertheless, evidence suggests that tPA solution is not diluted uniformly throughout the vitreous cavity because vitreous restricts the free circulation of intravitreal tPA. Possibly, tPA solution binds to components of the vitreous and creates a drug depot with prolonged local effects (45). Intravitreal tPA concentrations are high in the injected quadrant compared with the more distant sites (48). On the other hand, vitrectomized eyes can raise the toxic threshold for tPA (45,49). Moreover, the vitreous cortex may trap tissue plasminogen activator and limit its diffusion; the state of the posterior hyaloid must be studied in detail.
2. A coinjection of tPA and gas reduces the volume of vitreous that can pick up tPA solution. If 0.4 mL of gas is injected, the bubble enlarges to 0.8 mL within the first 6 hours, approximately 20% of the human vitreous cavity volume. Because of the reduced vitreous volume, the concentration of tPA is increased at the retina and the margin of safety is reduced (49).
3. The intravitreally injected dose of tPA must be sufficient to dissolve a subretinal hemorrhage to achieve a complete displacement of the blood underneath the retina. The half-life of intravitreally injected tissue plasminogen is about 4 to 6 hours without a fibrin clot, and about 10 to 12 hours in the presence of a fibrin clot.
4. There is no therapeutic benefit from the lysis of the clot using tPA without concomitant pneumatic displacement or surgical evacuation (50–52). In other words, the use of tPA must be followed by a intravitreal gas injection or surgical removal with the intent of avoiding damage to the retina.

Commercial recombinant human tPA solution (Activase; Genentech Inc, San Francisco, California) must be reconstituted as directed to a concentration of 1 mg/mL. The vehicle consists of L-arginine phosphate (34 mg/mL), phosphoric acid (10 mg/mL), and polysorbate 80 (<80 mg/mL). Small aliquots of tPA can be maintained at −70°C. Before using, the aliquot is warmed at room temperature and diluted in sterile balanced salt solution to the desired concentration (45).

The toxic dose of intravitreal commercial tPA has never been well defined, but based on animal studies and clinical experience, the currently recommended intravitreal total dose is 25 to 50 µg/0.1 mL (44).

As mentioned above, tPA administration can be dangerous. Adverse and toxic reactions that have been reported include:

1. Mild to moderate anterior chamber reactions (45).
2. Vitreous strand formation.
3. Inflammatory vitreous debris, usually clearing within the first 2 weeks (45).
4. Exudative retinal detachment (21).
5. Diffuse pigment alterations (21,45). These fundus changes are typically geographic and centered in the quadrant of injection, with the severity and extent of damage increasing with dose.
6. Widespread vascular attenuation (45).
7. Photoreceptor loss and vacuolization of the inner nuclear layer (45,46,49,53).
8. RPE necrosis and reproliferation with some pigment clumping areas (44,45,53).
9. Reduction of scotopic b-wave amplitude (44–46,49).
10. Recurrent hemorrhage (19,24,29).

Studies demonstrate that the L-arginine vehicle in the commercially available solution, rather than the tPA protein itself, is the toxic agent. The L-arginine may have toxic effects on the outer retina because of its structural similarity to lysine, an amino acid with known retinotoxic potential.

Unfortunately, L-arginine-free tPA for intravitreal applications is currently not commercially available (45).

Factors affecting the sensitivity of a given eye to toxic reactions by commercial tPA solution are unknown but may include (7):

1. Vitreous volume.
2. Extent of vitreous liquefaction.
3. Position of the needle tip relative to the retina.
4. Degree of fundus pigmentation.

MANAGEMENT

Several methods for treating SMH have been described.

Pneumatic Displacement

In 1996, at the pre-Academy Retina meeting, Dr. Wilson Heriot was the first to describe a technique for treating subretinal hemorrhage. This technique, now known as pneumatic displacement, involves the intravitreal injection of tPA and gas in an attempt to dissolve and displace subretinal blood. This first step of the technique is achieved with prone positioning, which the patient should adopt for several days. The therapeutic principle of this procedure is based on two synergistic effects: enzyme-induced lysis of the clot by tPA, and subsequent mechanical displacement of the liquefied blood through the gas bubble (21). The initial results suggested a high anatomic success rate with few complications (7,16,21, 23–25,29).

The crossing of intravitreal tPA into the subretinal space may be explained by mechanically induced microlesions of the retina. The microlesions would facilitate diffusion in

both directions (21). Additionally, the compressive effect of the gas bubble can force the tPA through the retina into the subretinal space. Further, tPA-induced subretinal plasmin can enter the vitreous cavity through microlesions and dissolved proteins of the vitreoretinal interface, thus facilitating a posterior vitreous detachment (21).

This technique can effectively and consistently displace relatively thick or medium sized SMH. Possible but unproven advantages include greater safety and better visual outcome (Figs. 20.1 and 20.2).

Candidates for this procedure are patients with recent, acute SMH in an eye with useful vision immediately before the hemorrhage. Because a thin layer of blood probably has minimal long-term deleterious effect on macular photoreceptors, the procedure should be reserved for thick blood beneath the fovea. To be classified as thick, the blood should be sufficient to cause an elevation of the retina from the RPE in the fovea. Table 20.2 summarizes the selection criteria (7). Typical clinical findings after tPA and gas injection (21) are depicted in Table 20.3.

Technique

The procedure is performed using expansible, inert gas, either sulfur hexafluoride (SF_6) or perfluoropropane (C_3F_8). After prepping the conjunctiva with 5% betadine solution, a tuberculin syringe with a 30-gauge needle is used to inject 0.3 to 0.5 mL of gas through the pars plana, 3.5 or 4 mm posterior to the limbus, and into the midvitreous cavity. Anterior chamber paracentesis is typically performed before the gas injection to compensate for the changes in volume and minimize the possibility of an intraocular pressure elevation. Also, intravitreal tPA can be injected before or after the gas. At this point, an unfolding

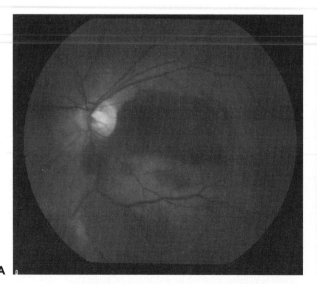
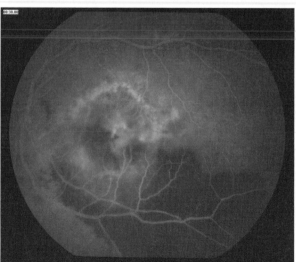

A

B

Figure 20.1 **A.** Red-free photograph of the left eye. Presence of a medium-large subretinal hemorrhage with subfoveal involvement. Some sub-RPE component. **B.** After pneumatic displacement. Fluorescein angiography shows occult subfoveal choroidal neovascularization and residual subretinal hemorrhage under the inferior vascular arcade.

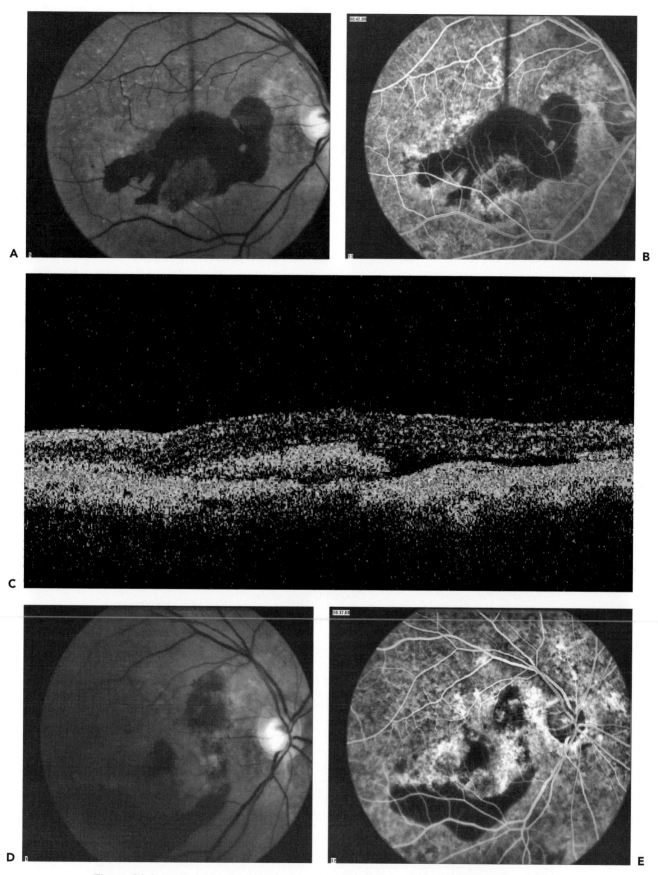

Figure 20.2 **A.** Red-free photograph of the right eye. Medium-sized subretinal hemorrhage with subfoveal involvement. **B.** Fluorescein angiography showing small area of hyperfluorescence under the hemorrhage. **C.** Optical coherence tomography showing photoreceptor detachment secondary to subretinal hemorrhage. **D.** Red-free photograph after the pneumatic displacement. **E.** Fluorescein angiography showing residual subretinal hemorrhage under the inferior vascular arcade.

TABLE 20.2
PATIENT SELECTION CRITERIA

1. Recent submacular hemorrhage.
2. Useful vision immediately before hemorrhage.
3. Thick blood beneath the fovea (foveal elevation off RPE)
4. Absence of thick sub-RPE blood centrally.
5. Hemorrhage not massive in size.
6. Presence of posterior vitreous detachment.

RPE, retinal pigment epithelium. (Modified from Johnson MW. Pneumatic displacement of submacular hemorrhage. *Curr Opin in Ophthalmol.* 2000;11:201–206.)

in the technique has been proposed (two-step technique) (7), in which initially only the intravitreal gas is injected and the patient is re-evaluated after 24 to 48 hours of prone positioning. If the blood displacement is inadequate, tPA can be injected in a second step and the patient is asked to resume a prone position for an additional 48 hours (two-step direct technique). With this variation in the technique, a second injection is reserved for those eyes in which the submacular blood is not displaceable with gas alone.

On the other hand, Hesse (27) suggest a two-step inverse technique, first injecting tPA in the vitreous cavity followed by 0.2 mL to 0.3 mL of gas 24 hours after the tPA injection. This approach has the theoretical advantage of a better distribution of the tPA before the gas injection (the tamponade effect of the gas bubble may obstruct the tPA's diffusion through the retina). However, other investigators feel that a delay of 3 to 6 hours should be sufficient to allow tPA migration across the retina (19). Obviously, positioning is crucial for successful displacement of the SMH. The patient is instructed to assume a prone position approximately 6 hours after the procedure and maintain it for 24 to 48 hours. Support devices, such as a foam doughnut device, facilitate positioning at home (3). Whenever blood displacement from under the fovea is not complete, prone positioning is continued for an additional 24 to 48 hours.

When the patient is positioned face down after the injection of gas, an additional benefit can be obtained from the tamponade effect. The bubble of gas is not only displacing the blood but also the subretinal fluid. If the scar is formed while the retina is attached, there is a greater chance of preserving useful macular function. Moreover, displacement of exudates and blood may improve the chances for successful laser ablation, PDT, or TTT (54).

Results

Table 20.4 summarizes the experience of different researchers with the pneumatic displacement of SMH, both with and without tPA.

TABLE 20.3
SUMMARY OF CLINICAL FINDINGS AFTER INTRAVITREAL GAS tPA AND GAS INJECTION

Time after Procedure	Clinical Observations
Day 1	Color of subretinal clot changes form dark to bright, lower parts of subretinal clot spontaneously shift towards inferior temporal arcade.
Day 2 and 3	Liquefied blood is pushed more distant to inferior retinal periphery, thin remnants of residual hemorrhage still cover macular region, visual acuity can improve depending on the underlying disease.
Day 4 to 7	Color of liquefied blood changes from light red to transparent. Posterior vitreous detachment evolves. Reddish vitreous haze may develop.
1–4 weeks	Spontaneous reabsorption of subretinal blood remnants. Hyperpigmentation of RPE in previously detached retina.

The liquefied blood dislodged through the periphery is reabsorbed within 2–4 weeks. However, remnants of subretinal blood in the macular area disappear in 3 month or more. The difference in time can be explained by malfunctioning of macular RPE in AMD.

AMD, age-related macular degeneration; RPE, retinal pigment epithelium; tPA, Human tissue type plasminogen activator. (Modified from Hesse L, Schmidt J, Kroll P. Management of acute submacular hemorrhage using tissue plasminogen activator and gas. *Graefe's Arch Clin Exp Ophthalmol.* 1999;237:273–277.)

Complications

Related to the gas bubble injection:

1. Rhegmatogenous retinal detachment (25,55).
2. Proliferative vitreoretinopathy.
3. Unplanned retinectomy.
4. Vitreous hemorrhage (19,23,24). When is mild it usually resolves in 2 weeks, but if it is more dense a vitrectomy is necessary (41).
5. Vitreous opacities (56). These opacities or clouds are formed by fragments of erythrocytes that infiltrate the retina and cross an intact internal limiting membrane, clouding the vitreous.
6. Elevated intraocular pressure.

Related to tPA injection:

1. Mild to moderate anterior chamber reactions.
2. Vitreous strand formation.
3. Inflammatory vitreous debris.
4. Exudative retinal detachment (21). Tends to resolve within 2 weeks and can represent a transitory dysfunction of the RPE.
5. Diffuse pigment alterations (44,45).

6. Widespread vascular attenuation (45).
7. Recurrent SMH (19,21,24,29). In such cases, pneumatic displacement with tPA can be repeated (19), but the risk of tPA retinal toxicity increases (44).

Related to the procedure:

1. Endophthalmitis (19,23).

Pneumatic displacement of subretinal hemorrhage out of the macula may be a valid alternative treatment, and has less associated trauma to the eye and retina than surgical removal. However, there are several theoretical limitations to the efficacy of subretinal fibrinolysis after intravitreal tPA injection (27):

1. Subretinal fibrinolysis may be ineffective because a large protein like tPA cannot cross retinal structures to accumulate in therapeutic concentrations in the subretinal space.
2. Fibrinolysis may be ineffective due to various inhibitors of fibrinolysis bound to the clot.
3. The ability of tPA to gain access to the center of the clot may be limited.
4. Because of tPA's short half-life, its therapeutic effect is limited to the first hours after the injection.

TABLE 20.4

VISUAL ACUITY AFTER PNEUMATIC DISPLACEMENT FOR SUBMACULAR HEMORRHAGE SECONDARY TO AGE-RELATED MACULAR DEGENERATION

Author	Number of Eyes	Initial Visual Acuity	Percentage of Improving	Percentage ≥20/100	Percentage of Successful Displacements
Natural History					
Bennet et al. (12)	12	20/1,300	25%	0%	—
Berrocal et al. (2)	20	20/200	40%	30%	—
Avery et al. (9)	41	20/125	26%	21%	—
Pneumatic Displacement with Intravitreal tPA					
Asan et al. (19)	13	HM to 20/200	92%	62%	100%
Hesse et al. (27)	13	HM to 20/40	69%	62%	70%
Meier, et al. (22)	22	—	82%	77%	100%
Handwerger et al. (25)	14	1/200 to 20/100	57%	36%	92%
Krepler et al. (28)	11	HM to 20/63	73%	82%	91%
Pneumatic Displacement without Intravitreal tPA					
Ohji et al. (41)	4	20/2,000 to 20/400	100%	50%	100%
Daneshvar et al. (43)	3	CF	67%	33%	67%
Surgical Evacuation Assisted with Subretinal tPA					
Lewis (31)	24	LP to CF	83%	21%	—
Ibañez et al. (34)	19	HM to 20/200	42%	0%	—
Lim et al. (35)	16	CF to 20/200	61%	31%	—
Moriarty et al. (36)	14	LP to 20/200	79%	30%	—
Pars Plana Vitrectomy, Subretinal tPA and Pneumatic Displacement					
Haupert et al. (32)	11	HM to 20/200	82%	26%	100%

CF, counting finger; HM, hand motion; LP, light perception; tPA, Human tissue type plasminogen activator.

Despite these theoretical limitations, several investigators have demonstrated a therapeutic effect after intravitreal tPA and gas injection (3,7,19,21,23–26,28,29,47).

Interestingly, other investigators have suggested that the intravitreous injection of gas alone may be effective in displacing subretinal blood (41–43).

Subretinal Hemorrhage Evacuation

Owing to the overall poor prognosis of massive SMH, surgical evacuation was proposed and in an attempt to achieve better outcomes (57–60). Of 21 patients in whom SMH was evacuated without the fibrinolytic effect of tPA, none attained visual acuity better than 20/200 postoperatively, and 48% of them attained visual acuity of counting finger or worse (57–60). Furthermore, the procedure resulted in a high rate of complications, including disciform scar, retinal detachment with proliferative vitreoretinopathy, and recurrent subretinal hemorrhage.

The poor results obtained with surgical removal, without tPA, of the submacular blood clot through a large-access retinotomy can be explained by the following factors:

1. Damage to the RPE and the outer retina caused by the hemorrhage (51).
2. The presence of CNV and the history of photocoagulation.
3. Mechanical damage to the RPE and outer retina during the surgical removal of the clot. Because fibrin interdigitates between the photoreceptor, the surgical traction at the submacular blood clot may damage the outer retina (14,61).

However, the intraoperative use of tPA lyses the clot, and the subretinal hemorrhages can be evacuated through small retinotomy minimizing the damage to photoreceptors (31,33–36).

These beneficial effects can be explained by the following (31,62):

1. The dilution of the toxic factors released by the red blood cells.
2. The reduction of the barrier to metabolic exchange caused by a contiguous blood clot in the subretinal space.
3. The lysis of interphotoreceptor fibrin.

Technique

The technique requires that a pars plana core vitrectomy be performed with careful removal of the posterior hyaloid face. A 33-gauge, sharp and bent subretinal cannula connected to a tuberculin syringe containing the fibrinolytic agent is inserted through the retina into the subretinal space, in an extramacular and elevated area into the hemorrhage. A temporal boarding to the macula seemed to be comfortable, simple, and sure. Approximately 0.1 to 0.3 mL of tPA is injected beneath neurosensory retina to cover the area of hemorrhage. Scleral plugs are placed into the sclerotomy sites and the eye is left undisturbed for 25 to 40 minutes to allow for clot lysis.

Afterward, the scleral plugs are removed and an extrusion cannula attended with active aspiration is placed over or into the retinotomy to aspirate the subretinal blood. The blood aspiration can be partial (63,64) or complete, depending on the difficulty of the aspiration and the degree of lysis achieved. Excessive traction should be avoided; the partial extraction of the clot can be enough to clean the subfoveal area or to create enough space to combine the mechanical extraction with a pneumatic displacement of the residual blood.

If a choroidal neovascular complex is identified, the surgeon may attempt to grasp and remove the neovascular net if he thinks that it can be beneficial.

No laser photocoagulation is required unless the retinotomy site is large and the surgeon believes it may contribute to retinal detachment formation.

The peripheral retina is inspected after the blood removal, searching for retinal breaks that could complicate the postoperative course with a rhegmatogenous retinal detachment. A complete air-fluid exchange follows. The decision to use air alone or a gas mixture is influenced by the experience of the surgeon. Prone positioning is mandatory.

Postoperatively, the eye is inspected to determine the presence of recurrent hemorrhage or any complication related to the surgery. The thin layer of subretinal hemorrhage remaining immediately postoperatively usually clears within 2 weeks. Visual acuity tends to improve by 4 to 6 weeks postoperatively, and can be influenced by the following situations:

1. Presence of subfoveal neovascularization.
2. Postoperative RPE atrophy.
3. Subretinal fibrosis.
4. Cataract formation.

Other Technique Modifications

Chaudhry et al. report injecting tPA directly into the subretinal space 24 hours prior to the vitrectomy. They injected 25 μg of tPA in 0.1 mL of balanced salt solution, using a 1.5 inch 30-gauge needle. The maneuver was done under direct visualization using a 20 D lens and indirect ophthalmoscopy. This procedure would be performed only in patients with a SMH height of 3 mm or more. With less thick hemorrhages, this procedure poses an increased risk of globe perforation and entering structures deep to the RPE (33).

Haupert et al. described an interesting technique to ensure adequate concentrations of tPA in the subretinal space: after a pars plana vitrectomy a posterior vitreous detachment is created if not present, the tPA is injected directly into the subretinal space using a 36-gauge cannula. The fibrinolytic agent is injected into the substance of the clot, rather than above or beneath it, to minimize contact with the retina and the RPE. Fluid-air gas exchange is then performed and the patient positioned face down for several days. There is no attempt to directly evacuate the hemorrhage intraoperatively (32).

Results

Table 20.4 compares the results of surgical evacuation with tPA to those obtained with other surgical techniques.

TECHNIQUE SELECTION

Based on the experience of different investigators and the experimental data, certain ocular characteristics have been determined to help identify patients most likely to benefit from one of this techniques. The most important are (16):

1. Hemorrhage of 2-weeks duration or less.
2. Acceptable visual acuity before the hemorrhage.
3. Relatively thick hemorrhage beneath the fovea.
4. Hemorrhage larger than 3 disc diameters in greatest linear dimension.

Figure 20.3 summarizes the different surgical alternatives for the management of SMH.

No prospective, randomized, comparative studies have been published for any previously discussed surgical modalities. Therefore, the best approach for a given SMH has not been determined. However, based on the variably sized retrospective, noncomparative case studies to date, some general management guidelines can be suggested (16):

1. Small Hemorrhage: For most small hemorrhages under the macula, such as those centered on the foveal avascular zone and measuring less than 3 disc diameters, or for larger ones mostly eccentric to the fovea, observation is probably the best course of action.
2. Moderately-sized Hemorrhages: Arbitrarily defined as larger than approximately 3 disc diameters but still mostly contained within the temporal arcades. Any of the interventions can potentially improve upon the natural history of the hemorrhage. The authors of this work favor the pneumatic displacement approach (with or without tPA)

in most of these cases. Other opinions include vitrectomy and subretinal tPA combined with pneumatic displacement or evacuation through a small retinotomy site.

3. Large Hemorrhage: Extending far beyond the arcades. Intervention may or may not be attempted depending on the status of the fellow eye and visual needs of the patient. If the goal is to recover peripheral or ambulatory vision, however, vitrectomy and tPA-assisted direct evacuation can be the choice.

Another important factor to evaluate before choosing a technique is the state of the posterior hyaloid. Lack of posterior vitreous detachment and syneretic vitreous may prevent an adequate interface between the gas bubble and the SMH. This may lead to inefficient blood displacement. Moreover, some reports suggest the involvement of the posterior vitreous membrane in the pathophysiology of AMD and the role of pars plana vitrectomy in the management of wet AMD (65,66).

SUBMACULAR HEMORRHAGE DISPLACEMENT AND CHOROIDAL NEOVASCULARIZATION TREATMENT

For most patients with SMH, the final visual outcome appears to depend in large part on the natural history of the underlying macular pathology. Previously asymptomatic patients who lose vision abruptly because of thick SMH commonly harbor otherwise inactive (nonleaking) fibrovascular pigment epithelial detachments. After pneumatic displacement or removal of blood, some of these lesions remain relatively quiescent, permitting visual recovery and stability over prolonged follow-up (19). On the other hand, if an active CNV is discovered, some therapeutic alternatives are available (PDT or TTT).

Intravitreal tPA and gas may constitute a useful treatment strategy in patients with thick contiguous subretinal

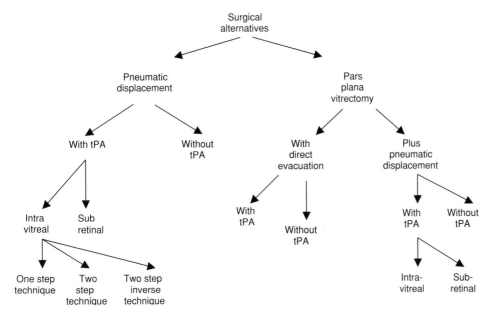

Figure 20.3 Surgical alternatives in the management of the submacular hemorrhage.

blood that obscures the boundaries of neovascular membranes amenable to further treatment. In particular, the ability to determine the proportion of the lesion that is classic CNV is important in PDT and TTT (24).

In order to improve the prognosis of SMH in AMD with subretinal CNV, in may be necessary to treat the consequence (SMH) *and* the cause (CNV). Using a limited posterior vitrectomy with removal of the posterior hyaloid, which improves the flexibility of the retina to obtain maximal blood displacement, an intravitreal injection of 100% SF_6 is performed, followed by a prone position for 8 hours (pneumatic displacement). Afterward, the patient is instructed to alternate prone positioning with short walks, allowing active and quick blood displacement. Days after, when the CNV can be identified, TTT can be performed (Goeminne P, et al. ARVO 2003).

SUMMARY

SMH is a serious condition that appears to benefit from treatment. Randomized, controlled trials comparing techniques are needed. For most patients, the final visual outcome appears to depend in large part on the natural history of the underlying macular disease. Pneumatic displacement, with or without tPA, is a quick, inexpensive, and relatively simple procedure for the management of SMH. For large hemorrhages, such as those that extend well beyond the temporal arcades, a combination of techniques may be necessary, such as pars plana vitrectomy, dissection of the posterior hyaloid, subretinal injection of tPA, and the pneumatic effect or direct evacuation.

REFERENCES

1. Lim JI. Subretinal hemorrhage. *Int Ophthalmol Clin.* 1995;35:95–104.
2. Berrocal MH, Lewis ML, Flynn HW. Variations in the clinical course of submacular hemorrhage. *Am J Ophthalmol.* 1996;122:486–493.
3. Borrillo JL, Regillo CD. Treatment of subretinal hemorrhage with tissue plasminogen activator. *Curr Opin Ophthalmol.* 2001;12:207–211.
4. Green WR, McDonnell PJ, Yeo JH, et al. Pathologic features of senile macular degeneration. *Ophthalmology.* 1985;92:615–627.
5. Scupola A, Coscas G, Soubrane G, et al. Natural history of macular subretinal hemorrhage in age-related macular degeneration. *Ophthalmologica.* 1999;213:97–102.
6. Nasrallah F, Jalkh AE, Trempe C, et al. Subretinal hemorrhage in atrophic age-related macular degeneration. *Am J Ophthalmol.* 1989;107:38–41.
7. Johnson MW. Pneumatic displacement of submacular hemorrhage. *Curr Opin Ophthalmolr.* 2000;11:201–206.
8. Chen WL, Liu JH, Lee FL. Natural course of submacular hemorrhage. *Zhonghua Yi Xue Za Zhi.* 1999;62:268–277.
9. Avery RL, Fekrat S, Hawkins BS, et al. Natural history of subfoveal subretinal hemorrhage in age-related macular degeneration. *Retina.* 1996;16:183–189.
10. Gillies A, Lahav M. Absorption of retinal and subretinal hemorrhages. *Ann Ophthalmol.* 1983;15:1,068–1,074.
11. El Baba F, Jarret WH II, Harbin TS Jr, et al. Massive hemorrhage complicating age-related macular degeneration: clinicopathologic correlation and role of anticoagulants. *Ophthalmology.* 1986;93:1,581–1,592.
12. Bennett SR, Folk JC, Blodi CF, et al. Factors prognostic of visual outcome in patients with subretinal hemorrhage. *Am J Ophthalmol.* 1990;109:33–37.
13. Chaudhry NA, Flynn HW, Lewis ML. Spontaneous resolution of submacular hemorrhage with marked visual improvement. *Ophthalmic Surg Lasers.* 1999;30:670–671.
14. Toth CA, Morse LS, Hjelmeland LM, et al. Fibrin directs early retinal damage after experimental subretinal hemorrhage. *Arch Ophthalmol.* 1991;109:723–729.
15. Glatt H, Machemer R. Experimental subretinal hemorrhage in rabbits. *Am J Ophthalmol.* 1982;94:762–773.
16. Tennant MT, Borrillo JL, Regillo CD. Management of submacular hemorrhage. *Ophthalmol Clin North Am.* 2002;15:445–452.
17. Hee MR, Baumal CR, Puliafito CA, et al. Optical coherence tomography of age-related macular degeneration and choroidal neovascularization. *Ophthalmology.* 1996;103:1,260–1,270.
18. Valencia M, Green RL, Lopez PF. Echographic findings of hemorrhagic disciform lesions. *Ophthalmology.* 1994;101:1,379–1,383.
19. Hassan AS, Johnson MW, Schneiderman TE, et al. Management of submacular hemorrhage with intravitreous tissue plasminogen activator injection and pneumatic displacement. *Ophthalmology.* 1999;106:1,900–1,907.
20. Haber E, Quertermouns T, Matsueda GR, et al. Innovative approaches to plasminogen activator therapy. *Science.* 1989;243:51–56.
21. Hesse L, Schmidt J, Kroll P. Management of acute submacular hemorrhage using recombinant tissue plasminogen activator and gas. *Graefe's Arch Clin Exp Ophthalmol.* 1999;237:273–277.
22. Meier P, Zeumer C, Jochmann C, et al. Management of submacular hemorrhage by tissue plasminogen activator and SF_6 gas injection. *Ophthalmologe.* 1999;96:643–647.
23. Buhl M, Scheider A, Schonfeld CK, et al. Intravitreal tissue plasminogen activator and gas in submacular hemorrhage. *Ophthalmologe.* 1999;96:792–796.
24. Hattenbach LO, Klais C, Koch FH, et al. Intravitreous injection of tissue plasminogen activator and gas in the treatment of submacular hemorrhage under various conditions. *Ophthalmology.* 2001;108:1,485–1,492.
25. Handwerger BA, Blodi BA, Chandra SR, et al. Treatment of submacular hemorrhage with low-dose intravitreal tissue plasminogen activator injection and pneumatic displacement. *Arch Ophthalmol.* 2001;119:28–32.
26. Hattenbach LO, Brieden M, Koch FH, et al. Intravitreal injection of rt-PA and gas in the management of minor submacular haemorrhage secondary to age-related macular degeneration. *Klin Monatsbl Augenheilkd.* 2002;219:512–518.
27. Hesse L, Schroeder B, Heller G, et al. Quantitative effect of intravitreal injected tissue plasminogen activator and gas on subretinal hemorrhage. *Retina.* 2000;20:500–505.
28. Krepler K, Kruger A, Tittl M, et al. Intravitreal injection of tissue plasminogen activator and gas in subretinal hemorrhage caused by age-related macular degeneration. *Retina.* 2000;20:251–256.
29. Leguay J, Gastaud P. Subretinal hematoma in age-related macular degeneration: treatment with intravitreal injection of tPA and gas. *J Fr Ophthalmol.* 2000;23:797–801.
30. Singh P, Singh R, Kishore KS, et al. Intravitreal tissue plaminogen activator in submacular haemorrhage. *Indian J Ophthalmol.* 1999;47:254–255.
31. Lewis H. Intraoperative fibrinolysis of submacular hemorrhage with tissue plasminogen activator and surgical drainage. *Am J Ophthalmol.* 1994;118:559–568.
32. Haupert CL, McCuenll BW, Jaffe GJ, et al. Pars plana vitrectomy, subretinal injection of tissue plasminogen activator, and fluid-gas exchange for displacement of thick submacular hemorrhage in age-related macular degeneration. *Am J Ophthalmol.* 2001;131:208–215.
33. Chaudhry NA, Mieler WF, Han DP, et al. Preoperative use of tissue plasminogen activator for large submacular hemorrhage. *Ophthalmic Surg Lasers.* 1999;30:176–180.
34. Ibañez HE, Williams DF, Tomas MA, et al. Surgical management of submacular hemorrhage. A series of 47 consecutive cases. *Arch Ophthalmol.* 1995;113:62–69.
35. Lim JI, Drews-Botsch C, Sternberg P, et al. Submacular hemorrhage removal. *Ophthalmology.* 1995;102:1,393–1,399.
36. Moriarty AP, McAllister IL, Constable IJ, et al. Initial clinical experience with tissue plasminogen activator (tPA) assisted removal of submacular hemorrhage. *Eye.* 1995;9:582–588.
37. Kamei M, Tano Y, Maeno T, et al. Surgical removal of submacular hemorrhage using tissue plasminogen activator and perfluorocarbon liquid. *Am J Ophthalmol.* 1996;121:267–275.
38. Lewis H. tPA and gas in submacular hemorrhage. *Ophthalmology.* 2002;109:824.
39. Boone DE, Boldt HC, Ross RD, et al. The use of intravitreal tissue plasminogen activator in the treatment of experimental subretinal hemorrhage in the pig model. *Retina.* 1996;16:518–524.
40. Kamei M, Misono K, Lewis H. A study of the ability of tissue plasminogen activator to diffuse into the subretinal space after intravitreal injection in rabbits. *Am J Ophthalmol.* 1999;128:739–746.
41. Ohji M, Saito Y, Hayashi A, et al. Pneumatic displacement of subretinal hemorrhage without tissue plasminogen activator. *Arch Ophthalmol.* 1998;116:1,326–1,332.
42. Ogawa T, Kitaoka T, Mera A, et al. Treatment for subretinal hemorrhage in the macula: pneumatic displacement of hemorrhages. *Retina.* 2000;20:684–685.
43. Daneshvar H, Kertes PJ, Leonard BC, et al. Management of submacular hemorrhage with intravitreal sulfur hexafluoride: a pilot study. *Can J Ophthalmol.* 1999;34:385–388.
44. Chen SN, Yang TC, Ho CL, et al. Retinal toxicity of intravitreal tissue plasminogen activator. *Ophthalmology.* 2003;110:704–708.
45. Hrach CJ, Johnson MW, Hassan AS, et al. Retinal toxicity of commercial intravitreal tissue plasminogen activator solution in cat eyes. *Arch Ophthalmol.* 2000;118:659–663.
46. Johnson MW, Olsen KR, Hernandez E, et al. Retinal toxicity of recombinant tissue plasminogen activator in the rabbit. *Arch Ophthalmol.* 1990;108:259–263.
47. Hesse L. Intravitreal injection of tissue plasminogen activator: four considerations. *Arch Ophthalmol.* 2001;119:456–457.

48. Egana BC, La Puente CR, Peyman GA. Intravitreal distribution of tissue plasminogen activator in nonvitrectomized and fibrin-filled vitrectomized eyes. *Invest Ophthalmol Vis Sci.* 1997;38(suppl):212.
49. Irvine WD, Johnson MW, Hernandez E, et al. Retinal toxicity of human tissue plasminogen activator in vitrectomized rabbit eyes. *Arch Ophthalmol.* 1991;109:718–722.
50. Morse LS, Benner JD, Hjelmeland LM, et al. Fibrinolysis of experimental subretinal haemorrhage without removal using tissue plasminogen activator. *Br J Ophthalmol.* 1996;80:658–662.
51. Johnson MW, Olsen KR, Hernandez E. Tissue plasminogen activator treatment of experimental subretinal hemorrhage. *Retina.* 1991;11:250–258.
52. Coll GE, Sparrow JR, Marinovic A, et al. Effect of intravitreal tissue plasminogen activator on experimental subretinal hemorrhage. *Retina.* 1995;15:319–326.
53. Benner JD, Morse LS, Toth CA, et al. Evaluation of a commercial recombinant tissue-type plasminogen activator preparation in the subretinal space of the cat. *Arch Ophthalmol.* 1991;109:1,731–1,736.
54. Averbukh E, Devenyi RG, Lam WC, et al. Letters to the editor. *Ophthalmology.* 2000;107:2,119.
55. Hejny C, Sternberg P. Retinal detachment after pneumatic displacement for subfoveal hemorrhage. *Retina.* 2001;21:260–262.
56. Lincoff H, Madjarov B, Lincoff N, et al. Pathogenesis of the vitreous cloud emanating from subretinal hemorrhage. *Arch Ophthalmol.* 2003;121:91–96.
57. Hanscom TA, Diddie KR. Early surgical drainage of macular subretinal hemorrhage. *Arch Ophthalmol.* 1987;105:1,722–1,723.
58. de Juan E Jr, Machemer R. Vireous surgery for hemorrhagic and fibrous complications of age-related macular degeneration. *Am J Ophthalmol.* 1988;105:25–29.
59. Vander JF, Federman JL, Greven C, et al. Surgical removal of massive subretinal hemorrhage associated with age-related macular degeneration. *Ophthalmology.* 1991;98:23–27.
60. Wade EC, Flynn HW, Olson KR, et al. Subretinal hemorrhage management by pars plana vitrectomy and internal drainage. *Arch Ophthalmol.* 1990;108:973–978.
61. Men G, Peyman GA, Kuo PC, et al. The effect of intraoperative retinal manipulation on the untherlying retinal pigment epithelium: an experimental study. *Retina.* 2003;23:475–480.
62. Lewis H, Resnick S, Flannery JG, et al. Tissue plasminogen activator treatment of experimental subretinal hemorrhage. *Am J Ophthalmol.* 1991;111:197–204.
63. Hesse L, Meitinger D, Schmidt J. Little effect of tissue plasminogen activator in subretinal surgery for acute hemorrhage in age-related macular degeneration. *Ger J Ophthalmol.* 1996;5:470–483.
64. Claes C, Zivojnovic R. Efficacy of tissue plasminogen activator (t-PA) in subretinal hemorrhage removal. *Bull Soc Belge Ophthalmol.* 1996;261:115–118.
65. Ondes F, Yilamaz G, Acar MA, et al. Role of the vitreous in age-related macular degeneration. *Jpn J Ophthalmol.* 2000;44:91–93.
66. Ikeda T, Sawa H, Koizumi K, et al. Pars plana vitrectomy for regression of choroidal neovascularization with age-related macular degeneration. *Acta Ophthalmol Scand.* 2000;78:460–464.

Submacular Surgery and the Submacular Surgery Trials

21

Nancy M. Holekamp   Matthew A. Thomas

INTRODUCTION

In the early 1990s, subfoveal choroidal neovascularization (CNV) due to age-related macular degeneration (AMD) was managed by observation with a generally poor outcome or, in some cases, subfoveal laser photocoagulation with its known destructive consequences (1–3). Submacular surgery evolved in an attempt to offer patients with subfoveal CNV an alternative treatment to observation or laser photocoagulation. Over the past decade, the surgical techniques of submacular surgery have been refined. They are now an established method in the vitreoretinal surgeon's armamentarium, and can be used to access the subretinal space to remove many types of CNV: subfoveal, juxtafoveal, extrafoveal, peripapillary, occult, and hemorrhagic. The appropriate indications for using submacular surgery in patient care are still being defined. The Submacular Surgery Trials are an important recent advance in determining who may or may not benefit from submacular surgery. The surgical techniques and their application in treating CNV due to AMD will be discussed in this chapter.

SURGICAL TECHNIQUE

Submacular surgery begins with a standard three-port pars plana vitrectomy. The locations of the right-handed and left-handed sclerotomies are chosen to provide comfortable access to the submacular pathology. It is helpful to have a preoperative angiogram available when choosing sclerotomy sites in cases of CNV. A sclerotomy site should provide a straight line through the proposed retinotomy site to the subretinal pathology. In selected cases, it may also be helpful to rotate away from the conventional 12:00 surgeon's position to either side, so that direct access avoids previous laser scars, the papillomacular bundle, and the optic nerve (4).

After a core vitrectomy, the posterior hyaloid membrane is stripped from the retinal surface out to the equator in eyes without a posterior vitreous detachment. This may be accomplished with a vitrector using active aspiration, a soft-tipped silicone cannula using active aspiration (Fig. 21.1) (5), or with a 130-degree angled flat-tipped pick, a hyaloid lifter (Fig. 21.2) (6). Using either method, a Weiss ring should be seen to confirm the surgical posterior vitreous detachment. This step is necessary because macular retinotomies are not treated with laser photocoagulation.

After a peripheral vitrectomy, the retinotomy site is chosen. Its location should provide a straight line to the subretinal pathology from the dominant-hand sclerotomy, be as far away from the foveal center while still allowing the CNV to be reached with angled subretinal instruments, and avoid major retinal vessels. Small retinotomies near the papillomacular bundle do not cause postoperative visual field loss (7). Therefore, a right-hand-dominant surgeon operating on a left eye can use a retinotomy superior nasal to the fovea for subfoveal CNV. The retinotomy is made by using a 36-gauge, 130-degree angled subretinal pick to perforate neurosensory retina (Fig. 21.3). Care must be taken not to scrape underlying retinal pigment epithelium (RPE) or choroid to avoid bleeding or subsequent

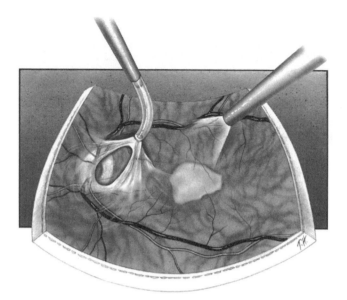

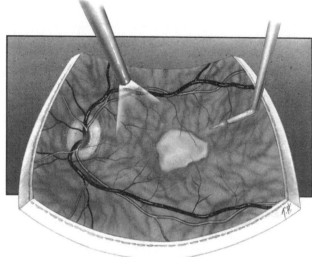

Figure 21.3 A 36-gauge angled subretinal pick is used to create a retinotomy.

Figure 21.1 A soft-tipped silicone cannula is used to separate the posterior hyaloid from the retinal surface.

development of CNV (8). Any retinal capillary hemorrhages can be easily controlled by temporarily raising intraocular pressure. Attention must be paid to the precise location of small, almost imperceptible retinotomies so that other instruments can be introduced into the subretinal space at the same site.

A limited neurosensory retinal detachment is created to provide working space in the area of the submacular CNV. A 130-degree angled 33-gauge cannula is introduced through the retinotomy, and a trace amount of balanced salt solution is slowly infused into the subretinal space by a surgical assistant (Fig. 21.4). A vigorous infusion can blow a hole through the fovea or create a retinal dehiscence at points of retinal-subretinal adhesion. The angled 33-gauge cannula and concomitant hydrodissection can be

used to gently separate the overlying retina from the underlying subretinal pathology. Scars from previous laser surgery, fibrotic CNV, chronic lipid from the CNV, and chorioretinal anastomoses can prove particularly adherent. It is important to release all attachments to the neurosensory retina so that removal of CNV does not result in macular tears.

The 130-degree angled subretinal pick is again introduced through the retinotomy and is used to bluntly dissect the CNV from surrounding tissue (Fig. 21.5). If the CNV lies anterior to the RPE (as in cases of ocular histoplasmosis, but rarely in cases of AMD), the pick is used to lift the edges of the CNV membrane off the underlying sheet of RPE. Often a rim of fibrin will also be elevated. All edges of the CNV can be dissected off the RPE so only the

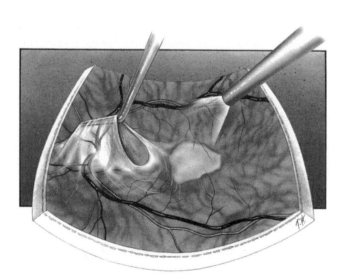

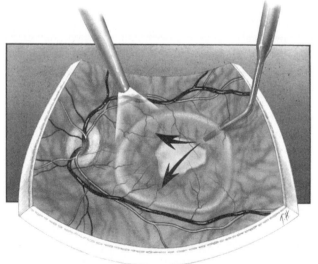

Figure 21.2 A hyaloid lifter is used to hook a Weiss ring and create a surgical posterior vitreous detachment.

Figure 21.4 A 33-gauge angled cannula is used to create a limited neurosensory retinal detachment.

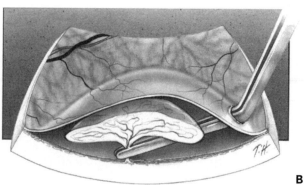

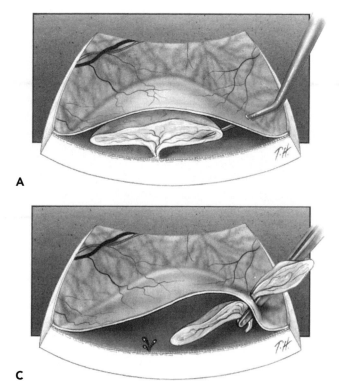

Figure 21.5 A. The angled subretinal pick is used to bluntly dissect the choroidal neovascularization from surrounding tissue. **B.–C.** The edge of the membrane can then be grabbed with horizontal subretinal forceps. Hemorrhage at the vascular ingrowth stalk is prevented by raising the intraocular pressure.

vascular ingrowth stalk remains attached to the choroid. If the CNV lies beneath or within the RPE layer (as is usually the case in AMD), the pick is used to dissect the CNV free from surrounding tissues to limit the area of lost RPE with extraction of the CNV. Pick dissection is carried out under normal intraocular pressure, but intraocular pressure is quickly elevated at the first indication of hemorrhage.

The 130-degree angled horizontal subretinal forceps are introduced through the retinotomy to grasp and slowly remove the CNV (Fig. 21.5). In cases where the CNV has been dissected free except for the vascular ingrowth stalk, the tissue is usually easily extracted, leaving behind intact RPE (rare in AMD). It is important to raise the intraocular pressure for hemostasis prior to disconnecting the vascular ingrowth stalk. When removed from the subretinal space, even large CNV complexes will mold to fit through small retinotomies. The intraocular pressure is slowly lowered, watching for any bleeding. In cases where the RPE is probably going to be extracted along with the CNV, one must carefully watch for the cleavage point of the RPE. If it appears that a large rim of healthy RPE not directly involved with CNV is going to be removed, horizontal subretinal scissors can cut healthy RPE from diseased tissue. This can also be done to cleave CNV from adherent laser scars. After removal from the subretinal space, the CNV complex is held in the mid vitreous cavity until adequate hemostasis is achieved, and is then vitrectomized or removed via the sclerotomy.

Indirect ophthalmoscopy is carried out to confirm that no iatrogenic retinal tears have occurred from passing sharp, angled instruments into the eye. A complete air-fluid exchange is carried out, aspirating over the optic nerve head with a soft-tipped extrusion cannula. A 33-gauge cannula can be used to aspirate at the retinotomy, removing any residual subretinal fluid or hemorrhage. The retinotomy site is not treated with laser photocoagulation unless circumstances indicate it is prudent to do so (large retinotomy, extensive subretinal blood present, extramacular location, etc.). Fluid is then reintroduced into the vitreous cavity with a soft-tipped cannula, pointed away from the macula and retinotomy, until only a 10% to 15% air bubble remains. One will see the fluid-air interface at the posterior surface of the lens in a phakic patient. The vitrectomy surgery is completed in the usual fashion. Postoperatively, the patient is instructed to be in a strict facedown position overnight so the small air bubble will close the retinotomy. A full air fill is indicated for patients who cannot be in a facedown position after surgery.

COMPLICATIONS OF SUBMACULAR SURGERY

Vitrectomy surgery to remove subfoveal CNV is prone to the same complications as other types of vitrectomy surgery. There is a small chance of endophthalmitis (less than 1%), retinal tear, and retinal detachment (both less than 5%). There is also a risk of progressive nuclear sclerotic cataract. In one study, this risk approached 80% two years after vitrectomy in individuals over the age of 50. This risk was less than 10% in individuals under the age of 50 (9).

Other types of complications are specific to submacular surgery. In most cases an active blood vessel is being severed, so there is a small chance of postoperative intraocular hemorrhage. This hemorrhage usually clears spontaneously in a vitrectomized eye. Problems may occur with the retinotomy. If facedown positioning does not adequately position the small air bubble over the retinotomy, on the first postoperative day there may be a persistent neurosensory detachment of the macula. This occurs frequently in children, and we now recommend a full air fill at the end of surgery in children's eyes. In adults, increased compliance with facedown positioning will flatten the retinotomy and the macula. The retinotomy is usually invisible by 1 postoperative month. However, in cases of a second submacular surgery, even with a different retinotomy site, the retinotomy may remain open. Mild epiretinal tissue may be present. Retinal detachment from an open retinotomy in the absence of proliferative vitreoretinopathy has not been seen. In addition, CNV has been reported to occur at the retinotomy site (8). This is most likely caused by scraping the RPE with the 36-gauge pick as the retinotomy is made. If CNV occurs, the retinotomy should be in an extrafoveal location and the CNV should be lasered. Finally, idiopathic peripheral visual field loss after vitrectomy with the removal of subretinal CNV has been described (10).

The most common complication of submacular surgery is recurrent CNV. Depending upon the underlying etiology of the CNV, recurrent neovascularization can occur in 18% to 100% of eyes (Table 21.1). In AMD, recurrence of CNV occurs in approximately one out of three cases. Because recurrent neovascularization following submacular surgery is common, it is recommended that the routine postoperative care include frequent fluorescein angiography (i.e., at least every 2 weeks for the first 6 weeks, then every month for the next 3 months) to detect early recurrent neovascularization. This allows for prompt laser photocoagulation or photodynamic therapy (PDT) to maintain a favorable visual result.

SUBMACULAR SURGERY RESULTS: AN IMPORTANT LESSON IN PATHOPHYSIOLOGY

Submacular surgery was pioneered for the removal of subfoveal CNV due to a variety of etiologies, including AMD, ocular histoplasmosis, multifocal choroiditis, high myopia, angioid streaks, and idiopathic causes, among others. Although the surgical technique in removing all types of subfoveal CNV is the same, the surgical success rate is not. Visual acuity results from the largest single-surgeon experience in removing subfoveal CNV due to a variety of etiologies, including AMD, are shown in Table 21.1 (Personal communication, Matthew A. Thomas, Macula Society Rosenthal Lecture, Palm Beach, Florida, 1995).

Surgical success after removing subfoveal CNV depends on the underlying disease. Eyes with subfoveal CNV due to focal disease of the RPE-Bruch's membrane-choriocapillaris complex have a good chance for better postoperative visual acuity (Table 21.2) (11). Postoperative visual acuity of 20/40 or better in 30% to 40% of eyes with subfoveal CNV due to ocular histoplasmosis, multifocal choroiditis, and idiopathic causes has been shown in several retrospective series (12–17). In contrast, eyes with subfoveal CNV due to diffuse or degenerative disease of the RPE-Bruch's membrane-choriocapillaris complex have little chance for better postoperative visual acuity (Table 21.2) (11). Postoperative visual acuity of 20/40 or better is rarely achieved in eyes with subfoveal CNV due to AMD, angioid streaks, or high myopia, as shown in numerous published series (15–18). In cases of AMD, the CNV lies anterior to

TABLE 21.1

SURGICAL RESULTS: A SINGLE SURGEON'S EXPERIENCE IN 247 CASES

Disease	Postoperative Visual Acuity, %			Postoperative Change in Visual Acuity			Recurrence Rate	Mean Follow-up, Mo
	≥20/40	20/50–20/100	≤20/200	Better ≥3 Lines	Same ±2 Lines	Worse ≤3 Lines		
Ocular histoplasmosis (n = 120)	35	30	35	40	44	16	42	13
Multifocal choroiditis (n = 17)	59	29	12	65	29	6	18	8
Idiopathic (n = 19)	21	26	53	42	53	5	37	10
Age-related macular degeneration (n = 60)	3	13	84	15	65	20	32	13
High myopia (n = 17)	12	41	47	12	65	23	53	10
Angioid streaks (n = 5)	0	20	80	0	100	0	100	6

TABLE 21.2
SUMMARY OF SURGICAL RESULTS

Better Surgical Results in Focal Disease[a]	Poor Surgical Results in Diffuse Disease[b]
Ocular histoplasmosis	Age-related macular degeneration
Idiopathic	High myopia
Multifocal choroiditis	Angioid streaks

[a] Often subfoveal retinal pigment epithelium is preserved.
[b] Usually subfoveal retinal pigment epithelium is lost.

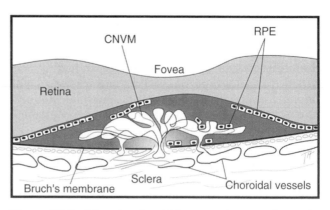

Figure 21.7 When the choroidal neovascularization has multiple ingrowth sites and lies beneath or within the disrupted retinal pigment epithelium, the surgical outlook is guarded (common in age-related macular degeneration). CNVM, choroidal neovascular membrane; RPE, retinal pigment epithelium.

the RPE (Fig. 21.6). When the CNV is surgically removed, subfoveal RPE is usually preserved. In the latter group, the CNV lies under or within the RPE (Fig. 21.7). When the CNV is surgically removed, subfoveal RPE is usually removed as well. Following submacular surgery, intact, native RPE is critical to foveal photoreceptor function and return of good visual acuity (17).

SUBMACULAR SURGERY FOR SUBFOVEAL CNV IN AMD

One may conclude that current surgical techniques can allow for safe removal of subfoveal CNV, but cannot adequately treat disease or degeneration of the RPE-Bruch's membrane-choriocapillaris complex that is characteristic of AMD. In addition to underlying diagnosis, factors that describe subfoveal CNV with a favorable surgical prognosis are listed in Table 21.3 (11). Eyes with AMD rarely have features that portend a favorable surgical prognosis. Consequently, with the advent of PDT, intravitreal antiangiogenic therapies, and other developments in the field, submacular surgery is now used infrequently in the management of subfoveal CNV due to AMD.

SUBMACULAR SURGERY FOR NON-SUBFOVEAL CNV IN AMD

It is possible to apply the surgical techniques for removing subfoveal CNV to other types of submacular CNV in AMD. This includes juxtafoveal, extrafoveal, peripapillary, occult, and hemorrhagic. In one such example, a large exudative macular detachment resolved after surgical removal of a poorly defined extrafoveal CNV due to AMD. Visual acuity improved from 20/200 to 20/25 within 18 months of follow-up (19). While juxtafoveal and peripapillary CNV due to AMD is usually treated with laser photocoagulation or PDT, many such lesions will fall outside current treatment guidelines. Recent reports suggest that submacular surgery can be considered a subset of these cases. Joseph et al. describe submacular surgery in nine eyes with juxtafoveal CNV due to AMD (20). Eight of nine eyes experienced stable or improved visual acuity. Six of nine eyes had final visual acuity of 20/80 or better. Bains et al. describe submacular surgery for six eyes with large peripapillary CNV due to AMD (21). Four of six eyes had final visual acuity of 20/80 or better. In actuality, these types of cases are rare and case selection is important, but submacular surgery can be considered as a viable treatment option.

Occult CNV in AMD falls outside current treatment guidelines for thermal laser photocoagulation, and study results of PDT for occult CNV are controversial. Similarly, thermal laser and PDT are rarely useful treatments for hemorrhagic CNV due to AMD. In select cases, submacular surgery can be considered in these two situations. If a CNV is poorly defined because of an occult component or overlying hemorrhage, but is thought to be extrafoveal in location based on fluorescein and/or indocyanine green angiography, it may be a reasonable candidate for submacular surgery if central visual acuity is threatened. If only extrafoveal RPE is removed with the CNV, then foveal function can be preserved, resulting in a good visual outcome. The following case is a good example.

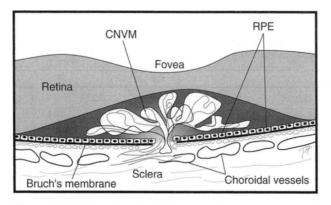

Figure 21.6 When the choroidal neovascularization has a single ingrowth stalk and lies anterior to the retinal pigment epithelium, there is a favorable surgical prognosis (rare in age-related macular degeneration). CNVM, choroidal neovascular membrane; RPE, retinal pigment epithelium.

TABLE 21.3

CHARACTERISTICS OF SUBFOVEAL CHOROIDAL NEOVASCULARIZATION (CNV) WITH A FAVORABLE SURGICAL PROGNOSIS

Patient younger than 50 years
Subretinal pigmented halo around the CNV
Sharply defined borders and plaque-like elevation to the CNV
No biomicroscopic or stereoscopic angiographic evidence of retinal pigment epithelial elevation
Fellow eye normal
Good visual potential (i.e. no prior subfoveal laser)
Short duration of foveal involvement
Origin of CNV away from the foveal center
Few adhesions of CNV to retina or adjacent scars

CASE 1

A 77-year-old gentleman presented with painless loss of vision to 20/200 in the right eye. He was found to have a large subfoveal hemorrhage associated with a choroidal neovascular membrane. Fluorescein angiography suggested an extrafoveal location of the choroidal neovascular mem-

brane, but due to overlying hemorrhage, its exact boundaries could not be identified (Fig. 21.8). The patient underwent vitrectomy surgery with removal of both the subfoveal hemorrhage and the subretinal neovascular membrane. At the time of surgery, the membrane was confirmed to lie entirely in the extrafoveal region. Postoperatively, a small recurrence occurred at the area of the extrafoveal CNV, and this was treated with laser photocoagulation according to MPS guidelines. Eighteen months following vitrectomy surgery, visual acuity is 20/40 (Fig. 21.9).

Occasionally, the techniques of submacular surgery can be used in cases of subfoveal CNV to stabilize visual acuity and limit scotoma size. The following is a good case example.

CASE 2

A 61-year-old gentleman presented with painless, sudden loss of visual acuity in the right eye. He was found to have a large, occult, subfoveal neovascular membrane associated with exudative macular detachment (Fig. 21.10). A preoperative Amsler grid showed a large area of central distortion (Fig. 21.11). Vitrectomy surgery with removal of the large, occult, subfoveal neovascular complex was performed. There was resolution of the exudative macular detachment. Although visual acuity remained limited to the 20/200 level,

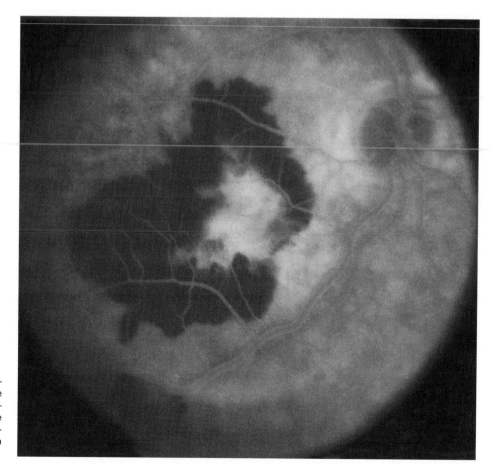

Figure 21.8 A fluorescein angiogram of the right eye shows a large hemorrhagic choroidal neovascularization (CNV) complex. Although the blood extends under the fovea, fluorescein angiography suggests an extrafoveal location of the CNV.

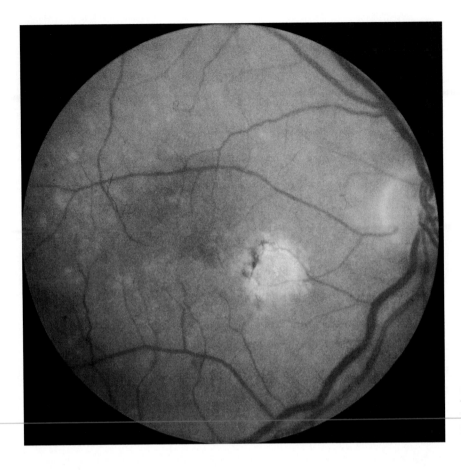

Figure 21.9 Following submacular surgery to remove the hemorrhagic choroidal neovascularization (CNV) complex, visual acuity returned to 20/40. A recurrent CNV resulted in the laser scar inferonasal to the fovea.

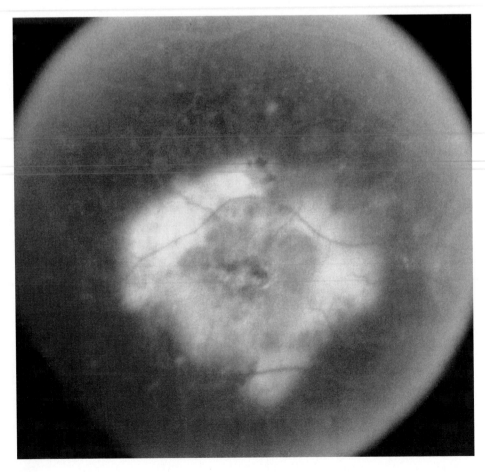

Figure 21.10 A fluorescein angiogram confirms a large occult subfoveal neovascular membrane in the right eye.

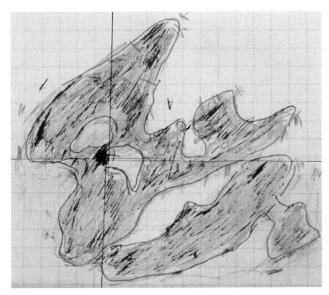

Figure 21.11 A preoperative Amsler grid shows a large area of central distortion.

there was a marked improvement in his postoperative Amsler grid (Fig. 21.12). Despite a central scotoma and a physiologic blind spot plotted on the Amsler grid, the patient noted a definite increase in visual function.

THE SUBMACULAR SURGERY TRIALS

It is important to emphasize that for many years vitrectomy surgery for removal of subretinal CNV, whether subfoveal or nonsubfoveal, has not been shown to be more beneficial over laser photocoagulation, PDT, or observation in any

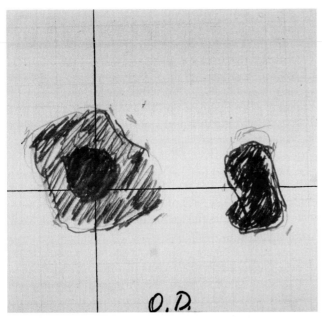

Figure 21.12 Although visual acuity remained limited to the 20/200 level, there was a marked improvement in the postoperative Amsler grid.

prospective clinical trial. Thus, while the surgical techniques were well defined, the indications for applying them are not.

The Submacular Surgery Trials are a group of three multicenter, randomized, clinical trials whose objective is to study the possible benefits of vitrectomy surgery in certain cases of subfoveal CNV in patients with AMD, ocular histoplasmosis, and idiopathic causes (22). The trials were initiated in 1997, prior to the advent of PDT and the use of intravitreal anti-angiogenic agents for subfoveal CNV. Sponsored by the National Institutes of Health, the three trials and their results are described here.

I. New Subfoveal CNV in AMD Trial (SST group N): The purpose of the SST group N was to evaluate surgical removal versus observation of subfoveal choroidal neovascularization due to age-related macular degeneration. Eligibility criteria for this trial are given in Table 21.4. Briefly, eyes were eligible if they had new-onset subfoveal CNV with some classic pattern on fluorescein angiography and best corrected visual acuity of 20/100 to 20/800. Any blood associated with the CNV had to account for less than 50% of the total lesion size. Eligible patients were randomized to either submacular surgery or observation. A successful outcome was defined to be either improvement of best-corrected visual acuity or visual acuity no more than 1 line worse at the 24 month examination compared to baseline.

Of 454 eligible patients, 228 eyes were randomized to observation and 226 to surgery. Forty-four percent of observed eyes and 41% of eyes assigned to surgery had a successful outcome as defined in the study. Median visual acuity loss from baseline to the 24-month examination was 2.1 lines in observed eyes and 2.0 lines in eyes assigned to surgery. Median visual acuity declined from 20/100 at baseline to 20/400 at 24 months in both groups. No subgroup of eyes was identified in which submacular surgery led to better visual acuity.

In summary, submacular surgery as performed in the SST group N clinical trial was not effective in improving or maintaining visual acuity compared to observation. Submacular surgery is not recommended for eyes with similar lesions due to AMD (23).

II. Hemorrhagic Subfoveal CNV in AMD Trial (SST group B): The purpose of the SST group B was to evaluate surgical removal versus observation of hemorrhagic subfoveal choroidal neovascularization due to age-related macular degeneration. Eligibility criteria for this trial are given in Table 21.4. Briefly, eyes were eligible if they had subfoveal CNV associated with blood accounting for more than 50% of the total lesion size with best-corrected visual acuity of 20/100 to light perception. Eligible patients were randomized to either submacular surgery or observation. A successful outcome was defined to be either improvement of best-corrected visual acuity or visual acuity no more than 1 line

TABLE 21.4
PATIENTS ELIGIBLE FOR ENROLLMENT IN SST

	Underlying Conditions	Eligible for Foveal Photoco-agulation Study	Lesion Size	Eligible Visual Acuity Range	Angiographic Features	Blood	Randomized Treatment Assignment
Group 1, AMD/ new–large	AMD	No	>3.5 MPS DA or poorly demarcated and ≤3.5 MPS DA	20/100– 20/800	New CNV (no prior laser; some classic)	None to <50%	Surgery vs. observation
Group 2, AMD/hem-orrhage	AMD	No–lesion >50% blood	CNV + blood: >3.5 MPS DA CNV: 0–≤9 MPS DA blood: If anterior to equator, at least 5 clock hours attached	20/100– light perception	New/Rec CNV; fluorescein angiographic leakage not required	>50% and obscures view of CNV borders	Surgery vs. observation
Group 3, histo/ idiopathic	Histo/idio-pathic CNV	No–Not AMD	≤9 MPS DA	20/50– 20/800	New/Rec CNV; must have some classic CNV or staining scar with serous detachment 2× size of scar (Blood in foveal avascular zone center excludes patients)	No restriction	Surgery vs. observation

AMD, age-related macular degeneration; CNV, chorodial neovascularization; MPS DA Macular Photocoagulation Study, disc areas.

worse at the 24 month examination compared to baseline.

Of 336 eligible patients 168 were randomized to observation and 168 to surgery. A successful outcome as defined by the study was achieved in 41% of observed eyes and in 44% of eyes assigned to surgery. Although severe visual acuity loss was not the primary outcome of interest, surgery more often prevented such loss: 36% in the observation arm versus 21% in the surgery arm. More eyes undergoing surgery required cataract surgery by the 24 month examination compared to observed eyes (44% compared to 6%). More eyes undergoing surgery experienced rhegmatogenous retinal detachment compared to observed eyes (16% compared to 2%).

In summary, submacular surgery as performed in the SST group B clinical trial was not effective in improving or maintaining visual acuity compared to observation. Submacular surgery was effective in reducing the risk of severe visual acuity loss compared to observation, but this surgical benefit should be weighed against the increased risk of cataract and retinal detachment (24).

III. Histoplasmosis/Idiopathic Subfoveal CNV Trial (SST group H): The purpose of the SST group H was to evaluate surgical removal versus observation of subfoveal choroidal neovascularization due to ocular histoplasmosis or idiopathic causes. Eligibility criteria for this trial are given in Table 21.4. Briefly, eyes were eligible if they had subfoveal CNV, either new or recurrent, with some classic pattern on fluorescein angiography and best-corrected visual acuity of 20/50 to 20/800. Eligible patients were randomized to either submacular surgery or observation. A successful outcome was defined to be either improvement of best-corrected visual acuity or visual acuity no more than 1 line worse at the 24 month examination compared to baseline.

Of 225 eligible patients, 113 study eyes were assigned to observation and 112 to surgery. Forty-six percent of the eyes in the observation arm and 55% in the surgery arm had a successful outcome as defined in the study (success ratio, 1.18; 95% confidence interval, 0.89–1.56). Median visual acuity at the 24-month examination was 20/250 among eyes in the observation arm and 20/160 for eyes in the surgery arm. A subgroup of eyes with visual acuity worse than 20/100 at baseline had more success with surgery; 76% in the surgery arm vs. 50% of eyes in the observation arm (success ratio, 1.53; 95% confidence interval, 1.08–2.16). Recurrent choroidal neovascularization developed by the 24-month examination in 58% of surgically treated eyes.

In summary, submacular surgery as performed in the SST group H clinical trial provided no benefit or a smaller benefit to surgery than the trial was designed to detect. The results do support consideration of surgery for eyes with subfoveal choroidal neovascularization and best-corrected visual acuity worse than 20/100 due to ocular histoplasmosis or idiopathic causes. However, the high rate of recurrent choroidal neovascularization suggests that additional treatment may be required after submacular surgery (25).

CONCLUSION

Submacular surgery was pioneered in the early 1990s as an innovative treatment for subfoveal CNV due to a variety of causes. The surgical technique has produced advances in both vitrectomy surgery and our understanding of CNV. The Submacular Surgery Trials were initiated in 1997 to better define the role of submacular surgery in treating subfoveal CNV due to AMD. The SST results demonstrated that submacular surgery provided no benefit for eyes with subfoveal CNV due to AMD and only modest benefit for selected eyes with hemorrhagic subfoveal CNV due to AMD and for selected eyes with subfoveal CNV due to ocular histoplasmosis and idiopathic causes. It seems likely that with more recent developments in the field, such as PDT and intravitreal anti-angiogenic agents, the role for submacular surgery in treating subfoveal CNV, will be a limited one. As for cases of nonsubfoveal CNV in AMD, laser photocoagulation should be performed in laser-eligible lesions according to MPS guidelines. For the rare case of non-laser-eligible CNV, careful case selection with a full understanding of the risks and benefits is the recommended guideline when considering the use of submacular surgery.

REFERENCES

1. Macular Photocoagulation Study Group. Laser photocoagulation of subfoveal neovascular lesions in age-related macular degeneration. Results of randomized clinical trial. *Arch Ophthalmol.* 1991;109:1,219.
2. Macular Photocoagulation Study Group. Laser photocoagulation of subfoveal recurrent neovascular lesions in age-related macular degeneration. Results of a randomized clinical trial. *Arch Ophthalmol.* 1991;109:1,232.
3. Fine SL, Wood WJ, Singerman LJ, et al. Laser treatment for subfoveal neovascular membranes in ocular histoplasmosis syndrome: results of a pilot randomized clinical trial. *Arch Ophthalmol.* 1993;111:19.
4. Jacobi FK, Pavlovic S. Temporal pars plana vitrectomy for submacular surgery. *Retina.* 1998;18(1):70.
5. Mein CE, Flynn HW Jr. Recognition in removal of the posterior cortical vitreous during vitreoretinal surgery for impending macular hole. *Am J Ophthalmol.* 1991;112:611.
6. Holekamp NM, Thomas MA. Surgical removal of choroidal neovascular membranes. In: Peyman GA, et al., eds. *Atlas of Vitreoretinal Surgery.* London: Martin Dunitz, in press.
7. Holekamp NM, Thomas MA. Subretinal Surgery. In: Guyer, et al., eds. *Retina-Vitreous-Macula: A Comprehensive Text.* Philadelphia: WB Saunders Company, in press.
8. McCannel CA, Syrquin MG, Schwartz SD. Submacular surgery complicated by a choroidal neovascular membrane at the retinotomy site. *Am J Ophthalmol.* 1996;122(5):737.
9. Melberg NM, Thomas MA. Nuclear sclerotic cataract after vitrectomy in patients younger than 50 years of age. *Ophthalmology.* 1995;102:1,466.
10. Melberg NS, Thomas MA. Visual field loss after pars plana vitrectomy with air-fluid exchange. *Am J Ophthalmol.* 1995;120:386.
11. Gass JDM. Biomicroscopic and histopathologic considerations regarding the feasibility of surgical excision of subfoveal neovascular membranes. *Am J Ophthalmol.* 1994;118:285.
12. Thomas MA, Kaplan HJ. Surgical removal of subfoveal neovascularization in the presumed ocular histoplasmosis syndrome. *Am J Ophthalmol.* 1991;111:1.
13. Holekamp NM, Thomas MA, Dickinson JD, et al. Surgical removal of subfoveal choroidal neovascularization in presumed ocular histoplasmosis: stability of early visual results. *Ophthalmology.* 1997;104:22.
14. Berger AS, Conway M, Del Priore LV, et al. Submacular surgery for subfoveal choroidal neovascular membranes in presumed ocular histoplasmosis. *Arch Ophthalmol.* 1997;115:991.
15. Berger AS, Kaplan HJ. Clinical experience with the surgical removal of subfoveal neovascular membranes. Short-term postoperative results. *Ophthalmology.* 1992;99:969.
16. Thomas MA, Grand MG, Williams DF, et al. Surgical management of subfoveal choroidal neovascularization. *Ophthalmology.* 1992;99:952.
17. Thomas MA, Dickinson JD, Melberg NS, et al. Visual results after surgical removal of subfoveal choroidal neovascular membranes. *Ophthalmology.* 1994;101:1,384.
18. Adelberg DA, Del Priore LV, Kaplan HJ. Surgery for subfoveal membranes in myopia, angioid streaks and other disorders. *Retina.* 1995;15:198.
19. Connor TB, Wolf MD, Arrindell EL, et al. Surgical removal of an extrafoveal fibrotic choroidal neovascular membrane with foveal serous detachment in age-related macular degeneration. *Retina.* 1994;14:125.
20. Joseph DJ, Uemura A, Thomas MA. Submacular surgery for juxtafoveal choroidal neovascularization. *Retina.* 2003;23:463.
21. Bains HS, Patel MR, Singh H, et al. Surgical treatment of extensive peripapillary choroidal neovascularization in elderly patients. *Retina.* 2003;23:469.
22. Holekamp NM, Thomas MA. The Submacular Surgery Trials. In: Kertes P, Conway MD, eds. *Clinical Trials in Ophthalmology: a Summary and Practice Guide.* Surgery for hemorrhagic choroidal neovasular lesions of age-related macular degeneration: ophthalmic findings: SST report no. 13. [Clinical Trial. Journal Article. Multicenter Study. Randomized Controlled Trial] *Ophthalmology.* 2004;111(11):1,993–2,006.
23. Hawkins BS, Bressler NM, Miskala PH, et al. Submacular Surgery Trials (SST) Research Group. Surgery for subfoveal choroidal neovascularization in age-related macular degeneration: ophthalmic findings: SST report no. 11. [Clinical Trial. Journal Article. Multicenter Study. Randomized Controlled Trial] *Ophthalmology.* 2004;111(11):1,967–1,980.
24. Bressler NM, Bressler SB, Childs AL, et al. Submacular Surgery Trials (SST) Research Group. Surgery for hemorrhagic choroidal neovascular lesions of age-related macular degeneration: ophthalmic findings: SST report no. 13. [Clinical Trial. Journal Article. Multicenter Study. Randomized Controlled Trial] *Ophthalmology.* 2004;111(11):1,993–2,006.
25. Hawkins BS, Bressler NM, Bressler SB, et al. Submacular Surgery Trials Research Group. Surgical removal vs observation for subfoveal choroidal neovascularization, either associated with the ocular histoplasmosis syndrome or idiopathic: I. Ophthalmic findings from a randomized clinical trial: Submacular Surgery Trials (SST) Group H Trial: SST Report No. 9 [see comment] [erratum appears in *Arch Ophthalmol.* 2005;123(1):28]. [Clinical Trial. Journal Article. Multicenter Study. Randomized Controlled Trial] *Archives of Ophthalmology.* 2004;122(11):1,597–1,611.

Limited Macular Translocation

22

Motohiro Kamei   Yasuo Tano

INTRODUCTION

Choroidal neovascularization (CNV) frequently leads to severe and irreversible loss of central vision and is associated with age-related macular degeneration (AMD), ocular histoplasmosis, and pathologic myopia, among others. AMD is the leading cause of irreversible, severe visual loss in individuals over age 50 in industrialized countries (1). Pathologic myopia is also a major cause of legal blindness in many developed countries, especially Asia and the Middle East (2).

Current treatments, including photocoagulation (3), surgical excision (4,5), and photodynamic therapy (PDT) (6,7), are effective in only a small number of patients with subfoveal CNV. The Macular Photocoagulation Study demonstrated that photocoagulation of certain patients with well-defined CNV is associated with a slightly better visual prognosis than observation. Surgical excision of CNV is reportedly effective, but the benefit is limited to patients with subfoveal CNV. The visual acuity (VA) of patients with subfoveal CNV, however, rarely improves after the procedure, and most patients lose central vision immediately after surgery or later. Immediate visual loss occurs because choroidal neovascular membranes develop posterior to the retinal pigment epithelium (RPE) in occult CNV, and to some degree even in classic CNV, and at the time of surgical removal the RPE and choriocapillaris are removed with the choroidal neovascular complex. Late visual loss is associated with atrophic creep in the RPE and choriocapillaris, which is commonly observed, especially in eyes with pathologic myopia (8). PDT has been widely applied, and the Treatment of Age-Related Macular Degeneration with Photodynamic Therapy Study and the Verteporfin in Photodynamic Therapy Study have both reported that PDT can stop the decrease of vision when compared with observation, but that the final VA decreases from the pretreatment baseline level (6,7). Macular translocation, therefore, may represent a better option for treating subfoveal neovascular maculopathy (9–15).

Three surgical techniques of macular translocation have been described: macular translocation with 360-degree retinotomy (9–11), translocation with partial retinotomy (12), and limited macular translocation (13–15). Each has advantages and disadvantages with respect to effectiveness and complications. Limited macular translocation is less invasive and has a lower complication rate, compared with macular translocation with 360-degree retinotomy or partial retinotomy. The disadvantages of limited macular translocation include a smaller degree of and less predictable foveal displacement (15,16), the development of foveal folds (15,17,18), and surgically induced astigmatism (19,20).

BASIC CONCEPT OF LIMITED MACULAR TRANSLOCATION

Macular translocation, proposed to improve vision in cases with subfoveal CNV, relocates the macula away from the CNV, enabling the macula to receive nourishment from healthier underlying RPE and choroid. To displace the macula, an iatrogenic retinal detachment is created in the two temporal quadrants including the macula, the sclera is shortened in the superotemporal quadrant, and the retina is reattached by gas tamponade superiorly to inferiorly. Inferior retinal folds develop as the result of retinal redundancy, resulting in downward macular displacement (Fig. 22.1). In limited macular translocation, no retinotomy is performed except for minute injection sites for balanced saline solution with a 39-gauge or 41-guage

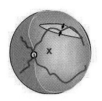

Figure 22.1 Limited macular translocation involves creation of an iatrogenic retinal detachment in the temporal two quadrants including the macula, shortening the sclera in the superotemporal quadrant, and retinal reattachment by gas tamponade from superior to inferior. An inferior retinal fold, the result of retinal redundancy, causes downward displacement of the macula. *X* indicates the displaced new fovea; *x* indicates the original fovea; *arrows* indicate scleral shortening, the direction of rotation of the gas bubble, and the track of displacement of the macula and redundant retina.

needle. This results in less severe complications such as postoperative proliferative vitreoretinopathy, which occurs at the rate of 10% to 40% after macular translocation with a 360-degree retinotomy.

HISTORY OF LIMITED MACULAR TRANSLOCATION

The original technique was developed and reported by de Juan and coworkers in 1998, to reduce surgical invasion of macular translocation with 360-degree retinotomy (13,14). To shorten the sclera, the investigators first performed a crescent-shaped scleral resection, consisting of the superficial two-thirds to three-fourths of the sclera. Subsequently, to reduce the complexity of the procedures, they performed scleral infolding with five or six circumferential scleral mattress sutures. To improve the results of limited macular translocation, we modified the technique of scleral shortening from infolding to outfolding of the sclera, choroid, and RPE. Our outcomes in an animal model (21) and an initial clinical trial (22,23) demonstrated that radial outfolding with clips represents a more predictable and effective method of limited macular translocation (Fig. 22.2). Because the radial outfolding technique carries the risk that the choroidal folds will affect the macula, and because it is technically difficult to create a sufficiently long radial fold, we modified the technique from radial to diagonal outfolding (24). Other techniques use radial-interrupted mattress sutures (25), scleral retraction sutures (26), or a twofold suture technique (8).

CASE SELECTION

The candidates for this surgery were patients with subfoveal CNV that did not extend more than 1 disc diameter inferior to the center of the fovea, acute visual loss of less than 6-months duration, VA worse than 20/40, and the absence of previous photocoagulation. The type of CNV or original disease does not affect the surgery criteria, whereas patients over 80 are not good candidates. Fujii et al. reported that eyes with stable and central fixation (without a dense central scotoma), good preoperative VA, and a short duration of symptoms are those with the greatest chance of achieving good vision after macular translocation (27).

SURGICAL TECHNIQUES

The current techniques of limited macular translocation include scleral infolding with mattress sutures, radial outfolding with clips, and scleral gathering with retraction sutures. While the techniques have a number of surgical maneuvers in common, the methods of scleral shortening differ. Essentially, the surgical procedure consists of four major steps:

1. Three-port standard vitrectomy with complete posterior vitreous detachment (PVD).
2. Iatrogenic retinal detachment.
3. Scleral shortening.
4. Partial fluid-air exchange.

Scleral Infolding Technique

Preplacing Mattress Suture, Vitrectomy, and Creation of PVD
After placing control sutures at the superior and lateral rectus muscles, five or six mattress sutures are placed through the partial thickness of the sclera 2 mm posterior to the rectus muscle insertion, with three or four sutures placed between the superior and the lateral rectus muscle, one suture just nasal to the superior rectus muscle, and one suture just inferior to the lateral rectus muscle. The distance between the anterior and posterior bites is 3.5 mm to 9.0 mm (14,20,27–32). For the scleral gathering technique, each mattress suture is placed in an S-shaped configuration 10 mm, 12.5 mm, and 15 mm from the limbus (26).

A standard three-port vitrectomy is performed with complete removal of posterior and anterior vitreous. An intravitreal triamcinolone injection helps visualization of residual vitreous cortex, which prevents retinal detachment.

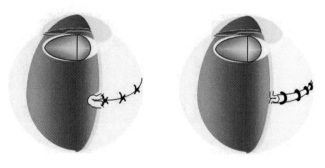

Figure 22.2 Various techniques of limited macular translocation.

Creation of Retinal Detachment

A retinal detachment is created in the temporal 180 degrees of the globe by injecting balanced saline solution into the subretinal space, using a 39-gauge or a 41-gauge needle that is connected to a pressure-controlled fluid injector. This is done by first forming two to three large retinal blebs adjacent to each other. These are then combined into one large continuous retinal detachment via fluid-air exchange with gentle rocking of the eye and, if necessary, use of a retinal manipulator. The retinal detachment extending from the optic nerve head to the ora serrata should be confirmed.

Scleral Shortening and Partial Fluid-Air Exchange

The scleral mattress sutures are secured, thus shortening the sclera. To prevent incarceration of the detached retina into the infusion cannula, infusion should be off during the scleral shortening procedure, and to make scleral outfolding easier, the intraocular pressure should be reduced by draining vitreous fluid through the sclerotomy. An approximately 40% fluid-air exchange is then performed.

Postoperative head positioning

After surgery, the patient lies on the temporal side for several minutes, then the head of the bed is gradually lifted with the patient remaining on his or her temporal side. The head should be raised to 90 degrees over the course of about 1 to 2 hours. Overnight, the patient sits face forward with the bed reclined slightly. The day after the surgery, the patient lies with the superotemporal side up (lying on the nasal side) with the head raised approximately 45 to 60 degrees for 12 hours, and finally with the temporal side up until the air bubble disappears (Fig. 22.3).

Scleral Outfolding Technique

In the scleral outfolding technique (22–24), a vitrectomy and iatrogenic retinal detachment is performed in the same way as during the infolding technique. For scleral shortening, titanium clips are used. With forceps, the sclera is outfolded in an area 2.0 mm to 2.5 mm wide, and 10 mm long diagonally from 4 mm posterior to the lateral rectus muscle to the insertion of the superior oblique

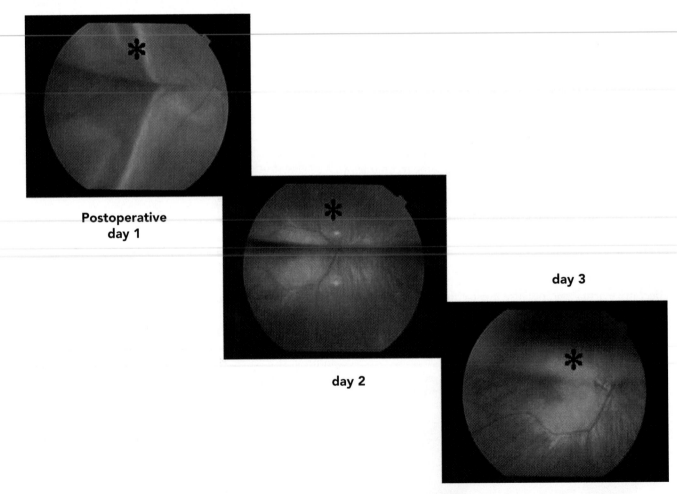

Postoperative day 1

day 2

day 3

Figure 22.3 Fundus changes in the early postoperative period. A bullous retinal detachment is observed in the lower two quadrants on postoperative day 1. The subretinal fluid is absorbed quickly, but a shallow localized retinal detachment remains in the inferior quadrant on postoperative day 2. The retina completely reattaches by postoperative day 3. A gas bubble is indicated by *.

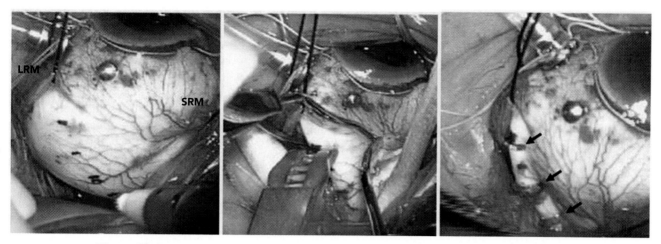

Figure 22.4 Intraoperative photographs of diagonal scleral outfolding. Four titanium clips are placed on a diagonal line from 4 mm posterior of the lateral rectus muscle insertion toward the superior oblique muscle insertion. The length of the outfolding is about 10 mm. LRM, lateral rectus muscle; SRM, superior rectus muscle.

muscle. The outfolded sclera is then fastened with titanium clips (DuraClose, Tyco Healthcare) (Fig. 22.4). The fluid-air exchange and postoperative head positioning is the same as described previously.

OUTCOMES AND COMPLICATIONS

Foveal Displacement

The mean foveal displacement reported previously ranged from 685 to 1,142 μm with the infolding technique (14,15,28–32), from 1,142 to 1,700 μm with the outfolding technique (Fig. 22.5) (22–24), and from 695 to 1,900 μm with the gathering technique (8,25,26). Including animal or cadaver eye studies, the outfolding or gathering technique seems to induce more scleral shortening, resulting in more foveal translocation (8,22–26,29). When comparing the displacement based on the original diagnosis, the foveal displacement seems greater in AMD than in myopia (24,28). In highly myopic eyes, the retina is generally stretched as retinal vessels appear straight. After retinal detachment and reattachment with scleral shortening, the

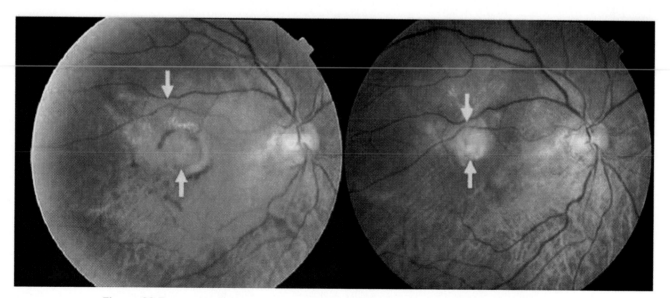

Figure 22.5 Preoperative and postoperative fundus of a patient who underwent limited macular translocation for subfoveal choroidal neovascularization (CNV). *Left*: Preoperatively, a choroidal neovascular membrane with a serous detachment, minimal subretinal hemorrhage, and hard exudates are seen. *Right*: Postoperatively, the CNV and fovea are displaced superiorly and inferiorly, respectively. There is a horizontal choroidal fold in the superotemporal quadrant. The fovea is totally displaced inferiorly by 1,860 μm. The vision improved from 20/200 to 20/30 1 year after surgery. The upper arrows indicate a vessel landmark vessel, and the lower arrows indicate the inferior edge of the CNV.

retina recovers a nearly normal appearance with curved vessels, which may result in reduced foveal displacement without apparent retinal folds.

Visual Outcomes

De Juan and coworkers reported the largest consecutive series of patients who underwent limited macular translocation (16,27). Of the 86 eyes followed for more than 1 year, 9.3% gained six or more lines of VA versus 8.1% that lost six or more lines, 4.6% gained and 8.1% lost four and five lines, 25.6% gained and 15.1% lost two or three lines, and 29.0% were within one line of baseline. Baseline VA before surgery was as good as 20/40 to

20/80 in 20% of eyes, and as poor as 20/400 or worse in 14% of eyes. A VA at 1 year of 20/40 or better was achieved in 5.8% of the eyes, and 20/40 to 20/80 in 30.2% of the eyes. Approximately two-thirds of the eyes achieved 20/160 or better.

VA improved by two or more lines in about 40% of the eyes (range of 30% to 100%) in the results reported in the literature (Table 22.1). There is no apparent difference among the infolding, the outfolding, and the gathering techniques. In our series, the mean preoperative and postoperative VA levels were 20/174 and 20/167 respectively, and the final VA was 20/100 or better in 52% of cases, which is equivalent to or better than the results of other reports (24).

TABLE 22.1
OUTCOMES AND COMPLICATIONS OF LIMITED MACULAR TRANSLOCATION

Technique	Foveal Displacement (μm) (mean or median)	Visual Outcome	Complications	CNV Recurrence Rate (%)
Scleral Infolding				
Pieramici et al.,[28] Fujii et al.[16,18] (n = 102)	1200 (range, 200–2,800)	>2 lines, 40% >20/100, 41%	Retinal tear, 10%; RD, 9%; MH, 9%; macular fold, 3%; SRH, 1%; CH, 1%	35
Lewis et al.[15] (n = 10)	1286 (range, 114–1,919)	>1 line, 40% ≥20/126, 30%	Retinal tear, 10%; RD, 10%; macular fold, 30%; diplopia, 10%	0
Glacet-Bernard et al.[29] (n = 23 of 32)	AMD, 1,105 (range, 200–2,160)	>2 lines, 30% >20/200, 39%	RD, 22%; macular fold, 9%; MH, 17%; diplopia, 26%	43
Ichibe[30] (n = 10)	Myopia, 1,560 (range, 600–2,600)	>3 lines, 100% >20/40, 60%	Macular fold, 10%; retinal tear, 20%	
Deramo et al.[31] (n = 10)	1,700 (range, 680–3,200)	>2 lines, 30% >20/200, 56%	MH, 11%; RD, 11%; ERM, 11%	
Chang et al.[32] (n = 8)	1,100 (range, 800–1,500)	>2 lines, 50% >6/12, 75%	Retinal tear, 13%; diplopia, 13%; RD, 0%	0
Scleral Gathering				
Glacet-Bernard et al.[29] (n = 9 of 32)	Myopia, 840 (range, 200–1,320)	>2 lines, 67% >20/100, 44%	RD, 22%; diplopia, 11%	11
Sullivan et al.[26] (n = 3)	2,033 (range, 1,400–2,400)	>2 lines, 67% >20/100, 67%		
Hamelin et al.[8] (n = 14)	Myopia, 695 (range, 100–1,520)	>3 lines, 50% >20/200, 79%	RD, 14%; MH, 7%; transient diplopia, 14%	14
Scleral Outfolding				
Lewis[22] (n = 25)	1,142 (range, 0–3,200)	>2 lines, 44% ≥20/126, 56%	RD, 0%	
Benner et al.[23] (n = 5)	1,276 (range, 852–1,620)	>2 lines, 20% ≥20/100, 40%	RD, 20%; diplopia, 20%; SRH, 20%	
Kamei et al.[24] (n = 27)	1,576 (range, 349–3,391)	>2 lines, 41% >20/150, 52%	MH, 15%; tear, 7%; RD, 4%; CH, 4%	Enlarged, 59

CH, choroidal hemorrhage; CNV, choroidal neovascularization; ERM, epiretinal membrane; RD, retinal detachment; MH, macular hole; SRH, subretinal hemorrhage.

Histologic evaluation

Histopathologic evaluation of a patient who underwent limited macular translocation showed that the fovea was translocated without causing apparent morphologic changes in the subfoveal RPE, Bruch's membrane, or the choriocapillaris with decreased cone density in the translocated fovea (33). An experimental study showed that the choroid is only minimally involved in the scleral outfolding using clips (21), and a postoperative indocyanine green angiographic study showed no obstruction of the choroidal circulation attributable to placement of the clips (24).

Complications

A large study with 153 cases demonstrated that at least one complication occurred in 35% of cases (18). The complications included retinal tears, retinal detachments, macular holes, retinal folds affecting the fovea, neovascularization at the injection site, and subretinal or choroidal hemorrhage. The rates of complication ranged from 3% to 20% (Table 22.1). Fujii et al. found that the incidence of any complication may decrease with the surgical learning curve (28).

Some patients complained of cyclotropia or diplopia after surgery, especially when a large amount of displacement was obtained. Although a patient who underwent strabismus surgery after limited macular translocation was reported (34), this complication is usually transient and resolves without further treatment as central suppression develops (15,22,35).

Surgically Induced Astigmatism

Postoperative corneal astigmatism is another serious problem associated with macular translocation surgery (19,20). Oshita et al. reported that in porcine eyes, corneal astigmatism induced by chorioscleral infolding ranged from 2.1 to 5.2 diopters (19). Kim et al. reported that surgically induced astigmatism ranged from 1.75 to 7.37 diopters (mean of 4.6) in patients who underwent macular translocation with placement of five or six mattress sutures of 3.5 mm anterior-posterior bite width (20). In contrast, the chorioscleral outfolding technique we used induced astigmatism ranging from 0 to 3 diopters (median of 0.5), and yielded visual improvement with less ocular deformity.

Postoperative CNV Recurrence

Persistence and recurrence of CNV are important causes of vision loss after successful limited macular translocation (16,24,28). Multiple logistic regression analysis revealed that a postoperative decrease in VA was associated with the postoperative enlargement of the CNV over other factors including age, diagnosis, preoperative VA, best postoperative VA, and foveal displacement.

Recurrence of CNV after surgical removal or laser photocoagulation after limited macular translocation surgery occurred in 14% to 63% of patients. Postoperative enlargement of the CNV in cases that did not receive any direct treatment during the limited macular translocation surgery occurred in 59% of patients, at an average of 4.8 months after surgery (24).

SUMMARY

Limited macular translocation surgery can produce improved or stabilized VA in approximately 70% patients with subfoveal CNV. This result can be superior to results achieved with other treatments including thermal laser and PDT, and new treatments including antivascular endothelial growth factor therapy. The problem associated with this surgery is a decrease in postoperative VA. Prevention of recurrence or enlargement of CNV is required to maintain the best possible postoperative VA.

REFERENCES

1. Bressler NM, Bressler SB, Fine SL. Age-related macular degeneration. *Surv Ophthalmol.* 1988;32:375–397.
2. Tano Y. Pathologic myopia: where are we now? *Am J Ophthalmol.* 2002;134:645–660.
3. Macular Photocoagulation Study Group. Five-year follow-up of fellow eyes of individuals with ocular histoplasmosis and unilateral extrafoveal or juxtafoveal choroidal neovascularization. *Arch Ophthalmol.* 1996;114:677–688.
4. Thomas MA, Grand MG, Williams DF, et al. Surgical management of subfoveal choroidal neovascularization. *Ophthalmology.* 1992;99:952–968.
5. Lambert HM. The management of subfoveal choroidal neovascular membranes and hemorrhage. *Semin Ophthalmol.* 2000;15:92–99.
6. Treatment of Age-Related Macular Degeneration with Photodynamic Therapy (TAP) study group. Photodynamic therapy of subfoveal choroidal neovascularization in age-related macular degeneration with verteporfin: one-year results of 2 randomized clinical trials—TAP report. *Arch Ophthalmol.* 1999;117:1,329–1,345.
7. Azab M, Benchaboune M, Blinder KJ, et al. Verteporfin therapy of subfoveal choroidal neovascularization in age-related macular degeneration: meta-analysis of 2-year safety results in three randomized clinical trials: treatment of age-related macular degeneration with photodynamic therapy and verteporfin in photodynamic therapy study report no. 4. *Retina.* 2004;24:1–12.
8. Hamelin N, Glacet-Bernard A, Brindeau C, et al. Surgical treatment of subfoveal neovascularization in myopia: macular translocation vs surgical removal. *Am J Ophthalmol.* 2002;133:530–536.
9. Machemer R, Steinhorst UH. Retinal separation, retinotomy and macular relocation. I: experimental studies in rabbit eyes. *Graefes Arch Clin Exp Ophthalmol.* 1993;231:629–634.
10. Machemer R, Steinhorst UH. Retinal separation, retinotomy, and macular relocation. II: A surgical approach for age-related macular degeneration. *Graefes Arch Clin Exp Ophthalmol.* 1993;231:635–641.
11. Fujikado T, Ohji M, Kusaka S, et al. Visual function after foveal translocation with 360-degree retinotomy and simultaneous torsional muscle surgery in patients with myopic neovascular maculopathy. *Am J Ophthalmol.* 2001;131:101–110.
12. Ninomiya Y, Lewis JM, Hasegawa T, et al. Retinotomy and foveal translocation for surgical management of subfoveal choroidal neovascular membranes. *Am J Ophthalmol.* 1996;122:613–621.
13. Imai K, Loewenstein A, De Juan E Jr. Translocation of the retina for subfoveal choroidal neovascularization I: experimental studies in rabbit eyes. *Am J Ophthalmol.* 1998;125:627–634.
14. De Juan E Jr, Loewenstein A, Bressler NM, et al. Translocation of the retina for management of subfoveal choroidal neovascularization. II: A preliminary report in humans. *Am J Ophthalmol.* 1998;125:635–646.
15. Lewis H, Kaiser PK, Lewis S, et al. Macular translocation for subfoveal choroidal neovascularization in age-related macular degeneration: a prospective study. *Am J Ophthalmol.* 1999;128:135–146.
16. Fujii GY, de Juan E Jr, Pieramici DJ, et al. Inferior limited macular translocation for subfoveal choroidal neovascularization secondary to age-related macular degeneration: 1-year visual outcome and recurrence report. *Am J Ophthalmol.* 2002;134:69–74.
17. Kadonosono K, Takeuchi S, Iwata S, et al. Macular fold after limited macular translocation treated with scleral shortening release and intravitreal gas. *Am J Ophthalmol.* 2001;132:790–792.
18. Fujii GY, Pieramici DJ, Humayun MS, et al. Complications associated with limited macular translocation. *Am J Ophthalmol.* 2000;130:751–762.

19. Oshita T, Hayashi S, Inoue T, et al. Topographic analysis of astigmatism induced by scleral shortening in pig eyes. *Graefes Arch Clin Exp Ophthalmol.* 2001;239(5):382–386.

20. Kim T, Krishnasamy S, Meyer CH, et al. Induced corneal astigmatism after macular translocation surgery with scleral infolding. *Ophthalmology.* 2001;108:1,203–1,208.

21. Kamei M, Roth DB, Lewis H. Macular translocation with chorioscleral outfolding: an experimental study. *Am J Ophthalmol.* 2001;132:149–155.

22. Lewis H. Macular translocation with chorioscleral outfolding: a pilot clinical study. *Am J Ophthalmol.* 2001;132:156–163.

23. Benner JD, Meyer CH, Shirkey BL, et al. Macular translocation with radial scleral outfolding: experimental studies and initial human results. *Graefes Arch Clin Exp Ophthalmol.* 2001;239:815–823.

24. Kamei M, Tano Y, Yasuhara T, et al. Macular translocation with chorioscleral outfolding: two-year results. *Am J Ophthalmol.* 2004;138(4):574–581.

25. Lin SB, Glaser BM, Gould D, et al. Scleral outfolding for macular translocation. *Am J Ophthalmol.* 2000;130:76–81.

26. Sullivan P, Filsecker L, Sears J. Limited macular translocation with scleral retraction suture. *Br J Ophthalmol.* 2002;86:434–439.

27. Fujii GY, de Juan E Jr, Sunness J, et al. Patient selection for macular translocation surgery using the scanning laser ophthalmoscope. *Ophthalmology.* 2002;109:1,737–1,744.

28. Pieramici DJ, De Juan E Jr, Fujii GY, et al. Limited inferior macular translocation for the treatment of subfoveal choroidal neovascularization secondary to age-related macular degeneration. *Am J Ophthalmol.* 2000;130:419–428.

29. Glacet-Bernard A, Simon P, Hamelin N, et al. Translocation of the macula for management of subfoveal choroidal neovascularization: comparison of results in age-related macular degeneration and degenerative myopia. *Am J Ophthalmol.* 2001;131:78–89.

30. Ichibe M, Imai K, Ohta M, et al. Foveal translocation with scleral imbrication in patients with myopic neovascular maculopathy. *Am J Ophthalmol.* 2001;132:164–171.

31. Deramo VA, Meyer CH, Toth CA. Successful macular translocation with temporary scleral infolding using absorbable suture. *Retina.* 2001;21:304–311.

32. Chang AA, Tan W, Beaumont PE, et al. Limited macular translocation for subfoveal choroidal neovascularization in age-related macular degeneration. *Clin Experiment Ophthalmol.* 2003;31:103–109.

33. Albini TA, Rao NA, Li A, et al. Limited macular translocation: a clinicopathologic case report. *Ophthalmology.* 2004;111:1,209–1,214.

34. Ohtsuki H, Shiraga F, Hasebe S, et al. Correction of cyclovertical strabismus induced by limited macular translocation in a case of age-related macular degeneration. *Am J Ophthalmol.* 2001;131:270–272.

35. Fujikado T, Ohji M, Saito Y, et al. Visual function after foveal translocation with scleral shortening in patients with myopic neovascular maculopathy. *Am J Ophthalmol.* 1998;125:647–656.

Macugen (Pegaptanib Sodium Injection)

Gene Ng   Emmett Cunningham   Anthony P. Adamis   David R. Guyer

INTRODUCTION

Ocular neovascularization and macular edema represent the leading causes of blindness in the United States. In the population over 50 years of age, age-related macular degeneration (AMD) is the leading cause of blindness (1–3), with the neovascular form being responsible for 90% of all AMD-related vision loss (4). In working-age Americans, the leading cause of new cases of blindness is diabetic retinopathy (5).

Pathologic angiogenesis, a subject of intense study over the last three decades, is central to the vision loss in these diseases (6–9). Although a combination of molecular regulators orchestrates the complex process (10–12), multiple lines of evidence have converged to support the role of vascular endothelial growth factor (VEGF) as a central signal in ocular neovascularization (Table 23.1) (13–23). This understanding has led to the successful development of Macugen (pegaptanib sodium injection; anti-VEGF aptamer) (24), the first anti-VEGF agent proved to be efficacious in patients with neovascular AMD (25). This major breakthrough represents a paradigm shift in the treatment of neovascular AMD, and opens an entirely new therapeutic vista for clinicians who treat retinal diseases.

Before the advent of Macugen, treatment options for neovascular AMD were limited (Table 23.2) (26–30). Thermal laser photocoagulation has been abandoned for subfoveal choroidal neovascularization (CNV) because of its destructive sequelae (26,31,32). Photodynamic therapy (PDT) with verteporfin has only been proven efficacious in predominantly classic angiographic subtypes of disease (29,30,33), which represent a minority of cases of subfoveal neovascular AMD. Studies have shown that patients with the predominantly classic lesion composition represent only approximately 25% of the overall neovascular AMD population (34–36). Additionally, these destructive therapies do not address the underlying pathophysiology of neovascular AMD.

By targeting VEGF, Macugen has enabled treatment of the entire spectrum of neovascular AMD patients (25) and has ushered in an era of targeted biological therapies for this largely unmet medical need. This chapter reviews the science of Macugen and the results of recently completed pivotal Phase III trials in patients with subfoveal CNV secondary to AMD.

MACUGEN CHEMISTRY

Macugen is a pegylated aptamer. Aptamers (Latin aptus—to fit, Greek meros—part or region) are an entirely new class of therapeutic agent (36), and Macugen is the first aptamer to demonstrate safety and efficacy in humans (25). Macugen is a chemically synthesized, 28-nucleotide RNA aptamer that is covalently linked to two polyethylene glycol (PEG) moieties (38). Its complex structure allows it to bind with high affinity and selectivity to extracellular VEGF, specifically the $VEGF_{165}$ isoform (24,39). Pegylation

TABLE 23.1
MILESTONES IN VEGF RESEARCH

1948–1958	Michaelson, Ashton, and Wise contribute to "factor X" hypothesis.
1971	Folkman publishes "tumor angiogenesis factor" hypothesis.
1983	Dvorak demonstrates tumor secretion of vascular permeability factor (VPF).
1989	Ferrara clones VPF and identifies it as an angiogenesis factor; VPF is rechristened VEGF.
1997	First clinical trials of antiangiogenic therapy in cancer patients initiated.
1999	First anti-VEGF therapy tested in humans with AMD.
2003	$VEGF_{164(165)}$ found to be required for pathologic, but not physiologic, retinal neovascularization.
2003	Optimal methods of long-term controlled delivery of an anti-VEGF agent evaluated in animal studies.
2004	First FDA-approved anti-VEGF therapy for colorectal cancer released.

of Macugen (i.e., adding two PEG anchors to Macugen) extends the bioavailability of the aptamer. Pegylation is commonly employed in pharmacology to retard the metabolism and extend the half-life of drugs (40).

APTAMERS AS THERAPEUTICS

Aptamers are chemically synthesized oligonucleotide (nucleic acid) sequences (40). They are an entirely new class of molecules that rivals antibodies for both therapeutic and diagnostic applications. The use of nucleic acid molecules for the treatment of disease was first conceptualized in the 1970s with the development of antisense compounds—single-stranded nucleic acids that inhibit protein production by hybridizing in a sequence-dependent man-

ner to encoding mRNAs (40). However, the basic mechanism of action of nucleic acid aptamers is different than that of antisense compounds. Although they are also single-stranded, nucleic acid aptamers directly inhibit a protein's function by folding into a three-dimensional structure that specifically binds with high-affinity to a target protein (Fig. 23.1) (40). They do not rely on Watson-Crick base pairing or intracellular access for their bioactivity, as do antisense-based and small interfering RNA-based (siRNA) agents (37,40,41).

Although aptamers are similar to monoclonal antibodies because they are highly targetable, they have advantages as therapeutic agents. Aptamers demonstrate remarkable target affinity and specificity. Typical dissociation constants range from the low picomolar to the low nanomolar range (37,40). Advances in in vitro selection techniques

TABLE 23.2
TREATMENT OPTIONS FOR SUBFOVEAL CHOROIDAL NEOVASCULARIZATION PRIOR TO THE ADVENT OF ANTI-ANGIOGENIC THERAPIES[26–30]

Treatment	Use	Limitations
Laser photocoagulation	Used in extrafoveal and juxtafoveal lesions, but not subfoveal lesions	Destroys photoreceptors overlying treatment area Immediate loss of vision High recurrence rate
Photodynamic therapy	FDA approved for predominantly classic lesions only	Only effective in predominantly classic subtype May not be effective in patients aged ≥75 years May damage healthy tissue Limited benefit in dark irides

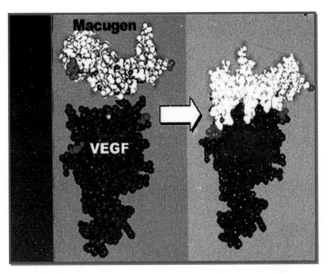

Figure 23.1 Aptamers bind with high affinity and specificity to their targets. VEGF, vascular endothelial growth factor.

have enabled the development of aptamers with sub-nanomolar affinities for their targets. High-specificity aptamer-protein interactions occur because the specific three-dimensional arrangements of complementary contact sites that mediate these interactions are unlikely to be recapitulated in other proteins (37,41). For example, Macugen binds with high specificity to $VEGF_{165}$ while leaving all other VEGF isoforms relatively unbound (39).

One major advantage of aptamers over monoclonal antibodies is that they are non-immunogenic. Aptamers are chemically synthesized and composed of single-stranded nucleic acids (RNA or DNA) (40). Thus, their small size and similarity to endogenous molecules renders them poorly antigenic (40). Immune responses to peptide-based therapeutics can result in inflammation and decreased efficacy. These sequelae are obviated with aptamers (37). Additionally, unlike antibodies, aptamers are highly stable given their chemical modifications, making them amenable to drug delivery (42). Moreover, because they are chemically synthesized, aptamers do not rely on bacterial or cell-based production and their attendant issues, such as endotoxin.

APTAMER SYNTHESIS

Aptamers are synthesized by a process named SELEX (systematic evolution of ligands by exponential enrichment). SELEX is in essence an extremely powerful purification method, in which short nucleic acid ligands with rare binding activities are isolated from a large combinatorial library of single-stranded nucleic acids (RNA, DNA, or modified RNA) using reverse transcription and PCR technologies. This iterative, in vitro selection and amplification technique allows fast and easy screening of very large combinatorial libraries (approximately 10^{14} to 10^{15} different sequences) of oligonucleotides (37,43). The process is illustrated in Figure 23.2.

VEGF IN OCULAR NEOVASCULARIZATION

VEGF is a family of peptide growth factors that acts primarily on blood vessels. The VEGF gene has been conserved throughout evolution, and codes for at least six distinct protein isoforms. The human VEGF isoforms are comprised of 121, 145, 165, 183, 189, and 206 amino acids (Fig. 23.3), with different isoforms appearing to serve different functions (44,45). For example, $VEGF_{165}$ appears to be the isoform responsible for pathological neovascularization in the eye (39,46–48). In contrast, $VEGF_{121}$ appears to be more essential for normal vascular function in the retina (39) and elsewhere in the body under normal physiological conditions (44).

VEGF is constitutively expressed in the retina, in particular by the retinal pigment epithelium (RPE) (11,49). $VEGF_{121}$ and $VEGF_{165}$ are the two prevalent isoforms expressed in the eye. VEGF plays a critical role in both physiological and pathological angiogenesis (Table 23.3) (39,50–53). VEGF is essential for normal blood vessel and embryonic development (54). In the normal eye, VEGF may be an important trophic factor for the choriocapillaris, thus maintaining adequate blood flow to the RPE and photoreceptors. VEGF may also be required to maintain choriocapillaris fenestrae. In addition, researchers are exploring the role of VEGF as a trophic factor for non-endothelial cells in the retina, such as retinal progenitor cells and photoreceptors (11). Emerging research in the field of neuroscience also suggests that VEGF may have neuroprotective properties (Table 23.4) (53,55,56).

The role of VEGF as an essential factor in the development of pathological neovascularization, both in the eye

TABLE 23.3
PROPERTIES OF VEGF

- Stimulator of angiogenesis
- Potent inducer of vascular permeability
- Proinflammatory effects
- Neuroprotective effects

TABLE 23.4
NEUROPROTECTIVE EFFECTS OF VEGF

- In neurodegenerative studies, VEGF displays neuroprotective effects under conditions of hypoxia, oxidative stress, and serum deprivation.
- VEGF reduces cell death in an in vitro model of cerebral ischemia.
- VEGF has a protective effect on neurons (hippocampal, cortical, cerebellar granule, dopaminergic, autonomic, and sensory) in vitro.

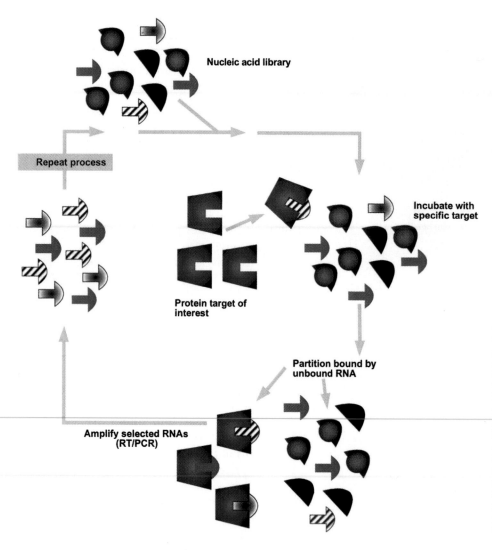

Nucleic acid library

Repeat process

Protein target of interest

Incubate with specific target

Partition bound by unbound RNA

Amplify selected RNAs (RT/PCR)

Figure 23.2 The systematic evolution of ligands by exponential enrichment (SELEX) process for generating therapeutic aptamers. An initial combinatorial library of nucleic acids is incubated with a protein target of interest. Ligands that bind to the target are separated from other sequences in the library. The bound sequences are then amplified to generate a library enriched in sequences that bind to the protein target. After several rounds that are increasingly stringent, the selected molecules are sequenced and evaluated for their affinity to the target. RT/PCR, reverse transcription-polymerase chain reaction.

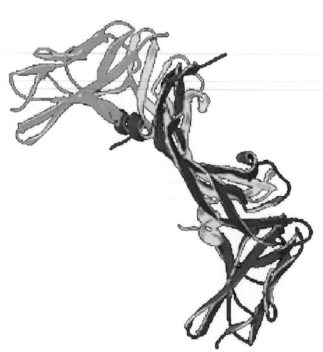

Figure 23.3 Vascular endothelial growth factor (VEGF) protein.

and elsewhere in the body, has been well validated over the last 20 years. VEGF stimulates angiogenesis (Table 23.5) and is a potent inducer of vascular permeability (Fig. 23.4) (13,22,39,51,57–60). More recently, VEGF has been shown to possess proinflammatory properties that may contribute to the pathogenesis of CNV (61–63).

Extensive experimental data suggest that VEGF is necessary and sufficient to produce all forms of ocular neovascularization (13–18,20). Proof-of-concept for anti-VEGF therapy in AMD has been well demonstrated in both a variety of animal models of ocular neovascularization (19,21–23), and most recently in replicate Phase III trials of Macugen in humans (25).

From examination of patient surgical specimens, VEGF has been shown to be present in all angiographic subtypes of CNV (Fig. 23.5) (64–67). The importance of VEGF as the common denominator in all angiographic subtypes of CNV cannot be overstated. This understanding represents a paradigm shift away from segmenting patients by angiographic subtype, and towards recognizing CNV patients as a common group that responds to a therapy targeting the underlying pathophysiological process at hand.

TABLE 23.5
VEGF STIMULATES ANGIOGENESIS

- Triggers degradation of basement membrane of endothelial cells.
- Endothelial cells then
    - change shape and invade surrounding stroma
    - proliferate and form migrating column
    - cease proliferating, change shape, and adhere to each other
    - form new capillary tube
- Sprouting tubes fuse into loops, creating circulation.

MECHANISM OF ACTION

Macugen binds with high affinity and specificity to extracellular VEGF—specifically $VEGF_{165}$—thus preventing it from binding to its cognate receptors (Fig. 23.6) (38). Macugen acts by selectively inhibiting $VEGF_{165}$, the isoform primarily associated with pathological neovascularization in the eye (39), and leaves the physiological isoform $VEGF_{121}$ unbound (39,68).

Preclinical evidence suggests that pathological, but not physiological, ocular neovascularization is characterized by overexpression of $VEGF_{165}$. In a rat model of proliferative retinopathy, the murine equivalent of human $VEGF_{165}$ ($VEGF_{164}$) was preferentially overexpressed. In these experiments, the expression ratio of $VEGF_{164}/VEGF_{120}$ was approximately 12 times higher in pathologic neovascularization than physiologic neovascularization in the retina (Fig. 23.7) (39). $VEGF_{164}$ was also the predominant isoform expressed when VEGF was up-regulated in experimentally induced CNV in rats (48).

In the proliferative retinopathy model, $VEGF_{164}$-specific neutralizing aptamer suppressed pathological neovascularization (Fig. 23.8) but had little or no effect on physiological neovascularization (Fig. 23.9). In contrast, blockade of all VEGF isoforms with a VEGFR-1/Fc fusion protein suppressed both pathological and physiological neovascularization (Figs. 23.8 and 23.9) (39). Another set of experiments demonstrated that $VEGF_{164}$-deficient mice exhibit no difference in physiological neovascularization

VEGF is a potent inducer of vascular permeability

- ❖ 50,000 times more potent than histamine in inducing vascular permeability

- ❖ Induces vessel leakage via multiple mechanisms

    - ▪ Leukocyte-mediated injury of endothelial cells

    - ▪ Formation of fenestrae

    - ▪ Dissolution of tight junctions and transcellular bulk flow

- ❖ Vascular permeability may be antecedent and necessary step for neovascularization

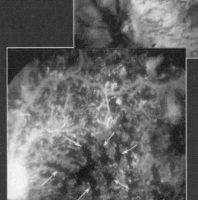

Fundus photo and FA of retina of primate eye injected with VEGF

Figure 23.4 Vascular endothelial growth factor (VEGF) is a potent inducer of vascular permeability.

VEGF—the common denominator in AMD

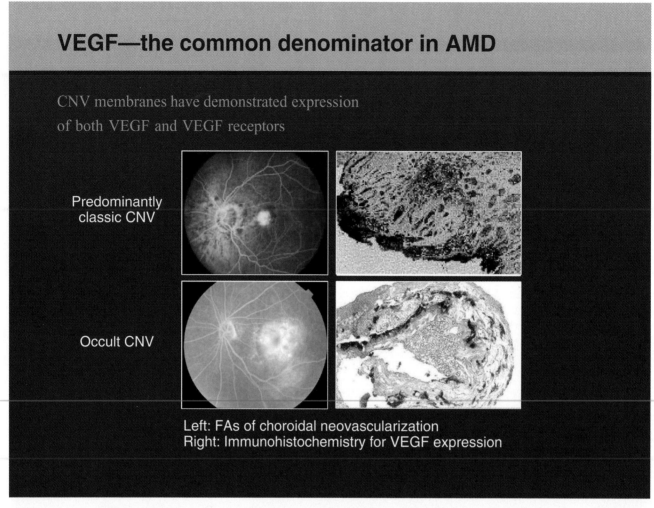

CNV membranes have demonstrated expression of both VEGF and VEGF receptors

Predominantly classic CNV

Occult CNV

Left: FAs of choroidal neovascularization
Right: Immunohistochemistry for VEGF expression

Figure 23.5 Vascular endothelial growth factor (VEGF)—the common denominator in age-related macular degeneration (AMD) (64). CNV, choroidal neovascularization; FAs, fluorescein angiograms.

compared with wild-type (VEGF$_{164}$-sufficient) controls (Fig. 23.10) (39). In summary, selective blockade of VEGF$_{165}$, compared with nonselective pan-isoform blockade, may prove to provide increased safety without compromising efficacy, and this hypothesis bears future examination as comparative clinical data become available.

PRECLINICAL STUDIES WITH MACUGEN

In preclinical studies, Macugen induced almost complete attenuation of VEGF-mediated leakage in the cutaneous vascular permeability (Miles) assay (a guinea pig model of vascular leakage). Similarly, in a model of diabetic blood-retinal barrier breakdown (BRB), Macugen led to almost complete suppression of BRB (47). In a rodent model of corneal neovascularization, systemic treatment with Macugen resulted in significant inhibition (65%) of VEGF-dependent angiogenesis compared with placebo. In a murine model of retinopathy of prematurity (ROP),

systemic treatment with Macugen resulted in an 80% reduction in retinal neovascularization compared with placebo (69).

VEGF INHIBITION STUDY IN OCULAR NEOVASCULARIZATION (VISION) STUDY DESIGN

Study Design and Enrollment Criteria

VISION consisted of two replicate pivotal Phase III trials (EOP1003 and EOP1004) that were identical in objectives and design. The trials evaluated the safety and efficacy of Macugen in patients with subfoveal neovascular AMD. Both were 54-week, randomized, sham-controlled, double-masked, multicenter, dose-ranging trials. A combined total of 1,208 patients from 117 centers were enrolled worldwide (Table 23.6). These patients displayed a very broad range of baseline characteristics (Table 23.7) (25).

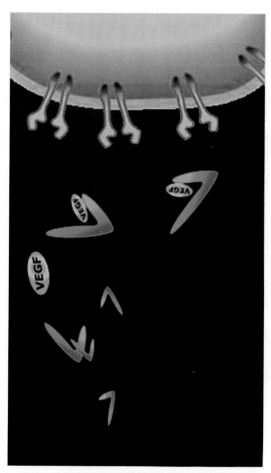

Figure 23.6   Macugen binds extracellular VEGF₁₆₅, the pathological isoform in ocular neovascularization.

End Points

Both clinical trials (EOP1003 and EOP1004) had identical efficacy and safety end points (25).

1. Primary End Point

   The primary end point for both trials was the number of patients losing <15 letters of visual acuity (responders) on the ETDRS chart at week 54 (25).

2. Secondary End Points

   The secondary end points were:
   - Proportion of patients gaining ≥15 letters at week 54.
   - Proportion of patients gaining ≥0 letters at week 54.
   - Mean change in visual acuity at 6, 12, and 54 weeks (25).

3. Other Prespecified End Points

   Additional prespecified end points were assessed, including:
   - Mean change in vision every 6 weeks through 54 weeks.
   - Proportion of patients with legal blindness (20/200 or worse) in study eye at baseline and at 6, 12, and 54 weeks.

4. Angiographic end points:
   - Mean change in total lesion size, CNV size, and leak size at 54 weeks.
   - Proportion of patients receiving PDT at any time during the study (25).

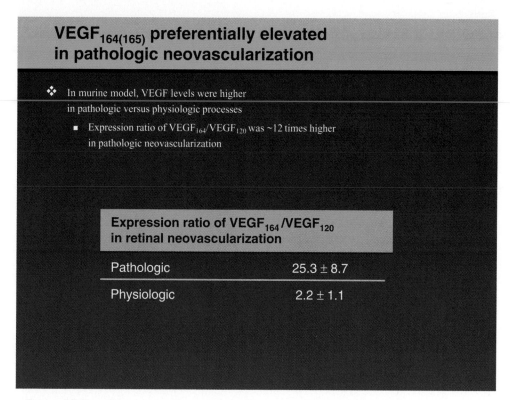

Figure 23.7   VEGF₁₆₄ ₍₁₆₅₎ preferentially elevated in pathologic neovascularization.

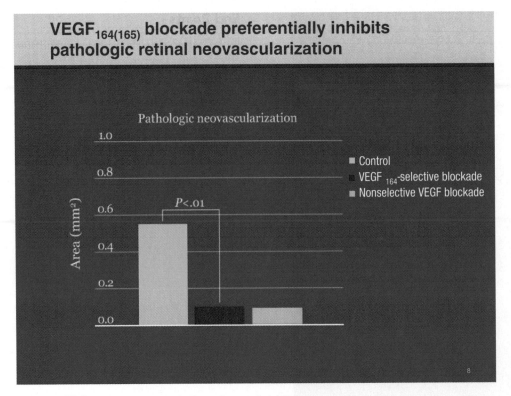

Figure 23.8   VEGF$_{164(165)}$ blockade preferentially inhibits pathologic retinal neovascularization.

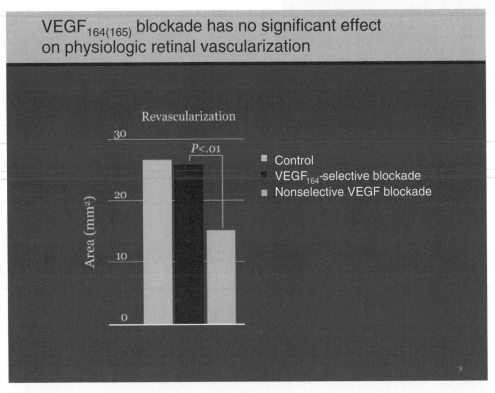

Figure 23.9   VEGF$_{164(165)}$ blockade has no significant effect on physiologic retinal vascularization.

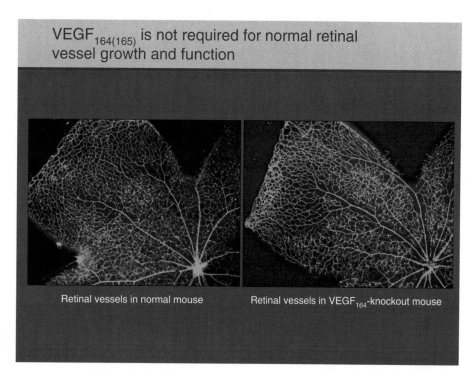

VEGF$_{164(165)}$ is not required for normal retinal vessel growth and function

Retinal vessels in normal mouse   Retinal vessels in VEGF$_{164}$-knockout mouse

Figure 23.10 VEGF$_{164(165)}$ is not required for normal retinal vessel growth and function.

POST HOC ANALYSES

Several post hoc analyses were performed:

- Mean changes in vision by baseline angiographic subtype, baseline lesion size, baseline vision (25), age, and iris color (38) at week 54 (from secondary end point analyses).
- Proportion of patients losing ≥30 letters (severe vision loss) at week 54.
- Proportion of patients gaining ≥5 letters at week 54.
- Proportion of patients gaining ≥10 letters at week 54 (25).

TREATMENT ARMS

The goals of VISION were twofold: determination of dose-ranging, as well as safety and efficacy. Patients were therefore randomized in a ratio of 1:1:1:1 to Macugen injection 0.3 mg, 1 mg, or 3 mg (N = 904), or sham injection (N = 304) every 6 weeks for 54 weeks (25).

All patients underwent a standardized preoperative antisepsis procedure. Patients receiving Macugen were injected via the pars plana into the vitreous cavity. Patients receiving sham had an identical, but needleless, syringe

TABLE 23.6
V.I.S.I.O.N. INCLUSION/EXCLUSION CRITERIA[25]

Selected V.I.S.I.O.N. Inclusion Criteria	Selected V.I.S.I.O.N. Exclusion Criteria
Ocular Subfoveal CNV secondary to AMD—all angiographic subtypes Total lesion size up to 12 disc areas Best corrected vision from 20/40 to 20/320 Subretinal hemorrhage composing ≤50% of total lesion size	Previous subfoveal thermal laser photocoagulation Any subfoveal scarring or atrophy Scarring or atrophy >25% of total lesion size More than one prior PDT with verteporfin or PDT <8 weeks or >13 weeks prior to baseline angiography Likelihood of cataract surgery within following 2 years
General Age ≥50 years Adequate hematologic, renal, and liver function	CNV due to causes other than AMD Previous or concomitant therapy with another investigational agent

TABLE 23.7

V.I.S.I.O.N. PATIENT CHARACTERISTICS AT BASELINE[25,38]

	Macugen (n = 892)	Usual Care (n = 298)
Gender		
Male	42%	40%
Female	58%	60%
Mean age (years)	76.0	75.7
Mean visual acuity (letters)		
In study eye	51.5	52.7
In fellow eye	55.7	55.9
Angiographic lesion subtype		
Predominantly classic	26%	26%
Minimally classic	36%	34%
Occult	38%	40%
Angiographic lesion size		
<4 disc areas	58%	52%
≥4 disc areas	41%	47%

pressed against the bulbar conjunctiva. To maintain investigator masking, different ophthalmologists performed injections or examinations (25).

PDT USAGE

In order to allow the trial to be as "real world" as possible, PDT with verteporfin was allowed at the physician's discretion for only predominantly classic lesions in all treatment arms, consistent with product labeling. Thus, sham patients were considered "usual care" for neovascular AMD. Fewer than 10% of all study patients received PDT prior to entry. Moreover, presence or absence of prior PDT was a stratification factor during randomization, so that patients with prior PDT were balanced across all groups (25).

STUDY COMPLIANCE

Patient compliance during the trials was very high, with a mean of 8.5 out of nine possible treatments administered to patients receiving Macugen 0.3 mg (25). This finding was a testament to how well-tolerated intravitreous injections were, and to how motivated this patient population was.

VISION RESULTS

VISION demonstrated that inhibition of $VEGF_{165}$ by Macugen provided a statistically significant and clinically meaningful visual benefit for patients with neovascular AMD, regardless of their angiographic subtype, baseline

vision, or lesion size (25). This result was accompanied by a strong safety profile and subsequent evidence of visual benefit that extended out to 2 years (38). The robustness of these data was evidenced by visual benefit observed by a variety of endpoints and over a wide range of patient characteristics. The summary data provided below are derived from analyses of the combined populations of both trials.

Primary End Point at 54 Weeks

Intent-to-treat (ITT) analysis of combined populations in VISION found that 70% of patients receiving Macugen 0.3 mg (206/294) lost <15 letters at 54 weeks, compared with 55% of patients receiving usual care (164/296). This represented a 27% relative difference between Macugen and usual care ($P <0.0001$) (25).

Mean Change in Vision Through 54 Weeks

Clinical benefit, as measured by mean change in vision, was observed as early as 6 weeks after initiation of therapy. This benefit continued to increase through 54 weeks and resulted in a 47% relative difference between Macugen 0.3 mg (mean loss of 7.93 letters) and usual care (mean loss of 15.05 letters) at week 54 ($P <0.05$) (Fig. 23.11) (25,38).

Angiographic End Points

Anatomical and biological correlation was provided by the effect of Macugen on CNV. Macugen-treated lesions grew less and leaked less compared with usual care (25).

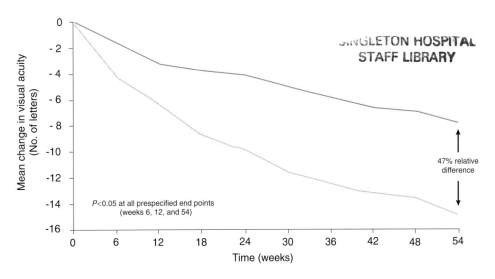

47% relative difference

P<0.05 at all prespecified end points (weeks 6, 12, and 54)

■ Macugen 0.3 mg (N=294)   ■ Sham (N=296)

Figure 23.11 Mean changes in visual acuity from baseline through week 54.

Subgroup Analyses

A number of post hoc analyses were performed to confirm that efficacy was not driven by any one subgroup. These analyses demonstrated that Macugen 0.3 mg was efficacious regardless of angiographic subtype, baseline lesion size, baseline vision (25), age, or iris color (38). Moreover, Macugen effect was independent of PDT use (25).

Macugen 0.3 mg was efficacious regardless of whether lesions were predominantly classic, minimally classic, or occult (Fig. 23.12) (25).

Macugen 0.3 mg was also efficacious over the range of baseline lesion sizes (Fig. 23.13) (25).

Macugen 0.3 mg was efficacious regardless of whether baseline vision was <54 letters (worse than 20/100) or ≥54 letters (20/100 or better) (Fig. 23.14) (25).

At week 54, PDT had been used in 20% of patients receiving Macugen and 25% of patients receiving usual care (38). Thus, Macugen demonstrated efficacy compared with usual care, despite increased PDT usage in the group of patients who did not receive Macugen. However, the numbers of patients who received combination therapy (PDT + Macugen) was too small to allow for subgroup analysis.

Fewer patients receiving Macugen 0.3 mg progressed to legal blindness (≤20/200) at 54 weeks, compared with usual care. A relative difference of 38% was present between Macugen and usual care at 54 weeks (*P* <0.0001) (Fig. 23.15) (25).

Severe vision loss (defined as losing ≥30 letters) was also lower in Macugen treated groups. Severe vision loss occurred in 10% of patients receiving Macugen 0.3 mg,

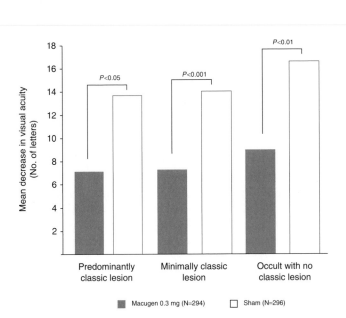

■ Macugen 0.3 mg (N=294)   □ Sham (N=296)

Figure 23.12 Mean changes in visual acuity by lesion subtype at week 54.

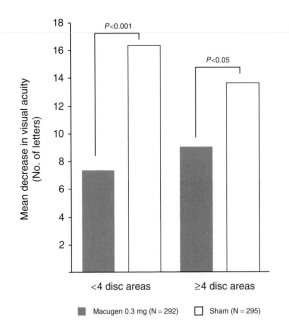

■ Macugen 0.3 mg (N = 292)   □ Sham (N = 295)

Figure 23.13 Mean changes in visual acuity by baseline lesion size at week 54.

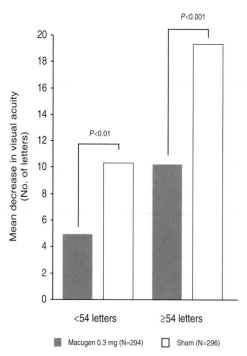

Figure 23.14 Mean changes in visual acuity by baseline visual acuity at week 54.

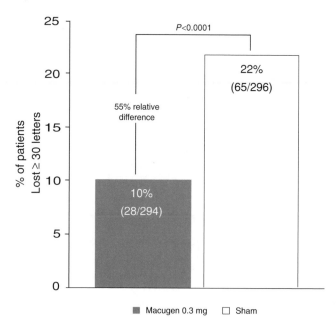

Figure 23.16 Percentage of patients losing ≥30 letters at week 54.

compared with 22% of patients receiving usual care. This represented a 55% relative difference (Fig. 23.16) (25).

In VISION, a greater proportion of patients maintained or gained vision with Macugen 0.3 mg, compared with usual care (Fig. 23.17) (25).

SAFETY AND TOLERABILITY

VISION demonstrated a strong safety profile for Macugen in the population of 1,190 patients who received at least

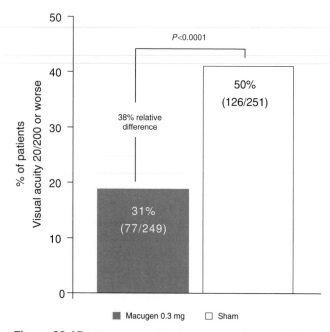

Figure 23.15 Percentage of patients progressing to 20/200 or worse in the study eye at week 54.

one dose during the trials. Adverse events were mostly mild, transient, and primarily attributed to the intravitreous injection procedure rather than the drug product. Of note, no severe ocular inflammation, persistent intraocular pressure changes, or nontraumatic cataracts attributable to the drug were observed. Of note, the discontinuation rate due to adverse events was very low (1%) in patients treated with Macugen 0.3 mg (25).

Serious adverse events were uncommon and comparable to rates identified in a comprehensive review of more than 15,000 intravitreous injections (70). These events included five cases of traumatic cataract (0.6%) and five cases of retinal detachment (0.6%). Infectious endophthalmitis occurred in 12 patients through 54 weeks, representing 1.3% of 892 patients who received Macugen during the first year of the trials. This incidence is equivalent to a per-injection incidence of 0.16%. Two-thirds of cases were culture positive, with coagulase-negative *Staphylococcus* being the most commonly implicated organism (25).

It is important to note that 75% of the endophthalmitis cases (9/12) were associated with protocol violations, such as failure to use an eyelid speculum (25). Had these protocol violations not occurred, the endophthalmitis incidence may have been lower. Despite this complication, most patients who developed endophthalmitis did well following conventional endophthalmitis care, which included intravitreous antibiotics (25).

Indeed, eight of 12 patients suffered only minimal vision loss (<15 letters from before the event), and patients with endophthalmitis on average still enjoyed better visual outcomes than patients in the sham control arm (38). Moreover, 75% of patients who developed endophthalmitis

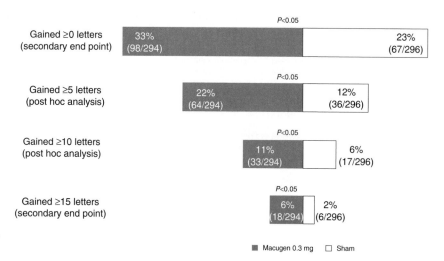

Figure 23.17 Percentage of patients who maintained or gained visual acuity at week 54.

■ Macugen 0.3 mg   □ Sham

(9/12) remained in the trials (25). Finally, reinforcement of proper aseptic injection technique of investigators during the second year of the trials resulted in a reduction in the endophthalmitis incidence (38).

PHARMACOKINETICS

Macugen is administered by intravitreous injection on a 6-weekly dosing schedule (25,71). The aptamer is highly stable (nuclease resistant) in the vitreous cavity (38). Preclinical data suggest that 6-weekly dosing achieves vitreous concentrations of Macugen that remain above the IC_{90} for VEGF inhibition. VISION demonstrated that the 0.3 mg dose was efficacious, and that 1 mg and 3 mg doses did not exhibit additional clinical benefit over and above the 0.3 mg dose (25). Thus, the 0.3 mg dose has been recommended for use in patients.

Systemic absorption of Macugen following intravitreous administration is the rate-limiting step for its disposition. The apparent plasma half-life for a 3 mg monocular dose (10 times the recommended dose) is approximately 10 days. However, Macugen only reaches low concentrations in the plasma following intravitreous injection. In animals receiving Macugen doses of up to 3 mg/eye in both eyes, plasma concentrations were 0.03% to 0.15% of that in the vitreous cavity (38).

For the 0.3 mg dose in humans, plasma concentrations of Macugen were below the lower limit of quantitation (8 ng/mL) for most of the dosing interval after intravitreous administration. Moreover, no accumulation of Macugen has been observed following multiple intravitreous doses (38). Collectively, these data support the systemic safety of Macugen in humans.

DOSING AND ADMINISTRATION

The recommended dose of 0.3 mg Macugen administered every 6 weeks by intravitreous injection is based on pharmacokinetic studies suggesting that this regimen results in

continuous VEGF inhibition (38). Neovascular AMD is a disease in which VEGF is constantly expressed throughout the life-cycle of the disease. This understanding suggests that continuous VEGF inhibition is required in treating the disease, akin to the course of therapy approach employed in antimicrobial and anticancer therapy. The hypothesis that continuous rather than intermittent VEGF inhibition is more beneficial for patients is supported by the VISION findings. The VISION data demonstrated that visual benefit extended to patients who were treated with 2 years of Macugen, compared with patients who were treated with only 1 year of Macugen (25,72).

The Macugen Phase III trials (VISION) also demonstrated that the majority of adverse events observed were due to the intravitreous injection procedure, rather than the aptamer itself (25). As such, proper aseptic technique for intravitreous injection is paramount for patient safety (73). In the trials, intravitreous injections were performed under aseptic conditions, which included the use of sterile gloves, sterile drape, and sterile eyelid speculum, as well as sterilization of the ocular surface with povidone-iodine preoperatively (25). Recent consensus discussions by thought-leaders in the fields of vitreoretinal surgery and ocular infectious diseases have been published in a peer-reviewed journal, and the reader is directed to these references for further information on best practices for intravitreous injections (74).

REFERENCES

1. Klein R, Wang Q, Klein BE, et al. The relationship of age-related maculopathy, cataract, and glaucoma to visual acuity. *Invest Ophthalmol Vis Sci.* 1995;36:182–191.
2. Bressler NM, Bressler SB, Fine SL. Age-related macular degeneration. *Surv Ophthalmol.* 1988;32:375–413.
3. Leibowitz HM, Krueger DE, Maunder LR, et al. The Framingham Eye Study monograph: an ophthalmological and epidemiological study of cataract, glaucoma, diabetic retinopathy, macular degeneration, and visual acuity in a general population of 2,631 adults: 1,973–1,975. *Surv Ophthalmol.* 1980; 24(Suppl):458–471.
4. Ferris FL, Fine SL, Hyman L. Age-related macular degeneration and blindness due to neovascular maculopathy. *Arch Ophthalmol.* 1994;102:1,640–1,642.
5. National Center for Chronic Disease Prevention and Health Promotion. Diabetes Health Resource. Available at: http://www.cdc.gov/diabetes/statistics/index.htm#prevalence. Accessed January 3, 2005.

6. Ferrara N. Vascular endothelial growth factor: basic science and clinical progress. *Endocrine Rev.* 2004;25:581–611.
7. Gass JD. Pathogenesis of disciform detachment of the neuroepithelium. *Am J Ophthalmol.* 1967;63(Suppl):S1–S139.
8. Green WR, Enger C. Age-related macular degeneration histopathologic studies. The 1992 Lorenz E. Zimmerman lecture. *Ophthalmology.* 1993;100:1,519–1,535.
9. Green WR. Histopathology of age-related macular degeneration. *Mol Vis.* 1999;5:27–36.
10. Folkman J, Klagsbrun M. Angiogenic factors. *Science.* 1987;235:442–447.
11. Witmer AN, Vrensen GFJM, Van Noorden CJF, et al. Vascular endothelial growth factors and angiogenesis in eye disease. *Prog Retin Eye Res.* 2003;22:1–29.
12. Ferrara N, Gerber H-P, Le Couter J. The biology of VEGF and its receptors. *Nat Med.* 2003;9:669–676.
13. Adamis AP, Miller JW, Bernal M-T, et al. Increased vascular endothelial growth factor levels in the vitreous of eyes with proliferative diabetic retinopathy. *Am J Ophthalmol.* 1994;118:445–450.
14. Adamis AP, Shima DT, Tolentino MJ, et al. Inhibition of vascular endothelial growth factor prevents retinal ischemia-associated iris neovascularization in a nonhuman primate. *Arch Ophthalmol.* 1996;114:66–71.
15. Aiello LP, Avery RL, Arrigg PG, et al. Vascular endothelial growth factor in ocular fluid of patients with diabetic retinopathy and other retinal disorders. *N Engl J Med.* 1994;331:1,480–1,487.
16. Aiello LP, Pierce EA, Foley ED, et al. Suppression of retinal neovascularization in vivo by inhibition of vascular endothelial growth factor (VEGF) using soluble VEGF-receptor chimeric proteins. *Proc Natl Acad Sci USA.* 1995;92:10,457–10,461.
17. Amano S, Rohan R, Kuroki M, et al. Requirement for vascular endothelial growth factor in wound- and inflammation-related corneal neovascularization. *Invest Ophthalmol Vis Sci.* 1998;39:18–22.
18. Krzystolik MG, Afshari MA, Adamis AP, et al. Prevention of experimental choroidal neovascularization with intravitreal anti-vascular endothelial growth factor antibody fragment. *Arch Ophthalmol.* 2002;120:338–346.
19. Leung DW, Cachianes G, Kuang WJ, et al. Vascular endothelial growth factor is a secreted angiogenic mitogen. *Science.* 1989;246:1,306–1,309.
20. Malecaze F, Clamens S, Simorre-Pinatel V, et al. Detection of vascular endothelial growth factor messenger RNA and vascular endothelial growth factor-like activity in proliferative diabetic retinopathy. *Arch Ophthalmol.* 1994;112:1,476–1,482.
21. Tolentino MJ, McLeod DS, Taomoto M, et al. Pathologic features of vascular endothelial growth factor-induced retinopathy in the nonhuman primate. *Am J Ophthalmol.* 2002;133:373–385.
22. Tolentino MJ, Miller JW, Gragoudas ES, et al. Vascular endothelial growth factor is sufficient to produce iris neovascularization and neovascular glaucoma in a nonhuman primate. *Arch Ophthalmol.* 1996;114:964–970.
23. Schwesinger C, Yee C, Rohan RM, et al. Intrachoroidal neovascularization in transgenic mice overexpressing vascular endothelial growth factor in the retinal pigment epithelium. *Am J Pathol.* 2001;158:1,161–1,172.
24. Ruckman J, Green LS, Beeson J, et al. 2'-Fluoropyrimidine RNA-based aptamers to the 165-amino acid form of vascular endothelial growth factor (VEGF$_{165}$). *J Biol Chem.* 1998;273:20,556–20,567.
25. Gragoudas ES, Adamis AP, Cunningham ET, et al., for the VEGF Inhibition Study in Ocular Neovascularization Clinical Trial Group. Pegaptanib for neovascular age-related macular degeneration. *N Engl J Med.* 2004;351:2,805–2,816.
26. Macular Photocoagulation Study Group. Visual outcome after laser photocoagulation for subfoveal choroidal neovascularization secondary to age-related macular degeneration. The influence of initial lesion size and initial visual acuity. *Arch Ophthalmol.* 1994;112:480–488.
27. Macular Photocoagulation Study Group. Recurrent choroidal neovascularization after argon laser photocoagulation for neovascular maculopathy. *Arch Ophthalmol.* 1986;104:503–512.
28. Macular Photocoagulation Study Group. Persistent and recurrent neovascularization after photocoagulation for subfoveal choroidal neovascularization of age-related macular degeneration. *Arch Ophthalmol.* 1994;112:489–499.
29. Visudyne [package insert]. Duluth, GA: Novartis Ophthalmics; 2003.
30. Treatment of Age-related Macular Degeneration with Photodynamic Therapy (TAP) Study Group. Photodynamic therapy of subfoveal choroidal neovascularization in age-related macular degeneration with verteporfin. One-year results of 2 randomized clinical trials—TAP report 1. *Arch Ophthalmol.* 1999;117:1,329–1,345.
31. Ciulla TA, Danis RP, Harris A. Age-related macular degeneration: a review of experimental treatments. *Surv Ophthalmol.* 1998;43:134–146.
32. Bressler NM, Maguire MG, Murphy PL, et al. Macular scatter ("grid") laser treatment of poorly demarcated subfoveal choroidal neovascularization in age-related macular degeneration. Results of a randomized pilot trial. *Arch Ophthalmol.* 1996;114:1,456–1,464.
33. Verteporfin in Photodynamic Therapy Study Group. Photodynamic therapy of subfoveal choroidal neovascularization in pathologic myopia with verteporfin. 1-year results of a randomized clinical trial—VIP report no.1. *Ophthalmology.* 2001;108:841–852.
34. Margherio RR, Margherio AR, DeSantis ME. Laser treatments with verteporfin therapy and its potential impact on retinal practices. *Retina.* 2000;20:325–330.
35. Haddad WM, Coscas G, Soubrane G. Eligibility for treatment and angiographic features at the early stage of exudative age-related macular degeneration. *Br J Ophthalmol.* 2002;86:663–669.
36. Bressler NM. Age-related macular degeneration. New hope for a common problem comes from photodynamic therapy. *BMJ.* 2000;321:1,425–1,427.
37. Jayasena SD. Aptamers: an emerging class of molecules that rival antibodies in diagnostics. *Clin Chem.* 1999;45:1,628–1,650.
38. Data on file. Eyetech Pharmaceuticals and Pfizer; 2004.
39. Ishida S, Usui T, Yamashiro K, et al. VEGF$_{164}$-mediated inflammation is required for pathological, but not physiological, ischemia-induced retinal neovascularization. *J Exp Med.* 2003;198:483–489.
40. White RR, Sullenger BA, Rusconi CP. Developing aptamers into therapeutics. *J Clin Invest.* 2000;106:929–934.
41. Hermann T, Patel DJ. Adaptive recognition by nucleic acid aptamers. *Science.* 2000;287:820–825.
42. Carrasquillo KG, Ricker JA, Rigas IK, et al. Controlled delivery of the anti-VEGF aptamer EYE001 with poly(lactic-co-glycolic) acid microspheres. *Invest Ophthalmol Vis Sci.* 2003;44:290–299.
43. Tuerk C. Using the SELEX combinatorial chemistry process to find high affinity nucleic acid ligands to target molecules. *Methods Mol Biol.* 1997;67:219–230.
44. Robinson CJ, Stringer SE. The splice variants of vascular endothelial growth factor (VEGF) and their receptors. *J Cell Sci.* 2001;114:853–865.
45. Neufeld G, Cohen T, Gengrinovitch S, et al. Vascular endothelial growth factor (VEGF) and its receptors. *FASEB J.* 1999;13:9–22.
46. McColm JR, Geisen P, Hartnett E. VEGF isoforms and their expression after a single episode of hypoxia or repeated fluctuations between hyperoxia and hypoxia: relevance to clinical ROP. *Mol Vis.* 2004;10:512–520.
47. Ishida S, Usui T, Yamashiro K, et al. VEGF$_{164}$ is proinflammatory in the diabetic retina. *Invest Ophthalmol Vis Sci.* 2003;44:2,155–2,162.
48. Yi X, Ogata N, Komada M, et al. Vascular endothelial growth factor expression in choroidal neovascularization in rats. *Graefes Arch Clin Exp Ophthalmol.* 1997;235:313–319.
49. Blaauwgeers HGT, Holtkamp GM, Rutten H, et al. Polarized vascular endothelial growth factor secretion by human retinal pigment epithelium and localization of vascular endothelial growth factor receptors on the inner choriocapillaris. Evidence for a trophic paracrine relation. *Am J Pathol.* 1999;155:421–428.
50. Alon T, Hemo I, Itin A, et al. Vascular endothelial growth factor acts as a survival factor for newly formed retinal vessels and has implications for retinopathy of prematurity. *Nat Med.* 1995;1:1,024–1,028.
51. Ferrara N, Houck K, Jakeman L, et al. Molecular and biological properties of the vascular endothelial growth factor family of proteins. *Endocrine Rev.* 1992;13:18–32.
52. Roberts WG, Palade GE. Increased microvascular permeability and endothelial fenestration induced by vascular endothelial growth factor. *J Cell Sci.* 1995;108:2,369–2,379.
53. Storkebaum E, Carmeliet P. VEGF: a critical player in neurodegeneration. *J Clin Invest.* 2004;113:14–18.
54. Ferrara N, Carver-Moore K, Chen H, et al. Heterozygous embryonic lethality induced by targeted inactivation of the VEGF gene. *Nature.* 1996;380:439–442.
55. Jin KL, Mao XO, Greenberg DA. Vascular endothelial growth factor rescues HN33 neural cells from death induced by serum withdrawal. *J Mol Neurosci.* 2000;14:197–203.
56. Shima DT, Nishijima K, Jo N, et al. VEGF-mediated neuroprotection in ischemic retina. *Invest Ophthalmol Vis Sci.* 2004;45:E-Abstract 3270.
57. Joussen A, Murata T, Tsujikawa A, et al. Leukocyte-mediated endothelial cell injury and death in the diabetic retina. *Am J Pathol.* 2001;158:147–152.
58. Dvorak HF, Sioussat TM, Brown LF, et al. Distribution of vascular permeability factor (vascular endothelial growth factor) in tumors: concentration in tumor blood vessels. *J Exp Med.* 1991;174:1,275–1,278.
59. Roberts WG, Palade GE. Neovasculature induced by vascular endothelial growth factor is fenestrated. *Cancer Res.* 1997;57:765–772.
60. Antonetti D, Barber AJ, Hollinger LA, et al. Vascular endothelial growth factor induces rapid phosphorylation of tight junction proteins occludin and zonula occluden 1. *J Biol Chem.* 1999;274:23,463–23,467.
61. Usui T, Ishida S, Yamashiro K, et al. VEGF$_{164(165)}$ as the pathological isoform: differential leukocyte and endothelial responses through VEGFR1 and VEGFR2. *Invest Ophthalmol Vis Sci.* 2004;45:368–374.
62. Sakurai E, Anand A, Ambati BK, et al. Macrophage depletion inhibits experimental choroidal neovascularization. *Invest Ophthalmol Vis Sci.* 2003;44:3,578–3,585.
63. Moromizato Y, Stechsculte S, Miyamoto K, et al. CD18 and ICAM-1-dependent corneal neovascularization and inflammation after limbal injury. *Am J Pathol.* 2000;157:1,277–1,281.
64. Matsuoka M, Ogata N, Otsuji T, et al. Expression of pigment epithelium derived factor and vascular endothelial growth factor in choroidal neovascular membranes and polypoidal choroidal vasculopathy. *Br J Ophthalmol.* 2004;88:809–815.
65. Kvanta A, Algvere PV, Berglin L, et al. Subfoveal fibrovascular membranes in age-related macular degeneration express vascular endothelial growth factor. *Invest Ophthalmol Vis Sci.* 1996;37:1,929–1,934.
66. Otani A, Takagi H, Oh H, et al. Expressions of angiopoietins and tie2 in human choroidal neovascular membranes. *Invest Ophthalmol Vis Sci.* 1999;40:1,912–1,920.

67. Lopez PF, Sippy BD, Lambert HM, et al. Transdifferentiated retinal pigment epithelial cells are immunoreactive for vascular endothelial growth factor in surgically excised age-related macular degeneration-related choroidal neovascular membranes. *Invest Ophthalmol Vis Sci*. 1996;37: 855–868.

68. Carmeliet P, Ng YS, Nuyens D, et al. Impaired myocardial angiogenesis and ischemic cardiomyopathy in mice lacking the vascular endothelial growth factor isoforms $VEGF_{164}$ and $VEGF_{188}$. *Nat Med*. 1999;5:495–502.

69. Eyetech Study Group. Preclinical and phase 1A clinical evaluation of an anti-VEGF pegylated aptamer (EYE001) for the treatment of exudative age-related macular degeneration. *Retina*. 2002;22:143–152.

70. Jager RD, Aiello LP, Patel SC, et al. Risks of intravitreous injection: a comprehensive review. *Retina*. 2004;24:676–698.

71. Macugen [package insert]. New York, NY: Eyetech Pharmaceuticals and Pfizer; 2004.

72. D'Amico DJ, VEGF Inhibition Study in Ocular Neovascularization (VISION) Clinical Trial Group. VEGF inhibition study in ocular neovascularization (VISION): second year efficacy data. *Invest Ophthalmol Vis Sci*. 2005:Submitted.

73. Ta CN. Minimizing the risk of endophthalmitis following intravitreous injections. *Retina*. 2004;24;699–705.

74. Aiello LP, Bruckner AJ, Chang S, et al. Evolving guidelines for intravitreous injections. *Retina*. 2004;24:S3–S19.

Lucentis (Ranibizumab Injection)

D. Virgil Alfaro, III   *Michelle Rothen*   *Rama D. Jager*   *Robert Kim*

INTRODUCTION

Vascular endothelial growth factor (VEGF) is a cytokine that has angiogenic and vascular permeability effects which have been implicated in the pathogenesis of macular diseases, including diabetic retinopathy and age-related macular degeneration (AMD) (Fig. 24.1). There are currently five known human isoforms of VEGF, based on alternate splicing of VEGF mRNA: $VEGF_{121}$, $VEGF_{145}$, $VEGF_{165}$, $VEGF_{189}$, and $VEGF_{206}$). Of these, $VEGF_{165}$ is the most predominant isoform. Inhibiting the actions of VEGF has been proposed as a possible treatment modality for macular disease, which results in visual loss secondary to ocular angiogenesis.

The use of VEGF inhibition as a treatment for human nonocular disease has been studied for more than a decade. In 1993, VEGF inhibition was described by Kim et al. through the effects of a murine anti-VEGF monoclonal antibody that was used to inhibit tumor growth in vivo (1). A humanized monoclonal anti-VEGF antibody known as bevacizumab (Avastin, Genentech, San Francisco, CA) was later developed and is currently approved by the FDA for the treatment of metastatic colon cancer.

Ranibizumab (Lucentis, Genentech, San Francisco, CA) is a recombinant, humanized, monoclonal anti-VEGF antibody fragment. The biologic was initially named rhuFab because it consists of one of the Fab (antigen-binding) portions of bevacizumab. The fragment consists of two parts: a nonbinding human sequence designed to render it less antigenic, and a high-affinity binding epitope, derived from the mouse, which serves to bind to VEGF, preventing it from binding to VEGF receptors. Ranibizumab is a smaller molecule (48 kD) compared to bevacizumab (148 kD), and consequently may penetrate the retina to a greater degree than bevacizumab when administered via intravitreal injection (2,3).

One advantage of ranibizumab is its ability to bind to all isoforms of VEGF, allowing complete inhibition instead of targeting only a single isotope of VEGF, as in the case of pegaptanib sodium (Macugen, Eyetech Pharmaceuticals, New York, NY). An additional benefit of the fragment is that its molecular weight is approximately one-third that of the full-length antibody (2,3). Animal studies show that the fragment penetrates the internal limiting membrane and subretinal space more easily upon intravitreal injection, presumably resulting in improved retinal and choroidal distribution (3).

BACKGROUND

In 1948, Isaac Michaelson theorized that a diffusable, vasoformative factor produced by the retina might be responsible for ocular neovascularization in proliferative diabetic retinopathy and retinal vein occlusions (4). The decades that followed have led to the discovery that VEGF plays a critical role in the development of ocular neovascularization. Numerous data now support the theory the VEGF is a potent cell mitogen that induces angiogenesis and increases vascular permeability. In 1994, Aiello et al. reported findings of elevated VEGF in various retinal disorders involving hypoxic conditions and ischemia (5). Studies by Kvanta et al. and Lopez et al. in 1996 reported elevated ocular VEGF levels in patients with AMD (6,7).

RATIONALE FOR VEGF INHIBITION

Significant experimental evidence exists which supports the theory that VEGF inhibition will lead to suppression of ocular angiogenesis. In experimental studies, retinal neo-

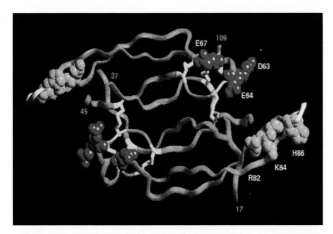

Figure 24.1 Vascular endothelial growth factor (VEGF) is a homodimeric glycoprotein that is secreted in response to hypoxia and ischemia. VEGF induces angiogenesis and vascular permeability. There are five isoforms in humans, with $VEGF_{165}$ being the most abundant.

vascularization has been suppressed by agents that bind VEGF or inhibit VEGF receptors. Aiello et al. evaluated in vitro and in vivo inhibition of VEGF and subsequent CNV suppression using VEGF-neutralizing chimeric proteins in a murine model of ischemic retinopathy (8).

Two different VEGF-receptor chimeric proteins were made using PCR and Pfu polymerase. The first molecule consisted of the entire human high-affinity VEGF receptor Flt bound to amino acids 216–443 of the human IgG1 heavy chain. The second protein was formed by joining the entire extracellular domain of the murine VEGF receptor Flk-1 to a mouse IgG(2Bγ) heavy chain. Testing determined that the VEGF-IgG chimeric receptors had the same affinity for VEGF as full-length native vascular endothelial cell VEGF receptors. The VEGF-IgG proteins bound to free VEGF and prevented it from binding to endothelial cell receptors. Control chimeric proteins were made using human CD4-IgG chimera instead of Flt-IgG, and a monoclonal anti-gp 120 antibody of the same IgG(2Bγ) isotope as the murine chimeric control.

The study consisted of two parts. In vitro inhibition of VEGF was evaluated by exposing confluently plated bovine retinal pericytes to hypoxic conditions (2% $O2/5\% CO_2/93\% N_2$) in a controlled CO_2 incubator. Pericytes from the same batch but grown under normoxic conditions (95% air/5% CO_2) served as controls. The media were collected and stored. The cells were plated and grown overnight in DMEM and 10% calf serum. VEGF was added to the media of some wells, while other media were removed and replaced with the "conditioned" media that had been collected from cells grown in hypoxic conditions or normoxic conditions, and with or without 10-fold molar excesses of one of the two chimeric proteins. On day 4, the cells were lysed and their DNA contents were measured and analyzed.

Bovine retinal endothelial cells that were exposed to VEGF underwent growth stimulation and increased in cellular DNA content by nearly 70% compared to cells that

were not exposed to VEGF. Cells in media containing VEGF and either the human Flt-IgG or murine Flk-1-IgG chimeric protein did not experience the VEGF-stimulating effect, while cells in media with VEGF and the control proteins not specifically directed toward VEGF did. Similarly, growth of retinal endothelial cells grown in media from the hypoxic conditions (which is known to stimulate expression of VEGF) was enhanced. Endothelial cell growth in the same media with the addition of human Flt-IgG or murine Flt-1-IgG chimeric proteins was suppressed by nearly 90% and 80%, respectively. Endothelial cell growth in the same media with control proteins had no effect, and growth of the cells was induced. The lack of cell growth in VEGF-rich media derived from cells in a state of hypoxia is the result of inhibition or neutralization of VEGF by human Flt-IgG or murine Flt-1-IgG chimeric protein in vitro.

The second part of the study investigated neutralization of VEGF by human Flt-IgG or murine Flt-1-IgG chimeric protein in vivo, and relied on the highly reproducible and much studied murine model of ischemia-induced retinal neovascularization (9,10). The mouse model closely resembles retinopathy of prematurity, where an infant is born before sufficient vascularization of the retina has occurred. This results in ischemia, production of VEGF, and subsequent neovascularization (5,11). The murine model follows this same principle.

Ischemia was induced by exposing newborn C57BL/6J mice and their mothers to 75% O_2 from postnatal day 7 to day 12, causing significant retinal capillary destruction. Upon returning to normal atmospheric conditions, the inner retinal layers became hypoxic, resulting in increased VEGF mRNA and protein production, and leading to retinal neovascularization by day 17 in 100% of the mice. Mouse eyes (left eyes) treated on day 12 with intraocular injections of either 200 ng to 500 ng of human Flt-IgG or 225 ng to 750 ng of murine Flt-1-IgG chimeric proteins showed a significant reduction in retinal neovascularization at day 17 (100% and 95% respectively). The contralateral eyes (right eyes) served as the control eyes; they received equivalent amounts of control protein and experienced 100% neovascularization. Inhibition of VEGF and subsequent neovascularization proved to be dosage-dependent and resulted in approximately 50% inhibition of neovascularization when utilizing the maximum dosage (250 ng) of Flt on day 12 and day 14. A single injection of Flk-1-IgG (225 ng) or dual injections also resulted in dose-dependent inhibition (37% and 46% respectively) of neovascularization.

On day 17 the mice were sacrificed. The eyes were enucleated, fixed, and embedded in paraffin. Eyes with retinal detachments or endophthalmitis were excluded. Six μm serial axial sections were obtained from the remaining eyes and stained with hematoxylin and periodic acid/Schiff reagent (9,10). Ten 300-μm-long sections, approximately 30 μm apart, were analyzed. Masked evaluators counted the numbers of retinal vascular cell nuclei anterior to the internal limiting membranes. Normal, unmanipulated mice lacked vascular cell nuclei anterior to the internal limiting membrane (10). Light microscopy of the paraffin-embedded cross sections did not reveal the presence of inflammation or any evidence of retinal toxicity.

The study by Aiello et al. was significant in several ways. It clearly demonstrated that stimulation of bovine retinal endothelial cell growth by both exogenous and hypoxia-induced VEGF was effectively suppressed with in vitro use of VEGF-receptor chimeric proteins. Furthermore, it demonstrated, using a highly reproducible murine model of ischemia-induced retinal neovascularization, that inhibiting VEGF with either human Flt-IgG or murine Flt-1-IgG chimeric proteins reduced retinal neovascularization in vivo.

The question of why the anti-chimeric proteins, while clearly effective, inhibited only approximately 50% of the retinal neovascularization remained. Aiello et al. theorized that while the remaining angiogenic activity could be the result of other growth-stimulating substances, it was probably due in part to the large size of the chimeric proteins. Human Flt-IgG and murine Flt-1-IgG chimeric protein both consist of the entire human or mouse VEGF-receptors bound to the human IgGγ1 or mouse IgG(γ2B) murine heavy chains. Penetration of the bulky final products into retinal tissues is unlikely, limiting the proteins' inhibitory actions to within the vitreous cavity, and targeting only the retinal capillaries on the inner retinal surface.

Anthony Adamis et al. determined that VEGF was necessary for retinal ischemia-associated iris neovascularization in a monkey model (12). Researchers occluded the branch retinal veins of both eyes in eight cynomolgus monkeys (*Macaca fascicularis*). One eye from each monkey was randomly assigned to an anti-VEGF monoclonal antibody treatment group, while the contralateral eye was assigned to the control group receiving control monoclonal antibody of the same isotype.

The monkeys received 20 μg injections of an anti-VEGF monoclonal antibody 4.6.1 (Fig. 24.2) or anti-gp 120 monoclonal antibody, a control antibody of the same isotype (IgG_1), every other day for 14 days beginning on the day of laser vein occlusion (day 0). Serial iris fluorescein angiograms were obtained and assessed by masked readers using a standardized grading system. The eyes were enucleated and the retinas were harvested for Northern Blot analysis.

The eight eyes receiving the anti-VEGF monoclonal antibody did not develop iris neovascularization, while neovascularization proceeded normally in five of the eight eyes receiving the control antibody. The difference was significant ($P = 0.3$). No evidence of biomicroscopic inflammation or toxicity was found in either treatment group. The ability of the ischemic retinas to increase expression of VEGF messenger RNA was not impaired in either group by the intravitreal antibody injections. The data revealed that VEGF was necessary for the iris neovascularization in the adult, nonhuman primate eye.

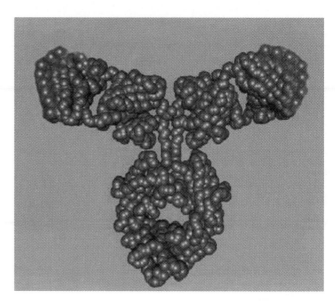

Figure 24.2 Mouse monoclonal antibody A4.6.1 was shown to bind and inactivate vascular endothelial growth factor.

HUMANIZATION AND AFFINITY-MATURATION

Despite the apparent success of murine antibodies in the primate model, their use as a human therapy was limited by the anti-globulin response (13,14). Chimeric molecules, where human constant (C) regions are fused with variable (V) rodent domains, are still capable of eliciting an immune response (23). Humanization of the monoclonal antibody (Mab) was an effective solution to overcome its clinical limitations (Fig. 24.3). The humanization of muMab VEGF A.4.6.1, as reported in Presta et al., involved the transfer of six complimentary-determining regions (CDR) from muMab VEGF A.4.6.1 to a human framework by site-directed mutagenesis, and subsequently reduced its binding to VEGF by over 1,000-fold (15). To achieve binding equivalent to the muMab A.4.6.1, seven framework residues in the humanized variable heavy (VH) domain chain and one in the humanized variable light (VL)

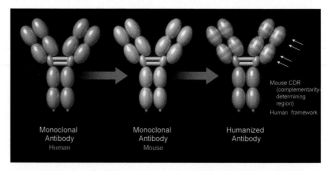

Figure 24.3 Mouse monoclonal antibodies are not useful as human therapies. Human anti-mouse antibodies form, leading to a loss of efficacy and potential allergic reactions. The humanization of muMab VEGF A.4.6.1 involves the transfer of six complimentary-determining regions from muMab VEGF A.4.6.1 to a human framework by site-directed mutagenesis.

domain were changed from human to murine. Comparison of the humanized and chimeric Fabs revealed similar off rates, but a twofold reduction in the on rate of the humanized molecule and consequentially a twofold reduction in binding. The two antibodies had the same activity.

Following humanization, the Fab part of rhuMab VEGF was affinity-matured through CDR mutation and affinity selection by monovalent phage display (2) (Fig. 24.4). High affinity variants were isolated from CDR-H1, H2, and H3 libraries after stringent binding selections at 37C. Dissociation selections lasted several days. Y0317, the final variant, had six mutations from the parental antibody. Four of the mutations yielded a 100-fold improvement in potency for inhibition of VEGF-dependent cell proliferation in in vitro cell-based assays. Radiography crystallography determined a high-resolution structure of the complex between VEGF and the affinity-matured Fab fragment. Superimposing the new Fab fragment over the original wild-type revealed that many of the contact residues remained in complete alignment, preserving the overall features of the binding interface. Locally, it was possible to improve the contact between the antibody and the antigen (Fig. 24.5). Two mutations improved the hydrogen bonding and van der Waals contact. The most favorable improvements, as determined by examination of the complex structure, were confirmed by site-directed mutants to have the most significant impact on the free energy of binding. Overall, the new affinity-improved Fab antibody had improved affinity for several variants of VEGF compared to the parent antibody, although some contact residues on VEGF vary in their contribution to the Fab binding energetics (2).

Mordenti et al. compared the safety, pharmacokinetic, and retinal distribution of [125]Iodine (I)-rhuMab HER2, the full-length humanized antibody, with ^{125}I-rhuMab VEGF Fab, the humanized Fab antibody, following bilateral intravitreal injections in Rhesus monkeys (3). RhuMab HER2

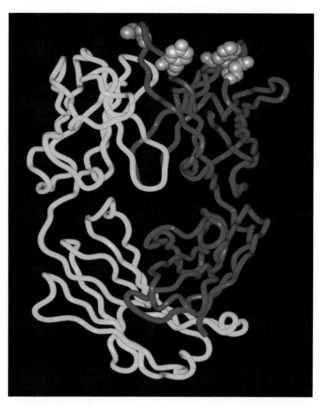

Figure 24.5 The vascular endothelial growth factor and the affinity-matured Fab fragment complex. Locally, it was possible to improve the contact between the antibody and the antigen through two mutations that improved the hydrogen bonding and van der Waals contact.

and rhuMab VEGF Fab (Fig. 24.6) (148 kD and 48.3 kD, respectively), chosen for their substantial size difference and the availability of in-house analyte and anti-analyte antibody assays, were radiolabeled with a modified chloramine-T iodination method. Each dose consisted of 25 μg in 50 μL of protein per eye.

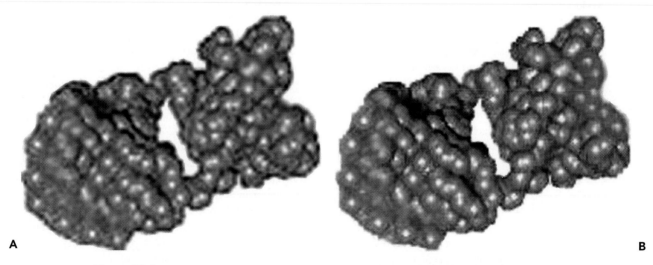

A   **B**

Figure 24.4   **A.** RhuFab **B.** RhuFab V2. RhuMab VEGF was affinity-matured through complementarity-determining region mutation and affinity selection by monovalent phage display (2). Superimposing the new Fab fragment over the original wild-type reveals that many of the contact residues remain in complete alignment, preserving the overall features of the binding interface.

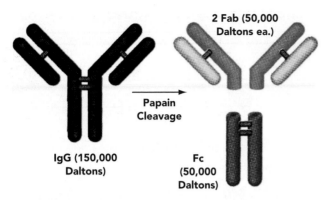

Figure 24.6 Papain cleavage of IgG antibody into two Fab fragments and the Fc fragment. The Fab portion is approximately one-third of the original IgG.

Ten healthy male Rhesus macaques, ranging in ages from 15 to 28 months, were selected for the study after completing ophthalmologic evaluations, physical exams, fecal cultures, clinical chemistry and hematology screens, and plasma analysis. The primates were randomly assigned to two treatments groups. Each animal received bilateral injections of either the full-length humanized antibody or the humanized Fab antibody on day 0. Ophthalmologic evaluations were conducted just before and just after injection. Plasma samples were also drawn prior to injection and 1 hour post-injection.

One animal in each group was euthanized on day 0 (1 hour post injection), day 1, day 4, day 7, and day 14, and safety assessments consisting of intraocular pressure measurements, directed ophthalmoscopy, body weight measurements, and hematology and clinical chemistry panels were conducted. Vitreous samples were collected from each eye and replaced with equivalent amounts of fixative. The eyeballs were carefully enucleated, fixed, and sectioned. One hematoxylin and eosin-stained section and three microautoradiographic exposures were made, and photomicrographs were taken.

As expected, intraocular pressures in all of the animals soared (three-fold to seven-fold in some cases) immediately following injection, and returned to baseline within the hour. The clinical and ophthalmologic findings for all of the animals with one exception were normal during the 14-day observation period. On day 5, one rhuMab VEGF Fab monkey developed acute intraocular inflammation, and moderate to severe aqueous flare by day 7. The inflammation, as well as a slight weight loss, mildly elevated white blood cell count, and low IOP, were thought to be a result of the injection procedure itself and not the rhuMab VEGF Fab injection. The clinical chemistry and hematology were normal for all of the animals with the exception of elevated serum CPK on days 0 to 4, which was thought to be related to the physical restraint and intramuscular injections of ketamine for dosing on day 0.

Retinal tissue distribution of ^{125}I-labeled rhuMab HER2 and rhuMab VEGF Fab was evaluated with microautoradi-

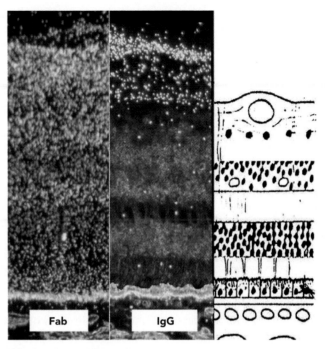

Figure 24.7 Histoautoradiograph of ^{125}I-rhuMab VEGF Fab, the humanized Fab antibody (Column A) and ^{125}Iodine (I)-rhuMab HER2, the full-length humanized antibody (Column B) following bilateral intravitreal injections in Rhesus monkeys (3). The Fab fragment penetrated all of the layers of the retina evenly, extending as far back as the retinal pigment epithelium, while the full-length antibody failed to penetrate farther than the inner limiting membrane at any point during the study.

ography (Fig. 24.7). The iodine-labeled proteins exposed silver grains, the locations of which where then detectable by light microscopy. At the 1-hour post-injection time point, rhuMab VEGF Fab was detected throughout the retinal layers, while rhuMab HER2 was found only in the vitreous cavity. RhuMab HER2 was finally detected at the inner limiting membrane (ILM) at day 1. Signals were highest on days 1 and 4, but were seen through day 14. RhuMab HER2 failed to penetrate ILM to any of the deeper layers, suggesting that the ILM might act as a physical barrier to the full-length protein.

In comparison, rhuMab VEGF Fab was detected throughout the retinal layers as far as the retinal pigment epithelium (RPE) in the medial and lateral portions as soon as 1 hour post injection. Protein in the posterior retina was found only through the outer nuclear layer (ONL) at the 1-hour mark, and may be attributed to the thicker nerve-fiber layer in this region. By day 1, rhuMab VEGF Fab was evenly distributed throughout all of the retinal layers, and remained so through day 4. Signals peaked to a maximum at day 1 and did not persist past day 7.

Diffusion of rhuMab HER2 and rhuMab VEGF Fab from the vitreous to the posterior and anterior chambers was noted from day 0 though day 4, and was consistent with known fluid flow throughout the eye.

The plasma samples and vitreal fluid collected from the primates through the course of the study were studied for antibody content and analyzed to determine pharmacokinetics of the study proteins in the vitreous. Plasma and vitreal fluid from the animals receiving ^{125}I-rhuMab HER2 were assayed using a human anti-human antibody (HAHA) HER2 Fc enzyme-linked immunosorbent assay (ELISA) and the HAHA HER2 Fab ELISA. Plasma and vitreal fluid from animals receiving the ^{125}I-rhuMab VEGF Fab was analyzed with a rhuMab VEGF Fab antibody ELISA. Antibodies to the test proteins were below the detectable limits, if present at all, for both treatment groups. Plasma levels of rhuMab VEGF Fab remained constant below the assay limit of detection (7.8 ng/mL) throughout the study. Plasma levels of rhuMab HER2 ranged from less than 4% to 30%.

Analysis of vitreous fluids revealed a half-life of 5.6 days for the full-length rhuMab HER2 antibody, and 3.2 days for the rhuMab VEGF Fab, supporting the conclusion that the rate of vitreous clearing is directly affected by the molecular size of the molecules. Microautoradiography showed Fab antibody's rapid progression into the layers of the retina, probably aided by its rapid clearance from the vitreous. The Fab fragment was able to penetrate all layers of the retina evenly, extending as far back as the RPE. Mordenti et al. suggested that Bruch's membrane may act as a barrier, preventing further diffusion into the choroids and resulting in an accumulation of rhuMab VEGF Fab in the RPE (3). The full-length antibody failed to penetrate farther than the ILM at any point in the study.

Mordenti et al. demonstrated that rhuMab VEGF Fab might be a more effective therapy for AMD than full-length rhuMab HER2 antibody because of its ability to diffuse to the retinal-choroidal boundary (3).

Krystolik et al. designed a two-phase study to evaluate the safety and efficacy of intravitreal rhuFab injections for choroidal neovascularization in 10 cynomolgus monkeys (16). The monkey model of retinal ischemia and iris neovascularization closely resembles human central vein occlusion (17–20). The laser-injury CNV model has been used in many experiments, including photodynamic therapy (PDT) studies.

Phase 1, the prevention phase, investigated the possibility of preventing the formation of significant CNV with intravitreal rhuFab VEGF injections. Each monkey was randomly assigned a prevention eye and a control eye. On day 0 and day 14, the prevention eyes were treated with intravitreal injections of 500 μg of reconstituted rhuFab per eye, while the control eyes received a vehicle with the same components as the reconstituted rhuFab minus the rhuFab VEGF protein. On day 21, nine CNV lesions were induced in the macula of each eye with argon green laser burns. At day 28, the prevention eyes were treated again with intravitreal injections of rhuFab, while the control eyes received intravitreal vehicles. Analysis of the CNV lesions using color photographs and fluorescein angiography at days 35 and 42 revealed that the rhuFab injected eyes had less chance of reaching grade 4 leakage than the vehicle treated

eyes, indicating that the formation of significant CNV can be prevented with intravitreal rhuFab VEGF injections.

Phase 2, the treatment phase, assessed the effect of intravitreal rhuFab therapy on existing CNV lesions. Phase 2 began 3 weeks after the laser treatments, at approximately the time when CNV lesions in the control eyes began to form. On day 42, the control eyes were switched over into a treatment group and received injections of 500 μg per eye of rhuFab VEGF. This was repeated on day 56. The effectiveness of treatment was determined by comparing the degree of grade 4 lesions on days 49, 56, and 63 with the number of lesions present on days 35 and 42. Analysis showed a significant decrease in the amount of leakage from already-formed CNV membranes after rhuFab treatment, although previous studies show that spontaneous regression of the lesions may have played a small role as well. The results from phase 2 suggest that rhuFab therapy is a beneficial treatment for established CNV lesions.

During the study, blood was collected from each animal prior to each treatment, 24 hours later, and 7 days later to test for antibodies to rhuFab VEGF. Blood serum was tested using the rhuFab VEGF antigen enzyme-linked immunosorbent assay method, and the antibodies were analyzed using the anti-rhuFab VEGF antibody immunosorbent assay method. Analysis determined one of the 10 primates developed antibodies to rhuFab VEGF with 32 ng/mL in the vitreous following the first injections and accumulating with subsequent treatments, as well as slightly elevated serum levels of rhuFab VEGF. The antibodies were generated toward the humanized rhuFab VEGF backbone (not the mouse-derived binding epitope), and are thereby not neutralizing.

Over the course of the study, researchers had the opportunity to evaluate the safety of intravitreal rhuFab VEGF through clinical examination and fundus photographs. No choroidal or retinal hemorrhages were found as a result of the intravitreal injections in either the rhuFab treated eyes

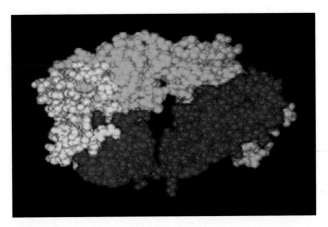

Figure 24.8   RhuFab V2 binds to all vascular endothelial growth factor (VEGF) isoforms and prevents VEGF from binding to cell receptors, leading to decreased vascular leakage and blocking angiogenesis.

rhuFabV2 – How it works

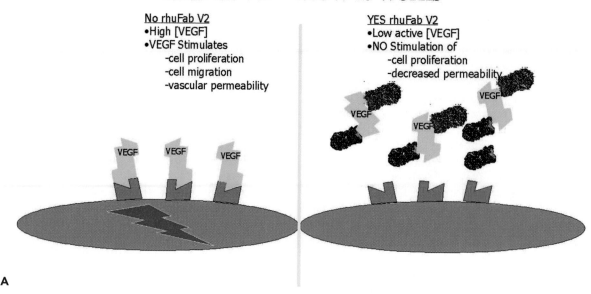

No rhuFab V2
- High [VEGF]
- VEGF Stimulates
  - -cell proliferation
  - -cell migration
  - -vascular permeability

YES rhuFab V2
- Low active [VEGF]
- NO Stimulation of
  - -cell proliferation
  - -decreased permeability

A

rhuFabV2 – What it does:

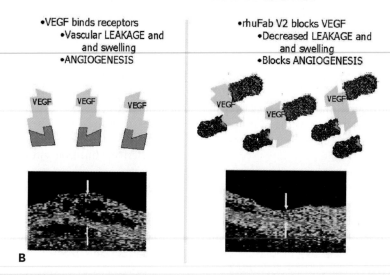

- VEGF binds receptors
  - Vascular LEAKAGE and and swelling
  - ANGIOGENESIS

- rhuFab V2 blocks VEGF
  - Decreased LEAKAGE and and swelling
  - Blocks ANGIOGENESIS

B

Figure 24.9 RhuFab V2 binds to vascular endothelial growth factor and inactivates it by blocking its binding sites.

or the vehicle receiving eyes. No perivascular lesions associated with higher rhuFab levels in some animals were noted. Consistent throughout phase 1 and phase 2 was the development of acute inflammation in each rhuFab-treated eye following the first injection with intravitreal rhuFab VEGF. Anterior chamber cells ranging in severity from one to four or more cells were noted 1 day after the first injections, and the inflammation resolved in all cases by day 7. Subsequent treatments resulted in less inflammation. Vehicle-treated eyes had little or no inflammation throughout the study (16). The ocular inflammation seen following intravitreal rhuFab VEGF was consistent with results from a previous study investigating rhuFab injections in cynomolgus monkeys, although in that study much higher concentrations were used (19).

In a monkey model of laser-induced CNV, prophylactic intravitreal injections of Lucentis prevented formation of clinically significant CNV (two doses were administered prior to laser induction of CNV). In eyes with established CNV, intravitreal treatment with Lucentis decreased leakage without significant toxic effects (12).

RHUFAB IN HUMANS

A Phase IA dose-escalation study (FVF 1770g) of single intravitreal injection of Lucentis (ranging from 50 µg to 1,000 µg) was performed on 27 patients with occult or mixed CNV to determine ocular and systemic safety (21). Visual acuity was measured at 3 months post injection.

While 11% of patients experienced a transient decline of three or more lines maximized by day 3, all 27 patients ended the study 3 months later with visual acuity similar to or improved from baseline. Dose-limiting toxicity resulting in ocular inflammation was reached at 1,000 μg/eye. A dose of 500 μg/eye was determined to be the maximum tolerated dose.

Furthermore, there was initial concern that the humanized protein containing the residual mouse sequences could elicit a human anti-mouse immunoresponse that might decrease Lucentis's efficacy. At the end of the 3-month trial, no serum antibodies against Lucentis were observed.

A Phase IB/II multicenter, randomized, controlled trial evaluating the safety and tolerability of multiple intravitreal Lucentis injections included both occult and classic patients, as well as patients previously treated by PDT (22). Patients were randomized to 300 μg/eye or 500 μg/eye regimes of Lucentis, or to observation or PDT therapy. The study lasted 3 months and patients received monthly injections.

Preliminary results of Phase IB/II studies were released at the 2003 21st Annual Meeting of the American Society of Retina Specialists in New York. These data have yet to be published. However, similar results to Macugen were noted at approximately 3 months. Of the 53 patients treated with Lucentis, 50 patients (94%) had stable or improved vision compared with baseline. Of these 50 patients, 14 patients (26%) improved 15 letters or more on the early treatment diabetic retinopathy study (ETDRS) chart, and 36 patients (68%) had stable vision at day 98 (defined as losing or gaining less than 15 letters on the ETDRS chart compared with baseline). The most common side effect of Lucentis was mild inflammation that appears to limit neither treatment nor outcome.

Based on these results, Genentech has initiated another Phase I/II study and two Phase III Lucentis trials. The FOCUS study (FVF 2428) is a single-masked, multicenter study evaluating the safety, tolerability, and efficacy of multiple-dose intravitreal injections of rhuFabV2 used in combination with verteporfin (Visudyne) PDT in patients with predominantly classic AMD. Patients are randomized 2:1 to receive PDT in combination with 500 μg of rhuFab V2, or PDT with a sham injection. Patients (N = 168) receive monthly intravitreal injections. The primary endpoint is based on the best corrected visual acuity by ETDRS at month 12. Investigators are interested primarily in safety and the percentage of patients losing less than 15 letters at the 12-month mark.

The first Phase III trial (FVF 2598g), MARINA, is a multicenter, randomized, double-masked, placebo-controlled trial for patients with minimally classic or occult subfoveal CNV secondary to AMD. Patients (N = 720) are randomized 1:1:1 to receive 300 μg of Lucentis, 500 μg of Lucentis, or a sham injection. Subjects receive monthly intravitreal injections for 2 years. The primary endpoint is the percentage of patients losing less than 15 letters in the best corrected

visual acuity score at month 12 compared to baseline using the EDTRS chart at 2 meters.

ANCHOR, the second Phase III trial (FVF 2587g) is a multicenter, randomized, double-masked, head-to-head comparison of Lucentis to Visudyne PDT. Patients (N = 428) with predominantly classic subfoveal CNV secondary to AMD are randomized 1:1:1 to receive either 300 μg of Lucentis plus sham verteporfin PDT, 500 μg of Lucentis with sham verteporfin therapy, or a sham intravitreal injection with real verteporfin PDT. Patients will receive monthly intraocular injections of Lucentis for 2 years. The primary endpoint is the percentage of patients losing less than 15 letters in the best corrected visual acuity score at month 12 compared to baseline using the EDTRS chart at 2 meters.

CONCLUSION

Based on the positive results from primate studies, it has been demonstrated that intravitreal injections of rhuFab V2 in cynomolgus monkeys were well tolerated, prevented the formation of clinically significant CNV, and may even be beneficial in treating established CNV. In light of these results and the results from preliminary human studies, Lucentis (rhuFab V2) may be a promising treatment for human choroidal neovascular lesions associated with neovascular AMD (Figs. 24.8 and 24.9).

REFERENCES

1. Kim KJ, Li B, Winer J, et al. Inhibition of vascular endothelial growth factor-induced angiogenesis suppresses tumour growth in vivo. *Nature.* 1993; 362:841–844.
2. Chen Y, Wiesmann C, Fuh G, et al. Selection and analysis of an OPTIMIZED anti-VEGF antibody: crystal structure of an affinity-matured Fab in complex with antigen. *J Mol Biol.* 1999;293(4):865–881.
3. Mordenti J, Cuthbertson RA, Ferrara N, et al. Comparisons of the intraocular tissue distribution, pharmacokinetics, and safety of ^{125}I-labeled full-length and Fab antibodies in rhesus monkeys following intravitreal administration. *Toxicol Pathol.* 1999;27(5):536–544.
4. Michaelson, IC. The mode of development of the vascular system of the retina, with some observations on its significance for certain retinal diseases. *Trans Ophth Soc UK.* 1948;68:137.
5. Aiello LP, Avery RL, Arrigg PG, et al. Vascular endothelial growth factor in ocular fluid of patients with diabetic retinopathy and other retinal disorders. *N Engl J Med.* 1994;334(22):1,480–1,487.
6. Kvanta A, Algvere PV, Berglin L, et al. Subfoveal fibrovascular membranes in age-related macular degeneration express vascular endothelial growth factor. *Invest Ophthalmol Vis Sci.* 1996;37(9):1,929–1,934.
7. Lopez PF, Sippy BD, Lambert HM, et al. Transdifferentiated retinal pigment epithelial cells are immunoreactive for vascular endothelial growth factor in surgically excised age-related macular degeneration-related choroidal neovascular membranes. *Invest Ophthalmol Vis Sci.* 1996;37: 855–868.
8. Aiello LP, Pierce EA, Foley ED, et al. Suppression of retinal neovascularization in vivo by inhibition of vascular endothelial growth factor (VEGF) using soluble VEGF-receptor chimeric proteins. *Proc Natl Acad Sci USA.* 1995;92(23):10,457–10,461.
9. Pierce EA, Avery RL, Foley ED, et al. Vascular endothelial growth factor/vascular permeability factor expression in a mouse model of retinal neovascularization. *Proc Natl Acad Sci USA.* 1995;92:574–584.
10. Smith LE, Wesolowski E, McLellan A, et al. Oxygen-induced retinopathy in the mouse. *Invest Ophthalmol Vis Sci* 1994;35:101–111.
11. Cryotherapy for retinopathy of prematurity cooperative group. *Arch Ophthalmol.* 1990;108:1,408–1,416.
12. Adamis AP, Shima DT, Tolentino MJ, et al. Inhibition of vascular endothelial growth factor prevents retinal ischemia-associated iris neovascularization in a nonhuman primate. *Arch Ophthalmol.* 1996;114:66–71.
13. Miller RA, Osseroff AR, Stratte PT, et al. Monoclonal antibody therapeutic trials in seven patients with T-cell lymphoma. *Blood.* 1983;62: 988–995.
14. Schroff RW, Foon KA, Deatty SM, et al. Human anti-murine immunoglobulin response in patients receiving monoclonal antibody therapy. *Cancer Res.* 1985;45:879–885.

15. Presta LG, Chen H, O´Connor SJ, et al. Humanization of an anti-vascular endothelial growth factor monoclonal antibody for the therapy of solid tumors and other disorders. *Cancer Res.* 1997;47:4,593–4,599.
16. Krzystolik MG, Afshari MA, Adamis AP, et al. Prevention of experimental choroidal neovascularization with intravitreal anti-vascular endothelial growth factor antibody fragment. *Arch Ophthalmol.* 2002;120:338–346.
17. Ferrera N, Dunting S. Vascular endothelial growth factor, a specific regulator of angiogenesis. *Curr Opin Nephrol Hypertens.* 1996;5:35–44.
18. Gaudreault J, Webb W, Van Hoy M, et al. Pharmacokinetics and retinal distribution of AMD rhuFab V2 after intravitreal administration in rabbits. *Am Assoc Pharm Sci Pharm Sci Suppl.* 1999;1:2,142.Abstract 3207.
19. O'Neill CA, Christian B, Murphy CJ, et al. Safety evaluation of intravitreal administration of rhuFab VEGF in cynomolgus monkeys for 3 months. *Invest Ophthalmol Vi. Sci.* 2000;41:S142.Abstract 732.
20. Ryan SJ. Subretinal neovascularization: natural history of an experimental model. *Arch Ophthalmol.* 1982;100:1,804–1,809.
21. Schwartz SD, et al. *Invest Ophthalmol Vis* Sci. 2002;42(4):5,522.Abstract 2807.
22. Presented at the American Academy of Ophthalmology, 2002.
23. Neuberger MS, Williams GT, Mitchell EB, et al. A hapten-specific chimaeric IgE antibody with human physiological effector function. *Nature (Lond.).* 1988;332:323–327.

Intravitreal Triamcinolone for Choroidal Neovascularization

D. Virgil Alfaro, III   Mónica Rodríguez Fontal   Elizabeth Rodríguez Méndez
Simón J. Villalba   Gene Ng   Francisco Gómez-Ulla
Alfredo Domínguez Collazo

BACKGROUND

Few treatment options are available for the treatment of occult subfoveal choroidal neovascularization (CNV) secondary to age-related macular degeneration (AMD). Data from the Macular Photocoagulation Study demonstrated that argon laser photocoagulation diminished the risk of significant visual loss in the treatment of predominately classic choroidal neovascular membranes (1).

In 2001, the Verteporfin in Photodynamic Therapy (VIP) Study Group published 2-year results of a randomized clinical trial that compared photodynamic therapy (PDT) to observation in eyes with occult or classic subfoveal CNV. The study found that PDT was only beneficial in certain subgroups of eyes determined to have presumed deterioration—namely, those with smaller lesions (four disc areas or less) or lower levels of visual acuity (an approximate Snellen equivalent of $20/50^{-1}$ or less). Moreover, 4.4% of eyes treated with PDT in the VIP Study had a severe decrease of vision (at least 20 letters compared with the visual acuity just prior to treatment). Therefore, the use of PDT for occult subfoveal CNV is limited and not without significant risks. In addition, 2-year results of a similar trial in patients with minimally classic subfoveal CNV (TAP Study Group) showed that PDT was ineffective, leaving a large group of patients with very limited treatment options.

Patients with occult CNV therefore have limited options, prompting the use of experimental approaches such as intravitreal triamcinolone injection. Other experimental therapies, such as transpupillary thermotherapy, external radiation therapy, and macular translocation surgery, have shown mixed results (2–5).

WHAT IS TRIAMCINOLONE?

Triamcinolone acetonide, chemically known as 9a-fluoro-11b,21-dihydroxy-16a,17a-isopropylidene-dioxy-1,4-pregnadiene-3,20-dione, exerts an anti-inflammatory effect due to the induction of the phospholipase A2 inhibitory proteins, collectively called lipocortins. It is postulated that these proteins control the biosynthesis of potent mediators of inflammation, such as prostaglandins and leukotrienes, by inhibiting the release of their common precursor, arachidonic acid. Arachidonic acid is released from membrane phospholipids by phospholipase A2.

TRIAMCINOLONE IN OPHTHALMOLOGY

In 1970, Smith and coworkers published a small clinical series demonstrating the efficacy of retrobulbar triamcinolone in patients with optic neuritis (6). Since then, the use of periocular triamcinolone has become commonplace. For example, posterior subtenon triamcinolone injection is often used for cystoid macular edema (CME), and intermediate and posterior uveitis (7–9). Triamcinolone injection has also been employed extraocularly, for example as a medical treatment option for chalazion (10).

INTRAVITREAL TRIAMCINOLONE

The first published report of intravitreal triamcinolone described the inadvertent injection of a corticosteroid preparation into the vitreous cavity in a patient undergoing treatment for a lid lesion. Perry, Cohn, and Auheim described intraocular injection via a Dermajet, a dermatologic device used to inject medical preparations intradermally (11). The authors followed the patient over a 3-year period, and noted no obvious harmful sequelae from the injection.

From 1978 to 1980, Drs. Yasuo Tano and Brooks McCuen served as vitreoretinal fellows under the mentorship of Dr. Robert Machemer at the Duke Eye Center in Durham, North Carolina. Interested in the pharmacologic treatment of proliferative vitreoretinopathy (PVR), they studied the safety profile and antiproliferative effects of intravitreal triamcinolone in animal models (12). The investigators used a rabbit model of PVR to test the benefits of intravitreal triamcinolone in ameliorating epiretinal membrane proliferation and traction retinal detachment. They found that eyes treated with triamcinolone did not develop traction retinal detachment, compared with untreated eyes.

As a follow-up study, the investigators evaluated the safety of intravitreal triamcinolone by injecting 1 mg of the drug into the vitreous cavities of rabbits, and then performing clinical examination, light microscopy, electron microscopy, and electroretinography. They found that the rabbit eye tolerated intravitreal triamcinolone well (13).

Hida and coworkers studied the intraocular toxicity of several commercial corticosteroid preparation vehicles, including Celestone Soluspan, Depo-Medrol, Decadron, Decadron L.A., Aristocort, and Kenalog. They found that only the vehicles in the latter two drugs, Aristocort and Kenalog, were non-toxic to intraocular structures. The other formulations caused retinal degeneration as evident on electron microscopy (14).

Kivilcim and coworkers studied the retinal toxicity of triamcinolone in silicone-filled eyes (15). The authors were motivated to perform their study by previously published experiments showing that intravitreal triamcinolone diminished PVR in a rabbit model. They performed pars plana vitrectomy and silicone oil injection in rabbit eyes and then injected 1, 2, or 4 mg of triamcinolone. Using electron microscopy and electroretinograms, they found that even the higher doses of triamcinolone were well tolerated in these eyes.

The intravitreal half-life and clearance of triamcinolone from the vitreous cavity has been studied in rabbits and humans. In 1982, Schindler and coworkers reported their findings in vitrectomized and nonvitrectomized rabbit eyes (16). Using direct visualization of the corticosteroid preparation in the vitreous cavity (they did not use an assay technique), it was estimated that triamcinolone was cleared in 6.5 days from vitrectomized and lensectomized eyes, in 16 days in vitrectomized eyes, and in 41 days in unoperated eyes. Three years later, Scholes et al. used HPLC analysis to determine that the half-life of intravitreal triamcinolone in rabbit eyes was 1.6 days, and that the drug was undetectable at 13 days post-injection (17). Beer and coworkers studied the ocular pharmacokinetics of triamcinolone after a single intravitreal injection in five patients (18). They found the elimination half-life was 18.6 days in nonvitrectomized eyes, and 3.2 days in eyes that had undergone previous vitrectomy.

The use of intravitreal triamcinolone was largely overlooked until Jonas published his findings on the beneficial effects of the triamcinolone on macular edema, ocular neovascularization, and during difficult surgical cases (19–23). Since that time, intravitreal triamcinolone therapy has gained worldwide popularity in the treatment of various retinal diseases, including intermediate uveitis, posterior uveitis, CME, diabetic macular edema, idiopathic parafoveal telangiectasis, and other conditions.

TRIAMCINOLONE FOR CHOROIDAL NEOVASCULARIZATION IN ANIMALS

Several studies in animals showed benefits of intravitreal triamcinolone in the treatment of experimental CNV. Ishibashi and coworkers at the Doheny Eye Institute in Los Angeles, California induced CNV in cynomolgus monkeys with argon laser (24). They then infused triamcinolone and or dexamethasone into the vitreous cavities of these animals. The authors noted that the development of CNV was significantly lower in treated animals compared with controls.

Ciulla and coworkers created CNV in rodents by applying krypton laser photocoagulation to the retina (a model previously developed by Ogata) (25). They noted that the animals failed to develop CNV if laser photocoagulation was followed by an intravitreal injection of triamcinolone. In contrast, nearly 70% of eyes that received intravitreal saline after laser photocoagulation developed CNV.

Recently, Ciulla and coworkers implanted intravitreal microimplants that slowly released triamcinolone in a rat model of CNV (26). Again, their findings supported the use of triamcinolone for the treatment of CNV. This innovative device, that releases triamcinolone in a sustained fashion, certainly merits further study.

INTRAVITREAL TRIAMCINOLONE IN THE TREATMENT OF CHOROIDAL NEOVASCULARIZATION IN HUMANS

Professor Alfredo Dominguez Collazo from Madrid, Spain is credited with the first publication describing the use of intravitreal triamcinolone in the treatment of various

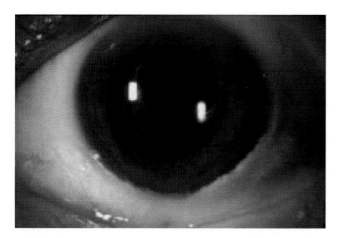

Figure 25.1 An eye with pseudoendophthalmitis, which presented 3 hours after injection. Here, triamcinolone has migrated into the anterior chamber after intravitreal injection. Courtesy of Harry Flynn, MD.

macular and vitreoretinal diseases. His work appeared in the Annals of Royal Society of Spanish Ophthalmology in 1994, and detailed the efficacy and safety of intravitreal triamcinolone in the treatment of exudative subfoveal CNV secondary to AMD (27).

In 1995, Penfold published results from a large series of patients (28). These data demonstrated the efficacy of a single dose of intravitreal triamcinolone in the management of occult subfoveal CNV secondary to AMD. Thirty eyes underwent an injection of 4 mg of triamcinolone. Follow-up fluorescein angiography showed significant reduction of dye leakage in these patients. The author also noted a significant improvement of visual acuity in treated eyes compared with control eyes. He noted progression of cataract in two patients, and increased intraocular pressure in four patients.

Challa and coworkers treated 30 eyes with occult subfoveal CNV with a single dose of intravitreal triamcinolone (29). All patients were treated with 4 mg and then followed

for 18 months. Overall, they noted that 15% of eyes had improvement of visual acuity, while 55% of eyes had stabilization of vision. Thirty percent of eyes suffered visual loss. In this series of patients, 23% of eyes suffered progression of cataract.

Danis, Ciulla, Pratt, and Anliker studied 27 eyes of patients who received one dose of intravitreal triamcinolone for occult subfoveal CNV (30). At 6 months, they noted significant improvement of subfoveal dye leakage. The authors discovered a high rate of glaucoma—approximately 25% of eyes developed high intraocular pressure. Topical antiglaucoma agents resulted in normalization of pressure in these patients.

Using his technique to obtain high concentrations of triamcinolone, Jonas and colleagues treated 71 eyes with 25 mg of intravitreal triamcinolone. Sixty-eight of the study eyes suffered from occult subfoveal CNV, and the other three eyes presented with classic lesions. Overall, 66% of eyes had visual improvement, while 15% of eyes suffered visual loss.

Gillies and coworkers performed a randomized, double-blind, placebo-controlled study in a relatively large study population (31). They treated patients with a single dose of intravitreal triamcinolone, and followed them for 1 year with clinical examination and fluorescein angiography. After 1 year of follow-up, they found that the 12-month risk of severe visual loss was 35% in both groups.

Spaide, Sorenson, and Maranan recently published their observations on the use of intravitreal triamcinolone in combination with PDT for the treatment of subfoveal occult CNV (32). Thirteen eyes received a combination of PDT and triamcinolone, and 13 patients were treated with triamcinolone alone. Both groups had minimal improvement in visual acuity, but fewer re-treatments with PDT were necessary in those eyes that had received combination therapy.

COMPLICATIONS OF INTRAVITREAL TRIAMCINOLONE

The use of intravitreal triamcinolone may cause complications involving the anterior and posterior segments of the eye (Figs 25.1–25.4). The most common complication of intravitreal injection is innocuous, namely subconjunctival hemorrhage. While the development of subconjunctival hemorrhages may be dramatic in certain patients, they resolve spontaneously and do not require treatment. It is our personal experience that patients more commonly develop subconjunctival hemorrhage during the injection of subconjunctival lidocaine, and not during the actual injection of intravitreal triamcinolone.

Elevation of intraocular pressure is a well-documented complication of periocular corticosteroid use. The exact mechanism of corticosteroid-induced glaucoma remains uncertain, although it is postulated that it results from the accumulation of glycosaminoglycans on the surface of the trabecular meshwork with secondary diminished outflow.

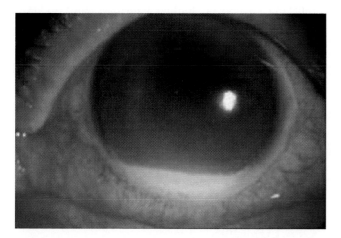

Figure 25.2 Noninfectious endophthalmitis 24 hours after intravitreal triamcinolone injection. Vision has diminished to hands motion, and inflammatory cells are seen in the anterior and posterior segments.

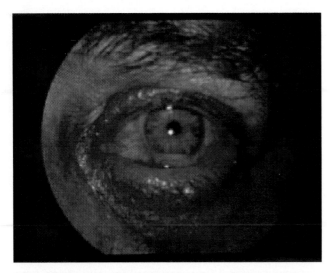

Figure 25.3 The eye developed endophthalmitis 5 days after intravitreal triamcinolone injection and was culture-positive for streptococcal species. The eye lost useful vision despite aggressive therapy with pars plana vitrectomy and intravitreal antibiotics.

It appears that patients develop increased intraocular pressure more commonly after intravitreal triamcinolone injection, compared with subtenon-injected Kenalog or topical corticosteroid therapy. The risk of glaucoma remains a serious concern in patients receiving intravitreal triamcinolone.

Vitreous hemorrhage is a relatively common complication of intravitreal triamcinolone injection, occurring in 3% to 5% of patients. Vitreous hemorrhage appears to be more commonly associated with injections performed with a 27-gauge versus a 30-gauge needle. Some clinicians prefer the use of a larger caliber needle because needle obstruction during injection is less likely.

Sterile endophthalmitis, pseudoendophthalmitis, and culture-positive infectious endophthalmitis have been documented after intravitreal triamcinolone injection (33–35). Pseudoendophthalmitis is seen in pseudophakic and aphakic patients, and results from the migration of triamcinolone particles from vitreous cavity into the anterior chamber. As the white particles settle in the inferior anterior chamber, a pseudohypopyon is formed, leading the clinician to suspect the diagnosis of endophthalmitis. Patients with pseudoendophthalmitis do not complain of pain, and visual acuity is not diminished below preinjection levels. Typically, the conjunctiva is quiet and without evidence of chemosis. Fundoscopy reveals a quiet vitreous cavity.

Patients with sterile endophthalmitis typically follow a course of self-resolution. They present 1 to 3 days after injection, complaining of painless visual loss. Their visual acuity may diminish to the light perception level, but in general they are devoid of the intense pain commonly seen in bacterial endophthalmitis. Slit lamp examination reveals a quiet or mildly injected conjunctiva in the setting of a 1+ to 4+ anterior chamber reaction. Many patients also develop a hypopyon, which is often white in color and sometimes contains crystals and precipitant. A moderate vitreous reaction is almost always seen, sometimes obscuring visualization of the posterior pole.

The exact mechanism of sterile endophthalmitis has not been determined. The phenomenon most likely results from a reaction to the triamcinolone preparation. Peyman and coworkers reported the presence of at least 10 different compounds present in a bottle of Kenalog (lidocainium chloratum, 5.0 mg; propylium parahydroxybenzoicum, 0.1 mg; methylium parahydroxybenzoicum, 0.9 mg; natrium chloratum, 4.1 mg; dinatrium hydrogenphosphoricum, 6.3 mg; polyvidonum, 10.0 mg; polysorbatum 5.0 mg; N,N dimethylacetamidum, 78.0 mg; purified water pro injection ad, 1.0 mg). They also postulated that para amino benzoic acid may represent the most noxious agent contained in a bottle of Kenalog, especially given its toxic effects when placed topically on the rabbit eye.

The presence of intraocular inflammation after intravitreal triamcinolone injection presents a dilemma for the treating ophthalmologist. It should be stated that in pseudophakic and aphakic patients, triamcinolone may migrate into the anterior chamber and settle inferiorly, mimicking a hypopyon. In these patients, careful slit lamp examination reveals the presence of the corticosteroid preparation in the anterior chamber.

In essence, the examining physician must rule out the presence of infectious endophthalmitis. These authors recommend that endophthalmitis treatment be initiated if one of the following symptoms or signs is present:

- Significant eye pain.
- Afferent papillary defect.
- Conjunctival chemosis.
- Retinal phlebitis.
- Vitreous abscess.

CONCLUSIONS

The exact role of intravitreal triamcinolone in the treatment of neovascular AMD remains to be determined.

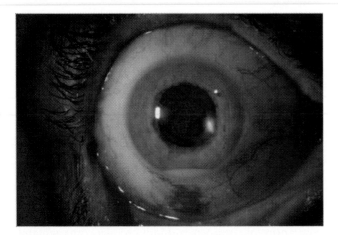

Figure 25.4 Pseudoendophthalmitis 12 hours after intravitreal triamcinolone injection. The conjunctiva is quiet except at the injection site. Intraocular inflammation cleared after 6 days on topical prednisolone acetate.

Several issues remain unresolved at the printing of this textbook:

- The type of subfoveal CNV that responds best to intravitreal triamcinolone.
- The role of PDT therapy as an adjunct to treatment.
- The dosing requirements for intravitreal triamcinolone.
- The frequency of injection of intravitreal triamcinolone.

Several multicenter, prospective clinical trials are underway to evaluate intravitreal triamcinolone in the management of macular edema secondary to diabetic retinopathy and branch vein occlusion. Additionally, a multicenter clinical trial is being planned to address the safety and efficacy of intravitreal triamcinolone in neovascular AMD.

REFERENCES

1. Macular Photocoagulation Study Group. Argon laser photocoagulation for neovascular maculopathy: five year results from randomized clinical trials. *Arch Ophthalmol*. 1991;109:1,109–1,114.
2. Reichel E, Berrocal AM, Ip M, et al. Transpupillary thermotherapy of occult subfoveal choroidal neovascularization in patients with age-related macular degeneration. *Ophthalmology*. 1999;106:1,908–1,914.
3. Ip M, Kroll A, Reichel E. Transpupillary thermotherapy. *Semin Ophthalmol*. 1999;14:11–18.
4. Valmaggia C, Ries G, Ballinari P. Radiotherapy for subfoveal choroidal neovascularization in age-related macular degeneration: a randomized clinical trial. *Am J Ophthalmol*. 2002;133(4):521–529.
5. Aisenbrey S, Lafaut BA, Szurman P, et al. Macular translocation with 360 degrees retinotomy for exudative age-related macular degeneration. *Arch Ophthalmol*. 2002;120(4):451–459.
6. Smith JL, McCrary JA, Bird AC, et al. Sub-tenon steroid injection for optic neuritis. *Trans Am Acad Ophthalmol Otolaryngol*. 1970;74(6):1,249–1,253.
7. Guex-Crosier Y, Othenin-Girard P, Herbort CP. Differential treatment of postoperative and uveitis-induced inflammatory cystoid macular edema. *Klin Monatsbl Augenheilkd*. 1992;200(5):367–373.
8. Tanner V, Kanski JJ, Frith PA. Posterior sub-tenon's triamcinolone injections in the treatment of uveitis. *Eye*. 1998;12(Pt 4):679–685.
9. Helm CJ, Holland GN. The effects of posterior subtenon injection of triamcinolone acetonide in patients with intermediate uveitis. *Am J Ophthalmol*. 1995;120(1):55–64.
10. Dua, HS; Nilawar, DV. Nonsurgical therapy of chalazion. *Am J Ophthalmol*. 1982;94(3):424–425.
11. Perry HT, Cohn BT, NAuheim JS. Accidental intraocular injection with Dermojet syringe. *Arch Dermatol*. 1977;113(8):1,131.
12. Tano Y, Chandler D, Machemer R. Treatment of intraocular proliferation with intravitreal injection of triamcinolone acetonide. *Am J Ophthalmol*. 1980;90(6):810–816.
13. McCuen BW II, Bessler M, Tano Y, et al. The lack of toxicity of intravitreally administered triamcinolone acetonide. *Am J Ophthalmol*. 1981;91(6):785–788.
14. Hida T, Chandler D, Arena J, et al. Experimental and clinical observations of the intraocular toxicity of commercial corticosteroid preparations. *Am J Ophthalmol*. 1986;101(2):190–195.
15. Kivilcim M, Peyman G, Elsaid E, et al. Retinal toxicity of triamcinolone acetonide in silicone-filled eyes. *Ophthalmic Surg Lasers*. 2000;31:474–478.
16. Schindler R, Chandler D, Thresher R, et al. The clearance of intravitreal triamcinolone acetonide. *Am J. Ophthalmol*. 1982;93:415–417.
17. Scholes G, O'Brien W, Abrams G, et al. Clearance of triamcinolone from the vitreous. *Arch Ophthalmol*. 1985;103:1,567–1,569.
18. Beer P, Bakri S, Singh R, et al. Intraocular concentration and pharmacokinetics of triamcinolone acetonide after a single intravitreal injection. *Ophthalmology*. 2003;110:681–686.
19. Jonas JB, Degenring R. Intravitreal injection of crystalline triamcinolone acetonide in the treatment of diffuse diabetic macular oedema. *Klin Monatsbl Augenheilkd*. 2002;219(6):429–432.
20. Jonas JB, Kreissig I, Degenring RF. Intravitreal triamcinolone acetonide as treatment of macular edema in central retinal vein occlusion. *Graefes Arch Clin Exp Ophthalmol*. 2002;240(9):782–783.
21. Jonas JB, Sofker A. Intravitreal triamcinolone acetonide for cataract surgery with iris neovascularization. *J Cataract Refract Surg*. 2002;28(11): 2040–2041.
22. Jonas JB, Sofker A, Degenring R. Intravitreal triamcinolone acetonide as an additional tool in pars plana vitrectomy for proliferative diabetic retinopathy. *Eur J Ophthalmol*. 2003;13(5):468–473.
23. Jonas JB, Sofker A, Degenring R. Intravitreal triamcinolone acetonide for pseudophakic cystoid macular edema. *Am J Ophthalmol*. 2003;136(2): 384–386.
24. Ishibashi T, Miki K, Sorgente N, et al. Effects of intravitreal administration of steroids on experimental subretinal neovascularization in the subhuman primate. *Arch Ophthalmol*. 1985;103(5):708–711.
25. Ciulla TA, Criswell MH, Danis RP, et al. Intravitreal triamcinolone acetonide inhibits choroidal neovascularization in a laser-treated rat model. *Arch Ophthalmol*. 2001;119(3):399–404.
26. Ciulla TA, Criswell MH, Danis RP, et al. Choroidal neovascular membrane inhibition in a laser treated rat model with intraocular sustained release triamcinolone acetonide microimplants. *Br J Ophthalmol*. 2003;87(8): 1,032–1,037.
27. Dominguez Collazo A. Devices and drugs introduced intraocularly for the treatment of eye diseases "in the office." *An R Acad Nac Med (Madr)*. 1994; 111(2):377–385.
28. Penfold PL, Gyory JF, Hunyor AB, et al. Exudative macular degeneration and intravitreal triamcinolone. A pilot study. *Aust NZJ Ophthalmol*. 1995;23(4)293–298.
29. Challa JK, Gillies MC, Penfold PL, et al. Exudative macular degeneration and intravitreal triamcinolone: 18-month follow up. *Aust NZJ Ophthalmol*. 1998;26:277–281.
30. Danis RP, Ciulla TA, Pratt LM, et al. Intravitreal triamcinolone acetonide in exudative age-related macular degeneration. *Retina*. 2000;20: 244–250.
31. Gillies MC, Simpson JM, Luo W, et al. A randomized clinical trial of a single dose of intravitreal triamcinolone acetonide for neovascular age-related macular degeneration: one-year results. *Arch Ophthalmol*. 2003;121(5): 667–673.
32. Spaide RF, Sorenson J, Maranan L. Combined photodynamic therapy with verteporfin and intravitreal triamcinolone acetonide for choroidal neovascularization. *Ophthalmology*. 2003;110(8):1,517–1,525.
33. Nelson ML, Tennant MT, Silvalingam A, et al. Infectious and presumed non-infectious endophthalmitis after intravitreal triamcinolone acetonide injection. *Retina*. 2003;23:686–691.
34. Moshfeghi DM, Kaiser PK, Scott IU, et al. Acute endophthalmitis following intravitreal triamcinolone acetonide injection. *Am J Ophthalmol*. 2003; 136(5):791–796.
35. Roth DB, Chieh J, Spirn MJ, et al. Noninfectious endophthalmitis associated with intravitreal triamcinolone injection. *Arch Ophthalmol*. 2003;121: 1,279–1,282.

Introduction to Gene Therapy and Related Techniques for Retinal Disorders and Age-Related Macular Degeneration

Alejandro J. Lavaque   *Peter E. Liggett*   *Alexander J. Brucker*
Joan Miller   *Hugo Quiroz-Mercado*

INTRODUCTION

Gene therapy involves the insertion of normal or modified genes into the somatic or germinal cells of a target organ in order to modify cell function as a means of treating or preventing pathological processes.

The delivery of foreign genes to ocular tissues to modify the genotype and phenotype of cells is enabling novel approaches to the understanding and treatment of many eye diseases.

Gene therapy received much of its early theoretical support by the early 1970s (before the recombinant DNA era) from knowledge of the mechanisms of cell transformation by tumor viruses. Classes of DNA and RNA tumor viruses have evolved that carry out precisely those functions crucial to gene therapy, that is, the heritable and stable introduction of functional new genetic information into mammalians cells. Thus it was proposed that such viruses or other similar agents, deprived of their own deleterious functions, could be used as vehicles to introduce normal and functional genes into human cells to correct cellular defects and cure genetic diseases (1).

In 1980, it was demonstrated that direct injection of foreign genes into the pronucleus of fertilized mouse eggs, followed by oviductal implantation of the surviving zygotes, resulted in the integration and apparent retention of exogenous genes in all cells of the newborn animal (2). Since that time, transgenic animals have become a major tool in the study of genetic disease, development genetics, immunology, oncology, and neurobiology.

The first human gene therapy trial was begun in September 1990 and involved transfer of the adenosine deaminase (ADA) gene into lymphocytes of a patient having an otherwise lethal defect in this enzyme, the disease produces immune deficiency. The results of this initial trial have been very encouraging and have helped to stimulate further clinical trials (3).

To be effective, gene therapy should follow certain steps. The defective gene must be identified and a normal counterpart isolated. An appropriate method must be found to put the normal gene into a cell where it can function. In order to obtain correct gene action, it may be necessary to put it into the correct site on the host cell chromosome, or even to delete the defective gene. An isolated, cloned gene can either be directly injected into a cell or be carried in by a virus to which it has been linked by recombinant DNA techniques. Once in the cell, it may became integrated into the nuclear DNA, or remain free in the cytoplasm as a self-replicating, extra-chromosomal element (4). The transferred DNA must be expressed by the host cells, resulting in a bioactive product. Some techniques of gene therapy require cells mitosis for efficient incorporation of the therapeutic gene into the host chromosome. Nevertheless, a new retroviral vector (lentivirus, a modified HIV vector) has proven its ability to transfect postmitotic adult retinal neurons.

Gene mapping is fundamental to successful gene therapy because knowledge of the structure, function, and regulation of the gene is essential for the design of the therapeutic strategy.

The eye is an excellent candidate for gene therapy, given its small size, its relative anatomical isolation, its numerous well-characterized genetic defects, and the ease with which vectors can be delivered to the immediate vicinity of cells involved in a particular disease. Moreover, the eye has distinct advantages as a target for virus-mediated gene therapy, such as easy accessibility, well-defined anatomy, and translucent media, allowing visualization of the transfer process. However, potential difficulties include problems in localizing and delivering genes to the retina, because retinal neurons are postmitotic.

RETINA CELL DIVERSIFICATION

Visual perception of our environment essentially depends on the correct assembly of six principal cell types into the functional architecture of the neuroretina. Briefly, visual stimuli are detected by the rod and cone photoreceptor cells and are, either directly or indirectly, transmitted via bipolar interneurons to retinal ganglion cells, which ultimately relay the signals to the brain. Further retinal processing in visual input, such as movement detection and contrast enhancement, is mediated by two types of interneurons: horizontal and amacrine cells (5).

In poikilothermic vertebrates, fishes, and amphibians, only a small part of the retina is generated in the embryonic period; most of the retina of the adult is produced during the larval period or in sexually mature animals; thus, new retina is continually formed at the margin of the eye and is seamlessly integrated into the previously generated and already functioning retina. Moreover, the retina of mature urodele amphibians and fish, as well as the retina of embryonic homeothermic vertebrates such as chickens and mammals, is capable of remarkable regeneration after damage. This is in part due to a highly conserved and well-

defined structure of the vertebrate retina, and to the development of cell-specific markers. Similarly, it has been known that the eye of fish and frogs continues to grow throughout their lifetimes. Several investigators demonstrated that the growth of the eye was due to the addition of new retinal cells. The new cells are primarily added at the peripheral margin, or ciliary margin, of the eye; the retina thus grows as concentric rings of new cells. The margin of the eye of fish and amphibians thus must contain stem cells capable of adding new retina for many years. These marginal cells have many features common to stem cells in other tissues. In addition, those cells at the far periphery give rise to clones containing both RPE cells and neural retina cells. A common precursor for both tissues at their border could explain how the growth of the retina and the RPE are coordinated during eye development. Moreover, the marginal progenitors cells can provide a source of new retina after damage. The retina marginal cells increase the production of new retina cells in response to mechanical or neurochemical retinal injury. For example, destruction of amacrine cells and bipolar cells by intraocular injection of kainic acid in *Rana pipiens* tadpoles causes an increase in the number of marginal cells during the weeks after the injury. The increased cell production specifically replaces those cells that were destroyed by the lesion. Destruction of the retina by transient ischemia causes a similar up-regulation in the marginal zone mitotic activity.

When stimulated to divide, stem cells undergo either symmetric divisions that amplify the population of stem cells or, more typically, asymmetric divisions that give rise to two intrinsically different daughter cells. In the latter case, one daughter cell replaces the original stem cell, and the other begins a progression down a path toward differentiation. This second cell, often referred to as a transit amplifying cell or progenitor cell, is capable of limited, but typically more frequent cell division and ultimately all of its daughter cells differentiate (6).

In others species of amphibians, the new retina cells arise from an unlikely source: the RPE. The RPE is derived from the outer layer of the optic cup, and several lines of evidence show that it has the capacity to develop either as neural retina or RPE, depending on local factors in the microenvironment. Following retina removal, the RPE cells begin to proliferate and quickly form two layers of cells instead of their normal single layer. These cells then begin to lose their pigmentation and genes normally expressed by RPE cells are down regulated. As they lose their pigmentation, the cells become more columnar in shape and more densely packed into a more typical-appearing neuroepithelium. The lamination of the neuroepithelium occurs much like that of normal development, and the sequence of generation of the different retinal cell types appears to be similar to normal retinal histogenesis (7).

Cell differentiation in the vertebrate retina is initiated in the inner layer of the central optic cup and progresses

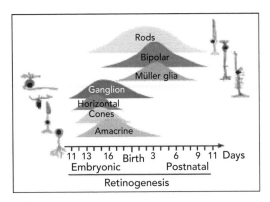

Figure 26.1 Retinal neurogenesis proceeds in a fixed histogenetic order. Retinal ganglion cells and horizontal cells differentiate first, followed in overlapping phases by cone photoreceptors, amacrine cells, rod photoreceptors, bipolar cells, and, finally, Müller glial cells. Note that the curves do not reflect the absolute, but rather the relative proportion of cells produced for each cell type. The numbers relate to embryonic and postnatal day of murine development. (With permission from Marquardt T, Gruss P. Generating neuronal diversity in the retina: one for nearly all. *Trends in Neurosciences.* 2002;25:32–38).

concentrically in a wave-like fashion until reaching the peripheral edges of the retina. These cells type derive from a common population of multipotent retinal progenitor cells (RPCs). Another characteristic feature of vertebrate retinogenesis is the relatively fixed chronological sequence after which the different retinal cells types are generated (Fig. 26.1). Retinal ganglion cells and horizontal cells differentiate first, followed in overlapping phases by cone photoreceptors, bipolar cells and, finally, Müller glial cells. These cells classes, which can be further subdivided, finally become incorporated into the local neural circuitry instrumental in the first steps in the processing of visual information. In mammals and amphibian, retinal progenitor cells are multipotent and retain their ability to generate different types up to the final cell's division. Several secreted factors are implicated in guiding RPCs towards different cells fates. Transforming growth factor-α (TGF-α), epidermal growth factor (EGF), and leukemia inhibitory factor, for instance, can stimulate the production of particular retinal cell types, while often leading to the suppression of others. Furthermore, the application of ciliary neurotrophic factor (CNTF) can redirect immature postmitotic rod photoreceptor towards the Müller glia fate well after cell cycle exit. From these experiments it could simply be assumed that during retinogenesis changing extrinsic signals promote the generation of the different retinal cell types from a homogeneous pool of multipotent RPCs. Following this notion, postnatal RPCs, for example, would be predicted to adopt cell fates predominantly generated during early retinogenesis by placing them into an embryogenesis retinal environment. Besides the action of extrinsic signals influencing cell fate, cell autonomous mechanisms must therefore operate in mediating changes in the intrinsic responsiveness of RPCs to particular extracellular signals (5). To account for these observations it was proposed that during the successive stages of retinogenesis RPCs switch

between different competence states. A possible mechanism therefore involves changes in the expression level of cell surface receptors, which thereby mediate intrinsic differences in the response of RPCs when challenged by the same extrinsic signals (8).

In all vertebral species a similar set of pivotal transcription factors initiate the eye development. These transcription factors are: Pax6, Rx1, Six3/6, and Lhx2. In the developing mouse retina, Pax6 is expressed in virtually all mitotic retinal progenitor cells during all states of retinogenesis, including postnatal stages shortly before the last retinal cells become postmitotic. The coexpression of such factors appears to be a defining feature of retinal progenitor cells and it is imaginable that the combinational action of these transcription factors controls the range of cell fates generated from retinal progenitor cells.

As described above, a unique aspect of the developing retina is that there are waves of differentiation of particular cell types occurring over a short period of time. Future studies could deliver viruses at defined fetal time points to decipher the specific roles of cellular receptors and the stage of differentiation in the final transgene expression patterns. Results of such a study would be relevant to development of fetal gene delivery techniques for every organ system.

There is currently no evidence for a neural/glial stem cell at the ciliary margin in the adult mammalian retina, and the retina of the mature mammals does not show regenerative capacity after damage. Nevertheless, the Müller glial and RPE cells, two sources of retinal progenitors in amphibians and fish, are able to proliferate in response to damage in mature mammalian retina. The fact that the RPE of embryonic chicks and mammals can be stimulated by several growth factors to regenerate neural retina shows potential conservation of a mechanism of phenotypic ability early in development that resembles the regeneration of amphibian retina. In the past years, there has been considerable progress made in the identification of the factors that control the proliferation and differentiation of the retinal progenitor cells in developing organisms, and the application of this information will soon provide tests of the possibility that neural/glial stem cell potential can be reinitiated in the adult mammalian retina (7).

THE RETINA AS A GENE TRANSFER TARGET

Retinogenesis is a developmental process that is tightly regulated both temporally and spatially and is therefore an excellent model for studying the molecular and cellular mechanisms of neurogenesis in the central nervous system (9).

The retina has many unique properties that make it particularly amenable for gene transfer. It is a thin laminar structure that is accessible by multiple routes; consequently, different areas of the eye and various cell types may be exposed to a therapeutic intervention. The fact that the eye is small and enclosed limits the dose of vector necessary to achieve a therapeutic effect and prevents exposure of other tissues to the vector. There are physical barriers in the retina, such as the blood-retinal barrier, that further protect a widespread diffusion of the vector to the systemic circulation. In particular, the subretinal space is separated from the blood supply by the retinal pigment epithelium (RPE) and an intracellular junction. These barriers provide a beneficial effect in protecting the retina from the immune response by sequestering antigens from the systemic circulation. Furthermore, the eye possesses experimental advantages for viral vector delivery; for example, due to the size of the globe, one can readily extrapolate a treatment dosage from an animal experiment to a human study. This extrapolation is more favorable than for other organ systems. In addition there are a number of sophisticated means to evaluate therapeutic efficacy over time. Retinal function can be monitored with noninvasive and quantitative tests, such as ophthalmoscopy, electroretinography, optical coherence tomography, the measurement of afferent papillary responses, and visual evoked potentials. Finally, a number of genes responsible for retinal disease have been identified, and many animal models resembling human retinal abnormalities exist (10).

RETINAL DEGENERATION AND REGENERATION

Retinal diseases amenable to gene therapies are generally characterized by neuronal degeneration (i.e., retinitis pigmentosa or Stargardt's disease) or by ocular neovascularization (i.e., age-related macular degeneration [AMD]).

Perhaps the most significant advance in the past few years has been the discovery of the ABCR (retina-specific, ATP-binding cassette transporter) gene and its mutation in autosomal recessive Stargardt's macular dystrophy and fundus flavimaculatus (11). The ABCR gene is expressed in rods; its gene product, rim protein, is thought to function in the recycling of rod outer segment components between the RPE and the retina (12).

Carriers of heterozygous gene defects may be at increased risk for AMD; several ABCR gene mutations have been identified in some populations of patients with AMD. In addition, mutations in TIMP3 lead to Sorsby's fundus dystrophy, a retinal disease that exhibits characteristics of AMD, including thickened Bruch's membrane, high risk for neovascularization, and photoreceptor degeneration (13).

There is some scientific basis for where it is possible to base regenerative strategies for the retina. The therapeutic use of cells for the correction of disease, generally referred to as cell therapy, is expected to provide an opportunity to cure untreatable disease caused by cell damage and dysfunction. An alternative choice of stem cells is embryonic stem cells isolated from the inner cell mass of the preimplantation embryo. As embryonic stem cells continue to proliferate in an undifferentiated state in vitro, an unlimited stem cell source or its derivates may be secured. It is also a potential benefit that embryonic cells may be genetically manipulated to permit the selective differentiation and/or isolation of a specific cell type. In these efforts, culture systems have been refined to selectively induce specific cell types, and not to generate other cell types, by using a combination of growth factors and forced expression of lineage-specific transcription factors. Efficient and reproducible induction of retinal cells including pigmented retina epithelium and photoreceptors cells from embryonic cells has great potential in cell replacement therapy for currently untreatable retinal disorders (14).

Regenerative biology has now been recognized as an emerging field with certain aims and goals. One direction of this new field is to understand the basic mechanisms by which tissue can be repaired and restored. The other direction examines the possibility of applying this basic knowledge to medicine with the goal of repairing damaged tissue. Regeneration tissues can be produced through the differentiation of stem cells (local or nonlocal) or through the transdifferentiation of local terminally differentiated cells (15). The terms *repair* and *regeneration* are sometimes used indiscriminately, and they basically refer to the same thing. They both can be used to describe how a particular tissue or part of an organ is reconstructed after damage. Regeneration occurs by primarily two strategies. One is by differentiated cells neighboring the site of damage. These cells restore the damaged tissue by proliferation or by transdifferentiation. In the latter, local cells are able to dedifferentiate (lose the characteristics of their origin) and subsequently redifferentiate in a different direction. This strategy is characteristic of epimorphic regeneration. The second strategy is by stem cells. Stem cells can be local (tissue-specific; reside in certain adult tissues) and upon damage they differentiate to reconstitute the lost part. Examples of tissue-specific stem cells include brain, skeletal muscle, cardiac muscle, liver, and cells of the mesenchymal lineage. Alternatively, there are stem cells that are not tissue-specific. These cells reside in the bone marrow and migrate to the site of damage and differentiate into many other cells types. The possibility that stem cells can be used to repair virtually all tissues has recently received enormous attention and has been heralded as the one technique that ultimately would lead to therapies for many diseases. The main challenge here is how to isolate and stimulate stem cells to differentiate as needed. This is very promising and, at the present time, is the major tenet of the field of regenerative biology and medicine.

Retina regeneration is also possible by transdifferentiation in urodele amphibians. Upon retinectomy, the neural RPE cells dedifferentiate, divide, and reconstruct the lost retina. Understanding the mechanism of retina regeneration would be of enormous importance in several degenerative diseases. Activating the appropriate cells to transdifferentiate to retina, for example, might lead to experimental or even clinical applications in cases of diseases such as macular degeneration (15).

For terminally differentiated cells to become involved in such regeneration, they must respond to specific signals in order to re-enter the cell cycle and change their genetic program to enable them to change their phenotype. The second avenue whereby renewal can be achieved is by stem cells, which can be local or derived from other tissue (mostly the bone marrow). Stem cells could be totipotent (capable of differentiating into many lineages, depending on the signals), or having the ability to differentiate to a particular cell lineage (progenitor cells). The existence of such cells in the body is of great promise for their use in tissue renewal. The existence of embryonal stem cells is of particular importance; these cells have been shown to differentiate to many cell types, and theoretically they can be pluripotent. Identification of stem cells and of the signals that stimulate their differentiation could, in principle, provide the means to repopulate damaged tissue with healthy cells.

DOMINANT AND RECESSIVE RETINAL DEGENERATIONS

Retinal diseases are rather complex. They may have a genetic or multifactorial cause. Inherited retinal degenerations may be basically sporadic, dominant, recessive, X-linked, or maternal (mitochondrial). In addition, they differ in onset, function of the gene product, pattern and level of gene expression, region of the retina affected, primary and secondary cells involved, and clinical manifestations. Ideally, it would be beneficial to develop a therapy that would permanently correct the defect at the genomic level. To date, researchers have focused on a gene replacement approach for recessive mutations and a gene inactivation approach for dominant mutations (10).

Recessively inherited retinal degenerations represent a group of retinal abnormalities whose phenotype is due to the lack of function of a gene; in other words, they are characterized by the inability to produce a functional gene product. The absence of the normal gene product, such as a structural protein of the outer segment or an enzyme of the phototransduction cascade, results in the expression of the mutant phenotype. The principle of gene therapy in recessive degeneration is to cure the disease by replacing the missing gene with a wild-type copy in each photoreceptor. The goal of photoreceptor rescue requires efficient transduction of most of the photoreceptor cells because, in theory, any cell expressing a wild-type gene will survive. Ali et al. (16) reported the first successful rescue in rds null mice. These animals fail to form outer segments, develop an early loss of retinal function, and their degeneration is characterized by progressive photoreceptor cell death. Following adeno-associated vector delivery of peripherin/RDS, functional and morphological studies revealed that there was outer segment restoration and proper disc

formation. Somatic therapies aimed at enhancing survival using growth factors and antiapoptosis genes have also been shown to improve photoreceptor cell survival in recessive degenerations, but are not curative.

On the other hand, autosomal dominant retinal degenerations are characterized by the production of abnormal protein in photoreceptor cells. The abnormal, mutant form of the protein is, in some way, toxic to the retina and causes progressive retinal degeneration, with the final common pathway being apoptotic cell death. For this reason, gene therapy for dominant disease is focused on inhibiting the translation of the mutant protein by direct cleavage of the mutant messenger RNA (mRNA) transcript.

Several animal models of dominant retinal diseases have been generated. These transgenic animals carry one copy of a mutated gene that encode a misfolded or mislocalized protein. The expression of these proteins in photoreceptors results in toxicity, which leads to cell death through an apoptotic mechanism. Therefore, it is necessary to eliminate or correct the mutated gene in order to restore function. The former has been successfully achieved with ribozymes in the P23H transgenic rat. Ribozymes are RNA-cleaving RNA molecules that specifically remove defective mRNAs or replace them with the correct sequence. The ribozymes were designed to target the mutant P23H transcript and be placed into an adeno-associated vector, under the regulation of a rhodopsin promoter. The treatment resulted in morphological and functional rescue (10).

In general, retinal degeneration varies from early and severe to late and progressive. Thus, slowly progressive diseases have a much wider therapeutic window than those with an earlier onset, such as Leber's congenital amaurosis. In the former case, it is critical to use a delivery vehicle that allows for sustained expression over time, and an eventual readministration could be necessary.

It is clear that it is still crucial to optimize these treatments. Consequently, it will be necessary to determine the mechanisms by which these molecules exert their protective function as well as the best route of administration (subretinal or intravitreal) and the therapeutic/toxic dose ratio. Continuing studies are assured.

TYPES OF POTENTIAL HUMAN GENETIC INTERVENTION

One framework for discussing human genetic intervention distinguishes four categories of procedures according to their goal and target cells (2).

Type 1 or somatic gene therapy: As applied to the treatment or prevention of disease, this type of intervention involves the correction of genetic defects in any cells of the body, with the exception of the germ or reproductive cells. Given the recent developments in the field of somatic gene therapy, it is appropriate to enlarge the definition to include the fact that genes can be introduced into cells to provide a new function. One example of such a approach involves the insertion of a cytokine gene, such as interleukin-2 or tumor necrosis factor, into a patient's malignant cells to produce an immune response against the tumor.

Depending on the location and orientation of the recombination targets, the recombination result could be the integration, excision, inversion, or translocation of the nuclear DNA (9).

Type 2 or germinal gene therapy: This genetic intervention involves the correction or prevention of genetic deficiencies through the transfer of properly functioning genes into reproductive cells. To achieve the desired results from this approach, it will probably be necessary to replace the faulty gene rather than add a new gene. In germ line alteration, gene addition would be unsatisfactory because it is not possible to predict the effects of a mixture of the normal gene and the mutated gene with respect to regulatory signals necessary for normal growth and development. Germ line genetic modification could be effected either before fertilization or in the early postfertilization stages of embryogenic development.

Type 3 and 4: These involve the use of somatic cell or germ line gene modification, respectively, to affect selected physical and mental characteristics, with the aim of influencing such features as physical appearance or physical abilities. A principal difference in these uses of genetic modification is that they could be directed toward healthy people who have no evidence of genetic deficiency disease. Further, type 4 genetic intervention, if successful, could assure that the enhancement would be passed-on to succeeding generations.

STRATEGIES IN GENE THERAPY

Basically, gene therapy can be carried-out in three different ways:

1. Ex vivo: a procedure in which the new gene is transferred to cells in the laboratory and the modified cells are then administered to the recipient. This technique overcomes the problem of intraocular cell targeting. This approach have several potential advantages. First, it improves the efficiency of transduction, selection, and cloning of transduced cells, which are more easily accomplished in vitro. Second, this approach permits assessment of safety profiles of modified cells prior to medical applications. The main disadvantages of ex vivo transduction is that certain cells, such as photoreceptors, cannot be removed and surgically reintroduced.
2. In vivo: this gene transfer relies on a vector to introduce a therapeutic gene into the target cell. The vector is generally delivered distant to the target cell; for instance, the vector is delivered intravenously and the target cells are the photoreceptors in the retina.
3. In situ: the gene or the vector is delivered in the vicinity of the target cells.

In these strategies, the transfer process is usually aided by a vector that helps deliver the gene to the intracellular site where it can function appropriately (17).

The choice of an ex vivo, in vivo, or in situ strategy and of the vector used to carry the gene is dictated by the clinical target.

Gene Replacement, Correction, or Augmentation

One form of gene therapy would involve specific removal of the mutant gene sequence and its replacement with normal, functional genomic material. An ideal approach, gene correction, would entail specific correction of a mutant gene sequence without any additional changes in the target genome (1). An alternative strategy is gene augmentation, which is modifying the content or expression of mutant genes in defective cells by introducing a foreign normal genetic sequence. During the past decade, a number of efficient methods have been developed to introduce functional new genes into mammalian cells. In many cases, it is possible to restore a genetic function by the addition of nontargeted but functional genetic information into nonspecific sites of the genome without the removal or correction of a resident, nonfunctional mutant gene.

During the creation of animal models for human genetic disease, inactivation of the target gene, so-called *gene knockout*, has been proven to be a successful methodology.

GENE THERAPY TECHNIQUES

A well-defined number of strategies for gene delivery have been proposed. They can be summarized as follows:

Adenovirus Vectors

Adenoviruses are nonenveloped, double-stranded DNA viruses that infect a broad range of human and nonhuman cells types by binding to specific cell-surface receptors. By a process of endocytosis, the virus gains access inside the target cell, then the virus binds to the nuclear envelope and enters the nuclear space. The virus is not incorporated into the host genome, but remains as a transcriptionally active episome within the nucleus (Fig. 26.2). Concerns about the infectious nature of adenoviral vectors has led to the development of replication-defective (helper-dependent) adenoviruses for gene transfer. Deletion of the replication-specific genes and nonessential DNA sequences from these viral vectors prevents viral replication. Adenoviral vectors can infect both dividing and nondividing cells, which makes them particularly useful to transfer genes to postmitotic cells. Adenoviruses have been effective in transducing retinal photoreceptors, ganglion cells, Muller cells, and RPE cells. Adenoviral vectors have some inherent limitations with respect to potential clinical application. For

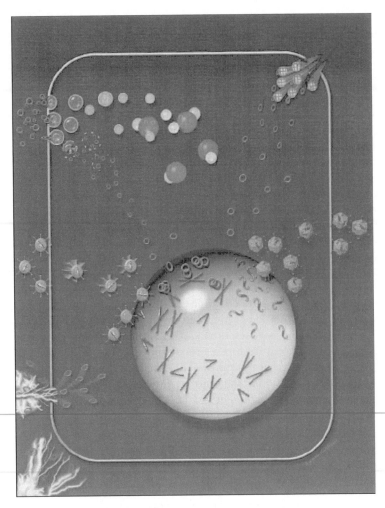

Figure 26.2 Gene transfer methods. Clockwise from upper left: *Lipid-mediated gene transfer:* Plasmid vectors are taken-up by endocytosis and are released into the cytoplasm by breakdown of the endosome. Plasmids migrate to the nucleus by passive diffusion through the cell. Many endosomes fuse with lysosomes where plasmid DNA is broken down. Plasmids that reach the nucleus may remain episomal or integrate into the host genome. *Mechanical delivery:* Gene guns deliver vector-coated particles directly through the cell wall into the cytoplasm. *Adenoviral gene transfer:* Adenoviruses are taken-up by a receptor-mediated mechanism and deliver viral DNA to the nucleus. The adenoviral DNA and any transgene contained in the viral vector remain as episomes within the nucleus. *Electroporation:* Vectors enter the cell through membrane pores opened in response to an electrical charge delivered to the cell. *Retroviral gene transfer:* Retroviruses are taken-up by a receptor-mediated mechanism. The virus is delivered to the nucleus, where the viral DNA and any transgene contained within it integrates into the host genome. (With permission from Chaum E, Hatton MP. Gene therapy for genetic and acquired retinal disease. *Surv Ophthalmol.* 2002;47:449–469).

instance, peak marker transgene expression is typically limited to a few weeks because there is no integration into the host DNA. The broad range of target cells is a potential disadvantage if only one cell layer or cell type is targeted for transduction. Adenoviral transduction can also cause tissue inflammation and a significant immune response to viral proteins in the host, limiting the duration of gene expression and exposing transduced cells to immunologic responses. Modified adenoviral vectors may improve the duration of gene expression by reducing the number of viral proteins presented to the host immune system (18).

Despite some limitations, the adenoviral DNA vectors have been shown to be effective. They are easy to apply experimentally in vitro and in vivo, and they may be particularly useful for gene therapy in which transgene expression of limited duration is sufficient to achieve the desired clinical effect (19).

Adeno-Associated Virus Vectors

The potential for gene delivery to the eye using adeno-associated virus (AAV) vectors has received much recent attention. AAV is a dependovirus from the parvovirinae subfamily of parvoviridae. It is nonenveloped, with icosahedral symmetry and a diameter of 18 to 26 nm. It was originally isolated as a contaminant of adenoviral cultures and thus given the name adeno-associated virus. This human nonpathogenic virus is replication defective in the absence of a *helper virus*. AAV is packaged as a 4.7 Kb single-stranded DNA molecule. In the absence of a helper virus or helper function, the AAV genome integrates in the host cell genome entering the latent phase of its cycle (10).

Different AAV serotypes have different virion shell proteins and, as a consequence, vary in their ability to bind to and transfect different host cell types. To date, eight different AAV serotypes have been isolated, and possibly many more may be harbored in the genome of different mammalian tissues. The most divergent AAV sequence belongs to serotype 5, which was isolated from a condylomatous lesion. AAV 7 and 8 sequences were isolated from rhesus monkey tissues. All others were isolated as contaminants of adenoviral cultures (10).

AAVs have a number of important advantages over other vectors that make them suitable for such studies; in particular, a relative lack of pathogenicity and their ability of induce long-term transgene expression in the eye. AAV vectors can be used to transfect a variety of ocular cell types including photoreceptors, RPE cells, Müller cells, retinal ganglion cells, trabecular meshwork cells, and corneal endothelial cells.

There are two main approaches by which therapeutic AAV-mediated gene transfer might be useful in the context of ocular disease. First, AAV-mediated gene therapy has the potential to correct the specific gene defect in conditions where the defect is well understood. Correction of an ocular genetic defect requires gene delivery to the defective cells and has been successfully used to slow photoreceptor loss in several rodent models of primary photoreceptor diseases. Nevertheless, there are many ocular conditions where no specific genetic defect has been characterized. It is likely that many of these diseases will turn out to involve pathology more complex than a well-characterized mutation in a single gene. In such circumstances, a second strategy for gene therapy may be useful. This involves not replacing a defective gene but using gene transfer to reduce loss of function by ameliorating the effect of the primary defect. For instance, AAV-mediated transfection of retinal cells with the gene for basic fibroblast growth factor (FGF-2), glial cell line-derived neurotrophic factor, and ciliary neurotrophic factor have been demonstrated to slow photoreceptor loss in rat models of retinitis pigmentosa (20).

Transduction of RPE cells and photoreceptors is most efficiently achieved by subretinal injection of AAV. Indeed, subretinal injection provides an almost ideal route for delivery of AAV to these cells. The subretinal space has a relatively high degree of immunoprivilege and typically very little evidence of inflammation is seen in the vicinity of the injection site. Subretinal injection induces a bleb of concentrated virus in intimate contact with photoreceptors and RPE cells. On the other hand, intravitreal injection can be used to transfect Muller cells and retina ganglions cells (21). Theoretically, the potential for a host immune response to AAV is greater following intravitreal injection and the possibility exists of an AAV-specific systematic antibody response.

Several developmental processes, including mitosis, migration, differentiation, cell death, and synaptic formation, may affect the cellular uptake of the virus vector, the distribution of the particles, and the persistence of transgene expression. On the other hand, the time of virus administration profoundly affects the tropism, efficiency, and distribution of the transgene (22).

One of the major limitations of AAV as a vector is the relatively small amount of passenger DNA that can be incorporated. Although genes up to 6.0 Kb have been packaged into AAV, these oversized viruses were not active. The usual packaging limit for AAV appears to be 5.1 to 5.3 Kb. Nevertheless, by exploiting the intermolecular rearrangement, it is possible to overcome this problem. Genes larger than 4.7 Kb can be split between two different AAV vectors (Fig. 26.3).

Herpes Simplex Virus Vectors

The herpes simplex virus (HSV) is a DNA virus that has natural tropism for neurons. Thus, it may be useful in applying gene therapy to diseases of the nervous system, including the retina. HSV can infect nonneuronal tissue as well, and does not require cell division to integrate into the host genome. Gene transfer using HSV utilizes either replication-defective mutants or multiple-deletion mutants that have a limited capacity for replication, but they may be able to deliver genes locally within tissue from a limited infection. The ability of HSV to exist in a latent state likely makes this vector efficacious in producing stable transgene expression within host neurons. Moreover, the HSV viral genome is large and has the capacity to carry more than 30 Kb of foreign DNA, significantly more than other vectors.

The HSV thymidine kinase gene (HSV-tk) has been used extensively in suicide gene therapy studies. The viral thymidine kinase has a markedly higher affinity for the prodrug ganciclovir than does the cellular thymidine kinase. Ganciclovir is converted to a cytotoxic metabolite with significantly higher efficiency by HSV-tk-transduced cells, and thus preferentially kills the transduced cell (19).

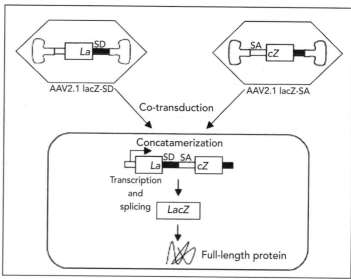

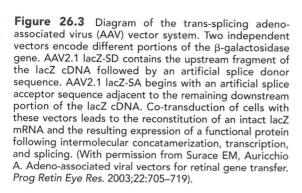

Figure 26.3 Diagram of the trans-splicing adeno-associated virus (AAV) vector system. Two independent vectors encode different portions of the β-galactosidase gene. AAV2.1 lacZ-SD contains the upstream fragment of the lacZ cDNA followed by an artificial splice donor sequence. AAV2.1 lacZ-SA begins with an artificial splice acceptor sequence adjacent to the remaining downstream portion of the lacZ cDNA. Co-transduction of cells with these vectors leads to the reconstitution of an intact lacZ mRNA and the resulting expression of a functional protein following intermolecular concatamerization, transcription, and splicing. (With permission from Surace EM, Auricchio A. Adeno-associated viral vectors for retinal gene transfer. *Prog Retin Eye Res.* 2003;22:705–719).

RNA Virus Vectors

Retroviruses are a family of RNA viruses that can infect cells and integrate into the genome of the host cell (Fig. 26.2). RNA viruses are surrounded by a lipid envelope. Upon entry into the target cell, the RNA is released and reverse transcribed into double-stranded DNA that is stably integrated into the host DNA. Transgenes delivered by retroviruses demonstrate long-term stable gene expression and may be vertically transferred to daughter cells. Most retroviral vectors cannot enter the nucleus directly; they require cell division to infect the host cell following breakdown of the nuclear envelope.

Lentivirus vectors are already used as effective gene delivery tools in cells from liver, retina, skeletal muscle, and the central nervous system (23).

Lentiviruses are a subclass of retroviruses that includes the HIV family. Like all retroviruses, lentiviruses integrate a DNA copy into the host genome, but they encode proteins that allow them to form a complex with the nuclear envelope and to transit the pores of an intact nuclear membrane. Thus, lentiviruses can infect dividing and nondividing cells.

The abilities of lentiviruses to integrate into nondividing cells relies on nuclear localization signals present in the preintegration complex that allow its entry into the nucleus without the need for nuclear membrane fragmentation (23).

Transgenes integrate into the host genome but viral genes do not; thus, there is less risk of generating recombinant retrovirus.

Despite modifications to render the virus replication-incompetent, there is appropriate concern about the clinical use of such vectors because of the theoretical possibility of generating a wild-type HIV virus during production or from viral recombination in the host (19).

Table 26.1 summarizes the characteristics of gene transfer with viral vectors.

Lipofection

Lipofection reagents are families of molecules composed of phospholipids and cholesterol, similar to those present in biologic membranes that contain both hydrophobic and hydrophilic domains. These reagents form complexes with the genetic material to be introduced in the target cell. The lipid/gene complexes fuse with the plasma membrane and are internalized into the cell by endocytosis (Fig. 26.2). The genetic material is released into the cytoplasm from the endosomes and makes its way to the cellular nucleus. In general, lipofection-mediated gene therapy uses plasmid vectors. Plasmids can carry larger DNA sequence than viral vectors and can be manufactured in high purity without the risk of generating infectious or recombinant viruses. Liposomes have many additional desirable qualities, including the ability to incorporate precise drug amounts over a wide range of desired concentrations, the ability to protect encapsulated drug per unit volume, and the ability to slowly release a drug without changing the drug's intrinsic characteristics (24). Disadvantages of lipofection include poor target selectivity, reduce efficiency compared with viral vectors, and short duration expression.

The efficiency of this technique may be improved by targeting specific cell-surface receptors, inhibiting lysosome digestion, and directing transport to the nucleus via a nuclear-localizing sequence.

TABLE 26.1

VIRAL VECTORS FOR GENE TRANSFER

Virus	Transduction	Infection of Nondividing Cells	Capacity (Kb)	Advantage	Disadvantages
Retrovirus	Stable	No	Up to 8	Integration. Many cell types	Instability. Insertional mutagenesis
Lentivirus (HIV)	Stable	Yes	Up to 10	Transduce both, quiescence and proliferating cells	Safety concerns from HIV-based vectors
Adenovirus (AV)	Transient	Yes	Up to 8	High titers	Immunogenic
Herpes simples virus (HSV)	Transient	Yes	>30	Natural tropism for neural cells	Safety concerns
Adeno-associated virus (AAV)	Stable	Yes	Up to 5	Low immunogenic	Production of high-titer stocks

(Modified from Pleyer U, Ritter T. Gene therapy in immune-mediated diseases of the eye. *Prog Retin Eye Res.* 2003;22:277–293.)

Mechanical Delivery

Using the "gene gun" strategy, the gene is introduced into the target cell using microinjections or microprojectiles. This technique is unlikely to have clinical applications soon due to cytotoxicity and the low efficiency of gene transfer in comparison with strategies such as viral vectors.

Electroporation

Generating an electrical potential across the target cell membrane, it is possible to transfect DNA material into the cell. Such approaches are effective in vitro but are limited, in part, by the ability to generate the electrical field in vivo. However, this approach may be effective for gene delivery to surface tissues such as cornea and conjunctiva.

Ribozyme Therapy

Ribozymes are RNA-based enzymes that can cleave specific mRNA sequences. Mutation-specific cleavage of the transcript functionally silences the mutant allele by preventing synthesis of the abnormal protein from the transcript (Fig. 26.4). The strategy used is to construct ribozymes that identify unique mutations or that permit binding to targeted, accessible sites in the mRNA transcript.

Ribozyme therapy is effective in delaying retinal degeneration in animal models of dominant retinal degeneration, even after the degenerative process has begun.

Growth Factor Gene Therapy

Gene therapy using trophic growth factors is another approach to enhancing the survival of retinal photoreceptors in dominant retinal generation. For instance, the intravitreal injection of basic fibroblast growth factor (bFGF) delays retinal degeneration in some animal models (25).

Successful treatment with growth factors may also be achieved by genetically modifying cells ex vivo and then implanting them within the eye to act as a reservoir of trophic factors that bathe the retina by slow release into the vitreous.

Apoptosis has been implicated in retinal development and degeneration, but the specific apoptotic pathways are incompletely understood. Apoptosis is a process of programmed cell death without an ensuing inflammatory

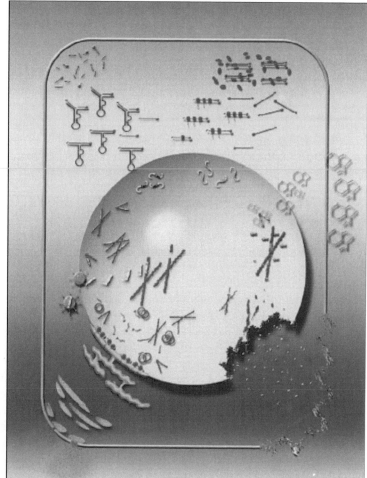

Figure 26.4 Therapeutic approaches to gene therapy. Clockwise from upper left: *Ribozyme therapy:* Ribozyme hybridize with mRNA from a mutated gene. The ribozyme enzymatically cleaves the mRNA and functionally silences the gene by preventing synthesis of the abnormal protein from the transcript. *Antisense therapy:* Complementary DNA molecules hybridize with the mRNA from the mutated gene. The ribosomes cannot bind to the double-stranded heteroduplex, preventing synthesis of the abnormal protein. *Suicide gene therapy:* Gancyclovir is converted to a cytotoxic nucleotide by a transfected viral thymidine kinase. The drug inhibits DNA synthesis, leading to cell death. Dying cells are also cytotoxic to nearby untransduced cells, causing the *bystander effect*. *Growth factor therapy:* Growth factors are synthesized and secreted from cells expressing growth factor transgenes. The growth factors have positive neurotrophic effects on surrounding retinal cells and also on the secreting cells via specific receptors. *Gene replacement therapy:* Mutated genes causing autosomal recessive retinal degeneration can be replaced using viral or nonviral methods. (With permission from Chaum E, Hatton MP. Gene therapy for genetic and acquired retinal disease. *Surv Ophthalmol.* 2002;47:449–469).

response. This neat packaging of cellular components allows for the precise removal of tissue during developmental remodeling, particularly in the retina. The retina develops from a single layer of undifferentiated ventricular neuroectoderm to a mature retina containing three cell layers of postmitotic, fully differentiated cells: the ganglion cell layer, the inner nuclear layer, and the outer nuclear layer. Extraneous cells unable to make functional neural connections are eliminated by apoptosis. Beyond this involvement in ocular development, apoptosis rarely occurs in a normal, healthy retina, but has been implicated in both inherited and acquired retinal degenerations. The molecular pathogenesis of these retinal degenerations is still unclear, but apoptosis is the final common pathway in many retinal diseases, ranging from glaucoma to AMD, retinitis pigmentosa, and retinal detachment (26). Several proapoptotic and antiapoptotic genes have been identified. The use of growth factor gene therapy could help in rescue and/or prevent the apoptotic phenomenon in the target cells.

Antisense Gene Therapy

Antisense gene therapy is based on the use of synthetic, short DNA sequences that are designed to be complementary to a targeted mRNA molecule. This short DNA sequence is capable of forming a stable DNA-mRNA heteroduplex that prevents the translation of the associated protein from the transcript.

Other techniques that warrant mention are the iontophoretic delivery of genes and the bioimplants. In the iontophoretic approach, the gene is delivered across the sclera (24). This technique may have practical applications in treating diseases of the retina and choroids. Bioimplants containing genetically modified cells have been demonstrated to deliver growth factors in the eye and to have a therapeutic effect on retinal degeneration.

GENE THERAPY AND AGE-RELATED MACULAR DEGENERATION

In wet AMD, a destabilization of the retinal and choroidal microenvironments leads to the formation of new blood vessels, which ultimately results in a decrease of visual acuity.

Degenerative changes of the RPE and Bruch's membrane are the primary factors responsible for the disease. The pathophysiology of the disease is still incompletely understood. The putative role of specific genes in the degenerative process in AMD is less clear. Although certain genes may predispose some patients to develop AMD, the genetic linkage remains controversial and, to date, the genetics of AMD are largely unknown. Genetic susceptibility to AMD is probably multifactorial and thus will not be amenable to gene therapy directed at the germinal line. In the absence of a well-defined genetic defect that gives rise to AMD, gene therapy will likely focus on somatic therapy using growth factors and antiapoptosis therapy to prolong the survival of the RPE and retinal photoreceptors.

Growth Factor Gene Therapy for AMD

There is experimental evidence that growth factors play an important role in maintaining the health of RPE cells and in enabling them to respond to injury. RPE cells express growth factors and their receptors demonstrate the autocrine and paracrine functions of these substance. Theoretically, it may be possible to enhance RPE cell survival by somatic modulation of growth factor gene expression in patients with AMD. For instance, age-related phagocytic dysfunction and incomplete digestion of photoreceptors membranes by the RPE result in loss of RPE cells and in geographic atrophy, perhaps due to the cytotoxicity of these deposits on the surrounding cells. Enhancing phagocytic activity in aging RPE cells using gene therapy is a potential approach to the treatment of AMD. bFGF has been shown to stimulate phagocytic activity and prolong retinal survival in animal models (19). An important number of other growth factors and secondary messengers of the intracellular signaling pathways have demonstrated protective effects on the retinal neurons in animal models of retinal degeneration. Gene transfer and expression of these growth factor proteins may similarly inhibit retinal degeneration by a neuroprotective effect in AMD (27).

The RPE synthesizes proteins that are antiangiogenic, such as tissue-inhibitors of metalloproteinases and pigment epithelium-derived factor (PEDF). Thus, potential gene therapy applications to choroidal neovascularization (CNV) include antiangiogenic growth factor gene therapy, antisense or ribozyme therapy directed at angiogenic factors, and suicide gene therapy directed at neovascular tissue. Moreover, recently it was demonstrated that expression of angiostatin in experimental CNV significantly reduces the size of CNV lesions (28).

Transplantation of Genetically Modified Iris Pigment Epithelial Cells

Submacular transplantation of autologous iris pigment epithelial (IPE) cells has been proposed to replace the damaged RPE following surgical removal of the CNV (29). The IPE is anatomically contiguous with the RPE and has the same embryonic origin. In vitro, IPE cells share functional properties with the RPE cells, such as phagocytosis, degradation of rod outer segments, and synthesis of trophic factors. However, autologous transplantation of IPE cells alone has not resulted in a prolonged improvement of vision in patients with AMD, potentially because the lack of expression of one or several factors that are an important part of RPE function. Semkova et al. (29) have suggested a treatment for AMD based on transplantation of genetically modified autologous IPE cells. The most significant findings are summarized as follows: first, IPE cells were readily transduced with a high-capacity adenovirus

(HC-ad) vector. Second, IPE cells secreted functionally active PEDF after HC-ad-mediated gene transfer. Third, subretinal transplantation of PEDF-expressing IPE cells inhibited neovascularization in models of retinal neoangiogenesis, and prevented photoreceptor degeneration.

Antiangiogenic Gene Therapy for AMD

Antiangiogenic gene therapy is a potential breakthrough therapy for ocular neovascular disease, including AMD.

Recognizing that the key pathogenic factor in AMD is aberrant neovascularization, strategies for curbing neovascularization by administration of antiangiogenic agents represent a compelling approach, and one that is currently being evaluated in numerous clinical trials. Many endogenous, as well as synthetic, factors have been shown to possess potent antiangiogenic activity, including endostatin, angiostatin, and soluble vascular endothelial growth factor receptor inhibitors. Several of these are currently in clinical trials.

AMD is a chronic disease; consequently, inhibition of the neovascular stimuli for prolonged periods of time is likely to be required. Oral administration of angiogenesis inhibitors carry with them the risk of systemic toxicity and chronic oral administration could potentially interfere with normal physiological functions that require angiogenesis, such as wound healing, collateral vessel formation, and menstruation. The two antiangiogenic drugs tested in randomized clinical trials for AMD, matrix metalloproteinase (MMP) inhibitor and interferon-α2a, both demonstrated nontrivial systemic toxicities. Furthermore, because of the blood-retina barrier, it is difficult with many proteins to achieve adequate therapeutic levels in the posterior part of the eye. One way to circumvent this is by direct intravitreal injection. Various antiangiogenic proteins have been administered in this way, including EYE001 and humanized anti-VEGF aptamer. However, these drugs have relatively short half-lives and require frequent intravitreous injections to maintain elevated levels.

Adenoviral Vectors Gene Therapy

Preclinical proof using either recombinant adenovectors to carry the genes encoding PEDF and endostatin, or recombinant adeno-associated viruses carrying the transgene encoding for angiostatin, have recently been published and demonstrate significant inhibition of CNV in various animals models. The intravenous administration of an adenoviral construct carrying the murine endostatin gene was recently tested in a murine model of CNV and found almost complete inhibition of neovascular activity. Similarly, subcutaneous injection of an AAV virus carrying a truncated angiostatin gene resulted in significant inhibition of retinal neovascularization. These encouraging results with endostatin and angiostatin suggest a potential role of antiangiogenesis in ocular disease.

Recently, PEDF has received major attention. PEDF was first described in 1989 by Tombran-Tink in conditioned medium from cultured, fetal RPE cells; it was found to be a potent neurotrophic factor (30). Subsequently, PEDF has been purified and cloned both from humans and mice (31). The gene is expressed as early as 17 weeks in human fetal RPE cells, suggesting that PEDF is intimately involved in early neuronal development. PEDF attracted even more attention when Dawson et al. demonstrated that PEDF is one of the most potent natural inhibitors of angiogenesis (32). In addition, PEDF is an inhibitor of endothelial cell migration. The amount of inhibitory PEDF produced by retinal cells was positively correlated with oxygen concentrations, suggesting that retinal cell loss plays a permissive role in ischemia-driven retinal neovascularization. Moreover, a correlation between changes in VEGF/PEDF ratio and the degree of retinal neovascularization in a rat model was demonstrated.

The AdVPEDF.11 is a replication-deficient adenovirus vector designed to deliver the human PEDF gene. Intravitreous injection of AdPEDF resulted in increased expression of PEDF mRNA in the eye, compared with AdNull (the same vector without the transgene) or with uninjected controls. PDEF trail was present not only in the retina but in other parts of the eye, including the iris, lens, and corneal epithelium. After subretinal injection of AdPEDF, it was strongly detected in the RPE cells compared with other ocular structures (31).

Ocular neovascularization is a key factor in the most common causes of blindness in humans in the developed word: AMD and proliferative diabetic retinopathy. Prevention of ocular neovascularization by development of antiangiogenic drugs represents a rational and appealing therapeutic approach. However, because these are chronic disease characterized by ongoing new vessels formation, long-term inhibition of the angiogenic stimuli is likely to be needed.

SAFETY AND OBSTACLES IN GENE TRANSFER

The theoretical safety concerns regarding human gene transfer are not trivial. For the individual recipient, there is the possibility of vector-induced inflammation and immune responses. There are also theoretical issues that are important to society, including concerns about modifying the human germ line and about protecting the environment from new infectious agents generated from gene transfer vectors carrying expression genes with powerful biologic functions.

There have been adverse events in human gene transfer trials, including inflammation induced by the administration of adenovirus vectors and by administration to the central nervous system of a xenogenic producer cell line releasing a retrovirus vector (17). However, compared with the total numbers of individuals undergoing gene transfer, adverse events have been rare and have been related mostly to the dose and the manner in which the vectors were administered.

Two potential problems with retroviral vectors warrant discussion: insertional mutagenesis and helper virus production. Problems with insertional mutagenesis, such activation of cellular oncogenes, are shared with any gene transfer technique that results in integration of new sequences into the cellular genome, with the possible exception of adeno-associated virus. Although there are many examples of retroviral activation of cellular oncogenes in mice, these events occur in the context of a spreading infection by replication-competent virus. On the other hand, the potential for production of replication-competent (helper) virus during the production of retroviral vectors remains a concern, although for practical purposes, this problem has been solved.

No novel infectious agents generated from recombination of the transferred genome and the host genome or other genetic information have yet been detected, nor has any replication-competent virus related to the vector. Cells modified ex vivo with retrovirus vectors have been infused repetitively without adverse effects. Finally, human gene transfer has not been implicated in initiating malignancy, although the number of recipients and time of observation will have to be much greater to allow definitive conclusions regarding this issue.

With the successes of the human gene transfer trials has come the sobering realities of the drug development process. Some of the following problems are generic for the field, and some are specific to the vector (17):

1. Inconsistent results: The majority of the human gene transfer studies have inconsistent results, and in some cases the bases for them are unclear. One of the more important problems is obtaining homogeneous results in the different studies.
2. Results extrapolation: There have been several surprise examples in which predictions from gene transfer studies in experimental animals have not been borne out in human safety and efficacy trials.
3. Production problems: There are some hurdles in vector production that must be overcome before large clinical trials can be initiated. Generation of replication-competent virus is observed in production of clinical-grade retrovirus and adenovirus vectors. Lack of reproducibility, aggregation, and contamination with endotoxin also complicate production of clinical-grade plasmid liposome complexes.
4. The perfect vector: The ideal gene transfer vector would be capable of efficiently delivering one or more genes of the size needed for the clinical application. The vector would be specific for its target, not recognized by the immune system, stable and easy to reproducibly produce, and could be purified in large quantities at high concentrations. It would not induce inflammation and would be safe for the recipient and the environment. Finally, it

would express the gene or genes it carries for as long as required in an appropriately regulated fashion. Clinical experience to date suggests that retrovirus, adenovirus, and plasmid-liposome vectors all need refinement. There is considerable interest in developing new vectors, but there is controversy as to which vector class is most likely to succeed, particularly for use in in vivo applications.

There are two philosophical camps in vector design: viral and nonviral. The viral proponents believe that the most efficient means to deliver an expression gene in vivo is to package it in a replication-deficient recombinant virus. The logic supporting this approach is the knowledge that viruses are masterful at reproducing themselves, and thus have evolved strategies to efficiently express their genetic information in the cells they infect. The nonviral proponents concede this argument, but believe that the redundant immune and inflammatory host defenses against viruses may be a risk to recipients, will limit the duration of expression as the infected cells are recognized by the immune system, and may hinder repeat administration of the vectors.

CONCLUSIONS AND FUTURE DIRECTIONS

Progress in gene therapy has offered patients the hope for treatment for retinal degeneration. Researches have identified candidate genes and suitable delivery vehicles. Over the last decade, viral vector technology has grown and the use of AAV as a delivery vehicle for gene therapy has been accepted for broad applications.

The development of novel technologies for gene delivery allows scientists to overcome a number of the limitations which were previously posed by the vector, such as packaging capacity and the ability to regulate gene expression, thus expanding the vector's applications.

In the retina, it will be important to track the different steps of the vector transduction, at both the cellular and molecular levels, to gain an understanding of the transduction entry pathways, intracellular trafficking, and mechanism of episomal expression and integration.

Viral delivery of secreted therapeutic proteins has also been used to provide a symptomatic cure for ocular neovascularization. Several clinical trials for the treatment of AMD are currently underway using an adenoviral vector encoding an antiangiogenic factor.

REFERENCES

1. Firedmann T. Progress toward human gene therapy. *Science*. 1989;244: 1,275–1,280.
2. Wivel NA, LeRoy W. Germ-line gene modification and disease prevention: some medical and ethical perspectives. *Science*. 1993;262:533–537.
3. Dusty Mieller A. Human gene therapy comes of age. *Nature*. 1992;357: 455–460.
4. Williamson B. Gene therapy. *Nature*. 1982;298:416–418.
5. Marquardt T. Transcriptional control of neuronal diversification in the retina. *Prog Retin Eye Res*. 2003;22:567–577.
6. Otteson DC, Hitchocock PF. Stem cells in the teleost retina: persistent neurogenesis and injury-induced regeneration. *Vision Res*. 2003;43: 927–936.

7. Reh TA, Levine EM. Multipotential stem cells and progenitors in the vertebrate retina. *J Neurobiol.* 1998;36:206–220.
8. Marquardt T, Gruss P. Generating neuronal diversity in the retina: one for nearly all. *Trends in Neurosceinces.* 2002;25:32–38.
9. Ashery-Padan R. Somatic gene targeting in the developing and adult mouse retina. *Methods.* 2002;28:457–464.
10. Surace EM, Auricchio A. Adeno-associated viral vectors for retinal gene transfer. *Prog Retin Eye Res.* 2003;22:705–719.
11. Allikmets R, Shroyer NF, Singh N, et al. Mutation of the Stargardt disease gene (ABCR) in age-related macular degeneration. *Science.* 1997;277:1,805–1,807.
12. Weng J, Mata NL, Azarian SM, et al. Insights into the function of Rim protein in photoreceptors and etiology of Stargardt's disease from the phenotype in abcr knockout mice. *Cell.* 1999;98:13–23.
13. Weber BH, Vogt G, Pruett RC, et al. Mutations in the tissue inhibitor of metalloproteinases-3 (TIMP3) in patients with Sorsby's fundus dystrophy. *Nat Genet.* 1991;8:352–356.
14. Hirano M, Yamamoto A, Yoshimura N, et al. Generation of structures formed by lens and retinal cells differentiating from embryonic stem cells. *Developmental Dynamics.* 2003;228:664–671.
15. Tsonis PA. Regenerative biology: the emerging field of tissue repair and restoration. *Differentiation.* 2002;70:397–409.
16. Ali RR, Sarra GM, Stephens C, et al. Restoration of photoreceptor ultrastructure and function in retinal degeneration slow mice by gene therapy. *Nat Genet.* 2000;25:306–310.
17. Crystal RG. Transfer of genes to humans: early lessons and obstacles to success. *Science.* 1995;270:404–409.
18. Pleyer U, Ritter T. Gene therapy in immune-mediated disease of the eye. *Prog Retin Eye Res.* 2003;22:277–293.
19. Chaum E, Hatton MP. Gene therapy for genetic and acquired retinal disease. *Surv Opthalmol.* 2002;47:449–469.
20. Martin KR, Klein RL, Quigley HA. Gene delivery to the eye using adeno-associated viral vectors. *Methods.* 2002;28:267–275.
21. Auricchio A. Pseudotyped AAV vector for constitutive and regulated gene expression in the eye. *Vision Res.* 2003;43:913–918.
22. Surace EM, Auricchio A, Reich SJ, et al. Delivery of adeno-associated virus vectors to the fetal retina: impact of viral capsid proteins on retinal neuronal progenitor transduction. *J Virol.* 2003;77:7,957–7,963.
23. Maurizio F. Lentiviruses as gene delivery vectors. *Curr Opin Biotech.* 1999;10:448–453.
24. Kurz D, Ciulla TA. Novel approaches for retinal drug delivery. *Ophthalmol Clin North Am.* 2002;15:405–410.
25. Faktorovich EG, Steinberg RH, Yasumura D, et al. Photoreceptor degeneration in inherited retinal dystrophy delayed by basic firbroblast growth factor. *Nature.* 1990;347:83–86.
26. Hahn P, Lindsten T, Ying G, et al. Proapoptotic Bcl-2 family members, Bax and Bak, are essential for developmental photoreceptor apoptosis. *Invest Ophthalmol Vis Sci.* 2003;44:3,598–3,605.
27. Garcia Valenzuela E, Sharma SC. Rescue of retinal ganglion cells from axotomy-induced apoptosis through TRK oncogene transfer. *Neuroreport.* 1998;9:165–170.
28. Lai CC, Wu WC, Chen SL, et al. Suppression of choroidal neovascularization by adeno-associated virus vector expressing angiostatin. *Invest Ophthalmol Vis Sci.* 2001;42:2,401–2,407.
29. Semkova I, Kreppel F, Welsandt G, et al. Autologous transplantation of genetically modified iris pigment epithelial cells: a promising concept for the treatment of age-related macular degeneration and other disorders of the eye. *Proc Natl Acad Sci USA.* 2002;99:13,090–13,095.
30. Tombran-Tink J, Johnson L. Neuronal differentiation of retinoblastoma cells induced by medium conditioned by human RPE cells. *Invest Ophthalmol Vis Sci.* 1989;30:1,700–1,709.
31. Rasmussen HS, Rasmussen CS, Durham RG, et al. Looking into anti-angiogenic gene therapies for disorders of the eye. *Drug Discov Today.* 2001;22:1,171–1,175.
32. Dawson DW, Volpert OV, Gillis P, et al. Pigment epithelium-derived factor: a potent inhibitor of angiogenesis. *Science.* 1999;285:245–248.

Human Retinal Transplantation

27

Suzanne Binder

INTRODUCTION

Transplantation of retinal cells has been performed in animal and human eyes during the last two decades, following the path of successful experimental neuronal transplantation (1,2). Despite evidence that transplantation was somewhat effective in animal models, its efficacy in humans has been confounded by various difficulties. One reason for this may be an overestimation of the efficacy of retinal transplantation. While vasodestructive methods (e.g., laser photocoagulation and photodynamic therapy) are widely used and accepted as successful (3–6), research within the field of retinal transplantation has not led, thus far, to a similar prevalence.

Retinal transplantation is expected to work in three different ways:

1. It should halt the disease process.
2. It should retain or improve visual function for an indefinite time.
3. It should reverse the condition of already damaged photoreceptors and choriocapillaris.

The expectations listed above are often difficult to meet in eyes in which retinal transplantation is attempted, as often, only eyes with very advanced pathology become candidates for subretinal surgery and thus, transplantation. In contrast, the requirements for successful transplantation are numerous.

Successful transplantation requires the following:

- A viable source of cells.
- A technique for safe delivery.
- Survival of the transplanted cells within the host.
- No transdifferentiation of the grafted cells from their normal retinal pigment epithelial (RPE) phenotype (i.e., ideally restoration of the RPE monolayer).

- A restoration of normal retinal architecture
- A stabilization or improvement in vision.

The following chapter describes the current state of human retinal transplantation and RPE transplantation. Some of the described results that have been achieved thus far are indeed encouraging. Our hope is that the achievements described within this chapter will foster more contributions that lead to the eventual success of retinal transplantation.

BACKGROUND: TRANSPLANTATION OF OCULAR TISSUES

Animal Experiments

The earliest experiments detailing the behavior of transplanted neural tissue were performed in 1946 by Tansley, who transplanted embryonic eyes into rat brains (7). Although the use of the anterior chamber as a tissue culture chamber to observe the behavior and growth of various transplanted tissues had already been reported previously, the first transplantation of fetal retina into the anterior chamber of maternal eyes in rats was performed by Royo and Quay in 1959 (8). No further experiments were reported for more than 20 years.

Retinal Pigment Epithelial Transplantation

The concept of RPE transplantation evolved from the successful culturing of RPE from donor eyes by Flood et al. in 1980 (9). In 1984 and 1985, cultured human retinal cells were transplanted in the eyes of monkeys, first by open sky techniques and later with closed eye methods by Gouras and others (10–13). Finally, the therapeutic potential of RPE transplantation was demonstrated in the Royal College of Surgeons (RCS) rat model when radiolabeled RPE suspension grafts delivered through a bleb detachment were fully capable of phagocytosing host outer segments (14,15). The retinal atrophy that occurred in the RCS rat within 2 months after birth as a result of the inherited phagocytosis defect of the photoreceptor outer segment was therefore prevented (16–18). These data were further confirmed by functional experiments on such transplanted animals (19–21).

The RPE is known to produce a variety of cytokines both in vivo and in vitro (22). In addition to the expected rescue effects observed over areas with transplanted RPE cells, fine cellular processes extending from the transplanted RPE over long distances were observed with electron microscopy. This suggested that trophic factors secreted from the graft may be involved in rescue of the overlying retina as well (14). It is well known that experimental debridement of Bruch's membrane in normal pigmented rabbits will lead to atrophy of the underlying choriocapillaris and the overlying neural retina (20,21). Interestingly, intravitreal administration of basic fibroblast growth factors (bFGF) in RCS rats also led to a transient effect of photoreceptor rescue, which therefore may support such a trophic factor interaction (23,24).

Neural Retinal Transplantation

Retinal degenerations often involve the entire sensory retina. It is therefore necessary to develop cell-biologic strategies to restore vision via transplantation of neuronal cells and/or tissues. Embryonic retinas have been aspirated, fragmented, and then injected via syringe as donor tissue into the subretinal space by Turner and Blair in 1986 (25). Although another group demonstrated that transplanted photoreceptors can survive for an extended period (26), most of the tissue lost its organization and degenerated after 4 to 5 months (27). In 1989, Del Cerro et al. (28) enzymatically dissolved suspensions of retinal cells intended for transplantation. Vision was restored with this technique in a light blinded rat model; however, the cell suspension showed less organization compared to the fragments (29,30). In an attempt to transplant the entire photoreceptor layer, a neural retinal graft embedded in gelatin was shaped with a vibratome by Silverman and Huges in 1989 (31). Good results were reported initially, but unfortunately they have not been reproduced. The latter two methods underwent clinical trials and were reported as clinically safe, but no visual improvement was demonstrated in these patients (32,33).

Thus far in animal experiments, full-thickness embryonic grafts have been demonstrated to be transplantable in adult rabbits with few complications. The grafts organize into laminated retinas and display most normal retinal morphology. Their mean survival time is at least 10 months and they have a lower immunogenicity compared to fragmented neuroretinal transplants (34). Aramant and Seiler have transplanted intact sheets of fetal tissue to the subretinal space using a special instrument (35). In adult rats with retinal degeneration, they have demonstrated that an area of damaged retina can be morphologically repaired by a sheet of fetal retina with or without the RPE (36,37). Recent research has also demonstrated that the host photoreceptor layer plays a role in limiting graft–host anatomical integration, and bridging of fibers between the subretinal graft and the host retina occurs only when the host photoreceptor layer is missing or severely damaged (38).

Although significant knowledge has been derived from the research described above, the central question as to whether retinal transplantation can transfer visual information has not been answered by these experiments.

THE RETINAL PIGMENT EPITHELIUM

Retinal Pigment Epithelium Physiology

The RPE was considered to be a logical starting point in any attempt to repair or reconstruct the retina through transplantation. The RPE is a self-contained hexagonal monolayer that allows access from the subretinal space and plays a key role in maintaining photoreceptor homeostasis, Bruch's membrane, and the choriocapillaris-choroid complex (14). In vivo, the RPE is well differentiated and mostly maintains the epithelioid appearance with an apical-basal polarity. RPE cells are postmitotic and under normal conditions do not divide. In response to a pathologic condition, however, they can proliferate and migrate, and can also dedifferentiate (39). The RPE cells in the macular region are small (about 10–14 μm), but broader and flatter towards the peripheral retina (60 μm). The number of photoreceptors overlying each RPE cell remains about the same: roughly 22 to 30 photoreceptors per RPE cell, and four-to-five-thousand RPE cells are generally present within 1 square millimeter of retina (40).

The functions of the RPE include: maintaining the blood-retinal outer barrier; playing a crucial role in the visual vitamin A cycle (41); phagocytosing outer segments; and performing the isomerization of visual pigment (42). In addition, the RPE secretes and responds to several growth factors that can also act by diffusion, including: platelet-derived growth factors (PDGF, types A and B), whose production is increased during RPE-related wound healing (43); vascular endothelial growth factor (VEGF), which plays a central role in angiogenesis during retinal ischemia and also may serve as a trophic factor for vascular endothelial cells (44,45); fibroblast growth factors bFGF (46), acidic FGF (47), and FGF-5 (48); the transforming growth factor β-family (TGF-β), with its isoforms (where TGFβ2 is predominant [49] and is likely to modulate inflammation and immune response) (50–52); and, insulin-like growth factors (IGFS), which, like insulin, stimulate RPE proliferation (53) and may play a role in retinal development (54) along with pigment epithelium-derived factor (PEDF) which also acts as a key coordinator of retinal neuronal and vascular functions and is a potent inhibitor of angiogenesis (55,56).

It is therefore conceivable from the above that the RPE may limit angiogenesis (57,58) and release trophic factors to maintain photoreceptor homeostasis (59–61). The RPE can also support choriocapillaris survival through the RPE-produced extracellular matrix and through the release of growth factors that bind to the extracellular matrix (62). Thus, the versatility of the RPE and its relative anatomic isolation render it an excellent candidate for transplantation.

RPE Pathophysiology

Dysfunction of the RPE may alter the extracellular environment for photoreceptors and contribute to a variety of sight threatening diseases, including: age-related macular degeneration (AMD) (63), serous retinal detachment (64), and genetic diseases such as gyrate atrophy (65) and choroideremia (66). Other dystrophies, which are considered to involve primarily the RPE (and choroid) in the macular area include Stargardt's disease (67), Best's disease or adult vitelliform dystrophy (68), basal laminar drusen (69), Doyenne's honeycomb dystrophy (70), and pattern dystrophies (71).

Age-Related Changes of the Retinal Pigment Epithelium

RPE cell loss occurs at a rate of approximately 0.3% per year (72). RPE density is highest in the foveal area and decreases gradually towards the periphery. RPE density was found to remain constant in the macula and decreases only in the periphery as an individual ages. In contrast, apoptosis of the RPE is confined primarily to the macula of older human eyes. It has been suggested that migration of peripheral RPE cells may compensate for the death of macular RPE cells (73).

AGE-RELATED MACULAR DEGENERATION

AMD is the leading cause of visual impairment in Western countries in people over 50 years of age. It is believed to be caused by progressive deterioration of RPE, Bruch's membrane, and the choriocapillaris, which consequently leads to damage of the photoreceptor cells (74–77). In AMD, the RPE cells are dysfunctional, which results either in progressive atrophy (dry AMD) or pigment epithelial detachment, choroidal neovascularization (CNV), exudation and hemorrhage (wet AMD) with subsequent scar formation (78,79). The natural course of AMD leads to visual loss of more than six lines within 2 years in more than 60% of patients (80,81). The prevalence of AMD increases with age, with 0.1% of individuals aged 43 to 54 years affected, and 7.1% of individuals aged 75 years of age or older with the disease (82). Approximately 100,000 individuals are newly diagnosed with AMD annually in the United States. As the population in the United States and Europe grows older and better quality of life is being expected by

patients, the morbidity resulting from AMD is becoming increasingly significant (78).

Treatment of Exudative (Wet) AMD

Treatment strategies for the neovascular form of AMD have thus far focused on the prevention of further progress of the CNV either with laser photocoagulation for extrafoveal CNV (81–83), or with photodynamic therapy (PDT) for either predominately classic (<50%) or smaller occult lesions with no classic component (84). Although PDT has become increasingly prevalent, its effect on the patient's vision is limited. Only 14% of patients treated with PDT have an improved visual acuity of one or more lines after 2 years. Another issue is the large number of CNV recurrences reported after laser photocoagulation and the unpredictable repetition of treatments in 3 months intervals in PDT (81–84). The decision to use either laser photocoagulation or PDT to treat CNV is dependent on the exact location, boundaries, size and nature (e.g., classic or occult) of the membrane as viewed by clinical examination and fluorescein angiography. As only 20% of CNV fulfills all of these requirements and as the greatest group of lesions consists of occult with some classic components, there is no indication for either treatment in 80% of cases. In addition, only 20% of patients suffer from the wet form of AMD (74,75), leaving the vast majority of patients untreated (76,77). Unfortunately, the sole use of vasodestructive methods without any attempt to restore normal retinal morphology does not provide the large group of patients with dry AMD with any visual improvement benefit.

Atrophic (Dry) AMD

Geographic atrophy of the RPE is the advanced form of atrophic AMD. It is responsible for about 20% of the legal blindness due to AMD. In addition, atrophic AMD is responsible for a much larger percentage of moderate visual loss in the elderly (85). For people age 75 and above, the prevalence of geographic atrophy is about 3.5% (half that of CNV) (86,87). Its prevalence increases with age and is more common than CNV in older groups (88,89). Geographic atrophy may also follow in about 20% of cases after flattening of a pigment epithelial detachment (90–92).

The pathophysiologic mechanism for the development of atrophic AMD is partially explained by the coincidence of RPE atrophy and choriocapillaris atrophy (93,94). Experimental studies have shown that RPE cell death precedes choriocapillaris atrophy (95,96). In addition, research has shown that the loss of the production of extracellular matrix, including soluble molecules and insoluble growth factors that bind to the extracellular matrix, was responsible for choriocapillaris atrophy (97). As mentioned previously bFGF, which was shown to rescue photoreceptors in the RCS rat, is one of the growths factors produced by the RPE (98,99) Part of the rational for RPE transplantation in atrophic AMD therefore also lies in the diffusion of soluble factors produced by healthy transplanted RPE cells to prevent the progression of this disease. The reason for the dearth of patients in which RPE transplantation has been performed with autologous tissue is partially explained by the delayed immune reactions that were observed in these eyes (although it was reported that the immune reactions were less severe or prevalent than those observed in patients with exudative AMD). This contributed to a reduction in damage of the blood-retinal barrier in these patients (100,101). Thus far, autologous transplantation of iris pigment epithelium or RPE has not been performed in human eyes with atrophic AMD; however, these patients may be better candidates for RPE transplantation because of minor inflammation and the lack of any other curative treatment against atrophic AMD today. Although there is some evidence that the combination of specific vitamins might slow progression of AMD, this seems to be the case in a rather small risk group of patients. The long-term tolerability and side effects of this treatment must also be carefully evaluated (102). Machemer and de Juan proved that foveal function can be regained on an intact extrafoveal pigment epithelium with their initial reports of retinal rotation (103,104). In contrast to this method, which can be fraught with rather high rates of intraoperative and postoperative complications (105–107), the procedure of retinal transplantation is a relatively simple procedure and has a lower likelihood of severe complications.

Subretinal Surgery

Removal of the CNV together with extensive hemorrhage in AMD was described first by De Juan and Machemer in 1988 (108). This surgery was successfully performed by Thomas and Kaplan in 1991 in patients with presumed ocular histoplasmosis syndrome (109). However, when performed in AMD patients, the visual results were generally disappointing and visual acuity improved in 0% to 33% of patients (110–115). In a retrospective meta-analysis we performed evaluating 26 different studies and a total of 647 cases of subretinal membrane excision in AMD patients, it was shown that improvement was achieved in about 33% and deterioration in 27%. A mean recurrence rate of the CNV in 25% (0% to 55%) was also found, which added to further visual loss in primary successful cases (116).

More disappointing, however, was the report about further progression of the atrophy after membrane excision by different groups. This was explained by the simultaneous removal of the RPE on and around the membrane during surgery, and the herewith associated subsequent photoreceptor and choriocapillaris dysfunction (117–119). In a prospective multicenter study comparing submacular surgery with laser photocoagulation, the two treatment options were found to be equivalent. After 2 years, 65% of laser-treated cases versus 50% of surgically treated eyes had a visual acuity that was better than or no more than one line worse than baseline (120).

RPE Transplantation in Human Eyes

RPE transplantation was performed by Peyman et al. in 1991 in two cases of terminal AMD (121). The first case used an autologous flap; in the second case, homologous material was used. In the first case, visual improvement was reported over several months. The second case reported no visual improvement. Along with the development of surgical techniques to remove subretinal membranes in eyes with presumed ocular histoplasmosis syndrome and neovascular AMD (109,122), a more controlled surgical approach for subretinal transplantation of cell suspensions or sheets became available. In addition, finer instruments for subretinal surgery were developed (123).

Photoreceptor transplantation was performed in human eyes in patients with retinitis pigmentosa by two groups. Human fetal neural cells were used in three patients by del Cerro and coworkers (124). One gained vision to 20/200 and the other two remained LP—no final followup results were given. A series of patients with terminal retinitis pigmentosa were treated and visual field improvements were reported by Das et al. (125). Kaplan and his group treated two patients that were NLP preoperatively with outer retinal sheet transplants derived from adult cadaver eyes. There were no complications, however no visual improvement was reported (126). More recently, another group has reported on human neural retinal transplantation in a series of patients with terminal AMD. There were no immune reactions, but also no visual improvement was observed (127).

The transplantation of RPE seemed to be a logical approach in restoring vision in patients with AMD. The disappointing visual results after membrane excision alone were explained by the mechanical removal of the RPE together with the membrane, as well as the primary dysfunction of the RPE in these cases. To compensate for the RPE deficit in AMD, five patients received a patch of previously cultured human fetal RPE placed in the foveal area after membrane excision. After 3 months, four of five cases lost fixation, macular edema developed, and fluorescein leakage was present, suggesting rejection. After 1 year, most of the patients had experienced mild visual loss compared to their preoperative vision (128). Then four eyes of atrophic (dry) macular degeneration received circular patches of 0.6 mm in diameter by the same group. This time the transplants were placed outside of the fovea. At 1-year follow-up, it was shown that the transplants did not adversely affect local visual function, and there was some evidence of growth but no visual improvement. A milder rejection was observed in these eyes and related to the more intact blood-retinal barrier in dry AMD eyes (100). Finally, to cover a larger area including the fovea, a cell suspension of concentrated dissociated fetal human RPE has been used in seven subsequent cases of advanced but dry AMD. With 50,000 RPE cells transplanted, rejection developed after 8 to 12 months, and with 500,000 cells, rejection developed after 3 months. Those two eyes, which received 20,000 and

200 cells respectively, did not show rejection at 1 year, but no visual improvement was observed (101).

Immune Reaction

Although the eye as a part of the central nervous system possesses the characteristics of an immunologically privileged site, it was demonstrated that RPE cell transplants sensitized their hosts to both alloantigens and RPE-specific autoantigens. Both of these effects can be considered potential barriers to successful transplantation and would make immune suppression regimens necessary (129). It was also demonstrated that the immunologic response is most likely related to the amount of transplanted cells and increases over time (130). In contrast to the initial reports where RPE allografts in the RCS rat were not rejected in eyes with up to 1 year followup (131), later reports have demonstrated evidence of rejection at different time intervals and of different severity (132,133). Cyclosporine has been given to rabbits receiving RPE allografts in order to suppress immunologic reaction, but it was not able to prevent RPE allograft destruction in the subretinal space (134). Comparing photoreceptor and RPE allografts may not be appropriate, however, because photoreceptors have been suggested to be less immunogenic than RPE (135). Conversely, RPE transplantation might be preferable over photoreceptor transplantation due to the important metabolic roles of the RPE and its relatively sequestered anatomic location.

An interesting strategy to eliminate rejection has been the use of autografts of iris pigment epithelium (IPE) to replace defective RPE (136,137). Several investigators have demonstrated the ability of IPE to phagocytose outer segments (138,139). However, compared to the RPE, the IPE has been demonstrated to digest outer segments much more slowly (140).

Autologous Transplantation

To circumvent the potential for graft rejection, transplantation of autologous tissue has been propounded. Full-thickness RPE-transplants taken from adjacent areas of the CNV performed in nine cases by Awylard demonstrated sequestration after a longer observation period (141), although some remaining functions were demonstrated on microperimetry (142).

Iris Pigment Epithelial Transplantation

Iris pigment epithelium cells have been used by groups in Japan and Germany (143,144). This concept is intriguing due to the ease by which the IPE can be harvested. The surgery can be performed in a one-step procedure or in two steps where iridectomy is performed in combination with cataract surgery and the IPE thereafter expanded in cell culture. Transplantation via subretinal surgery can then be scheduled at an optimal time, even years later, as it has been shown that cryopreserved IPE do not lose its function during long-term storage in liquid nitrogen (145). Some degree of visual improvement has been reported by Tamai and his group, and visual acuity was examined using a specially

developed low vision device (the L-O-V-E machine) (143). Prevention of further loss of vision or improvement along with a very low recurrence rate of the CNV has been reported in about 80% of 20 eyes with different neovascular diseases by Thumann and coworkers (144). The RPE has been shown on several occasions to be superior to IPE cells in its phagocytotic capacity. Further, after their initially common embryogenesis as the neuroepithelium of the optic vesicle, the RPE and IPE begin to develop relatively early distinct sets of molecular markers and thus functions, further contributing to their differing adult phenotype (140).

RPE Transplantation Technique

To restore more normal subretinal conditions, it is feasible to use autologous RPE to treat patients with neovascular AMD (146,147). Using a technique derived from silicone oil surgery during the pre-perfluorocarbon liquid era, RPE harvesting has been performed through a retinotomy nasal to the optic disc. Briefly, after pars plana vitrectomy and removal of the posterior hyaloid, a subretinal bleb was created nasal to the optic disc via a small retinotomy. The RPE cells were then gently mobilized with a soft tip bent cannula or a special instrument over an area of about 4 disc diameters. The RPE was slowly aspirated via a vitrectomy tube into a microsyringe. This technique guarantees full visual control during the surgery and a relatively low risk for surgical complications, because the retinotomy can be tamponaded together with the second central retinotomy (created for membrane removal) with a gas tamponade. While the aspirate is centrifuged and the RPE cells are counted and examined, the second retinotomy can be created superiorly from the CNV and the membrane gently removed. A small amount of perfluorocarbon liquid is injected immediately to prevent subretinal hemorrhage and to guarantee safe delivery of the transplanted RPE suspension. After transplantation of the RPE suspension (in 0.1–0.2 mL of BSS + solution) via a subretinal cannula directly connected to a microsyringe in the submacular area, the PFCL is left within the eye for a few minutes to allow the RPE to settle and prevent significant dispersion. An air-fluid exchange is then performed which is followed by a gas injection (Fig. 27.1). The patient is kept in a supine position for about 1 hour in an attempt to hold the RPE cells in place and improve adhesion to the residual layers of Bruch's membrane. Then the patient is asked to turn around and maintain a prone position overnight (148).

Harvesting Efficacy of RPE Cells in Aspirates from Posterior Retinal Areas

Harvesting enough highly viable reproducible cells within the inoculate is critical for successful autologous RPE transplantation. We applied the subretinal technique of gentle mobilization and aspiration of RPE cells from the nasal area of the retina in 14 cadaver eyes and analyzed the efficacy of RPE cell harvesting using this technique. Total cell numbers harvested ranged from 11,000 to 29,000 (mean of 19,976 ± 6,016) with a remarkably constant harvesting

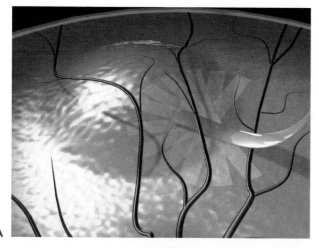

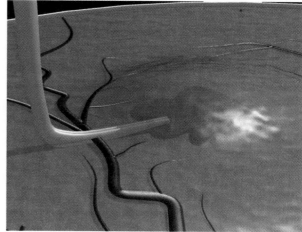

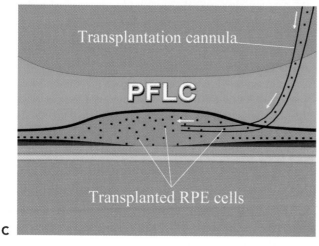

Figure 27.1 A. Harvesting of retinal pigment epithelium cells via a small retinotomy from an area of the retina that is medial to the optic disc. **B.** Removal of a foveal choroidal neovascularization membrane via a small retinotomy. **C.** Subretinal transplantation of the previously harvested retinal pigment epithelium cells into the area where the central neovascularization membrane had been removed. This step is performed under a layer of perfluorocarbon, which helps to avoid reflux and improves adherence of the retina. PFLC, perfluorocarbon; RPE, retinal pigment epithelial.

efficacy (6,165 ± 746 cells/DD). The cell viability was high (82.0% ± 6.9%). This demonstrated that reasonable numbers of highly viable RPE cells suitable for autologous RPE transplantation can be efficiently harvested even from small retinal areas (149). It must be noted, however, that in the clinical setting, lesser amounts of RPE will be harvested, as post mortem changes in cadaver eyes used in these experiments may not reflect the normal in vivo adherence of the RPE. A Ca^{++}–Mg^{++}-free solution is used to create the bleb detachment at the nasal location in order to prevent mechanical disruption of the RPE and facilitate RPE harvesting (150).

Transplantation of RPE after Debridement of Bruch's Membrane

Early animal studies involving RPE transplantation into areas where normal native RPE and undisturbed Bruch's membrane were present do not accurately reflect the clinical situation of most patients. For instance, in AMD, it is well known that Bruch's membrane is thickened and altered with basal linear deposits (151,152). Exudation and, most likely, some degree of inflammation with an aged and dysfunctional RPE are also present (153). After neovascular membrane removal during submacular surgery,

the RPE and Bruch's membrane have been mechanically manipulated. Repopulation of bare Bruch's membrane (wound healing) by the remaining native RPE is incomplete and a progressive atrophy of the choriocapillaris often ensues (154). Similarly, in the animal model, when Bruch's membrane is damaged, repopulation of the bare surface is also incomplete (154). While localized hydraulic (gentle) debridement of RPE was associated with a nearly complete Bruch's membrane resurfacing within 1 week by an RPE monolayer and nearly complete preservation of overlying photoreceptors and recovery of choriocapillaris after 4 weeks, it was shown that (mechanical) abrasive debridement, which damages Bruch's membrane was associated with incomplete RPE repopulation in the debrided zone. Areas that underwent mechanical debridement lacked a normal RPE monolayer and subsequently developed secondary photoreceptor degeneration and choriocapillary atrophy (156). Similar results were also obtained in another model where the resurfacing of the defect was inhibited by mitomycin C (157). It has been suggested by several investigators that the subretinal environment present after surgical removal CNV membranes may be simulated by abrasive debridement of RPE from the surface of Bruch's membrane (158–160). Transplantation of allogenic gelatin-embedded RPE sheets onto abrasively debrided Bruch's membrane has been shown to decrease atrophy of the choriocapillaris in the area of the RPE transplants. However, allogenic transplantation does carry the risk of tissue rejection (161–163). In an experimental study, Tezel and associates have shown that the fate of RPE seeded on Bruch's membrane is partially dependent on the layer on which the cells are seeded. The authors found that a much better cell survival rate can be expected with the presence of the basal lamina or outer collagenous layers rather than the deeper elastin layers (164). However, they also state that the microenvironment of RPE cells seeded onto Bruch's membrane in tissue culture may be different from the subretinal space in clinical situations, because the neurosensory retina, choriocapillaris, and choroid were not present their in vitro experiments. In general, the RPE did not settle well on all present laminae of Bruch's membrane explants. In subsequent studies from this group it was shown to be due to accumulations of age-related debris in different layers of Bruch's membrane (165).

In contrast to the previous work, however, Wang et al. performed a series of RPE wound healing experiments on Bruch's membrane explants which demonstrated that RPE basement membrane supports RPE resurfacing of localized RPE defects. The deeper portion of the ICL of aged submacular human Bruch's membrane was limited in its ability support RPE resurfacing when compared to RPE basement membrane (166).

Phillips et al. investigated whether autologous RPE transplantation (using our previously described surgical technique [148] where RPE is transferred from one subretinal area to another within the same eye in a single operation) would alter the fate of a site of abrasive debridement in an animal model (167). Compared with the surgical technique of debridement only, the technique utilizing debridement plus transplantation of RPE resulted in more complete repopulation of the bare Bruch's membrane surface with relative preservation of choriocapillaris and photoreceptor loss.

Light and transmission electron microscopy of the center of the debridement site revealed extensive disruption of the outer nuclear layer. Only remnants of inner segments (and no photoreceptor outer segments) remained. No choriocapillaris vessels were present. Some central areas had no RPE, while others had thickened Bruch's membrane in these areas. Extensive collagen deposition was present in the area previously occupied by the choriocapillaris.

In contrast, light and electron microscopy of the center of the transplanted site revealed the presence of RPE with normal shape, polarity, and pigmentation; monolayered in some and multilayered in others; with basal infoldings and with apical villi surrounding photoreceptor outer segments. Some photoreceptor outer segments were present but attenuated. The outer and inner nuclear layers, along with the ganglion cell layer, appeared normal. Bruch's membrane was present but thickened. In some areas, cell processes of RPE were present within Bruch's membrane. The choriocapillaris was present and appeared normal.

Placoid proliferation after injury of the RPE has been well described and is similar to the findings in subretinal scarring after CNV (152,168–170). It is possible that the RPE cells transplanted immediately after abrasive debridement preserve the outer retinal architecture by minimizing the proliferative stimulus that results in RPE plaque formation. Whether the poor repopulation of Bruch's membrane and RPE plaque formation after abrasive debridement is the result of choriocapillaris injury, physical barriers to cell migration, damage to Bruch's membrane, alterations in cell surface ligand expression or growth factor expression, or some other factor, is not yet clear. The results from the above-mentioned study show a morphologic recovery that is better with abrasive debridement followed by transplantation than with abrasive debridement alone (167).

Autologous RPE Transplantation in Neovascular AMD Patients: Pilot Study

In a pilot study (148), 14 eyes underwent subretinal surgery because of foveal CNV with simultaneous transplantation of RPE harvested from the nasal subretinal area of the same eye.

Between 5,000 and 50,000 cells/mL were transplanted in each case in this series; cell vitality was between 80% to 90% with trypan blue staining; the RPE phenotype was also confirmed by immunocytochemistry. After a mean observation of 17 months, best-corrected visual acuity improved two or more lines in 57.1% (8 eyes), remained the same ± one line in 35% (5 eyes) and decreased by more than two lines in 7.1% (one eye). In 21%, useful reading acuity between Jaeger 1 and 4 points was achieved. No significant intraoperative and postoperative complications occurred in any eye, no recurrence of CNV was observed during the observation period of 17 months. Indocyanine green angiography did not show further atrophic changes of the choriocapillaris and choroid during the postoperative observation period.

RPE Cultures from Excised Subretinal Membranes

To answer the question about RPE conditions in the area of the membrane and its surrounding regions, RPE cultures from excised subretinal membranes were performed. CNV specimens from 31 patients were obtained and subsequently cultured in DMEM H16 supplemented with 20% autologous serum. In 26/31 (82%) CNV membranes, cell proliferation could be initiated in several. Pancytokeratin staining confirmed the presence of a pure RPE culture. The latter grew to confluence and large cell numbers could be obtained by passage. Furthermore, postconfluent cultures could be maintained at confluence for up to 6 months with no loss of morphologic differentiation. Immunohistochemistry of confluent cells revealed a uniform expression of cytokeratin 18 and vimentin in all 26 cultures, even after 6 months (171). In a similar study by another group, expression of cytokeratin 18 and vimentin was also found, while factor 8, glial fibrillary acidic protein, and smooth muscle actin were absent in all cultures. The expression of RPE markers cellular retinaldehyde binding protein (CRALBP) and RPE65 was detected by RT–PCR in all cultures tested. An epithelial character of the cultures was supported by the presence of apical microvilli, as determined by electron-microscopic studies (172).

However, there are reports that the RPE in and around the area of the CNV is altered by having a higher secretion of growth factors (VEGF) along with stronger voltage currents in L-type calcium channels. It remains unclear as to whether this is the cause or the result of the disease. The question as to whether these RPE cells may be a useful source for RPE autotransplantation needs further investigation.

Excised Membranes—Histopathology

Although the created defect appears rather small during membrane excision, progressive atrophy develops quickly thereafter. Choriocapillaris atrophy advances further after membranectomy, although some damage might also exist prior to surgery that is difficult to evaluate even with indocyanine green angiography. Little bleeding usually occurs during membrane removal, indicating that layers of Bruch's membrane and choriocapillaris are still present. Clearly, more RPE and basal lamina will be removed in eyes with membranes located under the pigment epithelium (Type I—Gass classification) than in eyes with membranes located anterior to the pigment epithelium (Type II). As already stated with PDT applied for classic CNV in many countries, candidates for surgery today are generally those with mixed or mainly occult membranes, or large occult membranes (those with a worse prognosis).

The cleavage plane for membrane removal is considered either to be in the basal lamina or the inner collagenous layer of Bruch's membrane (117). This theory is supported by histologic and electron microscopic examinations in which various amounts of Bruch's membrane contents were observed in 30% to 70% of excised membranes (173–174). From this, one could suggest that in 30% to 70% of basal lamina, Bruch's membrane is still present immediately after surgery. While this would favor simultaneous transplantation of fresh cells, the presence of more or less inflammation might be a disadvantage. When we examined a series of mainly occult membranes excised prior to RPE transplantation, we observed parts of Bruch's membrane in most of the specimens, but the amounts differed greatly between cases. Compared with the fluorescein angiographic appearance (in which all cases of CNV were diagnosed as occult membranes either with no or minimal classic components), there was a significant histologic difference in the amount of inflammatory cells and vascularity. Of note, RPE cells were observed in all membranes in variable amounts (173–175).

Adult Human RPE and Minimal Cell Numbers Needed for Monolayer Formation In Vitro

The use of fetal tissue in retinal transplantation is confounded by ethical issues and technical difficulties.

Consequently, transplantation of adult RPE cells has been researched more thoroughly. Although it has been demonstrated that adult as well as fetal RPE can rescue photoreceptors in RCS rats (176,177), the rat RPE exhibits a significant age-dependent decline in its ability to rescue photoreceptors. Although younger cells grow more quickly when cultured, aged human RPE cells can also be cultured in sufficient numbers (178).

Building on the above experiments, in vitro experiments attempting to elucidate minimal cell densities necessary for monolayer reformation in a Petri dish were studied by various groups (179,180). These data provided clues about the minimal cell yield needed from the RPE biopsy for ex vivo expansion.

Third-passage adult human RPE cells were studied in vitro with low-Ca^{++} media to define minimal plating densities for confluence. The critical amount of 1,500 cells per 96-well dish (i.e., 0.35 cm^2) reached confluence on plastic with a success rate of 40%. Seeding densities below this value were not viable. Although the above data are comparable with published data from Kim and Tezel (179), they were achieved with relatively simpler culture conditions. Confluent cultures were not epithelioid due to low-Ca^{++} media.

Clinical Trial for Autologous RPE Transplantation in Patients with CNV Secondary to AMD

Based on the results of the pilot study, a prospective trial was conducted in which transplantation after membrane excision was compared with a control group in which membrane excision alone was performed (181,182). Only those patients who were not eligible for laser or photodynamic therapy were included in the study. After 12 months observation, the preliminary results of 54 cases showed that in the group of membrane excision with simultaneous transplantation (N = 40) visual improvement of two or more lines was achieved in 52.5%, remained the same (i.e., ± one line) in 32.5%, and decreased two or more lines in 15%. In the control group (N = 14) in which membrane excision was performed (without transplantation), visual improvement was documented in 21.5%, remained the same in 57.8%, and deteriorated in 21.5%. Statistical analysis showed a trend in favor of the transplanted group, but no significant difference between the two groups. However, a significant difference between the two groups was observed when measuring reading acuity (P = 0.0001) (Fig. 27.2). In addition, multifocal ERGs showed a significant difference between the two groups (P = 0.01) with median values of 90.58 mV preoperatively and 89.13 mV after 12 months in the transplanted group, and median values of 97.35 mV preoperatively and 71.55 mV after 12 months in the control group. No difference in the decrease of central visual field defects was observed between the two groups, but mean deviation values of the control group were smaller (19.91) than those of the transplanted group (20.33). Optical coherence tomography demonstrated that the mean postoperative retinal

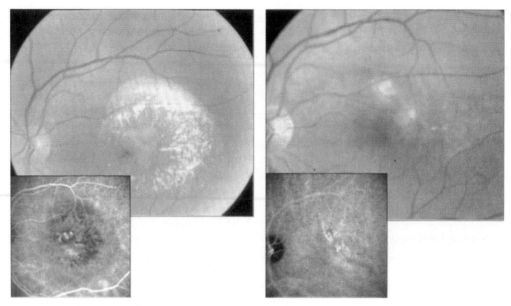

Figure 27.2 Preoperative and postoperative (12 months) photograph and late-phase angiogram (*insert*) of a patient after membrane excision and RPE transplantation. Visual acuity preop.: 0.22 Jg 14; postop.: 1.22 Jg 1. (With permission from Susanne Binder, ed. *The Macula*. Vienna: Springer-Verlag; 2004:81.)

thickness in the area of the lesions was higher in the transplantation group than in the control group (241.4 μm to 202.07 μm). Statistical analysis showed a trend but no significance between the two groups. Fluorescein and indocyanine green angiography demonstrated a recurrent membrane in two cases (5%) of the transplanted group and in one eye (7.8%) of the control group. Surgical complication rates were comparable to vitrectomy with subretinal surgery: in 8.7% (N = 5), a treatable retinal detachment developed.

These results clearly demonstrate for the first time that membrane excision combined with simultaneous transplantation of an autologous RPE suspension is superior to membrane excision alone. Given that only patients with large, mainly occult membranes underwent surgery, one might speculate that these results would improve if cases with a better prognosis (i.e., younger aged patients, smaller membranes, and classic membranes) underwent this procedure. Although the difference in reading acuity was significant between the two groups, useful reading vision was rarely achieved in the transplantation group (but absent in the controls). One has to acknowledge the limitations in the degree of visual rehabilitation that the outcomes represent. More sensitive tests like mERG show a clear difference between the two groups in favor of the transplants. Although these results are encouraging, the fate and function of the transplanted RPE is unclear. It may serve merely as a bystander in the digestion of cellular debris, secreting growth factors to facilitate reproliferation from the edges of the damaged areas; or it may settle/adhere as small islands and proliferate to confluence. Under ideal conditions, one would hope to achieve total RPE monolayer reformation without formation of discrete RPE clumps or multiple RPE layers (148).

RPE Wound Healing

Restoration of the RPE monolayer on the RPE basement membrane and inner collagenous layer in human submacular membrane explants of aged patients (mean age 71.9) was studied by Wang and coworkers (166). They were able to show that the presence of RPE basement membrane and superficial inner collagenous layers support wound healing of localized RPE defects, while deeper portions of the inner collagenous layer of aged submacular human Bruch's membrane do not support RPE resurfacing to the same extent. Similar observations were obtained in our group when the nasal RPE harvesting areas of patients were examined postoperatively. A reduction of the size of the debrided area was observed during the first 3 months after surgery in 50% of the examined cases (N = 14). The original extensions of the RPE defects were reduced in size between 10% to 20% after 3 months, then the borders of the areas remained unchanged until 24 months. Whether cell migration and/or proliferation occurred is unclear (D Rabenlehner and S Binder 2003, unpublished data).

Suspension versus Sheet

The use of RPE suspensions or RPE cells in microaggregates has previously demonstrated survival of transplanted RPE and photoreceptor rescue (11,13,184). The great advantage of its use is the ease with which it can be applied. Reflux of cells during transplantation can be prevented by using a gas or perfluorocarbon liquid tamponade under which the cells can be delivered safely.

However, transplantation of dispersed RPE and/or microaggregates may result in multilayers in the subretinal space and subretinal fibrosis (148,183). Uncovered areas of Bruch's membrane may result in localized photoreceptor atrophy (167,185). In contrast, transplantation of RPE sheets provides an organized monolayer with intact intercellular junctions and proper polarization. Further, the exposed Bruch's membrane can be covered more thoroughly. This technique is technically challenging, however. In the human setting, sheet transplantation has so far been associated with RPE multilayer formation and cell disorientation because of inadvertent folding or contraction of the sheet once the matrix was absorbed (186–189). Full-thickness transplantation of RPE-choroidal flaps showed sequestration after a longer observation period (141).

Carrier Substrates

The extracellular environment upon which transplanted RPE cells are seeded is often considered to be a rather hostile environment for attachment, growth, and differentiation of the transplant. As opposed to the previous section, where the RPE cells were transplanted without the provision of a matrix, the current section discusses various carrier substrates for the RPE graft, which have been proposed as a substitute for the likely damaged Bruch's membrane. Among them are cross-linked collagen (187), gelatin (188,189), fibrinogen (190), cryoprecipitate (191), poly-L-lactic acid (PLLA) (192), PLLA/PLGA (poly-DL-lactic-co-glycolic acid) film (193), hydrogel (194), the basement membrane-containing anterior lens capsule (195), epithelially denuded amniotic membrane (196), and even Bruch's membrane from human cadavers (197). There are many advantages and disadvantages associated with each of the prior art substrates used for transplantation of cultured RPE cells.

Cross-linked collagen, when used for transplantation, is damaging to the retina due to its thickness, poor permeability, and inability to degrade (187). However, cells seeded on non-cross-linked collagen were tolerated well in the subretinal space and did not produce atrophy of the neural retina (187). Yet, since such collagens are likely to cause immunologic reactions in situations where the outer blood retinal barrier is disturbed, and it is known that RPE cells require for proper phenotypic differentiation a specific mixture basal laminar components (198,199), these substrates are not ideal. Gelatin has been used as an embedding medium, but not as a substrate for attachment (188). Fibrinogen is also not suitable for transplanting RPE as a single sheet when transplanted to the subretinal space, despite monolayer outgrowth in the subretinal space (190). PLLA/PLGA films do provide an ideal RPE monolayer sheet for transplantation, but their neural-retinal toxicity and relative stiffness renders them unsuitable for transplantation (194). Hydrogel also provides the RPE monolayer sheet for transplantation, but the resultant cell density and the

cell tight junction determined by expression of ZO-1 is relatively low (194).

Although the lens capsule is a basement membrane-containing autologous material, when transplanted to the subretinal space, it impedes nutritional transport (195). Furthermore, the tendency of the capsule to curl has made this technique impracticable. Although it is thinner, the use of the posterior capsule has also been abandoned for a number of reasons. First, the posterior capsule is difficult to obtain during surgery without putting the patient at high risk for complications from such removal. Secondly, a lack of absorption or slow absorption of the lens capsule material may inhibit the survival of the transplanted RPE cells because of insufficient contact of the cells with Bruch's membrane and/or the choriocapillaris.

Recently, Bilbao and coworkers disclosed the use of PLGA coated on one side of a lens capsule to prevent curling and to facilitate its use for subretinal release. However, histological studies showed not only that the PLGA had completely dissolved after 4 weeks, but also that the overlying retinal layers were disrupted and were accompanied by a large amount of cell infiltration (200).

Cryoprecipitate, which can be produced from a blood sample, was tested as a possible autologous substrate for human fetal RPE by Farrokh-Siar and her group in 1999 (191). The growth and differentiation on this matrix appears promising. However this study was not carried further into animal experiments, which are necessary to demonstrate its subretinal delivery and tolerance.

As described above, there are many challenges with RPE transplantation that need to be overcome, including: maintenance of the morphology of the RPE phenotype in cultured and transplanted RPE cells; creation of a uniform monolayer of autologous RPE on a biocompatible substrate; improving the RPE cell transplant technique to better cover the defect; overcoming immune rejection of RPE transplants due to both alloantigens and RPE-specific autoantigens; and preventing subretinal fibrosis following RPE transplantation.

Amniotic membrane transplantation has been used for ocular surface reconstruction in the treatment of acute chemical and thermal burns of corneal tissue (201). In an in vitro study carried out by Stanzel and coworkers in 2002, amniotic membrane was found to support growth and differentiation of RPE cells seeded on the epithelially denuded basal lamina (202). Implantation of cryopreserved human amniotic membrane into rabbit subretinal space and the implantation of a homologous amniotic graft into a CNV model lesion in pigs (203) showed no rejection over 6 months and was even capable of suppression of inflammation.

Overall, the medical need for a viable method of culturing RPE cells suitable for transplantation into the subretinal space, yielding a suitable, functional RPE transplant with actions to maintain the epithelial phenotype and exert anti-inflammatory, antiscarring, and antiangiogenic effects to the underlying stroma, has not been met thus far.

Ex Vivo Expansion of an RPE Biopsy

The concept of having a delivery substrate further necessitates the development of clinically applicable techniques for a compound transplant of RPE cells and substrate, which is prepared in vitro and thereafter transplanted into the subretinal space. This will likely involve culture techniques including using media formulations that ideally yield an in vivo-like phenotype of RPE cells (204) and cryopreservation for long-term storage (205). Homologous transplants, even if HLA matched, will require long-term immunosupression (206). Furthermore, as already outlined above, these transplants will most likely be rejected. Therefore, effective RPE biopsy techniques need to be developed for the transplant to be of autologous origin. Such an approach will ensure transplant success.

FUTURE TRENDS FOR RETINAL TRANSPLANTATION TECHNIQUES

Future trends in retinal transplantation will lie in further improvement of surgical techniques as well as better case selection. Earlier timing for surgical intervention may result in more favorable results than obtained thus far. While the first positive results have been obtained in human eyes with AMD, these results must be strengthened and verified, and hopefully improved upon. Full-thickness or RPE sheet transplantation may be approached again because of less traumatic surgery today and better technology for sheet preparation (207).

In addition, providing better conditions for the transplanted RPE cells to enhance their chances for survival within the host bed will undoubtedly be important for visual restoration. If non-toxic in vivo markers can be used in a clinical trial, tracking of the transplanted cells may become possible. Finally, patients with dry AMD may be better candidates for retinal and pigment epithelial transplantation due to the lesser degree of inflammation and break down of the blood-retinal barrier.

ACKNOWLEDGMENTS

The author wishes to thank Boris Stanzel, CM for his technical assistance in the creation of this chapter. The author also thanks Rama D. Jager MD, MBA, for correcting the English and his editorial work with this chapter.

REFERENCES

1. Björklund A, Stenevi U. Growth of central catecholamine neurons into smooth muscle grafts in the rat mesencephalon. *Brain Res.* 1971.
2. Widner H, Rhencrona S. Transplantation and surgical treatment of Parkinsonian syndrome. *Curr Opin Neurol Neuroszrg.* 1993;6:344–349.
3. Macular Photocoagulation Study Group. Argon laser photocoagulation for neovascular maculopathy: five year results from randomised clinical trial. *Arch Ophthalmol.* 1991;109:1,109–1,114.
4. Macular Photocoagulation Study Group. Visual outcome after laser photo coagulation for subfoveal neovascularisation secondary to age related macular degeneration: the influence of initial lesion size and initial visual acuity. *Arch Ophthalmol.* 1994;112:480–488.
5. Treatment of Age Related Macular Degeneration with Photodynamic Therapy (TAP) Study Group. Photodynamic therapy of subfoveal choroidal neovascularisation in age-related macular degeneration with verteporfin: one year results of 2 randomized clinical trials—Tap report. *Arch Ophthalmol.* 1999;117:1,329–1,345.
6. Verteporfin therapy of subfoveal choroidal neovascularisation in age-related macular degeneration: two year results of a randomised clinical trial including lesions with occult with no classic choroidal neovascularisation: verteporfin in photodynamic therapy report 2. *Am J Ophthalmol.* 2001;131:541–560.
7. Tansley K. The development of the rat eye in graft. *J Exp Biol.* 1946;22:221–223.
8. Royo PE, Quay WB. Retinal transplantation from fetal to maternal mammalian eye. *Growth.* 1959;23:313–336.
9. Flood MT, Gouras P, Kjeldbye H. Growth characteristics and ultrastructure of human retinal pigment epithelium in vitro. *Invest Ophthalmol Vis Sci.*;19:1,309–1,320.
10. Gouras P, Flood MD, Eggers HM, et al. Transplantation of cultured human retinal cells to monkey retina. *An Acad Brasil, Ciencias.* 1984;56(4):431–443.
11. Gouras P, Flood MT, Kjeldbye H, et al. Transplantation of cultured human retinal pigment epithelium to Bruch's membrane of the owl monkeys eye. *Curr Eye Res.* 1985;4:253–265.
12. Lopez R, Gouras P, Brittis M, et al. Transplantation of cultured rabbit retinal epithelium to rabbit retina using a closed eye method. *Invest Ophthalmol Vis Sci.* 1987;28:1,131–1,137.
13. Li LX, Turner JE. Inherited retinal dystrophy in the RSC rat prevention of photoreceptor degeneration by pigment epithelial cell transplantation. *Exp Eye Res.* 1988;47:911–917.
14. Gouras P. Transplantation of retinal pigment epithelium. In: Marmor M, Wolfensberger Th, eds. *The Retinal Pigment Epithelium.* Oxford University Press; 1998;25:492–507.
15. Das SR, Bhardwaj N, Gouras P. Synthesis of retinoids by human retinal epithelium and transfer to rod outer segments. *Biochem J.* 1990;268:201–206.
16. Gouras P, Lopez R, Brittis M, et al. Transplantation of cultured retinal epithelium. In: Agarth E, Ehinger B, eds. *Retinal Signals System, Degenerations and Transplants.* Amsterdam: Elsevier; 1986:271–286.
17. Repucci V, Goluboff E, Wapner F, et al. Retinal pigment epithelium transplantation in the RCS rat. *Invest Ophthalmol Vis Sci.* 1988;29(Suppl):144.
18. Bourne M, Campell D, Tansley K. Hereditary degeneration of the rat retina. *Brit J Ophthalmol.* 1938;22:613–623.
19. Bok D, Hal M. The role of the pigment epithelium in the etiology of inherited dystrophy in the rat. *J Cell Bio.* 1971;49:664–682.
20. Heron WL. Retinal dystrophy in the rat. A pigment epithelial disease. *Inves Ophthal Vis Sci.* 1969;8:595–604.
21. Whiteley SJ, Lichfield TM, Tyers P, et al. Retinal pigment epithelium transplanted to the subretinal space improves the papillary light reflex in RCS rats. *Invest Ophthalmol Vis Sci.* 1995;36(4):212–219.
22. Mullen RJ, La Vail MM. Inherited retinal dystrophy: primary defect in retinal pigment epithelium determined with chimeric rats. *Science.* 1976;192:799–801.
23. Factorovich EG, Steinberg RH, Tasumura D, et al. Photoreceptor degeneration in inherited retinal dystrophy delayed by basic fibroblast growth factor. *Nature.* 1990;347:83–86.
24. Perry J, Du J, Kieldbye H, et al. The effects of bFGF on RSC rat eyes. *Curr Eye Research.* 1995;15:585–592.
25. Turner JE, Blair JR. Newborn rat retinal cells transplanted into a retinal lesion site in adult host eyes. *Brain Res.* 1986;391:91–104.
26. Gouras P, Du J, Kjeldbye H, et al. Long-term photoreceptor transplants in dystrophic and normal mouse retina. *Invest Ophthalmol Vis Sci.* 1994;35:3,145–3,153.
27. Bergström A, Ehinger B, Wilke K, et al. Transplantation of embryonic retina to the subretinal space in rabbits. *Exp Eye Res.* 1992;55:29–37.
28. del Cerro M, Notter MF, del Cerro C, et al. Intraretinal transplantation for rod-cell replacement in light damaged retinas. *J Neuro Transplant.* 1989;1:1–10.
29. del Cerro M, Ison JR, Bowen GP et a: Intraretinal grafting restores visual function in light blinded rats: Neuroreport. 1991;2:529–532.
30. Juliusson B, Bergström A, van Veen T, et al. Cellular organisation in retinal transplants using cell suspensions or fragments of embryonic retinal tissue. *Cell Transplant.* 1993;2:411–418.
31. Silverman MS, Huges SE. Transplantation of photoreceptors in light damaged retina. *Invest Ophthalmol Vis Sci.* 1998;30:1,684–1,690.
32. del Cerro M, Das TP, Lazar E, et al. Fetal neural retinal grafts into human retinitis pigmentosa. (RP). *Soc Neurisci.* 1996;22:319–328.
33. Kaplan H, Tetzel Th, Berger AS, et al. Human photoreceptor transplantation in retinitis pigmentosa. A safety study. *Arch Ophthalmol.* 1997;115:1,168–1,172.
34. Ghosh F, Ehinger B. Full thickness retinal transplants—a review. *Opthalmologica.* 2000;214:54–69.
35. Aramant RB, Seiler MJ. Organized embryonic retinal transplants to normal and light damaged rats. *Soc Neurisci.* 1995b; Abstr. 21, 1308.
36. Seiler MJ, Aramant RB. Intact sheets of fetal retina transplanted to restore damaged rat retinas. *Invest Ophthal Vis Sci.* 1998;39:2,121–2,132.
37. Seiler MJ, Aramant RB. Intact sheet transplants of human fetal retina with pigment epithelium develop normal lamination and survive long term in nude rats. *Exp Eye Res.* 2000;71(Suppl) 1-ICER Abstracts:60.

38. Zhang Y, Arner K, Ehinger B, et al. Limitation of anatomical integration between subretinal transplants and the host retina. *Inv Ophthal Vis Sci.* 2003;44:324–330.

39. Marmor M. The retinal pigment epithelium. In: Marmor, Wolfensberger, eds. *The Retinal Pigment Epithelium.* Oxford University Press; 1998:3–9.

40. del Priore LV, Kuo YH, Tezel Th. Age-related changes in human RPE cell density and apoptosis proportion in situ. *Invest Ophthalmol Vis Sci.* 2002;43:3,312–3,318.

41. Das Sr, Bhardwaj N, Gouras P. Synthesis of retinoids by human retinal epithelium and transfer to rod outer segments. *Biochem J.* 1990;268: 201–206.

42. Gouras P, Lopez R, Brittis M, et al. Transplantation of cultured retinal epithelium. In: Agarth E, Ehinger B, eds. *Retinal Signals System, Degenerations and Transplants.* Amsterdam: Elsevier:271–286.

43. Campochiaro PA, Hackett SF, Vinores SA, et al. Platelet derived growth factor is an autocrine growth stimulator retinal pigmented epithelial cells. *J Cell Sci.*;107:2,459–2,468.

44. Vinores SA, Küchle M, Mahlow J, et al. Blood-ocular barrier break down in eyes with ocular melanoma: a potential role for vascular endothelial growth factor/vascular permeability factor. *Am J Pathol.* 1995b;147: 1,289–1,297.

45. Vinores SA, Youssri AI, Luna JD, et al. Up regulation of vascular endothelial growth factor in ischemic and non-ischemic human and experimental retinal disease. *Histol Histopathol.* 1997;12:99–109.

46. Schweigerer L, Malerstein B, Neufeld G, et al. Basic fibroblast growth factor is synthesized in cultured retinal pigment epithelial cells. *Biochem Biophys Res Comm.* 1987;143:934–940.

47. Kitaoka T, Bost LM, Ishigooka H, et al. Increasing cell density down-regulates the expression of acidic FGF by human RPE cells in vitro. *Curr Eye Res.* 1993;12:993–999.

48. Bost LM, Aotaki-Keen AE, Hjelmeland LM, et al. Coexpression of FGF-5 and bFGF ba the retinal pigment epithelium in vitro. *Exp Eye Res.* 1992;55:727–734.

49. Kavanta A. Expression and secretion of transforming growth factor-beta in transformed and nontransformed retinal pigment epithelial cells. *Ophthalmic Res.* 1994;26:361–367.

50. Cousins SW, Trattler WB, Streilen JW. Immune privilege and suppression of immunogenic inflammation in the anterior chamber of the eye. *Curr Eye Res.* 1991;10:287–297.

51. de Boer JH, Limpens J, Orengo Nania S, et al. Low mature TGB-β2 levels in aqueous humor during uveitis. *Invest Ophthalmol Vis Sci.* 1994;35:3,702–3,710.

52. Gabrielan K, Osusky R, Sippy BD, et al. Effect of TGF-β on interferon-y induced HLA-DR expression in human retinal pigment epithelial cells. *Invest Ophthalmol Vis Sci.* 1994;35:4,253–4,259.

53. Lesche KH, Hackett SF, Singer JH, et al. Growth factor responsiveness of human pigment epithelial cells. *Invest Ophthalmol Vis Sci.* 1990;31:839–846.

54. Waldbillig RJ, Arnold Dr, Fletcher RT, et al. Insulin and IGF-1 binding in developing chick neural retina and pigment epithelium: a characterisation of binding and structural differences. *Exp Eye Res.* 1991a;53:13–22.

55. King GL, Suzuma K. Pigment-epithelium derived factor—a key coordinator of retinal neuronal and vascular functions. Clinical implications of basic research. *NEJM.* 2000;342:349–351.

56. Dawson DW, Volpert OV, Gillis P, et al. Pigment epithelium derived factor: a potent inhibitor of angiogenesis. *Science.* 1999;285:245–248.

57. Seaton AD, Turner JE. RPE transplants stabilize retinal vasculature and prevent retinal neovascularisation in the RSC rat. *Invest Ophthalmol Vis Sci.* 1992;33:83–91.

58. Seaton AD, Sheedlo HJ, Turner JE. A primary role for RPE transplants in the inhibition and regression of neovascularisation in the RSC rat. *Invest Ophthalmol Vis Sci.* 1994;35:162–169.

59. Li L, Turner JE. Inherited retinal dystrophy in the RSC rat: prevention of photoreceptor degeneration by pigment epithelial cell transplantation. *Exp Eye Res.* 1988a;47:911–947.

60. Li T, Turner JE. Transplantation of retinal pigment epithelium cells to immature and adult rat hosts: short and long-term survival characteristics. *Exp Eye Res.* 1988b;47:771–785.

61. Castillo BV, del Cerro M, White RM, et al. Efficacy of nonfetal human RPE for photoreceptor rescue. *Exp Neurol.* 1997;146:1–9.

62. Zhao MW, Jin ML, HE S, et al. A distinct integrin—mediated phagocytic pathway for extracellular matrix remodeling by RPE cells. *IOVS.* 1999;40 2,713–2,723.

63. Young RW. Pathophysiology of age–related macular degeneration. *Surv Ophthalmol.* 1987;31:291–306.

64. Marmor MF. New hypothesis on the pathogenesis and treatment of serous retinal detachment. *Graefes Arch Clin Exp Ophthalmol.* 1988; 226:548–552.

65. Mitchell GA, Brody LC, Sipila U, et al. At least two mutant alleles of ornithine-D-aminotransferase cause gyrate atrophy of the choroids and retina in Finns. *Proc Natl Acad Sci USA.* 1989;89:197–201.

66. Cremers FPM, van der Pol DJRK, van Kerkhof PM, et al. Cloning a gene that is rearranged in patients with choroideremia. *Nature.* 1990;347:674–677.

67. Noble KG, Carr RE. Stargardt's disease and fundus flavimaculatus. *Arch Ophthalmol.* 1979;97:1,281–1,285.

68. Malony WF, Robertson DM, Duboff SM. Hereditary vitelliform macular degeneration. *Arch Ophthalmol.* 1977;95:979–983.

69. Gass JDM, Fallow S, Davis B. Adult vitelliform macular detachment occurring in patients with basal lamina drusen. *Am J Ophthalmol.* 1985; 99:445–459.

70. Deutmann AF, Hansen LMAA. Dominantly inherited drusen of Bruch's membrane. *Br J Ophthalmol.* 1970;34:337–382.

71. Marmor MF, Byers B. Pattern dystrophies of the pigment epithelium. *Am J Ophthalmol.* 1799;84:32–44.

72. Panda–Jonas S, Jonas JB, Jacobczyk-Zmijy M, et al. Retinal epithelial cell count, distribution and correlations in normal eyes. *Am J Ophthalmol.* 1996;121:181–189.

73. del Priore LV, Kuo YH, Tezel T. Age related changes in human RPE cell density and apoptosis proportion in situ. *Invest Ophthalmol Vis Sci.* 2002; 43:3,312–3,318.

74. Bressler Nm, Bressler SB, Fine SL. Age related macular degeneration. *Surv Ophthalmol.* 1988;32:375–413.

75. Ferris FL, Fine SL, Hyman L. Age related macular degeneration and blindness due to neovascular maculopathy. *Arch Ophthalmol.* 1984;102:1,640–1,642.

76. Leibowitz HM, Krueger DE, Maunder LR, et al. The Framingham Eye Study monograph: an ophthalmological and epidemiological study of cataract, glaucoma, diabetic retinopathy, macular degeneration and visual acuity in a general population of 2631 adults, 1973–1975. *Survey Ophthalmol.* 1980;24(Suppl):335–610.

77. Vingerling JR, Dielemans I, Hofmann A, et al. The prevalence of age-related maculopathy in the Rotterdam Study. *Ophthalmology.* 1995;102:205–210.

78. Klein R, Klein BE, Jensen SC, et al. The five year incidence and progression of age-related maculopathy: the Beaver Dam Eye Study. *Ophthalmology.* 1997;104:7–21.

79. Freud KB, Januzzi LA, Sorenson JA. Age-related macular degeneration and choroidal neovascularisation. *Am J Ophthalmol.* 1993;115:789–791.

80. Fine SL, Berger JW, Maguire MG, et al. Age-related macular degeneration. *N Engl J Med.* 2000;342:483–492.

81. Macular photocoagulation study group. Laser photocoagulation of subfoveal neovascular lesions of age-related macular degeneration: update findings from two clinical trials. *Arch Ophthalmol.* 1993;111:1,200–1,209.

82. Macular photocoagulation study group. Persistent and recurrent neovascularisation after laser photocoagulation for subfoveal choroidal neovascularisation of age-related macular degeneration. *Arch Ophthalmol.* 1994; 112:489–499.

83. Macular photocoagulation study group. Subfoveal neovascular lesions in age related macular degeneration: guidelines for evaluation and treatment in the macular photocoagulation study. *Arch Ophthalmol.* 1991;109: 1,242–1,257.

84. Bressler NM. Treatment of Age related Macular degeneration with photodynamic therapy (TAP) Study Group. Photodynamic therapy of subfoveal choroidal neovascularisation in age-related macular degeneration with verteporfin: two-year results of 2 randomized clinical trials—TAP report 2. *Arch Ophthalmol.* 2001;119:198–207.

85. Sunness JS. Geographic atrophy. In: Berger JW, Fine St.L, Maguire MG, eds. *Age Related Macular Degeneration.* Mosby; 1999:155–172.

86. Klein R, Klein BEK, Franke T. The relationship of cardiovascular disease and its risk factors to age-related maculopathy. The Beaver Dam Eye Study. *Ophthalmology.* 1993;100:406–414.

87. Vingerling JR, Dielemans I, Hofman A, et al. The prevalence of age related maculopathy in the Rotterdam Study. *Ophthalmology.* 1995;102:205–210.

88. Hirvela H, Luukinen H, Laara E, et al. Risk factors of age-related maculopathy in a population 70 years of age or older. *Ophthalmology.* 1996; 103:871–877.

89. Quillen D, Blankenship G, Gardner T. Aged eyes. Ocular findings in individuals 90 years and older. *Invest Ophthalmol Vis Sci.* 1996;47:111–121.

90. Braunstein RA, Gass JM. Serous detachment of the retinal pigment epithelium in patients with senile macular disease. *Am J Ophthalmol.* 1979;88: 652–660.

91. Caswell AG, Kohen D, Bird AC. Retinal pigment epithelial detachment in the elderly: classification and outcome. *Br J Ophthalmol.* 1985:397–403.

92. Elman MJ, Fine SL, Murphy RP, et al. The natural history of serous retinal pigment epithelium detachment in patients with age-related macular degeneration. *Ophthalmology.* 1986;93:224–230.

93. Sarks JP, Sarks SH, Killingsworth MC. Evolution of geographic atrophy of the retinal pigment epithelium *EYE.* 1988;2:552–577.

94. Green WR, Key SN. Senile macular degeneration: a histopathologic study. *Trans Am Ophthalmol Soc.* 1977;75:180–254.

95. Leonard DS, Zhang XG, Panozzo G, et al. Clinicopathologic correlation of localized pigment epithelium debridement. *Invest Ophthalmol Vis Sci.*1997;38:1,094–1,109.

96. Korte GE, Repucci V, Henkind P. RPE destruction causes choriocapillaris atrophy. *Invest Ophthalmol Vis Sci.* 1984;25:1,135–1,184.

97. Liu X, Ye X, Yanoff M, et al. Extracellular matrix of retinal pigment epithelium regulated choriocapillaris endothelial survival in vitro. *Exp Eye Res.* 1997;65:117–126.

98. Schweigerer L, Malerstein B, Neufeld G, et al. Basic fibroblast growth factor is synthesized in cultured retinal pigment epithelial cells. *Biochem Biophys Res Commun.* 1987;143:934–940.

99. Sternfeld MD, Robertson JE, Shipley GD, et al. Cultured retinal pigment epithelial cells express basic fibroblast growth factors and its receptors. *Curr Eye Res.* 1989;8:1,029–1,037.

100. Algvere PV, Berglin L, Gouras P, et al. Transplantation of RPE in age-related macular degeneration: observations in disciform lesions and dry atrophy. *Graefes Arch Clin Exp Ophthalmol.* 1997;235:149–158.

101. Algvere PV, Dafgard Kopp EME, Gouras P. Long-term outcome of RPE allografts in non-immunosuppressed patients with AMD. *Eur J Ophthalmol.* 1999;9:217–230.

102. A randomized, placebo controlled, clinical trial of high dose supplementation with Vit C and E and beta carotene for age-related cataract and vision loss: AREDS report Nr 9. *Arch Ophthalmol.* 2001;119:1,439–1,452.

103. Machemer R, Steinhorst R. Retinal separation, retinotomy and macular relocation, a surgical approach for age related macular degeneration. *Graefes Arch Clin Exp Ophthalmol.* 1993;231:635–641.

104. de Juan E, Löwenstin A, Bressler N. Translocation of the retina for the management of subretinal neovascularisation. *Am J Ophthalmol.* 1998; 125:635–646.

105. Eckardt C, Eckardt U, Conrad HC. Macular rotation with and without counter rotation of the globe in patients with age related macular degeneration. *Graefes Arch Clin Exp Ophthalmol.* 1999;237:313–325.

106. Wiedemann P, Faude F, Jochmann C, et al. Begrenzte Translokation der Makula beoi subfovealer choroidaler Neovascularisation. *Spektrum d Augenheilk.* 2000;14:254–258.

107. Toth CA, Machemer R. Macular translocation. In: Berger JF, Fine St L Maguire, eds. *Age Related Macular Degeneration.* Mosby; 1999:353–362.

108. de Juan E Jr, Machemer R. Vitreous surgery for haemorrhagic and fibrous complications of age-related macular degeneration. *Am J Ophthalmol.* 1988;105:25–29.

109. Thomas MA, Kaplan HJ. Surgical removal of subfoveal neovascularisation in the presumed ocular histoplasmosis syndrome. *Am J Ophthalmol.* 1991;111:1–7.

110. Lambert HM, Capone A Jr, Aaberg TM. Surgical excision of subfoveal neovascular membranes in age-related macular degeneration. *Am J Ophthalmol.* 1992;113:257–262.

111. Berger AS, Kaplan HJ. Clinical experience with the surgical removal of subfoveal neovascular membranes: short term postoperative results. *Ophthalmology.* 1992;99:969–976.

112. Thomas MA, Grand MG, Williams DF, et al. Surgical management of subfoveal choroidal neovascularisation. *Ophthalmology.* 1992;99:952–968.

113. Thomas MA, Dickinson JD, Melberg NS, et al. Visual results after surgical removal of subfoveal neovascular membranes. *Ophthalmology.* 1994;101: 1,384–1,396.

114. Schachat AP. Should we recommend vitreous surgery for patients with choroidal neovascularisation? *Arch Ophthalmol.* 1994;112:459–461.

115. Scheider A, Gündisch O, Kampik A. Surgical extraction of subfoveal new vessels and submacular haemorrhage in AMD. Results of a prospective study. *Graefes Arch Clin Exp Ophthalmol.* 1998;237:10–15.

116. Falkner I Ch, Binder S, Leitich H, et al. Subretinal surgery for age-related macular degeneration: a meta-analysis. *Arch Ophthalmol*—submitted.

117. Nasir MA, Sugino I, Zarbin MA. Decreased choriocapillaris perfusion following surgical excision of choroidal neovascular membranes in age-related macular degeneration. *Brit J Ophthalmol.* 1997;81:481–489.

118. Castellarin AA, Nasir MA, Sugino IK, et al. Clinicopathologic correlation of primary and recurrent choroidal neovascularisation following surgical excision in age-related degeneration. *Brit J Ophthalmol.* 1998;82:480–487.

119. Ormenrod LD, Puklin JE, Frank RN. Long-term outcomes after surgical removal of advanced subfoveal neovascular membranes in age-related macular degeneration. *Ophthalmology.* 1994:102:1,201–1,210.

120. Submacular surgery trials randomised pilot trial of laser photocoagulation versus surgery for recurrent choroidal neovascularisation secondary to age-related macular degeneration: I. Ophthalmic outcomes submacular surgery trials pilot study report NR 1. *Am J Ophthalmol.* 2000;130: 387–409.

121. Peyman GA, Blinder KJ, Paris KJ, et al. A technique for retinal pigment epithelial transplantation for age related macular degeneration secondary to extensive subfoveal scarring. *Ophthalmol Surg.* 1991;22:102–108.

122. Thomas MA, Dickinson J, Melberg N, et al. Visual results after surgical removal of subfoveal choroidal neovascular membranes. *Ophthalmology.* 1996;101:1,384–1,396.

123. Thomas MA, Ibsanez HE. Instruments for submacular surgery. *Retina.* 1994;14:84–87.

124. del Cerro M, Das T, Reddy VI, et al. Human fetal neural cell transplantation in retinitis pigmentosa. *Vis Research.* 1995;35(Supp):140 Abstract .

125. Das T, del Cerro M, Jalali S, et al. The transplantation of human fetal neuroretinal cells in advanced retinitis pigmentosa: results of a long-term safety study. *Exp Neurol.* 1999;157:58–68.

126. Kaplan HJ, Tezel TH, Berger AS, et al. Human photoreceptor transplantation in retinitis pigmentosa: a safety study. *Arch Ophthalmol.* 1997;115: 1,168–1,172.

127. Humayun MS, de Juan E, del Cerro M, et al. Human neural retinal transplantation. *Invest Ophthalmol Vis Sci.* 2000;3,100–3,106.

128. Algvere PV, Berglin L, Gouras P, et al. Transplantation of fetal retinal pigment epithelium in age-related macular degeneration with subfoveal neovascularisation. *Graefes Arch Clin Exp Ophthalmol.* 1994;232:707–716.

129. Grisanti S, Misaki I, Kosiewitz M, et al. Immunity and immune privilege elicited by cultured retinal pigment epithelial cell transplants. *Invest Ophthalmol Vis Sci.* 1997;38:1,619–1,626.

130. Gabrielan K, Organesian A, Patel SC, et al. Cellular response in rabbit eyes after human fetal RPE transplantation. *Graefes Arch Clin Ophthalmol.* 1999;237:326–335.

131. Yamamoto S, Du J, Gouras P, et al. Retinal pigment epithelial transplants and retinal function in RCS rats. *Invest Ophthalmol Vis Sci.* 1993;34: 3,068–3,075.

132. He S, Wang H-M, Ogden T, et al. Transplantation of cultured human retinal pigment epithelium into rabbit subretina. *Graefes Arch Clin Exp Ophthalmol.* 1993;231:737–742.

133. Jiang IQ, Jorquera M, Malek TW. The neurobiological role of interleukin-2 expressed during rejection of intraocular RPE allografts. *Invest Ophthalmol Vis Sci.* 1995;36(4):212–222.

134. Craford S, Algvere P, Kopp ED, et al. Cyclosporine treatment of RPE allografts in the rabbit subretinal space. *Acta Ophthalmol Scan.* 2000;78: 122–129.

135. Kaplan HJ, Yu X-H, Zhang H, et al. Antigen specific CTL fail to recognize neoretinal antigen in vivo. *Invest Ophthalmol Vis Sci.* 1995;35(4): 201–210.

136. Gelance M, Breipohl W, Wiedemann P, et al. First experimental iris pigment epithelial transplantation in subretinal space of RCS rats. *Invest Ophthalmol Vis Sci.* 34(Suppl):1,097–1,006.

137. Gelance M, Meneses P, Rosenfeld MR, et al. Long-term results of autologous transplantation of iris pigmented epithelial cells into the subretinal space. *Invest Ophthalmol Vis Sci.* 1997;38(4):334–342.

138. Thuman G, Heimann K, Schraemeyer U. Quantitative phagocytosis of rod outer segments by human and porcine iris pigment epithelial cells in vitro. *Invest Ophthalmol Vis Sci.* 1997;38(4):330.

139. Bisantis F, Fregona I, Mancini A. Is phagocytosis in iris pigmented (IPE) cultures by human iridectomies a self limited and dose dependant mechanism? *Invest Ophthalmol Vis Sci.* 1997;38(4) 5,330.

140. Dintelman T, Heimann K, Kayatz P. Comparative study of ROS degradation by IPE and RPE cells in vitro. *Graefes Arch Clin Exp.* 1999;237: 830–839.

141. Awylard GW, Kyrchenthal A, Stanga PE, et al. RPE-transplantation. A new surgical technique for treatment of choroidal NV in AMD, 12th Annual Meeting of the Retinal Society, 1999, Regensburg, Germany.

142. Stanga PE, Kychenhal A, Fitzke F. Retinal pigment epithelium translocation after choroidal neovascular membrane removal in age-related macular degeneration. *Ophthalmology.* 2002;109:1,492–1,498.

143. Tamai M, Abe T, Tomita, et al. Autologous iris pigment transplantation in age related macular degeneration. In: Das T, ed. *RETINA, Current Practice and Future Trends.* Hyderabad, India: PARAS publishing; 1999:151–161.

144. Thumann G, Aisenbrey S, Schraemeyer U. Transplantation of autologous iris pigment epithelium after removal of choroidal neovascular membranes. *Arch Ophthalmol.* 2000;118(10):1,350–1,355.

145. Abe T, Yoshida M, Tomita H, et al. Auto iris pigment epithelial cell transplantation in patients with age related macular degeneration: short term results. *Tohoku J Exp Med.* 2000;191:7–20.

146. Binder S, Stolba U, Krebs I, et al. Zur Transplantation autologer Pigmentepithelzellen. *Spektrum f Augenheilk.* 2000;14(5):249–253. 44.

147. Verma L, Das T, Binder S, et al. New approaches in the management of choroidal neovascular membrane in age-related macular degeneration. *Indian J Ophthalmol.* 2000;48,263–48,278.

148. Binder S, Stolba U, Krebs I, et al. Transplantation of autologous retinal pigment epithelium in eyes with foveal neovascularisation resulting from age-related macular degeneration: A pilot study. *Amer J Ophthalmol.*; 133(2):215–225.

149. Assadolina A, Binder S, Stanzel B, et al. Harvesting efficacy and viability of retinal pigment epithelial cells in aspirates from posterior retinal areas—a study in human eyes. *Spectrum Augenheilk.* 2003;17(1):8–10.

150. Fang XY, Hayashi A, Cekie O, et al. Effect of Ca$^{(2+)}$-free and Mg$^{(2+)}$-free BSS plus solution on the pigment epithelium and retina in rabbits. *Am J Ophthalmol.* 2001;131:481–488.

151. Green WR, Enger C. Age-related macular degeneration histopathologic studies. The 1992 Lorenz E. Zimmerman Lecture. *Ophthalmology.* 1993; 100:1,519–1,535.

152. Grossniklaus H, Hutchinson AK, Capone A. Clinicopathologic features of surgically excised choroidal neovascular membranes. *Ophthalmology.* 1994;101:1,099–1,111.

153. Hageman GS, Luthert PJ, Victor Chong NH, et al. An integrated hypothesis that considers drusen as biomarkers of immune-mediated processes at the RPE-Bruch's membrane interface in aging and age-related macular degeneration. *Prog Retin Eye Res.* 2001;20:705–732.

154. Castellarin AA, Nasir M, Sugino IK, et al. Progressive resumed choriocapillaris atrophy after surgery for age-related macular degeneration. *Retina.* 1998;18:143–149.

155. Hayashi A. Majji S, Fujioka H, et al. Surgically induced degeneration and regeneration of the choriocapillaris in rabbit. *Graefe's Arch Clin Exp Ophthalmol.* 1999;237:668–677.

156. Leonhard DS, Zhang X, Panozzo G, et al. Clinicopathologic correlation of localized retinal pigment epithelium debridement. *Invest Ophthalmol Vis Sci.* 1997;38:1,094–1,009.

157. del Priore LV, Kaplan HJ, Hornbeck R, et al. Retinal pigment epithelial debridement as a model for the pathogenesis and treatment of macular degeneration. *Am J Ophthalmol.* 1997;122:629–643.

158. del Priore LV, Hornbeck R, Kaplan HJ, et al. Debridement of the pig retinal pigment epithelium in vivo. *Arch Ophthalmol.* 1995;113:939–944.
159. Valentino TL, Kaplan HJ, del Priore LV, et al. Retinal pigment epithelial repopulation in monkeys after submacular surgery. *Arch Ophthalmol.* 1995;113:932–938.
160. Heriot WJ, Machemer R. Pigment epithelial repair. *Graefes Arch Clin Exp Ophthalmol.* 1992;230:91–100.
161. del Priore LV, Tezel TH. Retinal pigment epithelial transplantation onto bare areas of Bruch's membrane prevents atrophy of the choriocapillaris. *Invest Ophthalmol Vis Sci.* 1998;39:76–84.
162. Gabrielan K, Oganesian A, Patel SC. Cellular response in rabbit eyes after human fetal RPE transplantation. *Graefes Arch Clin Exp Ophthalmol.* 1998;236:753–757.
163. Zhang Y, Bok D. Transplantation of retinal pigment epithelial cells and immune response in the subretinal space. *Invest Ophthalmol Vis Sci.* 1997;38:331–338.
164. Tezel T, Kaplan H, del Priore L. Fate of human retinal pigment epithelial cells seeded onto layers of human Bruch's membrane. *Invest Ophthalmol Vis Sci.* 1999;40:467–476.
165. Tezel TH, Oda J, Hornbeck RC, et al. RPE repopulation of aged inner collagenous layer (ICL) is inhibited by reversible alterations in Bruch's membrane. 2001;42:4,995. Conference Proceeding.
166. Wang H, Ninomiya Y, Sugino IK, et al. Retinal pigment epithelium wound healing in human Bruch's membrane explants. *Investigative Ophthalmology Visual Science.* 2003;44:2,199.
167. Phillips S, Sadda, Liu H, et al. Autologous transplantation of retinal pigment epithelium after mechanical debridement of Bruch's membrane. *Exp Eye Res.* 2003.
168. Lopez PE, Groosniklas HE, Lambert HM, et al. Pathologic features of surgically excised neovascular membranes in age-related macular degeneration. *Am J Ophthalmol.* 1991;118:285–298.
169. Tso MO. Photic maculopathy in rhesus monkeys: a light and electron microscopic study. *Invest Ophthalmol Vis Sci.* 1973;12:17–34.
170. Wallow IH, Tso MO. Repair after xenon arc photocoagulation: an electron microscopic study of the evolution of retinal lesions in rhesus monkeys. *Am J Ophthalmol.* 1973;75:957–972.
171. Jahn CH, Krugluger W, Binder S, et al. Cultivation of retinal pigment epithelium cells from excised human subretinal membranes and single cell suspensions in autologous serum. Submitted to *Graefes Arch Clin Exp.*
172. Schlunck G, Martin G, Agostini HT, et al. Cultivation of retinal pigment epithelial cells from human choroidal neovascular membranes in age related macular degeneration. *Exp Eye Res.* 2002;74:571–576.
173. Assadoulina A, Feichtinger H, Binder S, et al. Subfoveal neovascular membranes—membrane morphology and outcome after combined subretinal surgery and autologous RPE transplantation. In: Binder S, ed. *The Macula: Diagnosis, Treatment and Future Trends.* Wien—New York: Springer; 2004:95–100.
174. Assadoulina A, Feichtinger H, Binder S, et al. Subfoveal neovascular membranes—histopathologic features as a predictive factor. *Spektrum Augenheilk.* 2003.
175. Assadoulina A, Feichtinger H, Binder S. Comparison of fluorescein-angiography and histopathology of occult choroidal neovascular membranes. *Invest Ophthalmol Vis Sci.* 2003;44:4:20 Abstract.
176. Castillo BV. Efficacy of nonfatal human RPE for photoreceptor rescue: a study in dystrophic RCS rats. *Exp Neurol.* 1997;146:1–9.
177. Little C, Castillo BV, DiLoreto DA, et al. Transplantation of human fetal RPE rescues photoreceptor cells from degeneration in the RCS rat retina. *Invest Ophthalmol Vis Sci.* 1996;37:204–211.
178. del Monte M, Maumenee I. New techniques for in vitro culture of human RPE. *Birth Defects.* 1980;16:327–338.
179. Kim KS, Tezel TH, Del Priore LV. Minimum number of adult human retinal pigment epithelial cells required to establish a confluent monolayer in vitro. *Curr Eye Res.* 1998;17:962–969.
180. Stanzel BV, Huemer KH, Ahnelt PK, et al. Minimal plating density of adult human RPE cells using a Ca⁺⁺-adjusted DMEM/F12 culture medium. *Invest Ophthalmol Vis Sci.* 2002;43:3,437 Abstract.
181. Binder S, Krebs I, Feichtinger H, et al. Outcome after transplantation of autologous retinal pigment epithelium in eyes with foveal CNV due to AMD. *Invest Ophthalmol Vis Sci.* 2002;43:924 Abstract.
182. Binder S, Krebs I, Hilgrers HD, et al. Outcome after transplantation of autologous RPE in age related macular degeneration—A prospective trial. *Invest Ophthalmol Vis Sci.* 2004;45:4,151–4,160.
183. Li L, Turner J. Transplantation of RPE cells to immature and adult rat host. Short and long-term survival characteristics. *Exp Eye Res.* 1988;47:774–785.

183a. Anderson DH, Guerin CJ, Erickson PA, et al. Morphological recovery in the reattached retina. *Invest Ophthalmol Vis Sci.* 1986;27:168–183.
184. Lopez R, Gouras P, Kjeldbye H, et al. Transplanted retinal pigment epithelium modifies the retinal degeneration in the RCS rat. *Invest Ophthalmol Vis Sci.* 1989;30:586–588.
185. Majji AB, de Juan E. (Retinal pigment epithelial autotransplantation: morphological changes in retina and choroid. *Graefes Arch Clin Exp Ophthalmol.* 2000;238:779–791.
186. Sheng Y, Gouras P, Cao H, et al. Patch transplants of human fetal RPE in rabbit and monkey retina. *Invest Ophthalmol Vis Sci.* 1995;36:381–390.
187. Bhatt NS, Newsome DA, Fenech T, et al. Experimental transplantation of human retinal pigment epithelial cells on collagen substrates. *Am J Ophthalmol.* 1994;117:214–221.
188. Ho TC, Del Priore LV, Kaplan HJ. Tissue culture of retinal pigment epithelium following isolation with a gelatin matrix technique. *Exp Eye Res.* 1997;64:133–139.
189. Del Priore LV, Kaplan HJ, Tezel TH, et al. Retinal pigment epithelial cell transplantation after subfoveal membranectomy in age-related macular degeneration: clinicopathologic correlation. *Am J Ophthalmol.* 2001;131:472–480.
190. Oganesian A, Gabrielian K, Ernest JT, et al. A new model of retinal pigment epithelium transplantation with microspheres. 1999;117:1,192–1,200.
191. Farrokh siar L, Rezai KA, Patel SC, et al. Cryoprecipitate: An autologous substrate for human fetal retinal pigment epithelium. *Curr Eye Res.* 1999;19:89–94.
192. Lu L, Yaszemski MJ, Mikos AG. Retinal pigment epithelium engineering using synthetic biodegradable polymers. *Biomaterials.* 2001;22:3,345–3,355.
193. Hadlock T, Singh S, Vacanti JP, et al. Ocular cell monolayers cultured on biodegradable substrates. *Tissue Eng.* 1999;5:187–196.
194. Singh S, Woerly S, Mclaughlin BJ. Natural and artificial substrates for retinal pigment epithelial monolayer transplantation. *Biomaterials.* 2001;22:3,337–3,343.
195. Nicolini J, Kiilgaard JF, Wiencke AK, et al. The anterior lens capsule used as support material in RPE cell-transplantation. *Acta Ophthalmol Scand.* 2000;78:527–531.
196. Stanzel BV, Huemer KH, Ahnelt PK, et al. Minimal plating density of adult human RPE cells using a Ca⁺⁺-adjusted DMEM/F12 culture medium. *ARVO Meeting Abstracts.* 2002;43:3,437.
197. Tezel TH, Del Priore LV, Kaplan HJ. Photomelded Bruch's membrane patch grafts: a novel concept to treat Bruch's membrane defects in age-related macular degeneration. *ARVO Meeting Abstracts.* 2002;43:925.
198. Campochiaro PA, Hackett SF. Corneal endothelial cell matrix promotes expression of differentiated features of retinal pigmented epithelial cells: implication of laminin and basic fibroblast growth factor as active components. *Exp Eye Res.* 1993;57:539–547.
199. Burke JM. Determinants of retinal pigment epithelial cell phenotype and polarity. In: Marmor MF, Wolfensberger TJ, eds. *The Retinal Pigment Epithelium: Function and Disease.* New York: Oxford University Press; 1998:86–102.
200. Bilbao KV, Leng T, Fung AE, et al. A Biodegradable matrix facilitates the use of lens capsule as a substrate for subretinal cell transplantation. *ARVO Meeting Abstracts.* 2002;43:3,441.
201. Kim JC, Tseng SC. Transplantation of preserved human amniotic membrane for surface reconstruction in severely damaged rabbit corneas. *Cornea.* 1995;14:473–484.
202. Stanzel BV, Espanja E, Grueterich M, et al. *Experimental Eye Research.* 2004;5:1–10.
203. Kiilgaard JF, la Cour M, Scherfig E, et al. Can transplantation of amniotic membrane prevent subretinal choroidal neovascularization? *Invest Ophthalmol Vis Sci.* 2001;41(4):1,253.
204. Hu J, Bok D. A cell culture medium that supports the differentiation of human retinal pigment epithelium into functionally polarized monolayers. *Molecular Vision.* 2001;7:14–19.
205. Valtink M, Engelmann K, Strauss O, et al. Physiological features of primary cultures and subcultures of human retinal pigment epithelial cells before and after cryopreservation for cell transplantation. *Graefes Arch Clin Exp Ophthalmol.* 1999;237:1,001–1,006.
206. Richard G. Transplantation of cultured retinal pigment epithelium. Second International Conference on Vitreoretinal Diseases, September 7–8, 2002, Vienna.
207. Van Meurs JC, van den Biesen PR. Autologous retinal pigment epithelium and choroid translocation in patients with exudative age-related macular degeneration. *ARVO Meeting Abstracts.* 2003.

Artificial Vision, Visual Prosthesis, and Retinal Implants

28

Richard M. Awdeh   *Rohit R. Lakhanpal*   *James D. Weiland*
Mark S. Humayun

RELEVANCE OF PROBLEM

Nearly 42 million people worldwide are legally blind (1). Over one million Americans contribute to this population (2). With increased average lifespan, the number of Americans with age-related eye disease and resulting visual impairment is expected to double during the next three decades. While ophthalmologists have been relatively successful at treating some of the most prevalent causes of visual impairment, including cataract and refractive error, hereditary retinal degeneration (e.g., retinitis pigmentosa [RP]) and age-related macular degeneration (AMD) are two examples of blinding retinopathies that, until lately, have had limited treatment options.

Retinitis pigmentosa is the leading inherited cause of blindness, with 1.5 million people worldwide affected and an incidence of 1 per 3,500 live births (3). AMD is the leading cause of visual loss among adults older than 65, with 700,000 newly diagnosed patients annually in the United States, of whom 10% become legally blind each year (4). Photodynamic and conventional laser therapy are two methods of slowing the progression of AMD. New surgical interventions (including macular translocation surgery [5–7] and intraocular retinal prosthesis) are examples of approaches currently being investigated to restore function caused by retinal disease. Genetic therapy offers the possibility of preventing or reversing the development of blindness from these diseases.

Lesions affecting the visual pathways or occipital cortex, such as those due to trauma, cortical tumors, or infarctions,

have traditionally presented a challenge in therapeutically addressing the associated visual loss. Thus far, physicians have been limited to offering low-vision devices to enhance the remaining vision. During the past few decades research in artificial vision has sought to create an alternative to provide useful vision for these patients. Therapeutically targeting and reversing the visual defect by an artificial prosthesis is now becoming possible for those patients who are left with no alternatives. This chapter will briefly summarize the history and evolution of the artificial visual prosthesis, including retinal implants, and present the current state of the field with the remaining challenges that lie ahead.

BACKGROUND AND HISTORY OF ARTIFICIAL VISION

Normal physiologic vision is initiated when light, passing through the cornea and lens of the eye to the rods and cones of the photoreceptor layer on the outer surface of the retina, causes photochemical transduction. The cell bodies of these receptors synapse with horizontal and bipolar cells. Bipolar cells synapse either directly or indirectly via amacrine cells with the ganglion cells (Fig. 28.1). The axons of the ganglion cells converge to form the optic nerve, acquire myelin sheathing upon exiting the lamina cribrosa, and travel posteriorly, joining the contralateral optic nerve to form the optic chiasm. The visual pathway continues as the optic tracks around the cerebral peduncle,

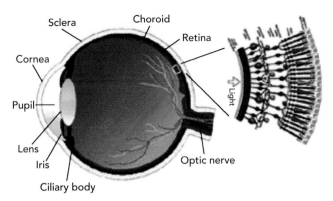

Figure 28.1 Human visual system I. Light travels through the tear film, cornea, aqueous, lens, and vitreous to activate the light-sensitive, multilayered neural network of cells and transsynaptic connections of the retina at the photoreceptor layer. Outer retinal degenerations, such as retinitis pigmentosa and age-related macular degeneration, primarily affect the photoreceptor layer and render millions legally blind.

to the lateral geniculate nucleus, and posteriorly via optic radiations to the primary visual cortex in the occipital lobe (Fig. 28.2). Visual information is then relayed from V1 to higher cortical association and processing areas.

Historically, several methods of supplementing remaining functional vision have been pursued via interventions at several points along the optic pathway, including the retina, optic nerve, and occipital cortex. The concept of electronically stimulating the nervous system to create artificial vision was first introduced in 1929. Foerster, a German neurosurgeon, observed that electrical stimulation of the visual cortex caused his subject to detect a spot of light (phosphene). He further demonstrated that the spatial psychophysical location of this phosphene depended upon the location of the electrical stimulation point over the cortex (8). Penfield and Rasmussen continued to experiment with electrical stimulation in creating visual sensations throughout the 1950s (9).

Advances in electrical engineering, computer sciences, and micromachining technology, including very large

scale integration (VLSI) microfabrications and microelectromechanical systems technology (MEMS), have all contributed to the evolution of the field of visual prostheses by allowing for the creation of both smaller electronics and smaller neural interfaces. These technological advancements, coupled with recent scientific investigations, have transformed the focus of the field from that of whether it is possible to create visual sensations through electrical stimulation to the more important question, whether this stimulation produces useful vision. Current issues being studied are the mechanical and electrical biocompatibility of the microelectronic implants and whether a whole visual image can be created by stimulation of many small areas of neuronal tissue.

Whether useful vision can be rendered via artificial visual prostheses depends on establishing a definition of useful vision, i.e., the minimum number of pixels required for human beings to accomplish activities of daily living. Several researchers have performed psychophysical experiments designed to determine the minimum acceptable resolution for useful vision. Brindley originally suggested that 600 points of stimulation (pixels) would be sufficient for reading ordinary print (10). More recent studies have tested humans with normal visual function by pixelating their vision. Using a small head-mounted video camera and monitor as via a portable phosphene simulator, patients walked through an obstacle course and read pixilated text. From this study it was concluded that 625 electrodes implanted in a 1 cm² area near the foveal representation in the visual cortex could produce a phosphene image producing approximately 20/30 acuity and reading rates near 170 words/minute with scrolled text and 100 words/minute with fixed text (11–13). Further, plasticity in the visual system was observed, as walking speeds increased 5-fold during 3 weeks of training (12). Other studies with electrodes placed over the entire macula, rather than a 1 cm² area, have assessed the ability of subjects to recognize faces through a pixilated square grid. Parameters included grid size, dot size, gap width, dot dropout rate, and gray scale resolution. The subjects achieved highly significant facial recognition accuracies in both high and low contrast, with a marked learning effect. These results suggest that reliable facial recognition is possible even with a crude visual prosthesis (14). The ability of subjects to read using a pixilated visual simulator, evaluated in a separate cohort, demonstrated that most subjects are able to read fonts as small as 36 point and all are able to read 57 point, using a 16×16 pixel array (15).

VISUAL PROSTHETICS

Occipital Cortex Prosthesis

Brindley and Dobelle continued to independently pioneer the field of artificial vision in the early 1970s, demonstrating the ability to evoke phosphenes and patterned perceptions

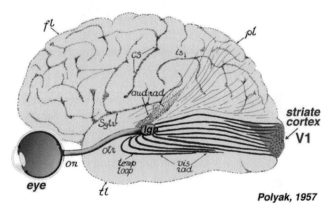

Figure 28.2 Human visual system II. Retinal ganglion cells merge to form the optic nerve, myelinate posterior to the orbit and merge with contralateral fibers to form the optic chiasm. The pathway terminates at the primary visual cortex in the occipital lobe.

by electrically stimulating the occipital cortex via implanted electrodes (10,16–22). Both researchers implanted arrays with over 50 electrodes subdurally over the occipital pole. These landmark experiments provided evidence of the ability to return the sensation of vision to individuals who had severed visual pathways, anterior to the visual cortex. Dobelle's 64 channel platinum electrode surface stimulation prosthesis allowed blind patients to recognize 6-inch characters at 5 feet (approximately 20/1200 acuity) (20,21,23). Problems identified from these experiments included: (1) controlling the number of phosphenes induced by each electrode; (2) interactions between phosphenes; (3) high currents and large electrodes that induced pain from meningeal stimulation; and (4) occasional focal epileptic activity following electrical stimulation (20,24,25). Patients in these initial experiments were unable to appreciate distinct phosphenes, but rather reported seeing "halos" surrounding each phosphene (26).

In order to address some of the shortcomings of surface cortical stimulation, intracortical stimulation was studied. Since most of the visual cortex is deep within the calcarine fissure and inaccessible to cortical surface electrodes, intracortical stimulation provided the ability to evaluate lower currents and effect higher fidelity (27). These intracortical devices employed smaller electrodes closer to the target neurons, thus requiring less current and resulting in a more localized stimulation. The stimulus threshold is 10 to 100 times lower for intracortical prostheses, as compared to surface stimulation. Further, this approach allows for closer spacing of electrodes at 500 μm (27). Initial studies of intracortical prosthesis, implanted in humans for a period of 4 months, demonstrated the ability to produce phosphenes which usually had color (27). Documented advantages of the intracortical versus surface cortical implants include: (1) predictable forms of elicited phosphenes; (2) absence of flicker phenomenon; (3) reduction in phosphene interactions: (4) increased number of electrodes; (5) reduced overall power requirement (25,27–29).

The Utah Electrode Array is a contemporary intracortical prosthesis, consisting of multiple silicon spikes, organized in a square grid measuring 4.2 mm by 4.2 mm (28). A platinum electrode is at the tip of each spike. A pneumatic system is employed to insert an array, consisting of 100 electrode devices, into the cortex in about 200 ms with minimal trauma (30). The cortical visual prosthesis is advantageous over other approaches because it bypasses all diseased visual pathway neurons rostral to the primary visual cortex. As such, this approach has the potential to restore vision to the largest number of blind patients.

There are some limitations to the cortical visual prostheses. First, histological changes from chronically implanted prosthetics need to be better understood (31–33). In the case of silicon doped penetrating electrodes, tissue reaction has ranged from none to gliosis and buildup of fibrotic tissue between the array and meninges (34). Second, the organization of the visual field is markedly more complex at the level of the primary cortex than at the retina or optic nerve and is not easily reproducible between patients (26). Next, the high level of specialization of every area of cortex for various parameters, including color, motion, and eye movement, make it unlikely to effect simple phosphenes from stimulation (35). Finally, surgical complications of this approach carry significant morbidity and mortality for the patient. The potential utility of the intracortical prosthesis requires further investigation in all of these areas.

Optic Nerve Prosthesis

The optic nerve has also been targeted as a potential site for the implementation of a visual prosthesis. Veraart et al. was one of the first groups attempting this, employing the concept of a spiral nerve cuff electrode (36–39). In this approach, an electrode cuff is surgically implanted circumferentially on the external surface of the optic nerve. As this device does not penetrate the optic nerve sheath, stimulation reflects the retinotopic organization within the optic nerve. Another group has recently implanted a chronic, self-sizing cuff with four electrodes in a human patient (40). Preliminary reports have demonstrated that electrical stimulation of the optic nerve produces colored phosphenes broadly distributed throughout the visual field (36–41).

The optic nerve is an appealing site for the implementation of a visual prosthesis as the entire visual field is represented in a small area. This area can be reached surgically and presents an accessible anatomic location for an implant. However, there are several challenges to address in this approach. First, the optic nerve is a densely consolidated neural structure, with approximately 1.2 million axons in a 2-mm-diameter cylinder. While this allows for the entire visual field to be represented in a relatively small area, it is difficult to achieve focal stimulation of neurons, and to appreciate the exact retinotopic cross-sectional profile of the optic nerve. The dense packing of neurons requires a large number of electrode contacts from the prosthesis in a small area, increasing the risk of damage to the nerve (42). Surgical manipulation of this area requires dissection of the dura, creating potentially harmful central nervous system effects, including interruption of blood flow to the optic nerve and infection. Fourth, intervention at this point within the optic pathway requires healthy retinal ganglion cells (RGC) and is, therefore, limited to the treatment of outer retinal (photoreceptor) degenerations. Last, the optic nerve and RGC represent higher order structures than the bipolar cells targeted by the retinal prosthesis. As such, much more image processing must be achieved by the implant rather than relying on the processing power of the lower order bipolar, horizontal, and amacrine cells in the visual physiologic pathways. Future development of this technology must address the above issues. Investigators have proposed intra-neuronal stimulation devices in order to more accurately target individual neurons within the optic nerve (43).

Retinal Prosthesis

Whereas the above prostheses are required for patients who have compromised visual pathways posterior to the retina, a microelectronic retinal implant may be suitable for cases in which the patient is affected by an outer retinopathy, as with RP or AMD. Nearly three decades ago, Potts demonstrated the concept of direct electrical stimulation of the retina by evoking an elicited response employing an electrode mounted on a corneal contact lens (44–46). This discovery was confirmed and expanded by Knighton, who demonstrated that inner retinal layers could be electrically stimulated and would elicit an electrical-evoked response (EER) (32,44–48). The more recent work of Humayun et al. has demonstrated that, even when there is profound photoreceptor loss in the above retinopathies, controlled electrical stimulation of the retina creates visual sensations in blind patients (49,50).

There is limited transsynaptic neuronal degeneration in RP and AMD, making it possible to electrically stimulate the remaining retinal neurons to elicit useful visual perceptions. This is supported by the post mortem morphometric analysis of the retina of patients with end-stage RP. This analysis has revealed that 78.4% of inner nuclear and 29.7% of ganglion layer cells were retained, compared to only 4.9% of photoreceptors (4,51–54). In legally blind neovascular AMD patients, 93% of RGC were spared (55,56). Furthermore, no statistical significance was noted in the ganglion cell density between non-neovascular eyes with geographic atrophy and age matched controls (55,56). This demonstrates limited transsynaptic neuronal degeneration in the aforementioned retinopathies, and supports the potential for the remaining retinal neurons to

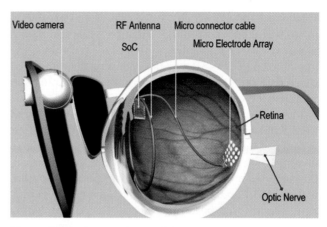

Figure 28.4 Illustrated view of the epiretinal prosthesis apparatus including the camera, connector cable, and microelectrode array is noted. Visual percepts are formed and transmitted through the optic nerve to the visual cortex.

elicit useful visual perceptions in response to a retinal prosthesis.

These initial observations have led to the development of an intraocular retinal prosthesis. This category of visual prostheses includes two different approaches: epiretinal and subretinal (Fig. 28.3).

Epiretinal Approach

The epiretinal prosthesis includes both an external, wearable component and an implantable, intraocular component (Fig. 28.4). The external portion is comprised of a lightweight camera built into spectacles, pocket batteries, and a small pager-sized visual processing unit. Power and data are sent wirelessly from this external unit to the internal portion of the prosthesis. The implanted portion of the device consists of a receiver/stimulating microelectronic chip and a microelectrode array. A current version includes 16 platinum electrodes of approximately 500 μm diameter (Fig. 28.5). This array is attached to the inner retinal surface.

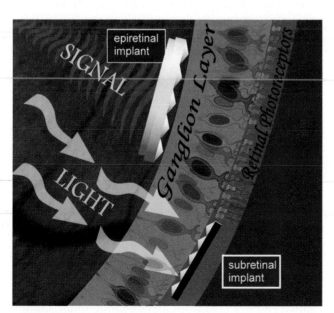

Figure 28.3 Illustrated topographic cross section of the retinal layers with epiretinal and subretinal implant locations, demonstrating the mechanism of light activation of both implants. The epiretinal implant is situated closer to the retinal ganglion cell layer and the subretinal implant is situated closer to the photoreceptor layers.

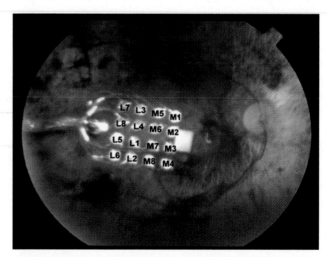

Figure 28.5 Fundus photograph of implanted epiretinal prosthesis in a patient with retinitis pigmentosa. Note that each platinum electrode is labeled with a unique designation for localization of percepts. This implant is located in the macula.

This model allows for digital video capture and translation to an external pixilated image. The final processed data is transferred to the implanted portion of the prosthesis. The implanted part of the device then converts the transferred visual data into controlled patterns of electrical pulses to stimulate the remaining retinal neurons.

Preliminary tests of epiretinal electronic stimulation were performed in humans (49,50,57). During these short periods of electrical stimulation, patients were able to identify crude forms such as letters or a box shape. Further, they reported no persistence of the image pursuant to stimulation (50). Based on these encouraging results, a permanent implant trial began in 2002 at the Doheny Retina Institute (DRI) as part of an FDA Investigational Device Exemption study. To date, three patients have received implants, each including 16-electrode, model 1 devices (Second Sight). During the follow-up period, objective (EERs recorded from the visual cortex) (Fig. 28.6) and subjective evidence of visual perception has been obtained. Patients report visual percepts in locations consistent with the implanted electrodes, the ability to discriminate between percepts created by different electrodes based on the locations of the percepts, the ability to discern brighter or dimmer percepts with varying levels of current, and the ability to distinguish the direction of motion of objects (58). Further, the subjects used the external imaging system to detect ambient light, being able to locate a flashlight carried by a person who was 120 cm away in 10/10 trials and also locating a dark object under normal room light conditions.

These preliminary patient tests are most encouraging because they provide further evidence of plasticity/learning curve of the visual pathway and demonstrate that epiretinal stimulation can be conducted in a retinotopic manner. While RGC are located in closest proximity to the microelectrode array and require less current, stimulation of these cells would require more image processing and complex stimulation patterns to account for lost retinal processing, and sub-optimal, larger, and ill-defined percepts (59,60). It is more desirable to stimulate the deeper bipolar cells, thereby utilizing the intact processing capability of

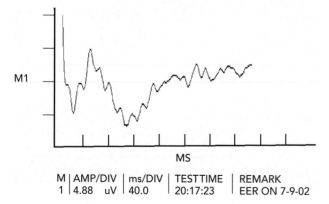

M	AMP/DIV	ms/DIV	TESTTIME	REMARK
1	4.88 uV	40.0	20:17:23	EER ON 7-9-02

Figure 28.6 Electrical-evoked response (EER) elicited from a patient with retinitis pigmentosa implanted with the epiretinal prosthesis during electrical stimulation.

inner retina cell layers. Experiments have found that higher pulse width stimulate RGC directly while photoreceptors and bipolar cells preferably respond to lower pulse width (61). Further, RGC responded to shorter pulse durations (<0.5 msec) while deeper retinal neural layers responded to longer pulse durations (>0.5 msec) (61). This evidence, coupled with the initial patient testing above, argues for the ability of the epiretinal prosthesis to create a visual perception with a maintained degree of retinotopy.

The advantages of the epiretinal approach include the following: (1) the epiretinal placement allows for the vitreous to act as a sink for heat-dissipation from the microelectronic device; (2) a minimal number of microelectronics are incorporated into the implantable portion of the device; (3) the wearable portion of electronics allows for easy upgrades without requiring subsequent surgery; and (4) the electronics allow the user and the doctor full control over every electrode parameter and digital signal processing involved in imaging objects.

The disadvantages to this approach include: (1) the requirement of techniques that will provide prolonged adhesion of the device to the inner retina; and (2) the increased current needed to stimulate the target bipolar cells using an epiretinal device when compared to a subretinal device, due to its closer proximity to these target cells.

Subretinal Approach

The subretinal approach to the retinal prosthesis involves implanting a microphotodiode array between the bipolar cell layer and retinal pigment epithelium. This is accomplished surgically either via an intraocular approach through a retinotomy site (ab interno) or a trans-scleral approach (ab externo). The subretinal prosthesis has two inherent advantages over the epiretinal prosthesis: (1) the implant is anatomically closer to the next surviving neuron in the visual pathway (bipolar cells) and therefore should require less current; and (2) the subretinal placement eliminates the need for adhesives to hold the implant in place. Further, prototype models of this design claim to not require external power sources or cameras, allowing the implant to be a stand alone, passive device. Current models incorporate 20 μm × 20 μm photodiodes which mimic the function of natural photoreceptor cells, absorbing photons of light 500 to 1,100 nm in wavelength and converting these stimuli to electrical impulses (26,62,63). These photodiodes are spaced 10 μm apart, allowing for over 1,000 photodiodes/mm², creating a density which rivals that of naturally occurring RPE cells (26).

As with the epiretinal prosthesis, the FDA approved a pilot study of the subretinal prosthesis. Chow et al. (64) reported subjective improvement in visual function in patients who received a subretinal implant placed approximately 20° superior and temporal to the macula (Fig. 28.7). However, these improvements in visual function have been attributed to an unknown, indirect effect of the implant rather from the activation of neurons by the prosthesis (60).

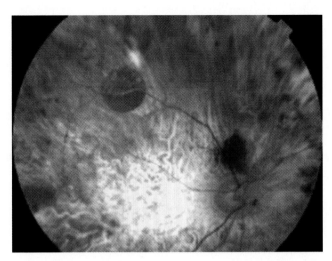

Figure 28.7 Fundus photograph of implanted subretinal prosthesis. Note that the implant is located outside the macula.

In theory, the subretinal prosthesis offers an attractive solution to enhance the vision of patients affected by RP and AMD. However, several limitations currently hinder this technology. Of primary concern is the inefficiency of current photodiode technology. The illumination levels required in order to achieve adequate electrical current generation are not realistically attainable as the solar cells will need to generate electrical energy many orders of magnitude greater than that which is currently available (26,62,65). This limitation jeopardizes the passive, all inclusive nature of the subretinal prosthesis, which more than likely will require active power supplementation from an external source in order to achieve threshold current levels.

Further, there are reports of histological changes to the surrounding retina including a decrease in the cellular density of the inner retina, expression of glial fibrillary acidic protein (GFAP) in Müller glia, and the presence of macrophages in the implant site (26,63,65). Finally, the anatomical location of the implant between two layers of retina does not allow for ample heat-dissipation. Research is ongoing to address these problems. The next generation of subretinal prostheses will include a porous architecture, allowing nutritional exchange between the retina and underlying choroids in an attempt to alleviate histological changes (66). Additionally, investigators are attempting to increase the spectrum of photodiode absorption to include infrared light in order to increase the energy delivery potential of current arrays (62,66,67).

FUTURE OF ARTIFICIAL VISION

Attempts to restore vision to the blind have been made throughout modern medicine and have most recently included cortical, optic nerve, and retinal prostheses. While each of these emerging technologies has the promise of restoring useful vision to these patients, there are still several hurdles to overcome. Advances in computer sciences and engineering technology, including VLSI and MEMS, will help researchers overcome these obstacles and develop prostheses which will incorporate more electrodes and generate denser pixel maps. Newer approaches, including the insertion of light-sensitive nanoparticles into the ganglion cell layer (68) or developing retinal prostheses using microfluid pumps to deliver neurotransmitters, such as GABA to activate neurons (60), may help play a role in the restoration of vision. Ultimately, these technologies will result in not only providing vision for unaided mobility, but also allow higher resolution vision that may enable reading and face recognition.

REFERENCES

1. WHO. *Blindness and Visual Disability: Seeing Ahead—Projections into the Next Century.* Geneva: WHO; 1997.
2. Ross RD. Is perception of light useful to the blind patient? [comment]. *Archives of Ophthalmology.* 1998;116(2):236–238.
3. Bunker CH, Berson EL, Bromley WC, et al. Prevalence of retinitis pigmentosa in Maine. *American Journal of Ophthalmology.* 1984;97(3):357–365.
4. Curcio CA, Medeiros NE, Millican CL, Photoeceptor loss in age-related macular degeneration. *Investigative Ophthalmology & Visual Science.* 1996;37(7): 1,236–1,249.
5. Fujii GY, Humayun MS, Pieramici DJ, et al. Initial experience of inferior limited macular translocation for subfoveal choroidal neovascularization resulting from causes other than age-related macular degeneration. *American Journal of Ophthalmology.* 2001;131(1):90–100.
6. Fujii GY, de Juan E Jr, Sunness J, et al. Patient selection for macular translocation surgery using the scanning laser ophthalmoscope. *Ophthalmology.* 2002;109(9):1,737–1,744.
7. Ng EW, Bressler NM, Boyer DS, et al. Iatrogenic choroidal neovascularization occurring in patients undergoing macular surgery. *Retina.* 2002; 22(6):711–718.
8. Foerster O. Beitrage zur pathophysiologie der sehbahn und der spehsphare. *J Psychol Neurol.* 1929;39:435–463.
9. Penfield WR, T. *The Cerebral Cortex of Man: A Clinical Study of Localization of Function.* New York: Macmillan; 1950.
10. Brindley G. The number of information channels needed for efficient reading. *J Physiol.* 1965;177:44.
11. Cha K, Horch KW, Normann RA. Simulation of a phosphene-based visual field: visual acuity in a pixelized vision system. *Annals of Biomedical Engineering.* 1992;20(4):439–449.
12. Cha K, Horch KW, Normann RA. Mobility performance with a pixelized vision system. *Vision Research.* 1992;32(7):1,367–1,372.
13. Cha K, Horch KW, Normann RA, et al. Reading speed with a pixelized vision system. Journal of the *Optical Society of America A-Optics & Image Science.* 1992;9(5):673–677.
14. Thompson RWB, D Humayun MS, Dagnelie G. Facial Recognition Using Simulated Prosthetic Pixelized Vision. In Press. 2003.
15. Hayes JSPD, Weiland JD, Humayun MS, et al. Visually guided performance of simple tasks using simulated prosthetic vision. *Journal of Vision.* 2003;In Press.
16. Brindley GRD. Implanted stimulators of the visual cortex as visual prosthetic devices. *Trans Am Acad Ophthalmol Otolaryngol.* 1974(78):741–745.
17. Brindley GS. Sensations produced by electrical stimulation of the occipital poles of the cerebral hemispheres, and their use in constructing visual prostheses. *Annals of the Royal College of Surgeons of England.* 1970;47(2): 106–108.
18. Brindley GS, Lewin WS. The sensations produced by electrical stimulation of the visual cortex. *Journal of Physiology.* 1968;196(2):479–493.
19. Brindley GS, Lewin WS. The visual sensations produced by electrical stimulation of the medial occipital cortex. *Journal of Physiology.* 1968;194 (2):54–5P.
20. Dobelle WH, Mladejovsky MG. Phosphenes produced by electrical stimulation of human occipital cortex, and their application to the development of a prosthesis for the blind. *Journal of Physiology.* 1974;243(2):553–576.
21. Dobelle WH, Mladejovsky MG, Evans JR, et al. "Braille" reading by a blind volunteer by visual cortex stimulation. *Nature.* 1976;259(5,539):111–112.
22. Dobelle WH, Quest DO, Antunes JL, et al. Artificial vision for the blind by electrical stimulation of the visual cortex. *Neurosurgery.* 1979;5(4): 521–527.
23. Dobelle WH. Artificial vision for the blind by connecting a television camera to the visual cortex. *ASAIO Journal.* 2000;46(1):3–9.
24. Pollen DA. Responses of single neurons to electrical stimulation of the surface of the visual cortex. *Brain, & Evolution.* 1977;14(1–2):67–86.

25. Schmidt EM, Bak MJ, Hambrecht FT, et al. Feasibility of a visual prosthesis for the blind based on intracortical microstimulation of the visual cortex. *Brain.* 1996;119(Pt 2):507–522.
26. Maynard EM. Visual prostheses. *Annual Review of Biomedical Engineering.* 2001;3:145–168.
27. Bak M, Girvin JP, Hambrecht FT, et al. Visual sensations produced by intracortical microstimulation of the human occipital cortex. *Medical & Biological Engineering & Computing.* 1990;28(3):257–259.
28. Maynard EM, Nordhausen CT, Normann RA. The Utah intracortical Electrode Array: a recording structure for potential brain-computer interfaces. *Electroencephalography & Clinical Neurophysiology.* 1997;102(3):228–239.
29. Uematsu S, Chapanis N, Gucer G, et al. Electrical stimulation of the cerebral visual system in man. *Confinia Neurologica.* 1974;36(2):113–124.
30. Rousche PJ, Normann RA. Chronic intracortical microstimulation (ICMS) of cat sensory cortex using the Utah Intracortical Electrode Array. IEEE *Transactions on Rehabilitation Engineering.* 1999;7(1):56–68.
31. McCreery DB, Yuen TG, Agnew WF, et al. A characterization of the effects on neuronal excitability due to prolonged microstimulation with chronically implanted microelectrodes. *IEEE Transactions on Biomedical Engineering.* 1997;44(10):931–939.
32. Agnew WF, Yuen TG, McCreery DB, et al. Histopathologic evaluation of prolonged intracortical electrical stimulation. *Experimental Neurology.* 1986;92(1):162–185.
33. Weiland JD, Anderson DJ. Chronic neural stimulation with thin-film, iridium oxide electrodes. *IEEE Transactions on Biomedical Engineering.* 2000;47(7):911–918.
34. Normann RA, Maynard EM, Rousche PJ, et al. A neural interface for a cortical vision prosthesis. *Vision Research.* 1999;39(15):2,577–2,587.
35. Margalit E, Maia M, Weiland JD, et al. Retinal prosthesis for the blind. *Survey of Ophthalmology.* 2002;47(4):335–356.
36. Veraart C, Raftopoulos C, Mortimer JT, et al. Visual sensations produced by optic nerve stimulation using an implanted self-sizing spiral cuff electrode. *Brain Research.* 1998;813(1):181–186.
37. Naples GG, Mortimer JT, Scheiner A, et al. A spiral nerve cuff electrode for peripheral nerve stimulation.[comment] *IEEE Transactions on Biomedical Engineering.* 1988;35(11):905–916.
38. Sweeney JD, Mortimer JT. An asymmetric two electrode cuff for generation of unidirectionally propagated action potentials. *IEEE Transactions on Biomedical Engineering.* 1986;33(6):541–549.
39. Ungar IJ, Mortimer JT, Sweeney JD. Generation of unidirectionally propagating action potentials using a monopolar electrode cuff. *Annals of Biomedical Engineering.* 1986;14(5):437–450.
40. Buckett JR, Peckham PH, Thrope GB, et al. A flexible, portable system for neuromuscular stimulation in the paralyzed upper extremity. *IEEE Transactions on Biomedical Engineering.* 1988;35(11):897–904.
41. Delbeke J, Oozeer M, Veraart C. Position, size and luminosity of phosphenes generated by direct optic nerve stimulation. *Vision Research.* 2003;43(9):1,091–1,102.
42. Cuoco FA Jr, Durand DM, Measurement of external pressures generated by nerve cuff electrodes. *IEEE Transactions on Rehabilitation Engineering.* 2000;8(1):35–41.
43. Branner A, Normann RA. A multielectrode array for intrafascicular recording and stimulation in sciatic nerve of cats. *Brain Research Bulletin.* 2000;51(4):293–306.
44. Potts AM, Inoue J. The electrically evoked response of the visual system (EER). 3. Further contribution to the origin of the EER. *Investigative Ophthalmology.* 1970;9(10):814–819.
45. Potts AM, Inoue J. The electrically evoked response (EER) of the visual system. II. Effect of adaptation and retinitis pigmentosa. *Investigative Ophthalmology.* 1969;8(6):605–612.
46. Potts AM, Inoue J, Buffum D. The electrically evoked response of the visual system (EER). *Investigative Ophthalmology.* 1968;7(3):269–278.
47. Knighton RW. An electrically evoked slow potential of the frog's retina. II. Identification with PII component of electroretinogram. *Journal of Neurophysiology.* 1975;38(1):198–209.
48. Knighton RW. An electrically evoked slow potential of the frog's retina. I. Properties of response. *Journal of Neurophysiology.* 1975;38(1):185–197.
49. Humayun MS, de Juan E Jr, Dagnelie G, et al. Visual perception elicited by electrical stimulation of retina in blind humans. *Archives of Ophthalmology.* 1996;114(1):40–46.
50. Humayun MS, de Juan E Jr, Weiland JD, et al. Pattern electrical stimulation of the human retina. *Vision Research.* 1999;39(15):2,569–2,576.
51. del Cerro M, Gash DM, Rao GN, et al. Retinal transplants into the anterior chamber of the rat eye. *Neuroscience.* 1987;21(3):707–723.
52. Humayun MS, Prince M, de Juan E Jr, et al. Morphometric analysis of the extramacular retina from postmortem eyes with retinitis pigmentosa. *Investigative Ophthalmology & Visual Science.* 1999;40(1):143–148.
53. Santos A, Humayun MS, de Juan E Jr, et al. Preservation of the inner retina in retinitis pigmentosa. A morphometric analysis. *Archives of Ophthalmology.* 1997;115(4):511–515.
54. Stone JL, Barlow WE, Humayun MS, et al. Morphometric analysis of macular photoreceptors and ganglion cells in retinas with retinitis pigmentosa. *Archives of Ophthalmology.* 1992;110(11):1,634–1,639.
55. Kim SY, Sadda S, Humayun MS, et al. Morphometric analysis of the macula in eyes with geographic atrophy due to age-related macular degeneration. *Retina.* 2002;22(4):464–470.
56. Kim SY, Sadda S, Pearlman J, et al. Morphometric analysis of the macula in eyes with disciform age-related macular degeneration. *Retina.* 2002;22(4):471–477.
57. Gerding H, HR, Eckmiller R, et al. Implantation, mechanical fixation, and functional testing of epiretinal multimicrocontact arrays (MMA) in primates [abstract]. *Invest Ophthalmol Vis Sci.* 2001;42 (Suppl):S814.
58. Humayun MSW, Fujii J, Greenberg GY, et al. Visual Perception in a Blind Subject with a Chronic Microelectronic Retinal Prosthesis. In Press. 2003.
59. Greenberg RJ, Velte TJ, Humayun MS, et al. A computational model of electrical stimulation of the retinal ganglion cell. *IEEE Transactions on Biomedical Engineering.* 1999;46(5):505–514.
60. Lakhanpal R, Yanai D, Weiland JD, et al. Advances in the development of visual prostheses. *Current Opinion in Ophthalmology.* 2003(14):122–127.
61. Greenberg R, Analysis of electrical stimulation of the vertebrate retina—work towards a retinal prosthesis in PhD Dissertation. Baltimore: The Johns Hopkins University; 1998.
62. Chow AY, Peachey NS. The subretinal microphotodiode array retinal prosthesis.[comment] *Ophthalmic Research.* 1998;30(3):195–198.
63. Peyman G, Chow AY, Liang C, et al. Subretinal semiconductor microphotodiode array. *Ophthalmic Surgery & Lasers.* 1998;29(3):234–241.
64. Chow AY, PG, Pollack JS, et al. Safety, feasibility and efficacy of subretinal artificial silicon retina prosthesis for the treatment of patients with retinitis pigmentosa [abstract]. *Invest Ophthalmol Vis Sci.* 2002;43(E-abstract 2,849).
65. Zrenner E, Stett A, Weiss S, et al. Can subretinal microphotodiodes successfully replace degenerated photoreceptors? *Vision Research.* 1999;39(15):2,555–2,567.
66. Schubert M, Lehner H, Werner J. Optimizing photodiode arrays for the use as retinal implants. *Sensors Actuators.* 1999(74):193–197.
67. Schubert M, Stelzle M, Graf M, et al. Subretinal implants for the recovery of vision. IEEE International Conf Systems Man Cybernetics. 1999, Tokyo, Japan. 376–381.
68. Greenbaum EH, MS Kuritz T, et al. Application of photosynthesis to artificial sight. 2001, Presented at 23rd Annual International Conference of the IEEE Engineering in Medicine and Biology Society, Istanbul, Turkey.

Neuroprotection in Macular Degeneration

29

Joyce Tombran-Tink   Colin J. Barnstable

INTRODUCTION

Age-related macular degeneration (AMD) is the most prevalent neurodegenerative disease in the world. It has a major impact on the health care system in many countries. Severe economic and quality of life dilemmas exist for AMD patients and their families. Less obvious are the costs of increased care needs of elderly patients, either by paid care providers or by family members who lose income in the process. Though it is not a life threatening disease, AMD can substantially increase the risk of fatal accidents. Early onset and juvenile forms of macular degeneration also represent a serious health issue. Since many specific forms of macular disease are grouped under the general heading of macular degeneration, important differences in causation and required therapy can be masked.

AMD is characterized by the death of cone photoreceptors, most noticeable in the macular region. The cellular and spatial variability of degeneration in this group of diseases has important implications for understanding the causes and progression of these entities, as well as for the types of therapy and drug delivery systems that are likely to be successful. Such variability makes research more difficult than that for rod-based photoreceptor diseases. Our understanding of rod photoreceptor degeneration, as in retinitis pigmentosa (RP), has developed rapidly because of the availability of good animal models (1) that mimic identical gene defects for many human forms of RP. Our knowledge of cone photoreceptor degeneration in AMD has been limited because few common experimental animals have a macula, making good models of this disease difficult to establish.

In this chapter, we will first consider the possible causes of AMD, since the different mechanisms and cell types involved will greatly influence the type of therapeutic agents

developed and the delivery methods used. The objective is not to present solutions to all the complex issues that surround the pathogenesis and treatment of MD. Rather, we look at what is currently known in the field of ocular neuroprotection, explore other possibilities for future MD treatment, perhaps provoke some new questions, and offer hope to those suffering from this condition.

Neuroprotection therapy can regulate cell death cascades triggered by a variety of intrinsic and extrinsic factors. The potential for use of polypeptide neuroprotective therapeutics to prevent or delay the progressive visual loss associated with AMD will be discussed. We predict that neuroprotective approaches will rapidly become major components of AMD therapy in the near future. The interrelationships between the various elements are shown diagrammatically in Figure 29.1.

CELLULAR TARGETS OF MACULAR DEGENERATION

Macular degeneration is defined as either wet or dry. The wet form is a neovascular disease (CNV) that affects approximately 10% of the AMD patient population. Cone loss is secondary to the abnormal growth of leaky blood vessels. CNV alone represents 80% of the legal blindness from AMD. The loss of vision is rapid and severe. Choroidal capillaries, the mainstay of nutritional support for the outer retina, proliferate and extend through defects in Bruch's membrane and junctional complexes of the RPE layer into the subretinal space. Disruption of the normal retinal architecture, serous and hemorrhagic detachment of the RPE and retina, pigment remodeling, and disciform scarring contribute to the death of photoreceptors in the macular region. In the absence of CNV, geographic atrophy

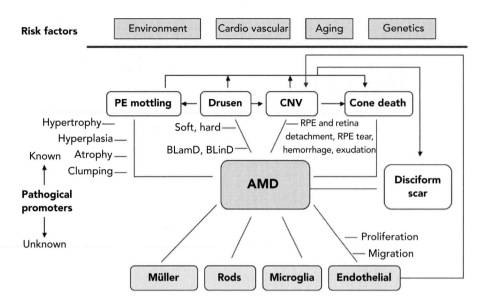

Figure 29.1 A diagrammatic representation of the risk factors and the pathological processes that can lead to macular degeneration. AMD, age-related macular degeneration; CNV, choroidal neovascularization; PE, pigment epithelium; RPE, retinal pigment epithelium.

of the RPE occurs as an end stage pathology in a specific type of advanced AMD (2).

The dry form of AMD can be considered a typical neurodegenerative disease where a primary defect disrupts the function and viability of a specific group of neurons: cone photoreceptors. Since dry AMD is one of the strongest risk factors for developing the wet form of AMD, treating dry AMD may be sufficient, in some cases, to prevent progression to the wet form, thereby preserving the remaining vision in these patients.

Photoreceptors

A number of cell types may be involved in the development and progression of AMD. Although death of cone photoreceptors and consequent loss of vision are endpoints of AMD, it is far from clear that the disease begins in these cells. Cones are closely associated with a number of other cell types, any of which could be the source of the primary defect in AMD. In fact, the survival and function of cones may be due to trophic influences from rod photoreceptors. There is one model suggesting that AMD begins in rod photoreceptors and that loss of cones is secondary (3). Among the lines of evidence supporting this idea are the dependence on rod development for final cone differentiation in many species and the later loss of cones seen in RP patients. A working hypothesis is that soluble factors secreted from rods are essential for normal cone physiology. The existence and identity of such factors have yet to be elucidated. The potential trophic, physical, or biochemical interdependence of retinal cells for survival is an interesting concept and one that is worthy of exploring in developing therapeutics for retinal degenerations.

The two other cell types in intimate contact with cones are retinal pigment epithelial (RPE) cells and Müller glial cells. These two cell types form the major components of

the blood-retinal barrier for the choroidal and retinal circulation, respectively. They regulate nutrient flow to photoreceptors and control the composition of the extracellular environment surrounding rods and cones.

Müller Glial Cells

These cells span the whole thickness of the retina and interact closely with all other retinal cell types. They clearly have a role in maintaining retinal structure because treatments that disrupt Müller cells lead to retinal folding and other abnormalities. The lateral processes of Müller cells surround synapses, including those of photoreceptors. This contact is critical even for foveal photoreceptors and serves to maximize the actions of neurotransmitters at appropriate postsynaptic sites. Müller processes also function to remove neurotransmitters at these sites rapidly to prevent them from diffusing to adjacent cells (4). In the outer retina, junctional complexes among Müller glial cells and between them and photoreceptor inner segments form the outer limiting membrane. Müller glial cells contain glycogen stores and presumably use them to regulate glucose availability to photoreceptors and other retinal cells. Disruption of any of these functions may put the retina at risk for retinal degenerations. In this context, a new conceptual framework is needed to address the role of Müller cells in cone degeneration. We discuss how Müller cells could serve as good targets for many of the agents that have shown promise in protecting photoreceptors in animal models of RP.

Retinal Pigment Epithelial Cells

Morphologically, RPE cells form a highly polarized epithelial sheet that separates the retina from the choroid. They secrete many growth factors that are important to survival of the adjacent retinal cells, and possibly cells of the choroid (5). RPE cells are responsible for phagocytosis of photoreceptor outer segments and contain key enzymes essential for the isomerization of retinoids in the visual cycle. The apical surface contains numerous microvilli that interdigitate between photoreceptor outer segments and provide a greatly expanded surface contact between the two cell types (Fig. 29.2). On the lateral faces of the RPE cells, a band of tight junctions creates a high resistance barrier to movement of ions and larger molecules in and out of the subretinal compartment. The basal RPE surface contains many infoldings that increase surface area. The whole RPE sheet sits on the extracellular material of Bruch's membrane. Defects in transport molecules at apical or basal surfaces, in junctional and other cell adhesion molecules, or in the secretion of trophic factors, could all compromise RPE cell function and lead to subsequent photoreceptor damage. One possible explanation for the infrequency of such defects may be that epithelial sheets in other parts of the body share the same molecules. A common defect involving multiple sites in the body might be lethal to the host.

The photoreceptor outer segments protrude into a unique compartment bounded by the RPE and Müller cells. The molecular composition of this compartment, the interphotoreceptor matrix (IPM), is also unique and contains components secreted by rod and cone photoreceptors, Müller cells, and RPE cells. In addition to transporting molecules among the cells bordering the IPM, various proteins and glycosaminoglycans provide a scaffold for the photoreceptor outer segments and regulate the water and ion content of their environment (6). Several trophic and neuroprotective factors have been identified in the IPM suggesting that this compartment serves as a dynamic neurotrophic reservoir that readily makes available molecules that are important to maintaining the health of cells in contact with it. Excessive stress on photoreceptors, either by strong light or other forms of metabolic stress, might cause release of neuroprotective factors from their matrix binding sites. Such a response could provide rapid protection that would not be possible if the signal had to be sent to either RPE or Müller glial cells to alter rates of expression of these factors. The function of many of the other IPM molecules remains unknown and the possibility that alterations in some of them may cause photoreceptor degeneration has yet to be fully explored.

Endothelial Cells

The proliferation and migration of endothelial cells can be thought of as the primary event causing the wet form of AMD because this condition is associated with neovascularization. Therefore, the effects of any therapies on these cells are of significance and should be carefully examined. For example, molecules that have the dual effects of promoting survival and differentiation of neurons need to be tested on endothelial cells to determine whether they have the added advantage of decreasing endothelial cell proliferation.

Microglial Cells

Microglia are a normal component of the retina. In the subretinal space, the number of these cells responds to metabolic conditions and stress. For example, the number of microglia in the subretinal space can be increased in experimental animals by increases in light exposure (7). In the brain, microglia play a major role in inflammatory processes that contribute to neuronal cell death by their secretion of cytokines that activate cell death signaling pathways. There is currently debate about the role of inflammatory processes in the development or progression of AMD (8,9). Whether microglia become activated and secrete factors that damage photoreceptors in AMD is not clear and thus, more research emphasis should be focused in understanding the role of microglia as a causative cell type in AMD.

Are Drusen a Target for AMD Therapy?

Finally, drusen, basal deposits external to the RPE which contain products of one or more of the cell types already discussed, should be included as a causative agent of AMD. Although the place of drusen in the development and progression of AMD is still debated, it is the earliest morphological feature of AMD. Drusen can be detected during fundoscopic eye examinations. They are described as hard,

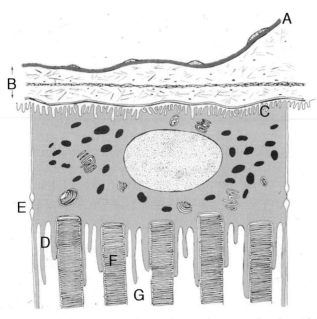

Figure 29.2   RPE cells form a barrier between the choroidal blood supply and the photoreceptor outer segments. Pathological changes in many of these structures are associated with the progression of macular degeneration. **A.** endothelial cells of the choroidal capillaries; **B.** Bruch's membrane; **C.** basal infoldings of the RPE cell; **D.** apical microvilli of the RPE cell; **E.** tight junctions between RPE cells forming a blood retinal barrier; **F.** photoreceptor outer segments; **G.** interphotoreceptor matrix.

soft, or diffuse, according to their size, matrix components, abundance, and shape. These deposits are further classified as distinct morphological classes. The basal laminar (BlamD) deposits are composed of a granular matrix with wide spaced collagen and are positioned between the plasma membrane and basal lamina of the RPE. The basal linear (BlinD) deposits contain membranogranular material and are located external to the basal lamina of the RPE in the inner collagenous zone of Bruch's membrane. Drusen contain a variety of lipids, polysaccharides, and glycosaminoglycans and numerous drusen proteins have been identified (10). Some of these molecules may be derived from RPE cells, some from photoreceptors and some from choroidal cells. It is not clear whether the presence of serum proteins in drusen represents a causative event or just a later stage of protein sticking.

Although the presence of soft drusen in the macular region is often called early AMD, the correlation between the presence of drusen and development of AMD is not strong enough to think of it as causative. Nevertheless, AMD is almost invariably accompanied by drusen formation, suggesting that they may be a contributing factor, if these deposits reach a certain size, frequency, or have a specific composition. The composition of drusen from normal and AMD eyes is very similar and there is little evidence yet of a unique component(s) in AMD drusen that could be used as a therapeutic target. It has, however, been noted that drusen from AMD eyes have a higher level of oxidative damage than those from normal and it has been proposed that oxidative modifications may be an initial step in drusen formation (10).

It is also likely that the presence of drusen can cause lateral stretching of the RPE monolayer and displacement of these cells from their vascular supply. Drusen may also exert pressure on photoreceptors and disrupt their architecture. Both effects could cause sufficient physical damage to initiate degeneration. In addition, these deposits could serve as a physical barrier between RPE cells and the choroidal circulation that would impede movement of nutrients, waste, the diffusion of oxygen, and other trophic factors that are required for retinal function. Drusen may exert a direct toxic action on surrounding RPE and photoreceptors.

While these can all be considered risk factors to the progression of AMD, they also offer potential AMD therapies. For example, the physical barriers created by drusen may also impede the movement of drugs from the choroidal circulation to the photoreceptors. Another important consideration for developing AMD therapies is whether drugs are selectively absorbed by drusen, thus changing the local pharmacokinetic profile. While we are beginning to understand the morphology and composition of drusen, little has been done to target these deposits in approaches to preserve vision. This is a wide open field for developing formulations to breakdown and remove drusen matrix as early intervention strategies to unclog the area between the RPE and basal vascular supply.

CELL DEATH IN MACULAR DEGENERATION

The current view of AMD is that most cases are caused by the confluence of multiple genetic and/or environmental factors, possibly in several different cell types. Whatever the causative factors, the end result is death of photoreceptors. There is general agreement that most of the photoreceptor cell death in AMD occurs through apoptosis. Some idea of the intensity with which apoptosis is being studied can be gained from the observation that there are over 10,000 papers per year published on this subject. In spite of this, there are still no good drugs that can therapeutically block apoptotic cell death.

Apoptosis has a distinct set of biochemical and morphological changes that occur in various cell compartments (11). The cells shrink and the endoplasmic reticulum vacuolates. In the nucleus, chromatin condenses to form compact masses and the DNA is fragmented by endonucleases. Eventually the cell disintegrates. Much of the cellular damage is initiated by the activation of a proteolytic cascade mediated by a set of enzymes called caspases. Although this cascade has been studied intensively, it is generally assumed that once the caspase cascade has been activated it is too late to save the cell. Thus, most therapies are designed to stop activation.

Caspase activation can occur by two pathways: a receptor-mediated or extrinsic pathway and a mitochondrial or intrinsic pathway. The two major membrane molecules that are linked to receptor-mediated apoptosis are Fas (CD95) and the tumor necrosis factor receptor (TNFR). Binding of ligands to these receptors activates initiating caspases (caspase-8 or caspase-10) that, in turn, activate the death cascade. It may be possible to block signals transduced by these receptors by activating lateral cell protective pathways, such as the NFkB cascade, that can intercept the direct vertical transmission of these signals to the nucleus and thus inhibit the flow of external cell death information.

The mitochondrial or intrinsic apoptotic pathway is activated by various stresses, most commonly oxidative stress. A protein complex forms a pore in the mitochondrial membrane through which cytochrome c leaks out. Cytochrome c forms a complex with the protein Apaf-1 and this can then activate the caspase cascade.

There are a large number of proteins that can promote or inhibit the formation of the mitochondrial pore. The effectiveness of proteins, such as Bad or Bax at promoting apoptosis, or of Bcl-2 or Bcl-X, at inhibiting apoptosis, has been amply demonstrated in animal models. These proteins have been overexpressed in transgenic mice or removed by gene knockout methods. However, effective pharmacologic modulation of their activity to regulate apoptosis has yet to be achieved.

Intracellular transduction pathways, leading to activation of the kinase Akt, can block apoptosis by decreasing the activity of Bad and by inhibiting the transcription factors necessary for the expression of other proapoptotic genes. Several of the neuroprotective factors described below cause activation of Akt. Thus part of their function may be as direct inhibitors of apoptosis.

A powerful method of protecting neurons from a variety of toxic insults has been to increase the activity of mitochondrial uncoupling proteins. These proteins allow a controlled leak of hydrogen ions across the inner mitochondrial membrane. Although this can decrease the driving force for ATP synthesis, it also decreases the driving force for calcium influx into the mitochondrion and decreases the endogenous production of reactive oxygen species (12). Activation of mitochondrial uncoupling proteins by genetic or dietary manipulations has shown protective effects on hippocampal neurons in models of epilepsy, on substantia nigra neurons in models of Parkinson's disease, and on retinal ganglion cells (13–15). Since the inner segments of photoreceptors contain an abundant population of mitochondria, it may be worthwhile to explore whether an increase of mitochondrial uncoupling protein activity or changing mitochondrial membrane potential could slow down intrinsic cell death signals at the onset of photoreceptor degeneration as it does for other neurons mentioned above.

NEUROPROTECTION

There are two overall approaches to therapeutic intervention for any degenerative disease arising from multiple causes. The first is to design and apply, in appropriate combinations, upstream therapies that counteract each of the causative factors or the receptors that transmit their signals. The second is to design a therapy that acts at a junctional point downstream that is common to all forms of the degenerating stimuli. It is the second of these that will be considered in the remainder of the chapter.

The goal of neuroprotective therapy is not only to prevent neurons from dying, but to maintain their functionality. While neuroprotective therapy could be directed toward any of the cell types mentioned above, our discussion will focus on factors that were originally thought to act directly on the affected neurons. As we shall see, direct actions on the target degenerating cells may not be necessary and the most effective factors may have additional actions that make them better suited for neuroprotective therapy.

Some success has been demonstrated by targeting excitotoxic damage in the central nervous system (CNS). Many of the agents in use serve as antagonists of glutamate receptors, particularly of N-methyl-D-aspartate (NMDA) receptors. By blocking excessive stimulation of the receptors from elevated concentrations of glutamate, these neuroprotective agents lessen depolarization of neurons, decrease calcium influx, and reduce the production of other potentially toxic compounds such as nitric oxide. This form of therapy may have potential in stroke and other brain trauma, as well as for ocular diseases, such as glaucoma. Other antagonists, particularly the α_2 antagonist brimonidine, show strong protection in a number of models of glaucoma, as well as in ischemia-reperfusion models of retinal damage (16,17). These studies indicate that application of brimonidine to the ocular surface can effect pharmacologically active concentrations in the retina.

This approach of blocking excessive neurotransmitter action may be less appropriate in AMD because photoreceptors are primary sensory neurons and receive no synaptic input. To prevent photoreceptor cell death, therefore, we need to devise neuroprotective therapies that work at some point between the initial toxic stimulus and the irreversible activation of a death cascade. These could be neuroprotective proteins, small molecules, or receptor antagonists/agonists.

The reported success of some of these approaches in neurodegeneration models has been associated with a recent resurgence of enthusiasm for neuroprotective therapy. As a cautionary note, the retina is a complex tissue, exposed to dozens of growth factors, cytokines, neurotrophic factors, and their respective receptors, with developmental, spatial, and pathological regulation of many of these molecules and their cognate receptors. In addition, there are issues of cell type specificity, interactions with other available factors in normal and pathological conditions, and multiple or sometimes opposing functions of a single factor. Until the biological responses to neuroprotective factors are fully understood, use of these factors may lead to a host of inadvertent side effects.

NEUROPROTECTIVE FACTORS AND THEIR RECEPTORS

Many neuroprotective molecules have been identified that show strong clinical protective effect for photoreceptors. For example, the small molecule, docosahexaenoic acid, promotes survival of rod photoreceptors in vitro, in part by increasing expression of anti-apoptotic genes such as Bcl-2 and decreasing expression of apoptotic genes such as Bax (18). Although this fatty acid is present at high levels in the retina and is clearly important for the development and normal function of photoreceptors, increasing dietary intake of docosahexaenoic acid does not correct a progressive rod-cone degeneration in dogs (19). The bulk of the evidence for such molecules is that they are essential for retinal health, but that they are unable to act as therapeutic neuroprotective factors by themselves.

We will, therefore, focus on four different proteins that show protection in a wide range of neurodegenerative models and which could be useful neuroprotective approaches for AMD. The factors are BDNF, CNTF, GDNF, and PEDF. The following short synopsis of the structure of each, their receptors, and their signal transduction pathways will provide a useful background for discussion of their role in retinal neuroprotective therapies.

Brain-Derived Neurotrophic Factor

Brain-derived neurotrophic factor (BDNF) is a member of the neurotrophins, a family of structurally and functionally related polypeptides that includes nerve growth factor (NGF), NT-3, and NT-4 (20,21). These are all small homodimeric polypeptides of 120 amino acids. BDNF was purified from pig brain as a factor that enhanced the survival and process outgrowth of neurons from many regions of the CNS, including retinal ganglion cells (22,23). There are sequence similarities between BDNF and NGF, the archetypal neurotrophic factor. Structural studies of the neurotrophins show that these factors consist of sheets of amino acids held together by a characteristic knot of disulphide linkages. The loops of amino acids extending from this structure contain the residues that give specificity to receptor binding. These loops of amino acids show extensive variability among the family members and may be responsible for the varying functions of the proteins. BDNF is expressed in regions that are targets for responsive neurons, suggesting that it serves as a target-derived neurotrophic factor. This is particularly true for retinal ganglion cells that appear to depend upon BDNF derived from target tissues.

BDNF binds to TrkB, one member of a family of high affinity tyrosine kinase neurotrophin receptors. BDNF may exert its neurotrophic activity, in part, by forming homodimers that bind to TrkB receptors to induce receptor dimerization and activation by phosphorylation. Phosphorylation of specific tyrosine residues on the cytoplasmic domain of TrkB creates docking sites for adapter proteins that, in turn, lead to activation of intracellular signaling cascades, most notably the extracellular-signal-regulated kinase (ERK)1,2 MAPK pathway, the PI3kinse/Akt pathway, and PLC-1 (24–26) that often constitute neuroprotective cascades.

Ciliary Neurotrophic Factor

Ciliary neurotrophic factor (CNTF) is a member of the family of IL-6-related cytokines (27). Closely related family members, leukemia inhibitory factor (LIF) and oncostatin M mimic many of the actions of CNTF. CNTF, derived from chick heart and embryo extracts, was described 25 years ago as a neurotrophin that improved survival of chick ciliary ganglion cells (28). Ten years later this cytokine was cloned and sequenced from rat tissue. The cloned cDNA predicted a 200 amino acid protein with a molecular mass of 22,800. CNTF has no detectable glycosylation site and contains a single cysteine residue, two properties rare in secreted proteins. Unlike the other factors described in this section, CNTF does not have a cleaved signal sequence characteristic of secreted proteins. It has been suggested that CNTF may, therefore, not function in the same way as most classical neurotrophic factors

because it is released only from tissues when they are damaged. The crystal structure of CNTF shows that it contains a core bundle of four α helices linked by loops of amino acids. Sequence variability in these loops give the different members of the IL-6 family of cytokines their unique properties and actions.

The neurotrophic activity of CNTF is linked to transduction cascades through a receptor that consists of three components. A CNTFR subunit binds only with relatively low affinity to CNTF alone. This interaction allows formation of a complex with two other polypeptides, Gp130 and LIFR. Gp130 is a common signal transducing receptor subunit for all of the IL-6 family of cytokines. IL-6 itself binds to two molecules of Gp130 whereas CNTF, LIF, and a few other members of the family bind to one Gp130 molecule and one LIFR subunit. The interactions of CNTF with its receptor subunits have been mapped to separate sites on the CNTF molecule, suggesting that it acts to cross link the receptor subunits as a mechanism to transduce its biological activity.

Activation of the CNTF receptor, in turn, activates two signal transduction pathways, the JAK/STAT pathway and the Erk1/2 MAPK pathway. Within the retina there is some evidence that activation of one or other of these pathways is restricted to specific cell types, although both can be activated in adult Müller glial cells. Although Müller glial cells are one of the strongest candidates to respond to and transmit CNTF signals to other cell types of the retina, there is still ongoing debate about which cells actually mediate CNTF neurotrophic actions in the retina.

Glial Cell Line-Derived Neurotrophic Factor

Glial cell line-derived neurotrophic factor (GDNF) is a member of a family of related neurotrophic factors that includes neurturin, persephin, and enovin/artemin (29). GDNF was originally isolated based on its potent and specific ability to promote the survival and morphological differentiation of dopaminergic neurons in embryonic midbrain cultures. This factor showed potent activity in reducing symptoms of Parkinson's disease, chemically induced in rodents or primates. It also promotes survival, neurite outgrowth, and choline acetyltransferase activity in motor neurons. GDNF is synthesized by a number of cell types in the retina, among them glial cells found at the optic nerve head (30). Like most other neurotrophic factors, GDNF is expressed outside the nervous system and exerts effects on the development of other organs such as the kidney.

The GDNF gene encodes a mature protein of 134 amino acid and is a distant member of the transforming growth factor family with about 19% sequence homology to other related members of this family. Like many secreted proteins, GDNF is produced as a pre-profactor. The signal sequence is first cleaved to yield a pro-GDNF that, in turn, is cleaved by further proteolysis to become the active factor. Functional studies using recombinant fragments of GDNF show that the C-terminus but not the N-terminus of the protein is essential for biological activity and that specific regions of the four helices and two pleated sheets that make up the molecule are necessary for receptor binding. GDNF interacts with heparin sulphate proteoglycans as a possible mechanism that allows it to localize and concentrate at sites of action. However, the precise functions of this binding is still unclear.

The receptors for the GDNF family of factors are multi-component complexes consisting of the c-Ret receptor tyrosine kinase and a glycosylphosphatidylinositol (GPI)-anchored accessory receptor (GFR). Four GFR subunits have been described, one for each member of the GDNF family. Binding of GDNF to its receptor is very avid with dissociation constants in the low picomolar range, suggesting that concentrations of GDNF below 1 ng/mL should be maximally effective. Actions of GDNF that are independent of c-RET may involve complexes of GFR with the cell adhesion molecule N-CAM. Thus, for the GDNF family of factors, there is the potential for activation of several different receptor pathways by a single factor.

GDNF triggers at least two transduction pathways. It activates Erk1/2 MAPkinase through a pathway involving phosphorylation of Ras and it activates PI3kinase and Akt through a pathway involving several intermediates.

PEDF

PEDF was first identified to have a neurotrophic activity in conditioned medium obtained from fetal human RPE cell cultures by Tombran-Tink and Johnson in 1987. The activity was subsequently purified and found in a single protein that migrated as a closely spaced doublet of 50 kD on SDS gels. At concentrations as low as 1 nM, purified PEDF effectively switched Y79 retinoblastoma cells from an actively growing suspension cell line to non-proliferating cells that attached to a substrate, extended neurites, and increased expression of molecules associated with differentiated neurons (31,32).

RPE cells synthesize and secrete PEDF into the interphotoreceptor matrix between the RPE layer and the photoreceptors. More recently other sites of PEDF expression in the eye have been found. These include the retinal ganglion cells, several cell types in the cornea and the ciliary epithelial cells, which are probably the major source of the human PEDF found in the vitreous overlaying the retina.

PEDF transcripts are also found in most regions of the brain and the protein is detected in the CSF as well (33). Ependymal cells are likely to be a major source of PEDF in human CSF, suggesting that, like the retina, much of the brain and spinal cord are bathed in this neurotrophic factor. In the spinal cord, PEDF is localized to motor neurons of the ventral horn and some neurons in the dorsal horn. Several non-neural tissues including skeletal muscle, bone, heart, placenta, and liver also synthesize PEDF.

The PEDF gene has been mapped to human chromosome 17p13.3, a hot spot for many retinal degenerative diseases and several severe brain disorders. The retinal diseases in this region of the chromosome include retinitis pigmentosa (RP13), Leber's congenital amaurosis, and a cone-rod dystrophy (CORD 5), all of which are characterized by loss of photoreceptor function and visual impairment. To date, no disease causing mutations have been detected in the PEDF gene.

The gene for this neurotrophic factor encodes a 418 amino acid protein with a hydrophobic signal characteristic of secreted proteins and a calculated molecular weight of 46.3 kD. The protein contains a single carbohydrate side chain that raises its apparent molecular weight to the 50 kD doublet seen on SDS gels. PEDF has structural and sequence homology to members of the serpin family of protease inhibitors. It contains a characteristic serpin reactive loop (RCL), but inhibitory activity against proteases has yet to be detected. The crystal structure of PEDF was recently determined at 2.85 resolution using recombinant human PEDF, expressed in and purified from hamster cells. The structure shows that the molecule contains two sites for interactions with extracellular matrix molecules. A concentration of aspartic and glutamic acid side chains in the N-terminal portion of PEDF promotes binding with high affinity to type I collagen and with lower affinity to type III collagen. Low affinity interactions between PEDF, heparin, and other glycosaminoglycans have been found and are probably mediated by a large surface on the PEDF protein that is rich in the basic amino acids, lysine and arginine. Whether a pool of bound PEDF exists and whether it can be released under specific conditions of activity or injury are not known.

Like most of the other neurotrophic factors discussed in this chapter, PEDF is likely to bind to cell surface receptors. It is unlikely that the intact protein is transported into the cells without cleavage because of its large size. However, it is the large, 50 kD doublet form that has been identified on western blots of cell extracts and cell conditioned medium, thereby challenging this presumption. While binding sites with an affinity in the nanomolar range have been detected, it is still unclear whether these represent a receptor for PEDF or regulatory proteins important for its function.

The current data on intracellular signaling pathways activated by PEDF are still very preliminary. Increased phosphorylation of IB, decreased levels of IB proteins, activation of NFB, nuclear translocation of p65 (RelA), and increased NFB DNA binding activity are all events triggered by PEDF during treatment of immature cerebellar granule cells (34). PEDF-induced activation of NFkB promotes survival of these cells by subsequent increases in the expression of the antiapoptotic genes, Bcl-2 and Bcl-X and the neurotrophic factors, BDNF, NGF, and GDNF. In retinal endothelial cells, PEDF alters activation of the ERK1,2 MAPK proteins by mechanisms that are not clear, especially since it can increase the detectable ERK1,2

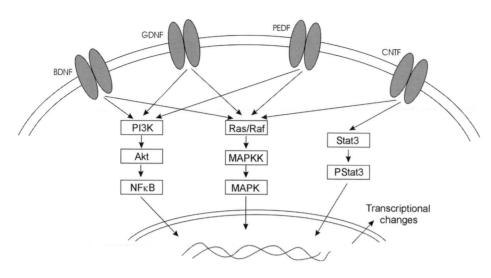

Figure 29.3 Diagrammatic representation of the major transduction pathways used by the neuroprotective factors discussed in this chapter. While novel transduction pathways may yet be defined for these factors, it is clear that most of them act in very similar ways and all four can influence the phosphorylation of the MAPK pathway.

phosphorylation in some cells and decrease the protein level in others (35).

PEDF differs from the other neuroprotective factors listed above in that it is also a potent antiangiogenic factor, an activity not described as yet for CNTF, BDNF, or GDNF (reviewed in reference 51). It inhibits endothelial cell migration and is described as being more effective than the well-studied angiogenesis inhibitor, angiostatin, even in the presence of the proangiogenic factor FGF (36). In ocular tissues and endothelial cells, PEDF expression is reduced while secretion of the angiogenic factor VEGF is increased under a strong stimulus for angiogenesis. In vitreous samples from patients, there is significant correlation between the ratio of PEDF and VEGF and the extent of neovascular disease. The lower the ratio the greater the outcome for neovascularization (37,38). Delivery of PEDF to the eye blocks neovascularization induced by one of several different methods. For some retinal diseases, including AMD, the dual properties of PEDF, neuroprotective and antiangiogenic, makes this protein an attractive candidate for neuroprotective therapy.

In summary, these four neuroprotective factors belong to different gene families and bind to different classes of receptors. Interestingly, however, they activate some common transduction pathways, as indicated diagrammatically in Figure 29.3. It is tempting to speculate that these common pathways are the major ones that lead to the neuroprotective effect and that other transduction pathways activated by these factors give them their unique properties.

EFFICACY OF NEUROPROTECTIVE FACTORS IN THE CNS

All four factors described above have been used in a wide range of in vitro and in vivo models from which their neuroprotective properties have been defined. At its simplest, neuroprotection reduces the cell death that occurs following presentation of a toxic insult. For example, when dissociated cultures of neurons are treated with micromolar concentrations of glutamate, cell death is proportional to the concentration of the excitotoxin present. Low nanomolar concentrations of PEDF prevents glutamate induced apoptotic cell death in cultures of cerebellar granule cells, hippocampal pyramidal cells, and spinal cord motor neurons (reviewed in reference 50). BDNF provides protection from glutamate excitotoxicity by several mechanisms, including down-regulation of NMDA receptors and subsequent reduction of calcium influx (39,40). Similarly, in cultures of cortical neurons, GDNF prevents excitotoxic neuronal death by reducing NMDA-receptor-mediated Ca^{2+} influx through an ERK-dependent pathway (41).

These factors also will protect against oxidative stress, one of the most common causes of neuronal death and a possible contributing factor to AMD. One way of experimentally inducing oxidative stress is by treating cells with low concentrations of hydrogen peroxide. When retinal neurons were pretreated with PEDF, they became more resistant to moderate concentrations of hydrogen peroxide (Fig. 29.4). The protection only occurred when cells were pretreated for at least an hour. Even after pretreatment, high concentrations of hydrogen peroxide were still toxic. This study emphasizes that the protection by these factors is finite, that strong toxic insults will still cause death, and that neuroprotective pathways must be activated before a rapidly acting toxic insult, like hydrogen peroxide, activates cell death cascades. Much work remains to be done to define the mechanism by which PEDF protects retinal neurons. BDNF protects against oxidative stress as well and it has been suggested that its mechanism of action is to reduce endogenous production of reactive oxygen species, possibly by actions at the level of the mitochondria (42,43).

It is well known that several neuroprotective factors can provide protection to photoreceptors in experimental animal models. FGF2 was the first of these to delay photoreceptor degeneration in the RCS strain of rats carrying an

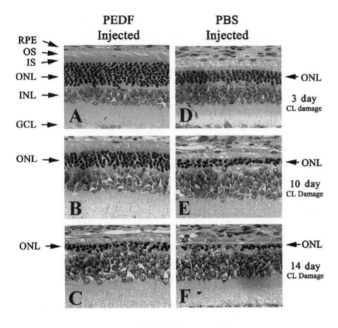

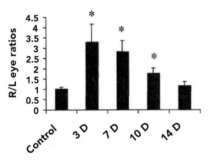

Figure 29.4 *Top Panel:* Rescue of photoreceptors by PEDF as a function of constant light-exposure. Animals were injected intravitreally with PEDF or PBS 2 days before light exposure. PEDF-injected eyes exposed to constant light for 3 (**A**), 10 (**B**), and 14 days (**C**). PBS-injected eyes exposed to constant light for 3 (**D**), 10 (**E**), and 14 (**F**) days. *Bottom panel.* Preservation of retinal function by PEDF. Mean right-to-left eye ratios of ERG B-wave amplitudes. *, $P = 0.05$ versus control group (*n* 56). CL, constant light; GCL, ganglion cell layer; INL, inner nuclear layer; ONL, outer nuclear layer; R/L, right/left. (Adapted from Cao et al., 1999.)

inherited retinal dystrophy (44). This effect of FGF2 on photoreceptor protection was seen following either intravitreal or subretinal injection. However, FGF2 also causes an increase in retinal microglia and cataracts. These observations, together with its known angiogenic potential on endothelial cells and its mitogenic effect on RPE cells and Müller glial cells, make FGF2 unsuitable as a candidate therapeutic agent for AMD.

On the other hand, intravitreally injected FGF2 protects rat photoreceptors against degeneration caused by constant light (45), a result that provides support for the idea that neuroprotective factors can inhibit a variety of insults to photoreceptors. In a larger study, a series of neuroprotective factors were injected intravitreally 2 days before a 1-week exposure of rats to constant bright light. FGF1, FGF2,

BDNF, CNTF, and IL-1b gave strong protection against damage induced by the constant light (46). Like the FGFs, IL-1b had a number of undesirable side effects including a large increase in the infiltration of macrophages and the induction of retinal folds and rosettes. BDNF and CNTF, on the other hand, showed promise as good candidates for photoreceptor protection without the side effects observed for FGF and IL-1b.

GDNF has not yet been fully tested in animal models of retinal disease but is effective in neuroprotective assays for other neurological models. GDNF has been shown to reduce motor neuron death and enhance axonal recovery after peripheral nerve injury in newborn or adult animals (47). It also modulates neuronal damage in models of epilepsy and in neurotoxin-induced models of Parkinson's disease. Unfortunately, in human trials for Parkinson's disease, patients given GDNF systemically experienced severe side effects, including weight loss. In both in vitro and in vivo models of ischemic damage, GDNF was shown to reduce excitotoxic neuronal cell death, not by directly preventing apoptosis, but rather by reducing calcium influx through NMDA receptors (41).

There is also substantial evidence that PEDF provides protection to neurons in vivo. In neonatal mice, axotomy by sciatic nerve section led to death of about 50% of motor neurons. Application of PEDF at the axotomy site reduced motor neuron death by 57% and prevented atrophy of the living neurons (48). Similarly, in an organotypic rat spinal cord culture model of chronic glutamate toxicity that mimics a defect in glutamate transport in ALS, PEDF was effective both in decreasing the slow degeneration of motor neurons and in preserving motor neuron processes (49). The potency of PEDF was comparable to gabapentin, riluzole, and IGF-1, all of which have been tested for clinical neuroprotective efficacy in this model and used clinically for chronic motor neuron diseases.

More relevant to AMD is the fact that PEDF stops the degeneration of rat photoreceptors after exposure to constant light (50). The effect is as potent as that described above for BDNF and CNTF. Similarly, progression of photoreceptor degeneration is delayed in *rd* mutant mice and apoptosis is reduced in photoreceptor cells in *rds* mutant mice treated with PEDF (51). These two mouse models have human counterparts in forms of retinitis pigmentosa. The death of photoreceptors arising from other insults also can be attenuated by PEDF. For example, those resulting from exposure of dissociated retinal cultures to oxidative damage caused by hydrogen peroxide (52) and those exposed to increased intraocular pressure from transient ischemia-reperfusion (53). Increased pressure within the eye is a major risk factor for glaucoma and its associated ganglion cell death.

Several general conclusions can be drawn from the efficacy studies described above. The first is that polypeptide neuroprotective factors are effective agents in protecting neurons against a wide range of insults. The second is that, for at least some of the factors, photoreceptors are protected equally as well as other neurons. The third is that the factors all show only temporary effects in chronic neurodegeneration models. The transience of this effect may be related to the experimental design, where a single application is given at the beginning of the experiment, the lack of stability of the neuroprotective agent, or its clearance over an extended period of time. It is likely that multiple treatments or the use of intraocular sustained release systems would be more effective in maintaining protection over a longer time frame.

Do Neuroprotective Factors Act Directly on the Degenerating Target Cells in the Retina?

In addition to direct effects on neurons, neuroprotective factors may also exert their effects by acting on other neighboring cell types that influence the activity of such neurons. Support for this hypothesis includes the findings that receptors for BDNF are not detected on normal rod photoreceptors, yet rods are protected from toxic damage by BDNF and the conflicting reports about the presence of receptors for CNTF on rod photoreceptors, with evidence for its presence better for some species than others. There are also inconsistent results about whether the intracellular signal transduction pathways for CNTF are present in photoreceptors and, if they are, whether they can be activated by CNTF.

Receptors for both BDNF and CNTF are found on Müller cells and, for CNTF, it is clear that the factors activate both known intracellular transduction pathways. It is possible that the primary neuroprotective effect of BDNF and CNTF is on Müller cells and that they, in turn, release neuroprotective factors that act on photoreceptors. For the other two neuroprotective factors discussed in this chapter, there is less information available. The primary cell target of GDNF in the retina is not known and PEDF acts on a variety of cell types including both neurons and glia. Its receptor has not yet been elucidated. PEDF also has autocrine actions on cells that secrete it, such as RPE. Thus, when considering AMD therapeutics, it may be worthwhile to develop strategies that influence both the target and supporting cells to maximize the effects of the treatment.

We pointed out earlier that several cell types, particularly the RPE cells, vascular endothelial cells, and microglia may all play important roles in the pathogenesis of AMD. BDNF is mitogenic for more than one microglial cell line and its receptors are found on these cells in primary culture (54). RPE cells express TrkB receptors and BDNF promotes differentiation and survival of these cells in several species. (55,56). There is general agreement that endothelial cells produce BDNF, but there is much less evidence that this factor can regulate endothelial cell function (57,58). This disparity in experimental results is, perhaps, due to variations in endothelial cells from different types of tissues. At present there is no information about the display of receptors or transduction cascades that these factors can stimulate on retinal endothelial cells.

Similarly, CNTF is produced by RPE and microglial cells, but there is no clear demonstration of its actions on these cells or on endothelial cells in the retina or choroid. GDNF, on the other hand, is produced by microglial cells and can enhance their survival and regulate the permeability of endothelial cell junctions (59,60). There is currently no evidence that GDNF is either synthesized by or acts on RPE cells.

PEDF is intimately involved in the physiology of most of the cell types that may be involved in the pathogenesis of MD. It is synthesized and secreted by the RPE and vascular endothelial cells. It protects photoreceptor cells, alters the morphology and properties of RPE and Müller glial cells, causes the production of other factors by microglial cells, and it has multiple inhibitory effects on endothelial cells during neovascularization (61–63).

PROTEINS OR PEPTIDOMIMETICS

Some of the problems encountered with using neuroprotective factors for treating retinal degenerations are that these factors are too large to diffuse easily into the eye, require multiple intraocular injections or they need to be delivered using viral vectors. To date, there have not been any systematic studies to identify smaller peptide fragments that mimic the neuroprotective functions of the whole molecule. There is limited information available for a large PEDF peptide that contains neurotrophic activity (reviewed in reference 63). The peptide is located in the N-terminal region of the molecule, although, from the crystal structure, much of it is buried in the interior of the molecule. It is possible that different functions of PEDF are mediated by separate epitopes on the protein. Whether each epitope is responsible for a specific effect on different cell types is currently unknown.

DELIVERY OF NEUROPROTECTIVE FACTORS

It is one thing to show that neuroprotective factors, or their peptide mimetics, are effective inhibitors of photoreceptor cell death. It is quite another to translate this finding into therapeutics for AMD. The indications from experimental models used so far suggest that the amounts of neuroprotective factors required for activity are relatively small, i.e., they work well in the low nanomolar-to-picomolar ranges. We will consider six strategies that have been used to make neuroprotective factors available to the photoreceptor layer of the retina. The first four represent physical delivery and the last two use viral vectors.

The simplest way of providing a neuroprotective factor is by systemic delivery. Since the factors under discussion are peptides, they are unlikely to survive the digestive tract. Thus, oral delivery is not likely to be effective. Systemic injection of neuroprotective factors is one option. In a mouse model of ischemia-induced retinopathy, daily injections of microgram quantities of PEDF prevented the retinal neovascularization seen in uninjected animals (64). The therapeutic threshold was determined to be 5 to 11 μg per day. Assuming there is a simple partition into the eye based on volumes only, the therapeutic dose in a mouse eye is approximately of the order of 1 ng. Given the restriction of PEDF movement by the blood retinal barrier, the binding of PEDF to other sites in the body and degradation of PEDF, the actual therapeutic dose may be much lower.

Although such experimental studies are encouraging there is still much work to be done to understand the activity of such molecules. We do not know how long injected neuroprotective factors remain intact in the body or how much reaches the target tissue. This is particularly an issue for factors such as PEDF that can bind to extracellular matrix molecules as well. Does this binding remove much of the diffusible factor? Can the extracellular matrix serve as a slow release reservoir? Is the injected factor the active agent or does it serve as a catalyst to stimulate the production of higher amounts of the same or a different protective factor.

Earlier, we discussed the possibility that CNTF and BDNF exert their protective effect on photoreceptors by primary actions on Müller glial cells. Perhaps systemically injected factors stimulate multiple cell types to produce a wide range of proteins that are involved in the protection effects. A further issue with systemic injection is that of unwanted side effects in other organs. One such example arose in the clinical trials of CNTF as a therapy for ALS where a substantial weight loss was observed among participants.

A second method of delivering neuroprotective factors is to inject them at the target site of action. For AMD, this means multiple intraocular or even subretinal injections. This strategy shows promise in several animal models. Injection of 1 μl of a 1μg/μl solution of BDNF, CNTF, or other potential neuroprotective factors into the vitreous of a rat eye provided protection against the damaging effects of 1 week of continuous light exposure. Although a number of diseases routinely require patients to carry out systemic injections at home, intraocular injections will require more careful administration by trained personnel and will most likely have greater risks of retinal damage. It is unclear how often such injections would be needed. If injections were needed once a week to provide an effective concentration of neuroprotective factor in the eye, this method would never become a widely used therapy.

A variant to this approach that holds promise is the development of long-term slow release pellets containing neuroprotective factors. Biodegradable polymers such as poly(lactide-co-glycolide) have been used to encapsulate proteins and peptides. These have been shown to release therapeutic doses of these molecules for extended periods (65,66). Examples of such studies using encapsulated neurotrophic factors have been shown in the brain and these have aided survival of transplants (67,68).

Finally, in attempts to target factors to the retina, we should not exclude application of such molecules to the ocular surface. For many years, application of eye drops containing drugs at pharmacologically active doses that diffused to the ciliary epithelium was used in the medical management of glaucoma. There is some evidence that drugs applied in this way can affect retinal physiology. Therefore, it is possible that therapies for AMD could be applied by eye drops. Unfortunately, the diffusion of neuroprotective proteins and peptides is slower than the small molecules currently used in eye drops and it is less likely that therapeutic doses could reach the retina by this route.

As an alternative, it may be possible to apply factors to the sclera overlying the retina. Experimental measurements of molecular diffusion across the sclera have found a rate inversely proportional to size. Proteins and nucleic acids large enough to be therapeutic agents can be induced to cross the sclera by application of a mild electric current (69). Although such methods have not yet been tested in animal models of retinal degeneration, it is easy to see how such treatments could be self administered or provided during simple office visits.

The other two methods of delivering neuroprotective vectors rely on delivery of a biological vector that carries the factor. Adenovirus and, more recently, adeno-associated viral constructs have been used to deliver therapeutic genes to localized target tissues. In the eye, a number of neuroprotective factors have now been delivered this way. Virally delivered CNTF can improve the survival of retinal ganglion cells and rod photoreceptors, as measured physiologically and anatomically (70–73). Similarly, viral delivery of PEDF into the vitreous or subretinal compartment can block retinal neovascularization. It is possible that virally vectored strategies could provide neuroprotective function as well. Six weeks after viral injections, levels of 20 to 70 μg PEDF per eye were measured (74) indicating that these vectors were able to produce therapeutic doses of PEDF over periods of at least 6 weeks. Similar results using PEDF DNA approaches have now been obtained by a number of other groups (75–78). Together they indicate that viral delivery of PEDF is effective in attenuating blood vessel growth.

Problems and patient risks are often encountered when using current DNA-mediated gene-transfer technologies. These include (1) obtaining clinically effective viral titers, (2) toxicity and immunogenicity as a result of the expression of viral genes, (3) stable transgene expression in individuals requiring long-term treatment, and (4) insertional mutagenesis by random viral integration into the host genome. Whether these problems prevent this approach from being generally acceptable to neuroprotective therapies for AMD remains to be seen.

In an effort to side step some of the problems associated with viral vectors, mammalian cells engineered to produce neuroprotective factors have been generated. Iris epithelial cells obtained from patients needing retinal protection can be engineered to produce high levels of a specific neuroprotective factors that, in turn, can be used to repopulate the diseased eyes (79). One AMD therapy under investigation is the transplantation of stem cells to replace lost photoreceptors. Such cells could also be engineered to produce neuroprotective factors and, when injected, would be at less risk from the microenvironment that led to loss of the photoreceptors. Engineered cells could also be encapsulated to lessen the probability that they will disperse from the site of injection or mount an immune response. These cells may provide implantable reservoirs of neuroprotective factors and are not restricted to autologous cells. Although the approach has been shown to work in several cases, it has yet to be applied to the eye and to diseases such as AMD. In a rat model, this approach of engineering cells to secrete PEDF was shown to be successful (79). Autologous iris epithelial cells, stably transfected to produce PEDF, were transplanted subretinally. The transplanted cells inhibited blood vessel growth in models of retinal neovascularization and inhibited photoreceptor death in a model of retinal degeneration. In both cases, higher levels of PEDF was expressed in the retina. It is possible that other types of cells, such as RPE cells from fetal or donor eye tissues, could be exploited for this form of neuroprotective strategy when autologous cells are not readily available. Such an approach may provide elevated levels of neuroprotective factors, as well as new RPE cells that could correct some of the pathologies resulting from the defective RPE cells associated with AMD.

Another approach, still in its infancy, is the use of stem cells genetically engineered to produce a target neuroprotective factor. In theory, after transplantation in the subretinal space, these cells would be given the appropriate retinal cues to undergo controlled differentiation and integration into the retina to replace lost photoreceptors. Such an approach would correct the visual deficits caused by AMD while, at the same time, allow adequate amounts of neuroprotective factor to become available to prevent more cells from dying.

SUMMARY AND PROSPECTS

There is now enough published evidence to conclude that neuroprotective factors can prevent cell death in models that mimic macular degeneration. Early findings of limited efficacy or short-term effects seem to be more related to issues of effective doses and sustained delivery. We still do not know if there are differences in the protective power of the various factors. This should become clearer as more information becomes available about the intracellular pathways activated by each factor. Although sustained delivery through gene transfer is a promising start, we predict that with continued improvement in long-term ocular drug delivery systems, pharmacological agents, developed from peptide derivatives of neuroprotective factors, will be the therapeutics of choice. Active mixtures of PEDF peptides offer a viable approach to controlling chronic diseases that have neovascular episodes, such as AMD, because of its additional anti-angiogenic properties. It is likely that a truly effective anti-angiogenic and neuroprotective therapy will require a mixture of agents and adjunctive strategies. The potency and multifaceted properties of PEDF suggest that it is likely to become one of the key elements in such a cocktail.

REFERENCES

1. Farrar GJ, Kenna PF, Humphries P. On the genetics of retinitis pigmentosa and on mutation-independent approaches to therapeutic intervention. *EMBO J.* 2002;21:857–864.
2. Sunness JS. The natural history of geographic atrophy, the advanced atrophic form of age-related macular degeneration. *Mol Vis.* 1999;5:25.
3. Mohand-Said S, Hicks D, Leveillard T, et al. Rod-cone interactions: developmental and clinical significance. *Prog Ret Eye Res.* 2001;20:451–467.
4. Buris C, Klug K, Ngo IT, et al. How Müller glial cells in macaque fovea coat and isolate the synaptic terminals of cone photoreceptors. *J Comp Neurol.* 2002;453:100–111.
5. Holtkamp GE, Kijlstra A, Peek R, et al. Retinal pigment epithelium-immune system interactions: cytokine production and cytokine-induced changes. *Prog Ret Eye Res.* 2001;20:29–48.
6. Hollyfield JG. Hyaluronan and the functional organization of the interphotoreceptor matrix. *Invest Ophthalmol Vis Sci.* 1999;40:2,767–2,769.
7. Ng TF, Streilein JW. Light-induced migration of retinal microglia into the subretinal space. *Invest Ophthalmol Vis Sci.* 2001;42:3,301–3,310.
8. Johnson LV, Leitner WP, Staples MK, et al. Complement activation and inflammatory processes in drusen formation and age related macular degeneration. *Exp Eye Res.* 2001;73:887–896.
9. Anderson DH, Mullins RF, Hageman GS, et al. A role for local inflammation in the formation of drusen in the aging eye. *Am J Ophthalmol.* 2002;134:411–431.
10. Crabb JW, Miyagi M, Gu X, et al. Drusen proteome analysis: an approach to the etiology of age-related macular degeneration. *Proc Natl Acad Sci USA.* 2002;99:14,682–14,687.
11. Lawen A. Apoptosis—an introduction. *BioEssays.* 2003;25:888–896.
12. Horvath TL, Diano S, Barnstable CJ. Mitochondrial uncoupling protein 2 in the central nervous system. *Biochem Pharmacol.* 2003;65:1917–1921.
13. Horvath TL, Diano S, Leranth C, et al. Coenzyme Q induces mitochondrial uncoupling and prevents dopamine cell loss in a primate model of Parkinson's disease. *Endocrinol.* 2003;144:2,757–2,760.
14. Diano S, Matthews RT, Patrylo P, et al. Uncoupling protein 2 prevents neuronal death including that occurring during seizures: a mechanism for preconditioning. *Endocrinology.* 2003;144:5,014–5,021.
15. Barnstable CJ, Li M, Reddy R, et al. Mitochondrial uncoupling proteins: regulators of retinal cell death. In: LaVail MM, Hollyfield JG, Anderson RE, eds. *Retinal Degeneration 2002.* New York: Kluwer Academic/Plenum Press; 2003:269–275.
16. Wheeler L, WoldeMussie E, Lai R. Role of alpha-2 agonists in neuroprotection. *Surv Ophthalmol.* 2003;48(Suppl)1:S47–S51.
17. Osborne NN, Chidlow G, Wood J, et al. Some current ideas on the pathogenesis and the role of neuroprotection in glaucomatous optic neuropathy. *Eur J Ophthalmol.* 2003;13:(Suppl)3:S19–S26.
18. Rotstein NP, Politi LE, German OL, et al. Protective effect of docosahexaenoic acid on oxidative stress-induced apoptosis of retina photoreceptors. *Invest Ophthalmol Vis Sci.* 2003;44:2,252–2,259.
19. Aguirre GD, Acland GM, Maude MB, et al. Diets enriched in docosahexaenoic acid fail to correct progressive rod-cone degeneration (PRCD) phenotype. *Invest Ophthalmol Vis Sci.* 1997;38:2,387–2,407.
20. Thoenen H. The changing scene of neurotrophic factors. *Trends Neurosci.* 1991;14:165–170.
21. Ibanez CF. Neurotrophic factors: from structure-function studies to designing effective therapeutics. *Trends Biotechnol.* 1995;13:217–227.
22. Leibrock J, Lottspeich FH, Holn A, et al. Molecular cloning and expression of brain-derived neurotrophic factor. *Nature.* 1989;341:149–152.
23. Barde YA, Davies AM, Johnson JE, et al. Brain derived neurotrophic factor. *Prog Brain Res.* 1987;71:185–189.
24. Cheng A, Wang S, Yang D, et al. Calmodulin mediates brain-derived neurotrophic factor cell survival signaling upstream of Akt kinase in embryonic neocortical neurons. *J Biol Chem.* 2003;278:7,591–7,599.
25. Han BH, Holtzman DM. BDNF protects the neonatal brain from hypoxic-ischemic injury in vivo via the ERK pathway. *J Neurosci.* 2000;20:5,775–5,781.
26. Nakazawa T, Tamai M, Mori N. Brain-derived neurotrophic factor prevents axotomized retinal ganglion cell death through MAPK and PI3K signaling pathways. *Invest Ophthalmol Vis Sci.* 2002;43:3,319–3,326.
27. Butte MJ. Neurotrophic factor structures reveal clues to evolution, binding, specificity, and receptor activation. *Cell Mol Life Sci.* 2001;58:1,003–1,013.
28. Varon S, Manthorpe M, Adler R. Cholinergic neuronotrophic factors: I. Survival, neurite outgrowth and choline acetyltransferase activity in mono-

layer cultures from chick embryo ciliary ganglia. *Brain Res.* 1979;173 (1):29–45.

29. Airaksinen MS, Saarma M. The GDNF family: signaling, biological functions and therapeutic value. *Nat Rev Neurosci.* 2002;3:383–394.

30. Wordinger RJ, Lambert W, Agarwal R, et al. Cells of the human optic nerve head express glial cell line-derived neurotrophic factor (GDNF) and the GDNF receptor complex. *Mol Vis.* 2003;9:249–256.

31. Tombran-Tink J, Johnson LV. Neuronal differentiation of retinoblastoma cells induced by medium conditioned by human RPE cells. *Invest Ophthalmol Vis Sci.* 1989;30:1,700–1,707.

32. Tombran-Tink J, Chader GG, Johnson LV. PEDF: a pigment epithelium-derived factor with potent neuronal differentiative activity. *Exp Eye Res.* 1991;53:411–414.

33. Tombran-Tink J, Mazuruk K, Rodriguez IR, et al. Organization, evolutionary conservation, expression and unusual Alu density of the human gene for pigment epithelium-derived factor, a unique neurotrophic serpin. *Mol Vis.* 1996;2:11.

34. Yabe T, Wilson D, Schwartz JP. NFkappaB activation is required for the neuroprotective effects of pigment epithelium-derived factor (PEDF) on cerebellar granule neurons. *J Biol Chem.* 2001;276:43,313–43,319.

35. Hutchings H, Maitre-Boube M, Tombran-Tink J, et al. Pigment epithelium-derived factor exerts opposite effects on endothelial cells of different phenotypes. *Biochem Biophys Res Commun.* 2002;294:764–769.

36. Dawson DW, Volpert OV, Gillis P, et al. Pigment epithelium-derived factor: a potent inhibitor of angiogenesis. *Science.* 1999;285:245–248.

37. Ogata N, Nishikawa M, Nishimura T, et al. Unbalanced vitreous levels of pigment epithelium-derived factor and vascular endothelial growth factor in diabetic retinopathy. *Am J Ophthalmol.* 2002;134:348–353.

38. Ohno-Matsui K, Morita I, Tombran-Tink J, et al. Novel mechanism for age-related macular degeneration: an equilibrium shift between the angiogenesis factors VEGF and PEDF. *J Cell Physiol.* 2001;189:323–333.

39. Courtney MJ, Akerman KE, Coffey ET. Neurotrophins protect cultured cerebellar granule neurons against the early phase of cell death by a two-component mechanism. *J Neurosci.* 1997;17:4,201–4,211.

40. Brandoli C, Sanna A, De Bernardi MA, et al. Brain-derived neurotrophic factor and basic fibroblast growth factor downregulate NMDA receptor function in cerebellar granule cells. *J Neurosci.* 1998;18:7,953–7,961.

41. Nicole O, Ali C, Docagne F, et al. Neuroprotection mediated by glial cell line derived neurotrophic factor: involvement of a reduction of NMDA-induced calcium influx by the mitogen-activated protein kinase pathway. *J. Neurosci.* 2001;21:3,024–3,033.

42. Iwata E, Asanuma M, Nishibayashi S, et al. Different effects of oxidative stress on activation of transcription factors in primary cultured rat neuronal and glial cells. *Brain Res Mol Brain Res.* 1997;50:213–220.

43. Yamagata T, Satoh T, Ishikawa Y, et al. Brain-derived neurotropic factor prevents superoxide anion-induced death of PC12h cells stably expressing TrkB receptor via modulation of reactive oxygen species. *Neurosci Res.* 1999; 35:9–17.

44. Faktorovich EG, Steinberg RH, Yasumura D. Photoreceptor degeneration in inherited retinal dystrophy delayed by basic fibroblast growth factor. *Nature.* 1990;347:83–86.

45. Faktorovich EG, Steinberg RH, Yasumura D, et al. Basic fibroblast growth factor and local injury protect photoreceptors from light damage in the rat. *J Neurosci.* 1992;12:3,554–3,567.

46. LaVail MM, Unoki K, Yasumura D, et al. Multiple growth factors, cytokines, and neurotrophins rescue photoreceptors from the damaging effects of constant light. *Proc Natl Acad Sci USA.* 1992;89:11,249–11,253.

47. Hottinger AF, Azzouz M, Deglon N, et al. Complete and long-term rescue of lesioned adult motoneurons by lentiviral-mediated expression of glial cell line-derived neurotrophic factor in the facial nucleus. *J Neurosci.* 2000;20: 5,587–5,593.

48. Houenou LJ, D'Costa AP, Li L, et al. Pigment epithelium-derived factor promotes the survival and differentiation of developing spinal motor neurons. *J Comp Neurol.* 1999;412:506–514.

49. Bilak MM, Corse AM, Bilak SR, et al. Pigment epithelium-derived factor (PEDF) protects motor neurons from chronic glutamate-mediated neurodegeneration. *J Neuropathol Exp Neurol.* 1999;58:719–728.

50. Cao W, Tombran-Tink J, Elias R, et al. In vivo protection of photoreceptors from light damage by pigment epithelium-derived factor. *Invest Ophthalmol Vis Sci.* 2001;42:1,646–1,652.

51. Cayouette M, Smith SB, Becerra SP, et al. Pigment epithelium-derived factor delays the death of photoreceptors in mouse models of inherited retinal degenerations. *Neurobiol Dis.* 1999;6:523–532.

52. Cao W, Tombran-Tink J, Chen W, et al. Pigment epithelium-derived factor protects cultured retinal neurons against hydrogen peroxide-induced cell death. *J Neurosci Res.* 1999;57:789–800.

53. Ogata N, Wang L, Jo N, et al. Pigment epithelium derived factor as a neuroprotective agent against ischemic retinal injury. *Curr Eye Res.* 2001;22: 245–252.

54. Zhang J, Geula C, Lu C, et al. Neurotrophins regulate proliferation and survival of two microglial cell lines in vitro. *Exp Neurol.* 2003;183: 469–481.

55. Hackett SF, Friedman Z, Freund J, et al. A splice variant of trkB and brain-derived neurotrophic factor are co-expressed in retinal pigmented epithelial cells and promote differentiated characteristics. *Brain Res.* 1998;789: 201–212.

56. Liu ZZ, Zhu LQ, Eide FF. Critical role of TrkB and brain-derived neurotrophic factor in the differentiation and survival of retinal pigment epithelium. *J Neurosci.* 1997;17:8,749–8,755.

57. Donovan MJ, Lin MI, Wiegn P, et al. Brain derived neurotrophic factor is an endothelial cell survival factor required for intramyocardial vessel stabilization. *Development.* 2000;127:4,531–4,540.

58. Ruprecht K, Stadelmann C, Hummel V, et al. Brain derived neurotrophic factor does not act on adult human cerebral endothelial cells. *Neurosci Lett.* 2002;330:175–178.

59. Igarashi Y, Utsumi H, Chiba H, et al. Glial cell line-derived neurotrophic factor induces barrier function of endothelial cells forming the blood-brain barrier. *Biochem Biophys Res Commun.* 1999;261:108–112.

60. Salimi K, Moser K, Zassler B, et al. Glial cell line-derived neurotrophic factor enhances survival of GM-CSF dependent rat GMIR1-microglial cells. *Neurosci Res.* 2002;43:221–229.

61. Tombran-Tink J, Barnstable CJ. PEDF: a multifaceted neurotrophic factor. *Nat Rev Neurosci.* 2003;4:628–636.

62. Bouck N. PEDF: anti-angiogenic guardian of ocular function. *Trends Mol Med.* 2002;8:330–334.

63. Tombran-Tink J, Barnstable CJ. Therapeutic prospects for PEDF: more than a promising angiogenesis inhibitor. *Trends Mol Med.* 2003;9:244–250.

64. Stellmach V, Crawford SE, Zhou W, et al. Prevention of ischemia-induced retinopathy by the natural ocular antiangiogenic agent pigment epithelium-derived factor. *Proc Natl Acad Sci USA.* 2001;98:2,593–2,597.

65. Saltzman WM, Olbricht WL. Building drug delivery into tissue engineering. *Nat Rev Drug Discov.* 2002;1:177–186.

66. Cypes SH, Saltzman WM, Giannelis EP. Organosilicate-polymer drug delivery systems: controlled release and enhanced mechanical properties. *J Control Release.* 2003;90:163–169.

67. Haller MF, Saltzman WM. Nerve growth factor delivery systems. *J Control Release.* 1998;53:1–6.

68. Mahoney MJ, Saltzman WM. Millimeter-scale positioning of a nerve-growth-factor source and biological activity in the brain. *Proc Natl Acad Sci USA.* 1999;96:4,536–4,539.

69. Davies JB, Ciavatta VT, Boatright JH, et al. Delivery of several forms of DNA, DNA-RNA hybrids, and dyes across human sclera by electrical fields. *Molecular Vision.* 2003;9:569–578.

70. Cayouette M, Gravel C. Adenovirus-mediated gene transfer of ciliary neurotrophic factor can prevent photoreceptor degeneration in the retinal degeneration (*rd*) mouse. *Hum Gene Ther.* 1997;8:423–430.

71. Cayouette M, Behn D, Sendtner M, et al. Intraocular gene transfer of ciliary neurotrophic factor prevents death and increases responsiveness of rod photoreceptors in the retinal degeneration slow mouse. *J Neurosci.* 1998;18: 9,282–9,293.

72. Liang FQ, Dejneka NS, Cohen DR, et al. AAV-mediated delivery of ciliary neurotrophic factor prolongs photoreceptor survival in the rhodopsin knockout mouse. *Mol Ther.* 2001;3:241–248.

73. van Adel BA, Kostic C, Deglon N, et al. Delivery of ciliary neurotrophic factor via lentiviral-mediated transfer protects axotomized retinal ganglion cells for an extended period of time. *Hum Gene Ther.* 2003;14: 103–115.

74. Raisler BJ, Berns KI, Grant MB, et al. Adeno-associated virus type-2 expression of pigmented epithelium-derived factor or Kringles 1–3 of angiostatin reduce retinal neovascularization. *Proc Natl Acad Sci USA.* 2002;99: 8,909–8,914.

75. Auricchio A, Behling KC, Maguire AM, et al. Inhibition of retinal neovascularization by intraocular viral-mediated delivery of anti-angiogenic agents. *Mol Ther.* 2002;6:490–494.

76. Duh EJ, Yang HS, Suzuma I. Pigment epithelium-derived factor suppresses ischemia-induced retinal neovascularization and VEGF-induced migration and growth. *Invest Ophthalmol Vis Sci.* 2002;43:821–829.

77. Mori K, Gehlbach P, Ando A, et al. Regression of ocular neovascularization in response to increased expression of pigment epithelium-derived factor. *Invest Ophthalmol Vis Sci.* 2002;43:2,428–2,434.

78. Takita H, Yoneya S, Gehlbach PL, et al. Retinal neuroprotection against ischemic injury mediated by intraocular gene transfer of pigment epithelium-derived factor. *Invest Ophthalmol Vis Sci.* 2003;44:4,497–4,504.

79. Semkova I, Kreppel F, Welsandt, G, et al. Autologous transplantation of genetically modified iris pigment epithelial cells: a promising concept for the treatment of age-related macular degeneration and other disorders of the eye. *Proc Natl Acad Sci USA.* 2002;99:13,090–13,3095.

Pigment Epithelium Endoscopic Laser Surgery: PEELS

30

Frank H. J. Koch   Hugo Quiroz-Mercado

BRIEF SUMMARY STATEMENT

A pars plana vitrectomy combined with pigment epithelium endoscopic laser surgery (PEELS) treats choroidal neovascularization (CNV) in age-related macular degeneration (AMD) for stabilization and/or improvement of vision. The initial retinal detachment is limited to the posterior pole. Serious complications like proliferative vitreoretinopathy (PVR) are unlikely. The CNV appears to be permanently quiet after PEELS.

INTRODUCTION

Due to poor visual prognosis and heterogenous clinical appearances of eyes with submacular CNV, several therapeutic modalities have been investigated (1–12).

The main objective of the various modalities of treatment is to preserve macular photoreceptors while closing the CNV.

The first treatment of subretinal CNV in the macula was transretinal laser photocoagulation. This induces non-specific damage to the CNV, including adjacent retinal structures. Depending on the involvement of the foveal area, eyes can experience a significant decline in vision immediately after treatment (1). The extraction of a subretinal CNV is also a potentially destructive strategy, mainly because of the potential loss of RPE cells and Bruch's membrane, which often significantly limits the visual outcome (3,4).

A non-invasive, photoreceptor-sparing treatment of subfoveal CNV is photodynamic therapy (PDT), which does not produce thermal damage to the neurosensory retina but does induce thrombosis of new vessels. However, it typically requires more than one treatment and is not available in all countries (2,13,14).

In the Macula Photocoagulation Study (MPS), the common method of transretinal photocoagulation was associated with thermal damage of the neurosensory retina and subsequent decline in vision.

Therefore, Thomas tested the strategy of laser delivered subretinally to the CNV in three cases (15). When following landmarks seen on a projected fluorescein angiogram, he created a small retinal detachment using BSS and performed the laser coagulation without direct visualization of the CNV. The procedure was evaluated to be potentially valuable as an adjunct to surgical removal of subfoveal choroidal membranes.

High-resolution gradient index solid rod lens (GRIN-ROD) endoscopic surgery in the subretinal space was introduced in 1997 (16–18). Endoscopic visualization is not limited by the clarity of the cornea or lens. The GRIN-ROD endoscope offers an excellent subretinal view of areas to be treated and also facilitates full control of all maneuvers performed behind the sensory retina.

If viscoelastic substances or heavy liquids are injected into the subretinal space during endoscopy, neither cell detritus or opaque serosanguinous subretinal fluid will interfere with the view.

There are two sites for introduction of the endoscope into the subretinal space: the retina for a pars plana–transretinal entry, or the sclera for a transscleral direct subretinal access. The latter appears to be a more logical approach (16,17) but requires a different and more complex surgical strategy. Whereas ample visualization was easily achieved to perform a variety of surgeries when the GRIN-ROD was introduced via the sclera through the choroid into the subretinal space, several aspects had to be considered as complex and cumbersome: the control of bleeding into the choroids and subretinal space and iatrogenic breaks during the hydraulic detachment of the retina. The latter may occur more frequently because the sensory retina above the CNV complex is very atrophic especially when performing surgery in advanced stages of the disease.

The transretinal entry is less demanding. It requires careful consideration of retinal hole management, which includes minimization of surgical trauma. Using the transretinal endoscopic approach, subretinal laser surgery requires less than 60 minutes with a minimal risk of causing PVR while maintaining full optical control over the subretinal pathology and all surgical maneuvers, e.g., laser, aspiration, or injection of liquids. Three international teams are evaluating the safety and efficacy of PEELS in treating wet AMD: a Mexican group (Asociacion para Evitar la Ceguera en Mexico, Mexico City), an Indian group (Aditya Jyot Eye Hospital, Mumbai) and a German group (University Eye Clinic, Frankfurt/M.).

With the GRIN-ROD endoscope, it is also possible to observe the action of instruments introduced through a second retinotomy into the subretinal space. Subretinal endoscopic erbium:YAG laser treatment of CNV by means of viscoelastic induction of a foveal retinal detachment was reported by Quiroz-Mercado et al. (Mexico City) (19–21). They showed that, in advanced stages of CNV complexes, the ablative power of the erbium:YAG laser flattens the complex, and may improve vision because of an increase of the oxygen supply from the choroids into the retina. Unfortunately, the erbium:YAG laser fiber cannot be coupled to the GRIN-ROD endoscope due to its thickness. Other laser fibers for the application of thermal laser energy (532 nm or 810 nm) do not have this limitation. The Frankfurt group started to treat CNV in AMD with thermal, subretinally supplied laser in 1999. The procedure was labeled PEELS, for pigment epithelium endoscopic laser surgery, which may include pigment epithelium stimulation, and has been performed exclusively since that time, as the current techniques mentioned above were disqualified. Since 2000, the Mexican group selected CNV in AMD and myopia (20), and in 2002 the Indian group reported on their first two PEELS cases (22).

PEELS combines several widely accepted procedures (PPV, standard laser, and iatrogenic retinal detachment). The purpose of the two main investigational procedures (by the Mexico City and Frankfurt/M groups) was to report on the treatment of CNV by direct subretinal delivery of 532 nm or 810 nm diode lasers using the high-resolution GRIN-ROD endoscope, after the creation of a retinal detachment in order to avoid thermal retinal damage of the photoreceptors. Two substances for providing and maintaining a sufficient elevated working space in the submacular areas were tested: sodium hyaluronate and perfluorooctane.

PATIENTS AND TECHNIQUES

Patients

Since the cases performed in India have a follow up of less than 1 year, we will not review their results, which are preliminarily good. Their patient selection and procedure is identical to the German group's setup.

Consecutive cases from Mexico (MEX) and Frankfurt University (FRA) were treated when patients with subfoveal CNV were not qualified for or rejected PDT or other current treatment modalities.

Risks and benefits of the technique were explained to all the patients and a signed informed consent form was obtained. Complete eye examinations were performed on all patients and fluorescein angiography confirmed the diagnosis and type of CNV.

Technique

The GRIN-ROD endoscope was initially reported by Rol et al. (23–25) and was further developed by Insight Instruments Inc. (Stuart, Florida). The whole unit is composed of a compact box (Fig. 30.1). It was used in all PEELS cases because of its advanced high-resolution and magnification capabilities.

Endoscope probes are available with a diameter of 19 or 20 gauge and include a working channel for the introduction of a laser fiber or for aspiration and infusion. Introduction of the endoscope probe through a tiny retinal hole is the optimal method for high-resolution visualization of the subretinal space, identifying CNV structures and delivering laser to them (Fig. 30.1). Since 1999, several significant improvements have been made to the IE-4000 GRIN-ROD micro/endoscope, including a lighter hand piece and a more powerful light source. The latest-generation micro/endoscope, with its crescent-shaped automatic light shutter, which reduces the amount of physical light introduced into the eye through specially designed software, significantly reduces the potential for light toxicity. As the light-emitting endoscope probe's distance to tissue decreases, so does the light output in the eye. The lens focusing system is controlled via a foot petal, which is capable of both high magnification near and distance viewing (Fig. 30.1).

Whereas in MEX, the surgeon used hyaluronic acid in the subretinal space to maintain a submacular retinal detachment, in FRA the PEELS procedure was performed with the aid of heavy liquids (26).

The preferred method of subretinal introduction is via a small retinotomy in the raphe. The ideal detachment is limited to the posterior pole inside or around the vascular arcades. The membrane can then be evaluated immediately after introduction through the retinotomy (Fig. 30.2).

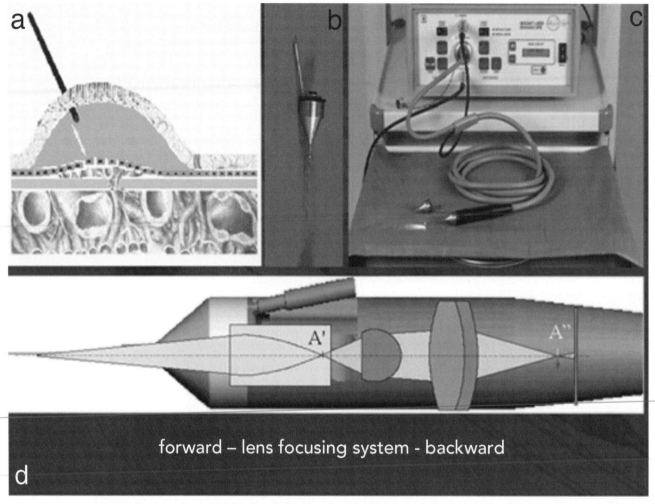

forward – lens focusing system - backward

Figure 30.1 **A.** Schematic drawing: introduction of endoscope shaft through small retinotomy. A bubble of hyaluronic acid or perfluorooctane is injected into the subretinal space to separate the neurosensory retina from the retinal pigment epithelium and CNM. Laser and endoscope are together in one 20-gauge tip. Three-mm working distance to the CNV-RPE level for laser ablation. **B.** Autoclavable 20-gauge probes with working channel for aspiration/infusion or laser coagulation. **C.** Insight Instruments, Inc. 4000 high-resolution GRIN-ROD endoscope box with 300-Watt xenon light, an automatic physical light-limiting shutter system, and foot pedal for focusing the GRIN-ROD endoscope. **D.** Integrated lens focusing system.

MEX PROCEDURE

In the present series, the surgeon performed a clear lens phacoemulsification in all AMD cases, as well as a posterior hyaloid separation. To initiate the retinal detachment, BSS solution was injected into the subretinal space through a small retinotomy followed by injection of low-viscosity viscoelastic solution.

After laser treatment of the CNV through the GRIN-ROD endoscope was accomplished, viscoelastic substances that were used to create the working space were extracted by either passive or active aspiration. Laser treatment (532 nm) was applied to the visible structures of the CNV as well as feeder vessels (when visible), until white laser burns were observed. Based on tests performed on rabbit eyes (27) it was determined that the energy setting should not be higher than 100 mW at a distance of approximately

1 mm and 0.2 sec of exposure. The use of endodiathermy of bleeding vessels on the edge of the retinotomy, laser photocoagulation around the retinotomy, and the use of a tamponade (gas or silicon oil) was decided at the time of the procedure according to the case and personal preferences of the surgeon.

For those eyes that had subretinal blood in the center of the macula at the end of the surgery, the patients were asked to maintain a specific position in order to displace the blood outside the macular area. Patients with gas-filled eyes maintained a face down position for at least 5 days, and patients with silicon-oil-filled eyes were asked to maintain an upright position. If not done initially, cataract surgery was performed 3 months later along with silicon oil removal. Complete eye examination (including linear Snellen visual acuity examination) was performed in all eyes 2 weeks, 4 weeks, 3 months, and 6 months

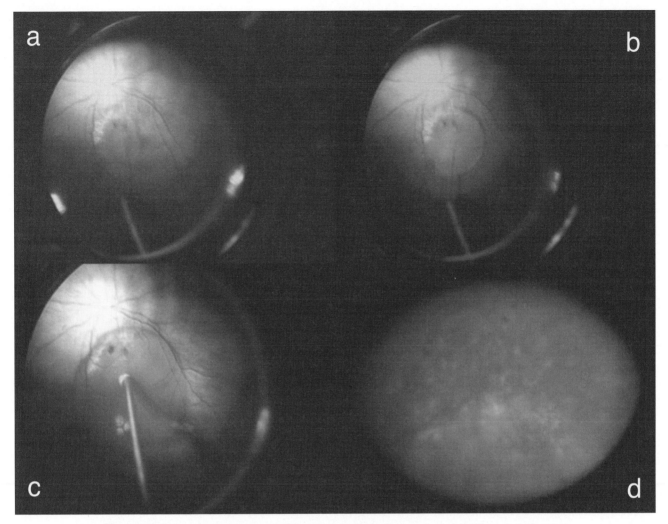

Figure 30.2 A. Microscopic view of PEELS with the endoscope introduced into the subretinal space via a small retinotomy. **B.** Slow injection of viscoelastic substances or heavy liquids to increase the detachment cavity at the posterior pole. **C.** Introduction of the endoscope via the raphe, focusing toward fovea. **D.** Intraoperative endoscopic aspect of an occult grayish membrane during PEELS surgery.

postoperatively. Fluorescein angiography was performed at 3 and 6 months postoperatively.

FRA PROCEDURE

The surgical technique included an initial three-port vitrectomy with complete detachment of the posterior vitreous cortex. The iatrogenic detachment was performed using a 39-gauge needle, and BSS plus solution was injected using the silicone oil pump system of the Accurus (Alcon, Fort Worth, Texas).

The size of the detachment ranged from 5 disc diameters up to a size of no more than 20% of the retina, centered on the posterior pole. If adhesions between the sensory retina, RPE, and CNV were very firm, we waited approximately 5 minutes before completing the detachment either with BSS or directly with heavy liquids (perfluorooctane).

It was important not to use too much force during the injection to avoid excessive hydraulic pressure, which usually leads to multiple RPE defects.

The surgeon's position relative to the raphe entry site and the CNV is essential and could be controlled via the microscope view (28). If a retinal detachment of the posterior pole did not occur at this time, either after delaying surgery or under PFC, we used a spatula to mechanically dissect permanent adhesions between the retina and underlying pathology. We endeavored to avoid any kind of retinal cauterization. In some cases, slight diathermization of the retina around the retinotomy where the endoscope probe entered the subretinal space was necessary when light bleeding started and did not stop spontaneously after waiting 2 minutes. The subretinal injection of perfluorooctane was performed slowly, either through a 25-gauge (with more destructive pressure) or a 20-gauge (with less destructive pressure) needle. BSS drained naturally through the retinotomy into the vitreous. An entry into the subretinal space was readily achieved with the 20/19-gauge probe of the GRIN-ROD endoscope, as was analysis and treatment of the CNV and the RPE. For laser treatment of the membranes and the surrounding RPE, we used the 810 nm or the 532 nm IRIS laser (Iridex, Mountain View, CA). Membranes required different energy and exposure times depending on their size, pigmentation, and thickness. Coagulation parameters had to be adjusted according to the direct visible response of mild test burns. Energy settings for the 532 nm laser setting ranged between 50 mW and 300 mW, with an exposure time of 200 ms to 500 ms. Energy settings for the 810 nm laser ranged between 300 mW and 1,500 mW with an exposure time between 500 ms and 1,000 ms. The laser energy was applied at an average distance of 3 mm between the tip of the endoscope and the surface of the membrane (200 μm spot diameter).

Since the 810 nm IRIS laser has a continuous wave mode as well as a minimal intensity setup (MIC) using duty cycles with on/off periods to limit the thermal effect, we chose MIC with a 10% duty cycle in two eyes. Since we could not see any response of the membranes to this MIC setup (membranes continued growing) we discontinued it. With the 810 nm IRIS laser it is possible to transfer the data from transpupillary thermal therapy (TTT) to the GRIN-ROD endoscope setup (endoscopic thermal therapy ETT). We applied the calculated energy over 45 min. and caused a limited but unacceptable amount of subretinal and epiretinal fibrosis with resulting shrinkage of the tissue. The same energy was applied for 20 sec instead of 45 sec in one other case, which caused some good results. Nevertheless we decided to discontinue with ETT.

The photoreceptor layer in the fovea showed some degree of transparency using the endoscopic view down to the subretinal RPE/CNV. Seven CNV cases showed varying RPE breaks, two were diagnosed preoperatively and five of them during surgery. Limited intraoperative RPE breaks with some small attachments of CNV could be repositioned with the laser-endoscope probe in two cases. When the RPE remained attached to the sensory retina, we treated the choroidal bed (two cases) and reattached the sensory retina with RPE to the choroid. When main portions of the CNV-RPE complex separated during surgery from both the sensory retina and the choroidal bed (two cases), we removed the already loose and free-floating complex and coagulated the bed. Both of these cases showed preoperative massive exudation, which cleared shortly (less than 4 weeks) after surgery, with limited but rapid visual improvement.

In four out of 15 eyes, we lowered the energies down to 50% of the threshold energy that we had used in the other 11 eyes (light grayish visible response). Preoperatively, all of the four eyes had shown increasing leakage over an observation period of at least 6 months. With this lower laser energy we treated the entire area that was proven to leak angiographically. Edema and exudates decreased dramatically after PEELS. Improvement of visual acuity resulted in some useful (two eyes) and some significant (two eyes) improvement of reading vision capabilities.

DISCUSSION

All surgeons involved in the present AMD study treated patients who had already suffered from advanced stages of the disease, that included poor visual acuity of ≤20/200 in 11 out of 15 cases. Four eyes had a preoperative vision between 20/200 and 20/100. The limited rate of improvement of visual acuity may be related to the poor preoperative conditions and the long history of CNV development. Interestingly, the endoscopic analysis in eight eyes showed some degree of transparency of the sensory retina and subretinal details could be visualized through the detached retina significantly better than what we have observed in eyes having a primary retinal detachment. So, this phenomenon, as well as the moderate visual acuity success rate, may also be related to some atrophy of the photoreceptors secondary to a history of CNV with continuous loss of vision for more than 6 months. The four best outcomes in the FRA group all had a history of increasing leakage over the observation period with no bleeding before PEELS surgery and a visual acuity of 20/200 and 20/100, and all of them were treated with lower energies (50% of threshold laser).

Endoscopes have been used in ophthalmic surgery for about 65 years (30–34). However, only with the development of the GRIN-ROD technology in 1995 has there been an endoscope that offers a high-resolution, non-pixilated video image. Its microscope-like focusing properties make this endoscope unique in the sense that focus may be achieved at any working distance with high resolution, unlike a pixilated endoscope, which cannot be focused.

Some of the optimal applications for this endoscope include: examining the outermost periphery (e.g., vascularization of the ciliary body); implanting drug delivery devices (35); controlling the peeling of inner limiting membrane-like translucent tissue; manipulation during sheathotomy in venous branch occlusion surgery; optical control in small cavities like the iatrogenically created subretinal space with a detachment limited to the posterior pole and vessel canalization; and visualization when the operating microscope cannot (as in endophthalmitis) (16–18).

We learned from the Macula Photocoagulation Study 1 that treatment of subfoveal CNV by standard laser photocoagulation causes significant damage of foveal photoreceptors followed by rapid loss of vision. We also learned that membrane extraction of subfoveal CNV may result in an unpredictable loss of pigment epithelium-Bruch's membrane complex with loss of vision (36).

Delivering thermal energy, as with TTT, may also result in loss of vision, whereas PDT has a high recurrence rate.

Limited macula translocation projects (5,6), as well as 360-degree macula rotation FHK (7,8), have a significant rate of complications and a high recurrence rate. Intravitreous injection of tissue plasminogen activator (tPA) and gas in the treatment of submacular hemorrhage may limit the loss of vision, but does not treat the cause of the disease (37).

By applying standard laser energy to the CNV behind the sensory retina, which is protected by a limited detachment at the posterior pole, we can avoid any kind of thermal effect on the photoreceptors. In case of potential recurrences, this procedure can be repeated.

MEX

Only two out of nine cases experienced a decrease of visual acuity. The remainder had improved vision without the need of additional treatment up to the last day of follow-up. Lack of recurrences may be explained by two factors: first, that the GRIN-ROD endoscope has better visualization (and therefore treatment) of the tissue requiring laser treatment; and second, as has been described in the literature, laser interaction with RPE to promote new RPE cell growth, as well as inhibition of growth factors. Other modalities of treatment such as PDT do not have these advantages. Although animal studies were performed to evaluate the best energy to stimulate RPE without inducing Bruch's membrane damage (27), we think submacular fibrosis in some cases was attributed to excessive laser treatment. The same conclusion may be reached for the subretinal strand observed in one other case. Even with this complication, visual acuity improved. Retinal scarring at the endoscope entry site observed in case 8, as well as in another reported set of cases (21), may be avoided by limiting the enlargement of retinotomy that is produced if the endoscope is not well oriented toward the CNV. When the GRIN-ROD endoscope was used along with erbium:YAG laser, the retinotomy had to be enlarged more than the usual 20-gauge diameter (21). If large retinotomies did not interfere with the center of the macula, an increase of visual acuity could be expected.

FRA

All cases FHJ reported in the current study reflect CNV in AMD with a history of from 6 months to several years. Almost 90% suffered from a minimally classic or occult without classic membrane complex and <20/200 vision. The membranes had remained in the subpigment epithelial space for a period of at least 6 months and did not develop the classic components suitable for PDT. Out of the two classic membranes we treated, one had poor vision preoperatively and remained quiet after PEELS treatment. The other, with 20/100, remained quiet and stable with subjective improvement probably related to the drying-out effect caused by PEELS surgery.

Preoperative bleeding and retinal pigment epithelium rips had the most negative impact on the postoperative visual outcome after PEELS.

Eyes which had subfoveal bleeding 21 days or less preoperatively, had a higher tendency to bleed during or shortly after PEELS surgery. For patients with these eyes, we decided to delay PEELS surgery for 4 weeks and perform a tPA injection first.

If RPE breaks occurred during surgery, most of them were related to progressive scarring over a period of at least 6 months or to the improper dissection of the sensory retina from the CNV complex.

In two cases, some RPE ripped off during dissection of the sensory retina and could be repositioned with the endoscope after laser treatment of the CNV.

Previous papers have shown that we should anticipate potential healing in RPE defects including larger rips in human eyes. In experimentally induced RPE defects, the pigment became pleomorphic about 1 month later when repigmentation occurred (38,39).

However, in our clinical series we found reproliferation of pigmented cells in only a few cases starting approximately 4 weeks after PEELS surgery. In all cases, cells lost their pigmentation gradually over the next 2 to 8 months, except in the four cases where lower energies (50% of threshold) had been applied.

In our series, the best results could be achieved when we successfully dried out the exudative type of disease and kept the CNV dry and flat. Postoperative fundus photography, fluorescein angiography, and the postoperative vision reminded us very much of our best PDT results in classic exudative membranes. However, until now, we have found only two cases with some degree of no response/early recurrence even after ≥12 months follow-up after PEELS (MIC group).

In the two eyes where the CNV had continued to grow, standard transretinal laser coagulation outside of the fovea stopped the CNV activity.

Obviously, our experience with preoperative exudations as well as with bleeding are consistent with the findings Thomas published in 1993 (15). Here he performed subretinal laser coagulation in three cases without endoscopic-controlled viewing.

The case with preoperative exudates and lipids improved from 20/200 to 20/80, whereas the case with preoperative subretinal hemorrhage got very fibrotic and did not improve in vision (20/300).

Today, with the availability of GRIN-ROD endoscopically controlled viewing, the laser effect can be adjusted to the individual membrane response. Different laser strategies are under consideration, mainly to determine how RPE function can be preserved and/or stimulated.

The potential of RPE migration and proliferation after experimental surgery in the subretinal space with or without subretinal laser, as well as the possible role of growth factors, are intensively discussed in the literature (40–53). Retinal pigment epithelial wound healing after experimental hydraulic debridement occurs rapidly and in a manner initially consistent with sliding migration. Progressive retinal pigment epithelial hyperplasia also occurs and may contribute to this repair process (39). In the rat retina on day 3 after laser coagulation, an intense gene expression of basic fibroblast growth factor (bFGF) and fibroblast growth factor receptor 1 (FGFR1) in the proliferating RPE cells was observed, as well as in macrophage-like cells. This effect decreased over time (42).

Intravitreal-injected bFGF increases the number of regenerated RPE cells in the rabbit over at least 3 weeks. It is speculated that this also may happen in human eyes (43).

In the adult primate, repopulation of retinal pigment epithelium can occur rapidly and support the repair of damaged photoreceptors following submacular surgery. Repopulation of RPE leads also to photoreceptor outer segment regrowth after 9 months (macaque monkey) (39). Principally, RPE cell-derived factors can be up-regulated in animals as well as in humans. Single growth factors as well as growth factor combinations are mentioned to be able to modulate RPE cell proliferation.

Interferon-β promotes proliferation to repair damaged RPE. After moderate dye laser photocoagulation in primate eyes (45), bFGF is found to stimulate cell proliferation in cultured human RPE cells. It may act as an autocrinic agent (48). DNA synthesis in human RPE cell cultures was found to be synergistically affected by certain growth factor combinations, such as pigment epithelial-derived growth factor (PDGF) and bFGF. PDGF and bFGF were more effective when given together. They were also more effective than other combination of factors, such as PDGF with tissue growth factor (TGF) or PDGF with tissue growth factor-β2 (TGF-β2) (49).

TGF-β produced by photocoagulated RPE cells, and also the down-regulation of angiogenic factors in repaired RPE cells, are obviously important after laser photocoagulation of human RPE cells in vitro (49). Pigment epithelial-derived factor (PEDF) showed its antiangiogenic activity in rat retinas as well as in cultured human retinal pigment epithelial cells after laser photocoagulation (50).

We tried to detect RPE migration and proliferation clinically after endoscopically guided subretinal laser coagulation. In four of the FRA membranes, we observed an increase in pigmented cell accumulation before these cells obviously decompensated and depigmented (4–6 months post PEELS).

Several reasons for the RPE behavior in our series may be hypothesized:

(a) Over-treatment of the RPE cells by using too many laser spots or too much energy. We know from other authors performing RPE coagulation through the iatrogenically detached retina that the energies used to close the CNV led to RPE cell decompensation (54–56). This hypothesis is obviously supported by the experience with our four cases, which showed good response and visual acuity after application of lower laser energies.

We are therefore involved in further studies to develop new techniques to enhance the response of the vasculature to laser and simultaneously save RPE cells. Different strategies are under investigation: thermal therapy (longer low-energy impulses), dye-enhancement techniques, and ablative laser energies. We are also considering the role of steroids and other drugs in the subretinal space. In primates, large doses of steroids seem to inhibit the migration and proliferation of RPE (57).

(b) The potential of RPE cells in AMD in humans may be different from those known from animal experiments. Studies combining laser and growth factors subretinally are already designed to determine the possibility of RPE regeneration after PEELS in humans.

(c) Irreversible damage of photoreceptors.

Direct observation of the fovea with the high-resolution GRIN-ROD endoscope revealed, that, in the majority of eyes a significant atrophy of the central retina occurs. In addition to the image we achieved with the endoscope in a retinal detachment case, the fovea shows a translucent lamellar-hole aspect in many AMD eyes. The atrophic condition of the sensory retina may accompany already severely damaged RPE. However, this does not explain why we could not find significant RPE migration/regrowth, since in the rabbit immature RPE cells can grow rapidly regardless of the presence of sensory retina up to 2 weeks after RPE removal. However, authors also mention that the regenerating RPE cells reconstruct a monolayer and their typical apical morphology under the influence of the sensory retina (40). The limited visual recovery of our patients at this time may be caused by the long symptomatic history and the irreversible damage that is caused to the photoreceptors. Modification of laser strategies will give us insight as to how we can influence the development of an AMD-related CNV complex. Due to the GRIN-ROD endoscopic optical properties, we are able to adjust the treatment modalities for each individual eye. Thermal therapy strategies and drug therapy concepts, as well as the potential of dye enhancements and the role of tissue ablation, need to be examined further.

We strongly believe that once a CNV complex in AMD has started to develop, we should avoid or stop any kind of leakage and stabilize the subretinal process without extracting it.

REFERENCES

1. Macular Photocoagulation Study Group. Laser photocoagulation of subfoveal neovascular lesions in age related macular degeneration: results of a randomized clinical trial. *Arch Ophthalmol.* 1991;109:1,220–1,231.
2. Treatment of Age-Related Macular Degeneration with Photodynamic Therapy Study Group. Photodynamic therapy of subfoveal choroidal neovascularization in age-related macular degeneration with verteporfin: one-year results of two randomized clinical trials—TAP report #1. *Arch Ophthalmol.* 1999;117:1,329–1,345.
3. de Juan E Jr, Machemer R. Vitreous surgery for hemorrhagic and fibrous complications of age-related macular degeneration. *Am J Ophthalmol.* 1988; 105:25–29.
4. Thomas MA, Grand MG, Williams DF, et al. Surgical management of subfoveal choroidal neovascularization. *Ophthalmology.* 1992;99:952–968.
5. de Juan E Jr, Lowenstein A, Bressler NM, et al. Translocation of the retina for management of subfoveal choroidal neovascularization in patients with age related macular degeneration. *Ophthalmology.* 1999;106: 1,908–1,914.
6. Machemer R. Macular translocation. *Am J Ophthalmol.* 1998;125:698–700.
7. Eckardt C, Eckardt U, Conrad HG. Macular rotation with and without counter-rotation of the globe in patients with age-related macular degeneration. *Graefes Arch Clin Exp Ophthalmol.* 1999;237:313–325.

8. Wolf S, Lappas A, Weinberger AW, Kirchhof B. Macular translocation for surgical management off subfoveal choroidal neovascularizations in patients with AMD: first results. *Graefes Arch Clin Exp Ophthalmol.* 1999;237:51–57.

9. Lappas A, Weinberger AW, Foerster AM, Kube T, Rezai KA, Kirchhof B. Iris pigment epithelial cell translocation in exudative age-related macular degeneration. A pilot study in patients. *Graefes Arch Clin Exp Ophthalmol.* 2000;238:631–641.

10. Bergink GJ, Deutman AF, Van Derk Brok JFCM. Radiation therapy for subfoveal neovascularization membranes in age-related macular degeneration. *Graefes Arch Clin Exp Ophthalmol.* 1994;232:591–598.

11. Stalmans P, Leys A, VanLimbergen E. External beam radiotherapy (20 y, 2 Gy fractions) fails to control the growth of choroidal neovascularization in age-related macular degeneration: a review of 111 cases. *Retina.* 1997;17:481–492.

12. Reichel E, Berrocal AM, Ip M. Transpupillary thermotherapy of occult subfoveal choroidal neovascularization in patients with age related macular degeneration. *Ophthalmology.* 1999;106:1,908–1,914.

13. Schmidt-Erfurth U. Photodynamic therapy: minimal invasive treatment of choroidal neovascularization. *Ophthalmologe.* 1998;95:725–731.

14. Iliaki OE, Naoumidi II, Tsilimbaris MK, Pallikaris IG. Photothrombosis of retinal and choroidal vessels in rabbit eyes using chloroaluminium sulfonated phthalocyanine and a diode laser. *Lasers Surg Med.* 1996;19(3):311–323.

15. Thomas MA, Ibanez HE. Subretinal endophotocoagulation in the treatment of choroidal neovascularization. *Am J Ophthalmol.* 1993;116:279–285.

16. Koch FHJ, Luloh KP, Grizzard WS, et al. *Vitreous Society Online Journal* [serial online] 1996 Jan-1997 Dec [cited 1998 Jun 1];1 (1) [10 screens and two videos].

17. Koch FHJ, Luloh KP, Augustin A, et al. Subretinal microsurgery with gradient index endoscopes. *Ophthalmologica.* 1997;211:283–287.

18. Frank HJ Koch, Hermann Gümbel. Subretinale Chirurgie. Mit Endoskopen auf dem Weg in die Zukunft. Der Ophthalmologe. *Das therapeutische Prinzip.* 1997;94:684–688.

19. Quiroz-Mercado H, Guerrero-Naranjo L, Ochoa-Contreras D, et al. Future investigations. In: Quiroz-Mercado H, Alfaro DV, Liggett PE, Tano Y, DeJuan E. *Macular Surgery.* Lippincott Williams & Wilkins; 2000.

20. Sanchez-Buenfil, Quiroz-Mercado H, Guerrero-Naranjo JL, et al. Viscoelastic foveal detachment and endoscopic subretinal laser ablation of subfoveal choroidal neovascularization. [ARVO Abstract]. *Invest Ophthalmol Vis Sci.* 2000;41(4):B329 Abstract. 954.

21. Quiroz-Mercado H, Yeshurun I, Sanchez-Buefil E, et al. Subretinal, viscoelastic-assisted, endoscope-guided photothermal ablation of choroidal neovascular membranes by erbium: YAG laser. *Ophthalmic Surg Lasers.* 2001;32:456–463.

22. Natarajan S, Koch FHJ. Endoscopic PEELS. 6th VRS Frankfurt-Marburg, June 2003, Frankfurt/M. Abstract.

23. Rol P, Jenny R, Beck D, et al. Optical properties of miniaturized endoscopes for ophthalmic use. *Optical Engineering.* 1995;34(7):2,070–2,077.

24. Rol P, Sasoh M, Manns F, Edney P, Niederer P, Parel J-M. Experimental intraocular laser surgery with a GRIN-ROD laser endoscope. *Proceedings of Ophthalmic Technologies VI.* 1996;2673:50–53.

25. Joos KM, Shen J-H, Parel J-M, Rol P. In vitro examination of the anterior chamber angle with a gradient-index (GRIN-ROD) lens endoscope. *Lasers in Ophthalmology.* 1994;II 2330.

26. Quiroz-Mercado H, Guerrero-Naranjo J, Yeshurum I, Rodriguez A, Perez-Reguera A, Koch F. Comparative Evaluation of different subretinal substances for submacular surgery. [ARVO abstract no.2313]. *Invest Ophthalmol and Vis Sci.* 2001;42:s429.

27. Romero RM, Rodriguez A, Yeshurun I, Guerrero-Naranjo JL, De-Barcia L, Quiroz-Mercado H. Evaluation of subretinal endoscopic photocoagulation with 532 nm laser in pigmented rabbit eyes. [ARVO abstract no.3506]. *Invest Ophthalmol Vis Sci.* 2002;43.

28. Greve MD, Peyma GA, Millsap, CM. Direction and location of retinotomy for removal of subretinal neovascular membranes. *Ophthalmic Surg.* 1995;26:330–333.

29. Koch FHJ, Quiroz-Mercado H, Hattenbach L-O, et al. PEELS. Pigment epithelium endoscopic laser surgery for treatment of choroidal neovascularization. *Ophthalmologica.* 2003.

30. Thorpe H. Ocular endoscope. An instrument for the removal of intravitreous non-magnetic foreign bodies. *Trans Am Acad Ophthalmol Otolaryngol.* 1934;39:422–424.

31. Koch F, Spitznas M. Video endoscopic vitreous surgery. *Ophthalmochirurgie.* 1991;2:71–78.

32. Koch F, Spitznas M. The video-endoscope as a useful adjunct to vitreous surgery. In: Stirpe M, ed. *Advances in Vitreoretinal Surgery.* Acta of the 3rd International Congress of Vitreoretinal Surgery. Fondazione G.B. Bietti per l=Oftalmologica. 1991.

33. Uram M. Ophthalmic microendoscope ciliary process ablation in the management of neovascular glaucoma. *Ophthalmology.* 1992;99:1,823–1,828.

34. Fisher YL, Slakter JS. A disposable ophthalmic endoscopic system. *Arch Ophthalmol.* 1994;112:984–986.

35. Koch FHJ, Gümbel HOC, Hattenbach LO, Ohrloff C. Endoskopische Kontrolle von Pars plana implantierten Ganciclovir Medikamententrägern zur Verbesserung der Langzeitprognose bei der Behandlung der Cytomegalievirusretinitis. *Klin Monatsbl Augenheilkd.* 1999;214:107–111.

36. Thomas MA, Ibanez HE. Surgical excision of subfoveal neovascular membranes and subretinal strands. In: Duane, *Clinical Ophthalmology*, Vol. 6. 1999.

37. Hattenbach LO, Klais, C, Koch FHJ, Gümbel, HOC. Intravitreous injection of tissue plasminogen activator and gas in the treatment of submacular hemorrhage under various conditions. *Ophthalmology.* 2001;108:1,485–1,492.

38. Heriot WJ, Machemer R. Pigment epithelial repair. *Graefes Arch Clin Exp Ophthalmol.* 1992;230:91–100.

39. Lopez, PF, Yan Q, Kohen L, et al. Retinal pigment epithelial wound healing in vivo. *Arch Ophthalmol.* 1995;113:1,437–1,446.

40. Valentino TL, Kaplan HJ, Del Priore LV, Fang SR, Berger A, Silverman MS. Retinal pigment epithelial repopulation in monkeys after submacular surgery. *Arch Ophthalmol.* 1995;113:932–938.

41. Del Priore LV, Kaplan HJ, Hornbeck R, Jones Z, Swinn M. Retinal pigment epithelial debridement as a model for the pathogenesis and treatment of macular degeneration. *Am J Ophthalmol.* 1996;122:629–643.

42. Yamamoto C, Ogata N, Matsushima M, et al. Gene expressions of basic fibroblast growth factor and its receptor in healing of rat retina after laser photocoagulation. *Jpn J Ophthalmol.* 1996;40:480–490.

43. Ozaki S, Kita M, Yamana T, Negi A, Honda Y. Influence of the sensory retina on healing of the rabbit retinal pigment epithelium. *Curr Eye Res.* 1997;16:349–358.

44. Kimizuha Y, Yamada T, Tamai M. Quantitative study on regenerated retinal pigment epithelium and the effects of growth factor. *Curr Eye Res.* 1997;16:1,081–1,087.

45. Tobe T, Takahashi K, Kishimoto N, Ohkuma H, Uyama M. Effects of interferon-beta on repair of the retinal pigment epithelium after laser photocoagulation. *Nippon Ganka Gakkai Zasshi.* 1995;99:792–805.

46. Pollack A, Korte GE. Repair of retinal pigment epithelium and choriocapillaries after laser photocoagulation: correlations between scanning electron, transmission electron and light microscopy. *Ophthalmic Res.* 1997;29:393–404.

47. Yamamoto C, Ogata N, Yi X, et al. Immunolocalization of basic fibroblast growth factor during wound repair in rat retina after laser photocoagulation. *Graefes Arch Clin Exp Ophthalmol.* 1996;234:695–702.

48. Schwegler JS, Knorz MC, Akkoyun I, Liesenhoff H. Basic, not acidic fibroblast growth factor stimulate proliferation of cultured human retinal pigment epithelial cells. *Mo Vis.* 1997;3:10.

49. Kaven CW, Spraul CW, Zavazava NK, Lang GK, Lang GE. Growth factor combinations modulate human retinal pigment epithelial cell proliferation. *Curr Eye Res.* 2000;20:480–487.

50. Ogata N, Ando A, Uyama M, Matsumura M. Expression of cytokines and transcription factors in photocoagulated human retinal pigment epithelial cells. *Graefes Arch Clin Exp Ophthalmol.* 2001;239:87–95.

51. Ogata N, Tombran-Tink J, Jo N, Mrazek D, Matsumura M. Up-regulation of pigment epithelium-derived factor after laser photocoagulation. *Am J Ophthalmol.* 2001;132:427–429.

52. Pollack A, Korte GE. Repair of retinal pigment epithelium and its relationship with capillary endothelium after krypton laser photocoagulation. *Invest Ophthalmol Vis Sci.* 1990;31:890–898.

53. Khaliq A, Jarvis-Evans J, McLeod D, Boulton M. Oxygen modulates the response of the retinal pigment epithelium to basic fibroblast growth factor and epidermal growth factor by receptor regulation. *Invest Ophthalmol Vis Sci.* 1996;37:436–443.

54. Roider J, Brinkmann R, Wirbelauer C, Birngruber R, Laqua H. Variability of RPE reaction in two cases after selective RPE laser effects in prophylactic treatment of drusen. *Graefes Arch Clin Exp Ophthalmol.* 1999;237:45–50.

55. Brinkmann R, Huttmann G, Rogener J, Roider J, Birngruber R, Lin CP. Origin of retinal pigment epithelium cell damage by pulsed laser irradiance in the nanosecond to microsecond time regimen. *Lasers Surg Med.* 2000;27:451–464.

56. Roider J. Retinal-sparing laser treatment of occult CNV by vitrectomy and localised detachment of the macula. *Graefes Arch Clin Exp Ophthalmol.* 2001;239:496–500.

57. Kishimoto N, Uyama M, Fukushima I, Yamada K, Nishikawa M, Ohkuma H. The effect of corticosteroid on the repair of the retinal pigment epithelium. *Nippon Ganka Gakkai Zasshi.* 1993;97:360–369.

Index

Pages followed by *f* indicate figures; pages followed by *t* indicate tables.